# Pulmonary and Critical Care Considerations of Hematopoietic Stem Cell Transplantation

Ayman O. Soubani
Editor

# Pulmonary and Critical Care Considerations of Hematopoietic Stem Cell Transplantation

Springer

*Editor*
Ayman O. Soubani
Pulmonary and Critical Care Medicine
Wayne State University
Detroit, MI, USA

ISBN 978-3-031-28796-1 ISBN 978-3-031-28797-8 (eBook)
https://doi.org/10.1007/978-3-031-28797-8



This Springer imprint is published by the registered company Springer Nature Switzerland AG
The registered company address is: Gewerbestrasse 11, 6330 Cham, Switzerland

*To my wife and kids who are the center of my love and the source of my inspiration and joy.*
*To my students and trainees who make what I do worth it.*
*To my patients whom I have the privilege of caring for and learning from every day.*

# Foreword I

In 1990, Dr. E Donnall Thomas received the Nobel Prize for the development of hematopoietic stem cell transplantation. In the more than three decades since, the procedure has become much more frequently used, far safer, and increasingly effective at eradicating disease. In 1990, roughly 10,000 transplants were performed annually worldwide. Today, that number has increased tenfold. Some of this increase is due to expanded donor availability, but equally important is the improved safety of the procedure, allowing its use in more settings and in older patients. When Thomas won the award, the risk of dying within 6 months from a complication of allogeneic transplantation approached 30%. Now, it is less than a third of that. As a result, cure rates for virtually every disease treated with transplantation have improved substantially. Much of this progress is the result of improved methods to prevent and treat the most feared complications of the procedure, including acute and chronic infections, organ failure, and graft-versus-host disease.

Part of Thomas's genius was his realization that the ultimate success of transplantation would require a team of experts from multiple disciplines focused on overcoming the various barriers to a successful outcome. Accordingly, he created his own multidisciplinary group, including pulmonologists, infectious disease experts, gastroenterologists, nephrologists, etc. Other transplant programs around the world followed suit. The result of their combined efforts is that over the last three decades the frequency of virtually every morbid complication of transplantation has dropped markedly, in most cases by 75% or more. While this progress is reason to celebrate, still too many of our patients die of the procedure or are left crippled because of a transplant-associated complication.

Now, Dr. Ayman Soubani, a pulmonary and critical care specialist who has long been a leader in conducting research and caring for hematopoietic stem cell transplant patients, has assembled an outstanding group of colleagues to create a textbook addressing pulmonary and critical care issues in stem cell transplant patients. While most transplant textbooks focus on the diseases being treated, Soubani and colleagues instead orient this book around the prevention and treatment of transplant-associated complications. Limiting the scope of the book to transplant complications allows the editor to broaden the range of complications included in the text, including some significant ones that are often ignored, such as sleep disturbances and caregiver burnout. The focus also allows each chapter to go deeper into its respective subject.

The authors of the individual chapters come from the leading transplant centers worldwide, thus providing a diverse, global voice.

By combining their expertise, Soubani and his coauthors have created a book that will be an extremely valuable resource for researchers and caregivers from all the multiple disciplines who come together to care for patients undergoing hematopoietic stem cell transplantation. But it goes further than that. The history of transplantation is now being echoed as a tsunami of novel immunotherapies and gene therapies are upon us. These new technologies offer enormous promise, but they also come with significant, sometimes fatal complications. Some of these toxicities overlap with those of transplantation while others are unique to the specific intervention. In either case, the approach first taken by Thomas and now detailed by Soubani and coauthors of the creation of a multidisciplinary group of experts focused on overcoming the complications of new technologies will be vital for the ultimate success of these new therapies and others yet to come.

Frederick R. Appelbaum
Division of Medical Oncology
University of Washington
Seattle, WA, USA

# Foreword II

It is a privilege to have been asked to write the foreword for this textbook, *Pulmonary and Critical Care Considerations of Hematopoietic Stem Cell Transplantation*, edited by Professor Ayman O. Soubani, a leading expert in this field. Hematopoietic stem cell transplantation (HSCT) has a long history, with first use in humans dating back to the 1950s. Since then, the number of patients receiving this therapy has increased rapidly, with more than 22,000 transplants performed in the USA in 2020 for both malignant (e.g., multiple myeloma, acute myeloid leukemia, and non-Hodgkin lymphoma) and non-malignant (e.g., aplastic anemia and sickle cell disease) conditions. Many of these patients will develop acute complications affecting multiple organ systems, some of which may be predicted and limited or prevented with careful patient assessment and management. Often such complications require admission to an intensive care unit for specialized care. With the increasing numbers of patients with HSCT, it is thus essential that all acute care physicians are aware of the possible complications.

In this comprehensive textbook, Professor Soubani has brought together, for the first time, 37 chapters covering all possible aspects of HSCT, from pulmonary, renal, neurological, and cardiac effects, through different infectious complications, including COVID, to sleep disturbance in patients, ICU organization for HSCT recipients, and burnout in healthcare providers. Each chapter is written by international experts in the field, providing readers with expertise in the care of HSCT patients from around the world. Appropriate and relevant Figures and Tables are included in each chapter.

This textbook provides the very latest advances in the care of this specific, increasingly large patient population and I am sure it will be of value to all involved in the direct management of HSCT recipients and all who may be responsible for dealing with any associated acute complications.

Department of Intensive Care
Erasme University Hospital
Brussels, Belgium

Jean-Louis Vincent

# Preface

Hematopoietic stem cell transplantation (HSCT) is an important treatment that is increasingly offered around the world for a variety of malignant and nonmalignant conditions. The survival of HSCT recipients has been steadily improving because of advances in conditioning regimens, supportive measures, and management of complications. However, HSCT recipients continue to have issues related to pancytopenia, side effects of conditioning regimens, and GVHD and its management. These complications range from infectious to noninfectious and affect almost every organ, occasionally leading to critical illness requiring admission to the intensive care unit.

This book focuses on the spectrum of pulmonary conditions that may develop following HSCT. These conditions continue to be a major cause of mortality and morbidity in this patient population and range from infectious—including bacterial, fungal, and viral—to noninfectious—such as diffuse alveolar hemorrhage, idiopathic pneumonia syndrome, interstitial lung disease, and bronchiolitis obliterans syndrome. The chapters also provide an overview of the major complications associated with other organs that may lead to critical illness including cardiac, neurologic, gastrointestinal, and renal complications. Experts from around the world discuss risk factors, clinical presentations, and advances in the diagnosis and management of these conditions.

This book is unique in several ways. It is the first work that is solely devoted to the topic of pulmonary and critical care complications of HSCT. While there are a limited number of works that address pulmonary and critical care issues following HSCT as part of the global discussion about transplant, there is no comprehensive textbook that provides such an in-depth, state-of-the-art presentation of the significant complications in this patient population. The authors represent a panel of international experts in this field who were able to successfully bridge the scientific basis of the conditions that lead to pulmonary and critical illness in HSCT recipients with the clinical knowledge necessary to provide the best care for this unique group of patients, both in the clinic and the intensive care unit. The chapters are written in a way that benefits all clinicians involved in the care of these patients including pulmonologists, intensivists, oncologists, and transplant specialists. It also informs specialists who are commonly involved in the management of HSCT recipients such as those in the fields of infectious disease, neurology, gastrointestinal, and nephrology. It provides insight on matters that arise during the care of patients such as provider burnout, nursing care, intensive care unit organization, nutritional support, and pulmonary and physical rehabilitation. Researchers, students, trainees, and allied healthcare providers involved in the care of HSCT recipients will find comprehensive information about this patient population as well.

I am grateful for the willingness of these experts to share their experience and knowledge in this field. I also would like to thank Ms. Anila Vijayan and Margaret Moore with the Springer Publishing Group for their support throughout the process.

Detroit, MI, USA Ayman O. Soubani

# Contents

# Editor and Contributors

## About the Editor

**Ayman O. Soubani, MD** is Professor of Medicine at Wayne State University School of Medicine in Detroit, Michigan, USA. He also serves as Medical Director, Medical ICUs, Detroit Medical Center Adult Central Campus; Service Chief, Pulmonary and Critical Care, Karmanos Cancer Center; and Medical Director, Critical Care Service, Karmanos Cancer Center.

## Contributors

**Vivek N. Ahya** Division of Pulmonary, Allergy, and Critical Care, University of Pennsylvania Perelman School of Medicine, Philadelphia, PA, USA

**Abinet Aklilu** Section of Nephrology, Yale University School of Medicine, New Haven, CT, USA

**Ali Alahmari** Oncology Center, King Faisal Specialist Hospital and Research Center, Riyadh, Saudi Arabia

**Amal Albeihany** Oncology Center, King Faisal Specialist Hospital and Research Center, Madinah, Saudi Arabia

**Mansour Alkhunaizi** Department of Medicine, Baylor College of Medicine, Houston, TX, USA

**Mohammed Almakadi** Oncology Center, King Faisal Specialist Hospital and Research Center, Madinah, Saudi Arabia

**Amin M. Alousi** Stem Cell Transplant and Cellular Therapy, The University of Texas MD Anderson Cancer Center, Houston, TX, USA

**Sammar R. Alsunaid** Department of Cardiothoracic and Vascular Surgery, Montefiore Medical Center, The University Hospital of the Albert Einstein College of Medicine, Bronx, NY, USA

**D. Martin Ashley** Division of Pulmonary and Critical Care Medicine, University of Texas McGovern Medical School, Houston, TX, USA

**Elie Azoulay** Critical Care Department, Saint Louis Hospital, Assistance Publique Hôpitaux de Paris (APHP), Paris Cité University, Paris, France

**Diwakar D. Balachandran** Department of Pulmonary Medicine, The University of Texas MD Anderson Cancer Center, Houston, TX, USA

**Lara Bashoura** Department of Pulmonary Medicine, The University of Texas MD Anderson Cancer Center, Houston, TX, USA

**Philippe R. Bauer** Division of Pulmonary and Critical Care Medicine, Department of Internal Medicine, Mayo Clinic, Rochester, MN, USA

**Lauryn Benninger** Department of Pulmonary and Critical Care Medicine, Respiratory Institute, Cleveland Clinic, Cleveland, OH, USA

**Anne Bergeron** Faculty of Medicine, University of Geneva, Geneva, Switzerland

Service de Pneumologie, Hôpitaux Universitaires de Genève, University of Geneva, Genève, Switzerland

**Michael Boeckh** Vaccine and Infectious Disease Division, Fred Hutchinson Cancer Center, Seattle, WA, USA

Clinical Research Division, Fred Hutchinson Cancer Center, Seattle, WA, USA

Division of Allergy and Infectious Disease, Department of Medicine, University of Washington, Seattle, WA, USA

**Zeinab El Boghdadly** Division of Infectious Diseases, The Ohio State University Wexner Medical Center, Columbus, OH, USA

**Louise Bondeelle** Faculty of Medicine, University of Geneva, Geneva, Switzerland

**Stefano Botti** Hematology Unit, Azienda USL-IRCCS di Reggio Emilia, Reggio Emilia, Italy

**Kyle R. Brownback** Division of Pulmonary, Critical Care and Sleep Medicine, University of Kansas School of Medicine, Kansas City, KS, USA

**Pranatharthi H. Chandrasekar** Division of Infectious Diseases, Wayne State University, Detroit, MI, USA

**Roy F. Chemaly** Department of Infectious Diseases, Infection Control and Employee Health, Unit 1460, The University of Texas MD Anderson Cancer Center, Houston, TX, USA

**Guang-Shing Cheng** Clinical Research Division, Fred Hutchinson Cancer Center and Division of Pulmonary, Critical Care and Sleep Medicine, Department of Medicine, University of Washington School of Medicine, Seattle, WA, USA

**Jessica Cheng** Nutrition Support WG, Asia-Pacific Blood and Marrow Transplantation Group, Chiang Mai, Thailand

Bone Marrow Transplant and Haematology, St Vincent's Public Hospital Sydney, Sydney, Australia

**Kenneth R. Cooke** Department of Oncology, Pediatric Blood and Marrow Transplantation Program, The Sidney Kimmel Comprehensive Cancer Center, The Johns Hopkins University School of Medicine, Baltimore, MD, USA

**Cassondra Cramer-Bour** Division of Pulmonary, Critical Care and Sleep Medicine, Wayne State University School of Medicine, Detroit, MI, USA

**Rachel N. Criner** Department of Thoracic Medicine and Surgery, Lewis Katz School of Medicine at Temple University, Philadelphia, USA

**Abhinav Deol** Department of Oncology, Wayne State University/Karmanos Cancer Institute, Detroit, MI, USA

**Rajat Dhar** Department of Neurology (Division of Neurocritical Care), Washington University in St. Louis School of Medicine, St. Louis, MO, USA

**Scott E. Evans** Department of Pulmonary Medicine, University of Texas MD Anderson Cancer Center, Unit 1462, Houston, TX, USA

**Saadia A. Faiz** Department of Pulmonary Medicine, The University of Texas MD Anderson Cancer Center, Houston, TX, USA

**Rachael A. Fornwalt** Division of Pulmonary and Critical Care Medicine, Department of Medicine, Johns Hopkins University, Baltimore, MD, USA

Oncology Intensive Care Unit, Johns Hopkins Sidney Kimmel Comprehensive Cancer Center, Johns Hopkins Hospital, Baltimore, MD, USA

**Alexander Franklin** Department of Infectious Diseases, Infection Control and Employee Health, Unit 1460, The University of Texas MD Anderson Cancer Center, Houston, TX, USA

Section of Infectious Diseases, Baylor College of Medicine, Houston, TX, USA

**Tomás Franquet** Department of Radiology, Hospital de Sant Pau, Universidad Autónoma de Barcelona, Barcelona, Spain

Hospital de Sant Pau, Barcelona, Spain

**Shigeo Fuji** Department of Hematology, Osaka International Cancer Institute, Osaka, Japan

Nutrition Support WG, Asia-Pacific Blood and Marrow Transplantation Group, Chiang Mai, Thailand

**Shruti Gadre** Department of Pulmonary and Critical Care Medicine, Respiratory Institute, Cleveland Clinic, Cleveland, OH, USA

**Ana Giménez** Department of Radiology, Hospital de Sant Pau, Universidad Autónoma de Barcelona, Barcelona, Spain

**Raffaella Greco** Hematology and Bone Marrow Transplantation Unit, IRCCS San Raffaele Scientific Institute, Milano, Italy

**Cristina Gutierrez** Division of Anesthesiology, Critical Care and Pain Medicine, Department of Critical Care, The University of Texas M.D. Anderson Cancer Center, Houston, TX, USA

**Salim S. Hayek** Department of Internal Medicine, Division of Cardiology, University of Michigan, Ann Arbor, MI, USA

**Sarah Hemstetter** Division of Pulmonary and Critical Care Medicine, Department of Medicine, Johns Hopkins University, Baltimore, MD, USA

Oncology Intensive Care Unit, Johns Hopkins Sidney Kimmel Comprehensive Cancer Center, Johns Hopkins Hospital, Baltimore, MD, USA

**Ann A. Jakubowski** Adult Bone Marrow Transplant Service, Department of Medicine, Memorial Sloan Kettering Cancer Center, New York, NY, USA

**Ryohei Jinbo** Department of Rehabilitation, Kita-Fukushima Medical Center, Fukushima, Japan

**Ricardo José** Department of Respiratory Medicine (Host Defence), Royal Brompton Hospital, Chelsea, London, UK

**Ryuichi Kasahara** Department of Rehabilitation, Kita-Fukushima Medical Center, Fukushima, Japan

**Carol A. Kauffman** Division of Infectious Diseases, Department of Internal Medicine, LTC Charles S. Kettles Veterans Affairs Medical Center, University of Michigan Medical School, Ann Arbor, MI, USA

**Partow Kebriaei** Department of Stem Cell Transplant and Cellular Therapy, The University of Texas M.D. Anderson Cancer Center, Houston, TX, USA

**Yiouli Ktena** Department of Oncology, Pediatric Blood and Marrow Transplantation Program, The Sidney Kimmel Comprehensive Cancer Center, The Johns Hopkins University School of Medicine, Baltimore, MD, USA

**Antoine Lafarge** Critical Care Department, Saint Louis Hospital, Assistance Publique Hôpitaux de Paris (APHP), Paris Cité University, Paris, France

**Naser Mahmoud** Section of Pulmonary Medicine, Department of Internal Medicine, King Hussein Cancer Center, Amman, Jordan

**Sandra Mazzini** Department of Radiology, Hospital de Sant Pau, Universidad Autónoma de Barcelona, Barcelona, Spain

**Rohtesh Mehta** Stem Cell Transplant and Cellular Therapy, The University of Texas MD Anderson Cancer Center, Houston, TX, USA

Clinical Research Division, Fred Hutch and the University of Washington School of Medicine, Seattle, USA

**Marisa H. Miceli** Division of Infectious Diseases, Department of Internal Medicine, Transplant Infectious Diseases Program, University of Michigan, Ann Arbor, MI, USA

**Dipenkumar Modi** Department of Oncology, Barbara Ann Karmanos Cancer Institute, Wayne State University, Detroit, MI, USA

**Shinichiro Morishita** Department of Physical Therapy, School of Health Sciences, Fukushima Medical University, Fukushima, Japan

**Laveena Munshi** Interdepartmental Division of Critical Care Medicine, Mount Sinai Hospital, Sinai Health System, University of Toronto, Toronto, ON, Canada

**Chikara Ogimi** Division of Infectious Diseases, Department of Medical Subspecialties, National Center for Child Health and Development, Tokyo, Japan

Vaccine and Infectious Disease Division, Fred Hutchinson Cancer Center, Seattle, WA, USA

**Chiara Oltolini** Clinic of Infectious Diseases, Division of Immunology, Transplantation and Infectious Diseases, IRCCS San Raffaele Scientific Institute, Milano, Italy

**Oren Pasvolsky** Department of Stem Cell Transplant and Cellular Therapy, The University of Texas M.D. Anderson Cancer Center, Houston, TX, USA

Institute of Hematology, Davidoff Cancer Center, Rabin Medical Center, Petah-Tikva, Israel

**Stephen M. Pastores** Critical Care Center, Department of Anesthesiology and Critical Care Medicine, Memorial Sloan Kettering Cancer Center, New York, NY, USA

**Steve G. Peters** Division of Pulmonary and Critical Care Medicine, Mayo Clinic, Rochester, MN, USA

**Chithra Poongkunran** Divisions of Critical Care, Pulmonary and Sleep Medicine, McGovern Medical School at UTHealth, Houston, TX, USA

**Amanda DeMauro Renaghan** Division of Nephrology, University of Virginia Health System, Charlottesville, VA, USA

**Frédéric Schlemmer** Pulmonology Unit—Medical ICU, Assistance Publique-Hôpitaux de Paris, Henri Mondor University Hospitals, Créteil, France

Faculty of Medicine, Paris-Est Créteil University (UPEC), Créteil, France

**Matteo Seligardi** Intensive Care Unit, Azienda USL-IRCCS di Reggio Emilia, Reggio Emilia, Italy

**Ajay Sheshadri** Stem Cell Transplant and Cellular Therapy, The University of Texas MD Anderson Cancer Center, Houston, TX, USA

Department of Pulmonary Medicine, The University of Texas MD Anderson Cancer Center, Houston, TX, USA

**Aryan Shiari** Division of Pulmonary, Critical Care and Sleep Medicine, Wayne State University School of Medicine, Detroit, MI, USA

**Nancy Cruz Sitner** Adult Bone Marrow Transplant Service, Memorial Sloan Kettering Cancer Center, New York, NY, USA

**Geetha Sivasubramanian** Division of Infectious Diseases, University of California, San Francisco, Fresno, CA, USA

**Ayman O. Soubani** Division of Pulmonary, Critical Care Medicine and Sleep Medicine, Wayne State University School of Medicine, Detroit, MI, USA

**Amy Spallone** Department of Infectious Diseases, Infection Control and Employee Health, Unit 1460, The University of Texas MD Anderson Cancer Center, Houston, TX, USA

**Thomas R. Spitzer** Department of Medicine, Massachusetts General Hospital, Boston, MA, USA

**Maria Teresa Lupo Stanghellini** Hematology and Bone Marrow Transplantation Unit, IRCCS San Raffaele Scientific Institute, Milano, Italy

**Dekel Stavi** Critical Care Medicine, Tel Aviv Sourasky Medical Center, Tel Aviv University, Tel Aviv, Israel

**R. Scott Stephens** Division of Pulmonary and Critical Care Medicine, Department of Medicine, Johns Hopkins University, Baltimore, MD, USA

Oncology Intensive Care Unit, Johns Hopkins Sidney Kimmel Comprehensive Cancer Center, Johns Hopkins Hospital, Baltimore, MD, USA

**Caroll C. Tipian** Adult Bone Marrow Transplant Service, Memorial Sloan Kettering Cancer Center, New York, NY, USA

**Joseph Uberti** Department of Oncology, Barbara Ann Karmanos Cancer Institute, Wayne State University, Detroit, MI, USA

**Kiddy Levente Ume** Department of Neurology (Division of Neurocritical Care), Washington University in St. Louis School of Medicine, St. Louis, MO, USA

**Alexi Vasbinder** Department of Internal Medicine, Division of Cardiology, University of Michigan, Ann Arbor, MI, USA

**Hemang Yadav** Division of Pulmonary and Critical Care Medicine, Mayo Clinic, Rochester, MN, USA

**Zhenmei Zhang** Division of Pulmonary and Critical Care Medicine, Mayo Clinic, Rochester, MN, USA

# Hematopoietic Stem Cell Transplantation: An Overview

1

Dipenkumar Modi and Joseph Uberti

## Introduction

Hematopoietic stem cell transplantation (HSCT) is an important therapeutic modality for several hematologic malignancies and benign conditions. It is the only curative treatment for many patients. There are two major types of stem cell transplant: autologous which uses patient's own hematopoietic stem cells to reconstitute the bone marrow and allogeneic in which hematopoietic stem cells from a donor (family member, unrelated donor, or umbilical cord blood) are used. According to the Center for International Blood and Marrow Transplant Research (CIBMTR) estimates, 11,557 autologous and 8326 allogeneic stem cell transplants were performed in the USA in 2020 [1]. The most common indications for HSCT in the USA in 2020 were multiple myeloma and lymphoma accounting for 58% of all HSCT [1].

## Autologous Stem Cell Transplant

The most common indications for autologous stem cell transplant (SCT) are hematologic malignancies such as multiple myeloma, amyloidosis, and Hodgkin and non-Hodgkin lymphoma. Testicular cancer is the only solid tumor where autologous SCT is used as a curative modality. The mechanism of cure relies on the delivery of higher doses of chemotherapy (conditioning regimen) to overcome tumor cell resistance. The chemotherapy chosen for transplant is usually one or more agents which have nonoverlapping toxicities and provide appropriate antitumor activity. Hematopoietic stem cells are infused after conditioning regimen to restore hematopoietic reconstitution as the high dose chemotherapy eliminates patients' marrow. The timing of autologous SCT depends on the disease and disease status. In multiple myeloma, autologous SCT is most often performed as consolidation after initial myeloma therapy. In 2019, 7663 autologous SCT were performed for multiple myeloma. In other diseases such as Hodgkin lymphoma and diffuse large B cell lymphoma (DLBCL), autologous SCT is offered after failure of initial therapy. A thorough pretransplant evaluation is performed to assess fitness for SCT which include bone marrow biopsy, EKG, echocardiogram, pulmonary function test, chest X-ray, and assessment of liver and kidney function.

### Collection of Stem Cells

Hematopoietic stem cells are harvested prior to transplant from either bone marrow (BM) or

D. Modi (✉) · J. Uberti
Department of Oncology, Barbara Ann Karmanos Cancer Institute, Wayne State University, Detroit, MI, USA
e-mail: modid@karmanos.org



A. O. Soubani (ed.), *Pulmonary and Critical Care Considerations of Hematopoietic Stem Cell Transplantation*, https://doi.org/10.1007/978-3-031-28797-8_1

peripheral blood. Peripheral blood stem cells (PBSC) are now more commonly used due to ease of collection, rapid engraftment, less contamination of infused cells with tumor cells, improved quality of life, and lower transplant-associated costs [2, 3]. No difference in disease-free survival was noted with PBSC compared to BM grafts [2, 4, 5]. Due to low concentration of stem cells in the peripheral blood, hematopoietic growth stimulating agents such as granulocyte colony stimulating factor (G-CSF) (10 μg/kg/day) alone or G-CSF plus cyclophosphamide are administered for stem cell mobilization. A minimum of $2 \times 10^6$ CD34+ cells/kg of recipient body weight is necessary for one transplant [6–8]. Most stem cell collection occurs in a single apheresis session. However, some patients require additional apheresis session(s) to achieve the stem cell goal. In patients with multiple myeloma, the most common practice is to collect enough stem cells for two transplants ($4 \times 10^6$ CD34+ cells/kg). The combination of cyclophosphamide 2 to 4 g/m$^2$ with G-CSF 10 μg/kg may also be used for stem cell mobilization. Although cyclophosphamide provides additional cytoreduction, this approach is associated with an increased rate of complications including febrile neutropenia, hemorrhagic cystitis, and pancytopenia. Most centers commonly administer G-CSF for 5 days prior to stem cell collection.

## Risk Factors of Poor Mobilization

Exposure to multiple prior lines of chemotherapy, prior radiation to marrow sites, and older age affect stem cell mobilization [9, 10]. In patients who fail mobilization with either G-CSF or G-CSF plus chemotherapy, plerixafor may be administered the evening prior to PBSC collection [11–15]. Plerixafor inhibits the interaction between stromal cell-derived factor 1 (SDF-1) and its receptor CXCR4, which plays a key role in the "trafficking" of PBSC [16, 17]. Interruption of this interaction results in the mobilization of highly functional PBSC into the circulation [18–21]. Plerixafor is currently approved for use in multiple myeloma and non-Hodgkin lymphoma.

## Conditioning Regimen

The conditioning regimen used prior to autologous SCT is based on the underlying disease. Melphalan 200 mg/m$^2$ is the most commonly used conditioning regimen for multiple myeloma. For lymphoma, the conditioning regimen usually consists of multiple agents with nonoverlapping extramedullary toxicities. BEAM (BCNU, etoposide, cytarabine, melphalan) and CBV (cyclophosphamide, BCNU, etoposide) are commonly used regimens for Hodgkin and non-Hodgkin lymphoma. Side effects related to conditioning regimens include pancytopenia and direct organ toxicity. Patients are usually pancytopenic for 10–12 days after transplant and usually require blood and/or platelet transfusions. The resultant neutropenia and profound immunosuppression from chemotherapy increase the susceptibility to infections. Patients frequently require systemic antibiotics. In addition, the chemotherapy may cause damage to the normal barriers of the gastrointestinal tract, oral mucosa, and skin which allows translocation of various pathogens into the circulation. Nausea, vomiting, and diarrhea are common during the conditioning regimen and immediate posttransplant period. These side effects are generally temporary, and management consists of symptomatic and supportive care.

## Allogeneic Stem Cell Transplant

Acute leukemias [acute myeloid leukemia (AML), acute lymphoblastic leukemia (ALL)] and myelodysplastic syndrome (MDS) [combined with myeloproliferative neoplasm (MPN)] are the most common indications for allogeneic HSCT accounting for 76% of allogeneic transplants [1]. The procedure differs from autologous SCT in that it requires use of a donor hematopoietic stem cell to replace and reconstitute patients' hematopoietic system after administration of the conditioning regimen. The mechanism of cure from this type of transplant is more complex than the autologous SCT. Conditioning regimen is given to overcome tumor resistance. In addition, the administration of donor cells provides an immunologically directed antitumor activity known as "graft-versus-tumor effect."

## Donor Selection for Allogeneic HSCT

The most important requirement for successful allogeneic HSCT is to find a human leukocyte antigen (HLA) matched donor for the patient. In general, the donor and recipient are matched for HLA class I (HLA-A, HLA-B, and HLA-C) and class II (HLA-DRB1 and HLA-DQB1) loci. The standard criterion for a perfect match is currently an 8/8 match which indicates that the patient and donor are matched on the antigen and allele level at the A, B, C, and DRB1 locus. Donor and recipient matching minimizes the development of acute and chronic graft versus host disease (GVHD), which is often the most difficult complication of donor transplants.

Historically, an HLA matched sibling donor was the only source of stem cells with each sibling having only a 25% chance of matching the patient. To overcome the lack of an HLA matched sibling donor, the National Marrow Donor Program (NMDP) was established in 1986 as a repository for unrelated stem cell donors. Subsequently, many registries have developed around the world to allow search for appropriate donors, and now all registries are linked as a common donor pool. With the growth of this registry, our ability to find HLA matched donors for patients who do not have sibling donors has increased dramatically. At present, the NMDP provides access to more than 39 million donors around the world. This has resulted in a dramatic change in the use of donors. As an example, HLA-identical sibling donors were most commonly used until 2013 when the use of unrelated donors increased, and now they represent the most common type of donors in the USA in 2020 [1]. Compared to matched sibling donors, matched unrelated donors (MUD) provide similar overall survival (OS), relapse-free survival (RFS), and non-relapse mortality (NRM) [22–26]. Three factors have driven the use of unrelated donors: First, more transplants are being performed in patients older than 65 years of age. In this setting, sibling donors are difficult to use as they are older and have comorbidities often making it difficult to go through stem cell collection. Second, more data has accumulated showing that younger donors provide a better overall outcome than older donors. This suggests that in the situation where we have an older HLA matched sibling donor and a younger HLA matched unrelated donor, the outcomes favor using the unrelated donor. Finally, in the USA and most developed countries, families are becoming smaller with less siblings making it harder to find HLA matched sibling donors.

Unfortunately, finding an unrelated donor typically takes 2–3 months. Our ability to find a fully MUD in the current registries depends on the ethnic and racial background of the patient with the highest possibility among whites of European descent at 75% and the lowest possibility among blacks of South or Central American descent at 16% [27]. The lower possibility of finding an optimal donor for African Americans and Asian Americans could be related to underrepresentation in the registry or polymorphic HLA repertoire. In situations where urgent transplantation is required and/or MUD is not available, umbilical cord blood (UCB) grafts and haploidentical donor (4/8 HLA match) are considered. Unrelated UCB grafts offer certain advantages over unrelated donors which include less requirement of HLA matching and decreased risk of GVHD. However, UCB grafts are associated with delayed engraftment, increased risk of infections, and graft failure. Previously, haploidentical donor transplants were associated with high rates of graft failure, acute and chronic GVHD, and NRM. Recently, Johns Hopkins University has pioneered a GVHD prevention strategy involving tacrolimus, mycophenolate, and cyclophosphamide which has allowed patients to undergo transplants using haploidentical donors [28–30]. The use of these multiple HLA-mismatched family donors provides excellent outcomes equivalent in some cases to using a fully matched sibling or unrelated donors. Use of haploidentical donors is increasing since 2012 and represented 21% of transplants in the USA in 2019. Umbilical cord blood (UCB) was the fourth common source of transplant in the USA in 2019 [31].

In addition to HLA matching, other donor characteristics including CMV serostatus, age, sex, and parity in female donors may influence transplant outcomes. Young donors [32], male donors, and nulliparous female donors are typically preferred. CMV-seropositive recipients experience worse survival, while CMV-seronegative recipients with CMV-seronegative donors have improved transplant outcomes. If the recipient is CMV-seronegative, a CMV-seronegative donor is preferred. If the recipient is CMV-seropositive, some centers advocate for the use of a CMV-seropositive donor. ABO and Rh compatibility are not typically required between the donor and recipient and may not affect survival [33].

## Sources of Hematopoietic Stem Cells

### Bone Marrow

Historically, donor stem cell collection was done harvesting bone marrow from the posterior iliac crest under regional or general anesthesia. Approximately 500–1000 cc of marrow is harvested from the donor to collect enough stem cells necessary for engraftment. The goal is to collect 2–4 × $10^6$ CD34+ cells/kg of patient weight which is associated with rapid hematopoietic recovery, reduced transplant-related mortality, and improved long-term survival [34–36].

In adult populations, donor bone marrow harvest is performed generally for patients with benign hematologic conditions such as thalassemia or aplastic anemia to minimize chances of GVHD and NRM. In pediatric population, however, there is still reliance on the bone marrow over PBSC. Bone marrow grafts represented 87% of matched related donor transplants and 52% of unrelated donor transplants among pediatric recipients in 2019 [31].

### Peripheral Blood

Among adults, PBSC is frequently used as the source of allograft for hematologic malignancies and accounted for 79% of unrelated donor transplants in 2019. In children, PBSC accounted for only 13% of matched related and 18% of unrelated donor transplants [31]. As mentioned above, hematopoietic growth factor stimulating agents are commonly used to mobilize stem cells from bone marrow.

### Umbilical Cord Blood (UCB)

UCB grafts accounted for 29% of pediatric unrelated transplants and 7% of unrelated donor grafts among adult recipients in 2019 [31]. UCB contains high concentration of HSC at the time of delivery. These cells can be cryopreserved and stored in cord blood banks. It can be used at any time for allogeneic stem cell transplantation upon request.

## Conditioning Regimen

Conditioning regimen plays an important role in allogeneic HSCT. They are divided into three subtypes based on intensity and toxicity (Table 1.1):

1. Myeloablative conditioning (MAC) regimen
2. Reduced intensity conditioning (RIC) regimen
3. Nonmyeloablative (NMA) regimen

MAC regimens provide intense cytoreduction to maximize antitumor activity prior to

**Table 1.1** Conditioning regimens for allogeneic HSCT

| Myeloablative conditioning regimen | Reduced intensity conditioning regimen | Nonmyeloablative conditioning regimen |
|---|---|---|
| Busulfan/fludarabine | Busulfan/fludarabine | Fludarabine/TBI |
| Cyclophosphamide/TBI[a] | Fludarabine/melphalan | Low dose TBI |
| Busulfan/cyclophosphamide | Fludarabine/cyclophosphamide | |
| VP16/TBI | | |

[a]*TBI* total body irradiation

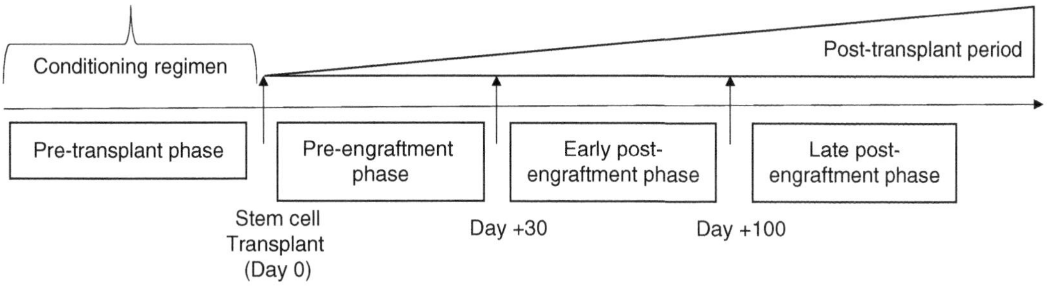


**Fig. 1.1** Timeline of stem cell transplant

allogeneic HSCT. Conversely, RIC and NMA rely on graft-versus-tumor effect by donor stem cells and less on the cytotoxicity of the chemotherapy [37]. RIC and NMA regimens are better tolerated in patients with advanced age and multiple comorbidities resulting in less NRM compared to MAC regimens. Selection of the conditioning regimen is influenced by the age and comorbidity of the patient and disease characteristics.

MAC regimens are associated with nausea, vomiting, pancytopenia, diarrhea, mucositis, and infertility. Initial busulfan containing regimens used high dose oral busulfan, which led to variable pharmacokinetics, high rate of sinusoidal obstructive syndrome (SOS), and seizures [38]. Subsequently, busulfan given intravenously led to better pharmacokinetic properties and reduced rates of toxicity [39]. Carmustine (BCNU) is a part of BEAM regimen and is associated with high rates of pulmonary toxicity, particularly in those who received radiation therapy to the chest [40].

TBI-containing MAC regimens use a TBI dose of 12–15 Gy, typically given over 4 days to reduce toxicity and improve tolerability. Although higher TBI dose (16 Gy) has been shown to reduce relapse rates compared to lower TBI dose (12 Gy), radiation induced pulmonary toxicity and NRM were significantly higher compared to lower TBI dose [41]. Long-term complications of TBI-containing conditioning regimens are pulmonary toxicity, cataracts, sicca syndrome, hypothyroidism, and thyroiditis [42]. The timeline of HSCT is shown in Fig. 1.1.

## Complications of Stem Cell Transplantation

### Early Complications

#### Graft-Versus-Host Disease (GVHD)

Graft-versus-host disease is a common complication occurring after allogeneic HSCT. It is an immune reaction driven by the donor stem cells. It is one of the most common causes of morbidity and mortality among allogeneic HSCT survivors. GVHD prophylaxis focuses on inhibition of donor T-cell activation using immunosuppressive medications. They are usually initiated prior to allogeneic HSCT and tapered around 6 months after HSCT in the absence of GVHD symptoms. GVHD prophylaxis varies with HLA mismatch, graft source, and institutional preference. It mainly consists of calcineurin inhibitors (CNI) such as tacrolimus or cyclosporine in combination with antimetabolites such as methotrexate or mycophenolate. The combination of CNI and antimetabolite has shown to reduce incidence of acute GVHD and improve survival compared to CNI or antimetabolite alone [43]. Antithymocyte globulin (ATG), an in vivo T-cell depleting agent, is often used in MUD allogeneic HSCT. The addition of ATG to standard GVHD prophylaxis has shown to reduce incidence of acute and chronic GVHD without any impact on survival in MUD allogeneic HSCT [44–48]. Abatacept, a T-cell costimulation inhibitory agent, is the first drug approved by the FDA for acute GVHD prophylaxis. The combination of abatacept with CNI and methotrexate was associated with significantly lower rate of acute GVHD and severe acute GVHD-free survival compared to CNI and methotrexate [49].

For patients undergoing haploidentical donor transplants, high dose cyclophosphamide in combination with tacrolimus and mycophenolate is used for GVHD prophylaxis. Cyclophosphamide 50 mg/kg when given on day +3 and +4 selectively depletes alloreactive T cells and spares memory T cells. It has significantly reduced acute and chronic GVHD rates and improved NRM and survival in haploidentical donor transplants [30].

The incidence and severity of GVHD depends on the degree of HLA mismatch between the donor and the recipient and intensity of the conditioning regimen. Based on the timing of onset, GVHD is divided into two types: acute GVHD and chronic GVHD.

*Acute GVHD:* Acute GVHD manifests early, typically within the first 100 days posttransplant. It is thought to be initiated by profound gastrointestinal mucosal injury caused by the conditioning regimen leading to release of cytokine storm and inflammatory cascade reactions. It primarily affects the skin, GI tract, and liver. Based on the degree of involvement of the skin, GI tract, and liver, acute GVHD is graded by the Glucksberg criteria [50]. Moderate to severe acute GVHD occurs in approximately 40% of allogeneic HSCT recipients.

*Chronic GVHD:* Chronic GVHD occurs in 40% of HLA-identical siblings and more than 70% of MUD transplants. Its onset is beyond day 100 posttransplant. It resembles autoimmune disorders such as Sjogren syndrome, scleroderma, primary biliary cirrhosis, and immune cytopenias and is characterized by fibrosis of several organs including the skin, GI tract, joints, eyes, lungs, and other organs. Fibrosis and collagen deposition lead to irreversible tissue damage. It is a major cause of late onset morbidity and mortality after allogeneic HSCT. It is graded by the National Institutes of Health (NIH) consensus criteria [51].

### Infectious Diseases

Autologous transplant patients are at increased risk of infections during the cytopenic period. Once neutrophil count recovers, risk of infection reduces significantly. In allogeneic HSCT recipients, the risk of infection is more prolonged extending into the post-engraftment period. Antibacterial prophylaxis has been shown to reduce fever, infections, NRM, and infection-related mortality. Therefore, we routinely initiate antibacterial prophylaxis with fluoroquinolones during conditioning regimen and continue until engraftment in both autologous and allogeneic HSCT.

Furthermore, patients undergoing HSCT are susceptible for *Candida* spp. and *Aspergillus* spp. during the pre-engraftment period. Thus, we administer antifungal and antimold prophylaxis with fluconazole and other azoles such as posaconazole. We also offer antiviral prophylaxis to prevent reactivation of herpes simplex virus (HSV), varicella-zoster virus (VZV), cytomegalovirus (CMV), and Epstein-Barr virus (EBV). Prophylaxis against *Pneumocystis jirovecii* pneumonia (PJP) is initiated for allogeneic HSCT patients after neutrophil engraftment and continues until immunosuppressive medications are discontinued [52]. Allogeneic HSCT recipients are at increased risk of CMV reactivation, and the risk is particularly high in the CMV-seropositive recipients. The use of letermovir prophylaxis significantly reduced clinically significant CMV infection (37.5 vs. 60.6%) and all-cause mortality at week 24 compared to placebo (10.2 vs. 15.9%) [53].

## Pre-engraftment: From HSCT to Engraftment (Day 0 to +30)

Patients are typically neutropenic during pre-engraftment period. Disruptions of mucosal barriers from chemotherapeutic agents, impaired cellular and humoral immunity, and functional asplenia from TBI-containing conditioning regimen increase the risk of systemic infections. Patients develop cellulitis, pneumonia, sinusitis, and urinary tract infections. Gram-positive and gram-negative bacteria, *Candida* spp., and HSV are the most common organisms responsible for infections. Endogenous flora in the GI tract is the common source of gram-negative bacteria, whereas the presence of exogenous device such as vascular catheter is the source of gram-positive bacteria. Only 30%–35% of febrile episodes in neutropenic patients can be documented microbiologically.

### Early Post-engraftment: Day +30–100

Neutropenia and mucositis have been resolved during this period. However, patients receive systemic immunosuppressive medications for GVHD, which affect immunity and predispose to CMV, adenovirus, BK polyomavirus, *Pneumocystis jirovecii*, *Candida* spp., *Aspergillus* spp., and other mold infections.

### Late Post-engraftment: Beyond Day +100

Patients are at high risk of infections from encapsulated bacteria (*Streptococcus pneumoniae*, *Haemophilus influenzae*, and *Neisseria meningitidis*), *Aspergillus* spp. and other molds, *Pneumocystis jirovecii*, and VZV due to impaired cellular and humoral immunity from chronic GVHD. To prevent such infections, vaccination against encapsulated bacteria is employed starting 6 months after transplant.

### Oral Mucositis

The incidence of oral mucositis is approximately 68% in autologous SCT and 98% in allogeneic HSCT [54, 55]. It is caused by the severe mucosal damage from the conditioning regimen. Its manifestations range between mild inflammation and mucosal ulceration, resulting in pain and difficulty swallowing. It typically occurs between 6 and 12 days after HSCT and resolves with engraftment. Breakdown of mucosal barrier increases chances of systemic infections and sepsis. Mucositis-related pain and infection cause significant morbidity and mortality among SCT recipients. There is no optimal approach for prevention of oral mucositis. For patients receiving high doses of melphalan containing myeloablative conditioning regimen, oral cryotherapy (ice chips swished around the mouth for 30 minutes) has been shown to prevent mucositis [56]. Although photo-biomodulation (laser therapy) and palifermin (recombinant human keratinocyte growth factor) are available for prevention of oral mucositis [57], they are not widely utilized due to the cost and inconvenience with use. Treatment of oral mucositis consists of supportive care. In severe mucositis, narcotic pain medications, sometimes in the form of patient-controlled analgesia (PCA), and systemic dexamethasone are considered.

### Hemorrhagic Cystitis

Hemorrhagic cystitis (HC) is a serious complication occurring in 5%–30% of HSCT recipients [58]. Patients typically present with urinary urgency and frequency, burning urination, painful urination, suprapubic pain, nocturia, or urinary incontinence. Hematuria is graded as microscopic (grade 1), macroscopic (grade 2), with clots (grade 3), and requiring instrumentation for clot evacuation or leading to urinary retention or requiring surgical intervention (grade 4). Its onset can be early within 2 weeks after conditioning regimen or late beyond 2 weeks after HSCT. Early onset HC is usually caused by direct toxicity of chemotherapeutic agents of the conditioning regimen. Cyclophosphamide, ifosfamide, busulfan, etoposide, and TBI are most common agents implicated in HC. It is mediated by the active metabolite of cyclophosphamide and ifosfamide, acrolein, which causes direct toxicity to the inner lining of the urothelium. Late onset HC is caused by BK polyomavirus infection and sometimes by adenovirus or CMV infection. Damaged urothelium provides a milieu for virus replication, and immunosuppression leads to virus reactivation and viruria.

*Prophylaxis:* Hydration with forced diuresis 3 $L/m^2/day$ with a goal of diuresis of >250 mL/h during and until the day after administration of alkylating agent is a commonly employed preventive strategy. For patients receiving cyclophosphamide or ifosfamide, mesna 1–1.5×, the daily dose of cyclophosphamide is used.

*Treatment:* Aggressive hydration and continuous bladder irrigation is commonly used. If HC is related to BK or adenovirus, administration of systemic or intravesical cidofovir, ciprofloxacin, or ribavirin can be considered. In refractory cases, selective embolization of the bladder arteries or cystectomy may be considered.

### Sinusoidal Obstruction Syndrome (SOS)

SOS is characterized by jaundice, fluid retention, and tender hepatomegaly occurring in the first 35–40 days after HSCT. The incidence of SOS is reported at 8% in allogeneic HSCT and 3% in autologous SCT [59]. The incidence is 10–15% after MAC and <5% after RIC allogeneic HSCT. It is caused by the damage and inflammation of the endothelial cells of the hepatic sinusoids. This leads to loss of fenestrae in sinusoidal endothelial cells (SEC) and formation of gaps within and between SEC. Subsequently, SEC dissects off and activates coagulation cascade and clot formation resulting in narrowing of the sinusoids. Preexisting liver disease, busulfan or TBI based conditioning regimen, HLA-mismatched donor, inotuzumab, and gemtuzumab are known risk factors of SOS. Seattle [60] and Baltimore criteria [61] are commonly used to diagnose SOS.

***Prophylaxis:*** Avoidance of hepatotoxic agents and busulfan containing conditioning regimen and use of NMA/RIC regimen may reduce risk of SOS. Prophylaxis with ursodeoxycholic acid is frequently used as prophylaxis and has shown to reduce incidence of SOS and SOS-related mortality without any impact on overall survival [62].

*Treatment:* It mainly consists of supportive care measures including close monitoring of fluid status in mild to moderate SOS. Defibrotide remains the only FDA approved drug for the treatment of SOS [63, 64].

### Transplant-Associated Microangiopathy (TMA)

TMA is a life-threatening complication caused by the endothelial dysfunction leading to small vessel thrombosis in the microcirculation. Its incidence is 3% among allogeneic HSCT recipients [65]. TBI based conditioning regimen, CNI, GVHD, infections (CMV), and unrelated donors are risk factors for TAM. It is characterized by microangiopathic hemolytic anemia with schistocytes and thrombocytopenia from platelet consumption. TMA is a multisystem disease involving the kidneys, gastrointestinal system, CNS, and pulmonary systems. Defects in the complement system leading to formation of C5b-9 complex are likely etiology of this disorder. It usually occurs within 1 and 2 months after HSCT. The diagnosis requires evidence of hemolytic anemia. Patients with renal TMA experience uncontrolled hypertension and proteinuria, and those with pulmonary involvement present with hypoxia, chest pain, tachycardia, and pulmonary hypertension. Intestinal TMA often simulates acute GVHD symptoms such as abdominal pain, diarrhea, vomiting, and GI bleeding. Cause of GI bleeding is ischemia in the bowel walls due to microangiopathy. X-ray shows ileus and thick mucosal walls. Polyserositis with pericardial and pleural effusion and ascites can occur due to diffuse vascular injury. Treatment consists of total plasma exchange and eculizumab.

## Late Complications

Majority of transplant survivors experience at least one late complication of HSCT. The 5-year cumulative incidence of nonmalignant late effect was 45% after autologous and 79% after allogeneic HSCT [66]. Late complications can affect any organ systems and impair quality of life and mortality. Transplant recipients with late complications had a higher rate of hospitalization and all-cause mortality than the general population [67]. The most common late complications are shown in Table 1.2.

In summary, HSCT has gone through a remarkable transformation over the past few decades including expansion of donor pool, availability of different sources of stem cells, and development of effective GVHD and infectious disease prophylaxis strategies. Nevertheless, disease relapse, non-relapse mortality from conditioning regimen toxicity, opportunistic infections, and acute and chronic GVHD are major impediments to survivorship.

**Table 1.2** Late complications of stem cell transplant

| Organ system | Type of complications | Incidence | Risk factors | Reference |
|---|---|---|---|---|
| Cardiovascular | | 5% at 5 years | Hypertension, dyslipidemia, diabetes, metabolic syndrome, chronic GVHD, prior cancer treatment, and clonal hematopoiesis of indeterminate potential (CHIP) | [68–71] |
| | Cardiomyopathy | 6% | | |
| | Ischemic heart disease | 3.8% | | |
| | Stroke | 3.5% | | |
| | Arterial disease, i.e., cerebrovascular, coronary artery, or peripheral artery disease | 22% at 25 years | | |
| Pulmonary | Chronic lung disease—bronchiolitis obliterans syndrome and restrictive lung disease | | Lung injury from TBI, chemotherapy, infections, and GVHD | |
| Hepatic | | | Iron overload, medications, chronic GVHD, hepatitis, infections | [72–74] |
| Renal | Chronic kidney disease (CKD) | 4.4% at 5 years | Old age, multiple myeloma | |
| | Thrombotic microangiopathy (TMA) | | Kidney disease, radiation, CNI, medications, GVHD | |
| | Nephrotic syndrome | | | |
| | Membranous glomerulopathy | | | |
| Endocrine | Diabetes/metabolic syndrome | 30% at 2 years | CNI, steroids | [69, 75] |
| | Hypothyroidism | One-third of patients by 25 years | TBI | [76] |
| | Hypogonadism/fertility disorder, premature menopause | | MAC regimen | [77–81] |
| | Hypoadrenalism | 13% in allogeneic HSCT; 1% in autologous SCT | Chronic glucocorticoids | [66] |
| Bone and joints | Osteopenia, osteoporosis | Up to 50% of recipients | Chronic GVHD | [82–84] |
| | Avascular necrosis | 4–19% | Steroids, male, TBI | [85–88] |
| Dermatology | Skin GVHD | | | |
| Ocular | Cataracts | | TBI-containing regimen | [89] |
| | Keratoconjunctivitis sicca | 20% at 15 years after allogeneic HSCT; 40% after GVHD | Chronic GVHD and TBI | |
| | Ischemic microvascular retinopathy | | | |

(continued)

**Table 1.2** (continued)

| Organ system | Type of complications | Incidence | Risk factors | Reference |
|---|---|---|---|---|
| Oral | Xerostomia, oral cancer | | Chemotherapy, radiation therapy, chronic GVHD of oral cavity | |
| Malignancy | Solid tumors | 1–2% at 10 years | | [90–93] |
| | Basal cell and squamous cell carcinoma of the skin | 6.5% and 3.4% at 20 years, respectively | TBI and GVHD | [94] |
| | Breast cancer | 11% at 25 years | Young age, TBI | [95] |
| | Secondary AML and MDS | 4.5% at 10 years among autologous transplant recipients | Prior cytotoxic chemotherapy, radiation | [96, 97] |
| | Posttransplant lymphoproliferative disorder (PTLD) | 1% at 10 years | EBV, T-cell depleting conditioning regimen | [98] |

## References

1. Auletta JJ Kou J, Chen M, Shaw BE. Current use and outcome of hematopoietic stem cell transplantation: CIBMTR US summary slides: CIBMTR; 2021. http://www.cibmtr.org
2. Vellenga E, van Agthoven M, Croockewit AJ, Verdonck LF, Wijermans PJ, van Oers MH, et al. Autologous peripheral blood stem cell transplantation in patients with relapsed lymphoma results in accelerated haematopoietic reconstitution, improved quality of life and cost reduction compared with bone marrow transplantation: the Hovon 22 study. Br J Haematol. 2001;114(2):319–26.
3. Brice P, Marolleau JP, Pautier P, Makke J, Cazals D, Dombret H, et al. Hematologic recovery and survival of lymphoma patients after autologous stem-cell transplantation: comparison of bone marrow and peripheral blood progenitor cells. Leuk Lymphoma. 1996;22(5–6):449–56.
4. Ottinger HD, Beelen DW, Scheulen B, Schaefer UW, Grosse-Wilde H. Improved immune reconstitution after allotransplantation of peripheral blood stem cells instead of bone marrow. Blood. 1996;88(7):2775–9.
5. Vose JM, Sharp G, Chan WC, Nichols C, Loh K, Inwards D, et al. Autologous transplantation for aggressive non-Hodgkin's lymphoma: results of a randomized trial evaluating graft source and minimal residual disease. J Clin Oncol. 2002;20(9):2344–52.
6. Bensinger WI, Longin K, Appelbaum F, Rowley S, Weaver C, Lilleby K, et al. Peripheral blood stem cells (PBSCs) collected after recombinant granulocyte colony stimulating factor (rhG-CSF): an analysis of factors correlating with the tempo of engraftment after transplantation. Br J Haematol. 1994;87(4):825–31.
7. Negrin RS, Kusnierz-Glaz CR, Still BJ, Schriber JR, Chao NJ, Long GD, et al. Transplantation of enriched and purged peripheral blood progenitor cells from a single apheresis product in patients with non-Hodgkin's lymphoma. Blood. 1995;85(11):3334–41.
8. Tricot G, Jagannath S, Vesole D, Nelson J, Tindle S, Miller L, et al. Peripheral blood stem cell transplants for multiple myeloma: identification of favorable variables for rapid engraftment in 225 patients. Blood. 1995;85(2):588–96.
9. Koenigsmann M, Jentsch-Ullrich K, Mohren M, Becker E, Heim M, Franke A. The role of diagnosis in patients failing peripheral blood progenitor cell mobilization. Transfusion. 2004;44(5):777–84.
10. Visani G, Lemoli RM, Tosi P, Martinelli G, Testoni N, Ricci P, et al. Fludarabine-containing regimens severely impair peripheral blood stem cells mobilization and collection in acute myeloid leukaemia patients. Br J Haematol. 1999;105(3):775–9.
11. Bilgin YM, Visser O, Beckers EA, te Boome LC, Huisman C, Ypma PF, et al. Evaluation of Dutch guideline for just-in-time addition of plerixafor to stem cell mobilization in patients who fail with granulocyte-colony-stimulating factor. Transfusion. 2015;55(5):1021–7.
12. Giralt S, Stadtmauer EA, Harousseau JL, Palumbo A, Bensinger W, Comenzo RL, et al. International myeloma working group (IMWG) consensus statement and guidelines regarding the current status of stem cell collection and high-dose therapy for multiple myeloma and the role of plerixafor (AMD 3100). Leukemia. 2009;23(10):1904–12.
13. Tricot G, Cottler-Fox MH, Calandra G. Safety and efficacy assessment of plerixafor in patients with multiple myeloma proven or predicted to be poor mobilizers, including assessment of tumor cell mobilization. Bone Marrow Transplant. 2010;45(1):63–8.
14. Vishnu P, Roy V, Paulsen A, Zubair AC. Efficacy and cost-benefit analysis of risk-adaptive use of plerixafor for autologous hematopoietic progenitor cell mobilization. Transfusion. 2012;52(1):55–62.
15. Worel N, Rosskopf K, Neumeister P, Kasparu H, Nachbaur D, Russ G, et al. Plerixafor and granulocyte-colony-stimulating factor (G-CSF) in patients with lymphoma and multiple myeloma previously failing mobilization with G-CSF with or without chemotherapy for autologous hematopoietic stem cell mobilization: the Austrian experience on a named patient program. Transfusion. 2011;51(5):968–75.
16. Fruehauf S, Seggewiss R. It's moving day: factors affecting peripheral blood stem cell mobilization and strategies for improvement [corrected]. Br J Haematol. 2003;122(3):360–75.
17. Papayannopoulou T. Current mechanistic scenarios in hematopoietic stem/progenitor cell mobilization. Blood. 2004;103(5):1580–5.
18. Calandra G, McCarty J, McGuirk J, Tricot G, Crocker SA, Badel K, et al. AMD3100 plus G-CSF can successfully mobilize CD34+ cells from non-Hodgkin's lymphoma, Hodgkin's disease and multiple myeloma patients previously failing mobilization with chemotherapy and/or cytokine treatment: compassionate use data. Bone Marrow Transplant. 2008;41(4):331–8.
19. Devine SM, Flomenberg N, Vesole DH, Liesveld J, Weisdorf D, Badel K, et al. Rapid mobilization of CD34+ cells following administration of the CXCR4 antagonist AMD3100 to patients with multiple myeloma and non-Hodgkin's lymphoma. J Clin Oncol. 2004;22(6):1095–102.
20. Devine SM, Vij R, Rettig M, Todt L, McGlauchlen K, Fisher N, et al. Rapid mobilization of functional donor hematopoietic cells without G-CSF using AMD3100, an antagonist of the CXCR4/SDF-1 interaction. Blood. 2008;112(4):990–8.
21. DiPersio JF, Micallef IN, Stiff PJ, Bolwell BJ, Maziarz RT, Jacobsen E, et al. Phase III prospective randomized double-blind placebo-controlled trial of plerixafor plus granulocyte colony-stimulating factor compared with placebo plus granulocyte colony-stimulating factor for autologous stem-cell mobilization and transplantation for patients with non-Hodgkin's lymphoma. J Clin Oncol. 2009;27(28):4767–73.

22. Alousi AM, Le-Rademacher J, Saliba RM, Appelbaum FR, Artz A, Benjamin J, et al. Who is the better donor for older hematopoietic transplant recipients: an older-aged sibling or a young, matched unrelated volunteer? Blood. 2013;121(13):2567–73.
23. Gupta V, Tallman MS, He W, Logan BR, Copelan E, Gale RP, et al. Comparable survival after HLA-well-matched unrelated or matched sibling donor transplantation for acute myeloid leukemia in first remission with unfavorable cytogenetics at diagnosis. Blood. 2010;116(11):1839–48.
24. Moore J, Nivison-Smith I, Goh K, Ma D, Bradstock K, Szer J, et al. Equivalent survival for sibling and unrelated donor allogeneic stem cell transplantation for acute myelogenous leukemia. Biol Blood Marrow Transplant. 2007;13(5):601–7.
25. Walter RB, Pagel JM, Gooley TA, Petersdorf EW, Sorror ML, Woolfrey AE, et al. Comparison of matched unrelated and matched related donor myeloablative hematopoietic cell transplantation for adults with acute myeloid leukemia in first remission. Leukemia. 2010;24(7):1276–82.
26. Weisdorf DJ, Anasetti C, Antin JH, Kernan NA, Kollman C, Snyder D, et al. Allogeneic bone marrow transplantation for chronic myelogenous leukemia: comparative analysis of unrelated versus matched sibling donor transplantation. Blood. 2002;99(6):1971–7.
27. Gragert L, Eapen M, Williams E, Freeman J, Spellman S, Baitty R, et al. HLA match likelihoods for hematopoietic stem-cell grafts in the U.S. registry. N Engl J Med. 2014;371(4):339–48.
28. Jones RJ. Haploidentical transplantation: repurposing cyclophosphamide. Biol Blood Marrow Transplant. 2012;18(12):1771–2.
29. Luznik L, Bolanos-Meade J, Zahurak M, Chen AR, Smith BD, Brodsky R, et al. High-dose cyclophosphamide as single-agent, short-course prophylaxis of graft-versus-host disease. Blood. 2010;115(16):3224–30.
30. Luznik L, O'Donnell PV, Symons HJ, Chen AR, Leffell MS, Zahurak M, et al. HLA-haploidentical bone marrow transplantation for hematologic malignancies using nonmyeloablative conditioning and high-dose, posttransplantation cyclophosphamide. Biol Blood Marrow Transplant. 2008;14(6):641–50.
31. Phelan R, Arora M, Chen M. Current use and outcome of hematopoietic stem cell transplantation: CIBMTR summary slides. 2020. http://www.cibmtr.org.
32. Kollman C, Spellman SR, Zhang MJ, Hassebroek A, Anasetti C, Antin JH, et al. The effect of donor characteristics on survival after unrelated donor transplantation for hematologic malignancy. Blood. 2016;127(2):260–7.
33. Kanda J, Ichinohe T, Matsuo K, Benjamin RJ, Klumpp TR, Rozman P, et al. Impact of ABO mismatching on the outcomes of allogeneic related and unrelated blood and marrow stem cell transplantations for hematologic malignancies: IPD-based meta-analysis of cohort studies. Transfusion. 2009;49(4):624–35.
34. Bahceci E, Read EJ, Leitman S, Childs R, Dunbar C, Young NS, et al. CD34+ cell dose predicts relapse and survival after T-cell-depleted HLA-identical haematopoietic stem cell transplantation (HSCT) for haematological malignancies. Br J Haematol. 2000;108(2):408–14.
35. Bittencourt H, Rocha V, Chevret S, Socie G, Esperou H, Devergie A, et al. Association of CD34 cell dose with hematopoietic recovery, infections, and other outcomes after HLA-identical sibling bone marrow transplantation. Blood. 2002;99(8):2726–33.
36. Zubair AC, Zahrieh D, Daley H, Schott D, Gribben JG, Alyea EP, et al. Engraftment of autologous and allogeneic marrow HPCs after myeloablative therapy. Transfusion. 2004;44(2):253–61.
37. Bacigalupo A, Ballen K, Rizzo D, Giralt S, Lazarus H, Ho V, et al. Defining the intensity of conditioning regimens: working definitions. Biol Blood Marrow Transplant. 2009;15(12):1628–33.
38. Slattery JT, Clift RA, Buckner CD, Radich J, Storer B, Bensinger WI, et al. Marrow transplantation for chronic myeloid leukemia: the influence of plasma busulfan levels on the outcome of transplantation. Blood. 1997;89(8):3055–60.
39. Schuler US, Renner UD, Kroschinsky F, Johne C, Jenke A, Naumann R, et al. Intravenous busulphan for conditioning before autologous or allogeneic human blood stem cell transplantation. Br J Haematol. 2001;114(4):944–50.
40. Peters WP, Shpall EJ, Jones RB, Olsen GA, Bast RC, Gockerman JP, et al. High-dose combination alkylating agents with bone marrow support as initial treatment for metastatic breast cancer. J Clin Oncol. 1988;6(9):1368–76.
41. Clift RA, Buckner CD, Appelbaum FR, Bearman SI, Petersen FB, Fisher LD, et al. Allogeneic marrow transplantation in patients with acute myeloid leukemia in first remission: a randomized trial of two irradiation regimens. Blood. 1990;76(9):1867–71.
42. Gopal R, Ha CS, Tucker SL, Khouri IF, Giralt SA, Gajewski JL, et al. Comparison of two total body irradiation fractionation regimens with respect to acute and late pulmonary toxicity. Cancer. 2001;92(7):1949–58.
43. Storb R, Deeg HJ, Whitehead J, Appelbaum F, Beatty P, Bensinger W, et al. Methotrexate and cyclosporine compared with cyclosporine alone for prophylaxis of acute graft versus host disease after marrow transplantation for leukemia. N Engl J Med. 1986;314(12):729–35.
44. Arai Y, Jo T, Matsui H, Kondo T, Takaori-Kondo A. Efficacy of antithymocyte globulin for allogeneic hematopoietic cell transplantation: a systematic review and meta-analysis. Leuk Lymphoma. 2017;58(8):1840–8.
45. Theurich S, Fischmann H, Shimabukuro-Vornhagen A, Chemnitz JM, Holtick U, Scheid C, et al. Polyclonal anti-thymocyte globulins for the prophylaxis of graft-versus-host disease after allogeneic stem cell or bone

marrow transplantation in adults. Cochrane Database Syst Rev. 2012;(9):CD009159.
46. Finke J, Schmoor C, Bethge WA, Ottinger H, Stelljes M, Volin L, et al. Long-term outcomes after standard graft-versus-host disease prophylaxis with or without anti-human-T-lymphocyte immunoglobulin in haemopoietic cell transplantation from matched unrelated donors: final results of a randomised controlled trial. Lancet Haematol. 2017;4(6):e293–301.
47. Kroger N, Solano C, Wolschke C, Bandini G, Patriarca F, Pini M, et al. Antilymphocyte globulin for prevention of chronic graft-versus-host disease. N Engl J Med. 2016;374(1):43–53.
48. Walker I, Panzarella T, Couban S, Couture F, Devins G, Elemary M, et al. Pretreatment with anti-thymocyte globulin versus no anti-thymocyte globulin in patients with haematological malignancies undergoing haemopoietic cell transplantation from unrelated donors: a randomised, controlled, open-label, phase 3, multicentre trial. Lancet Oncol. 2016;17(2):164–73.
49. Watkins B, Qayed M, McCracken C, Bratrude B, Betz K, Suessmuth Y, et al. Phase II trial of costimulation blockade with abatacept for prevention of acute GVHD. J Clin Oncol. 2021;39(17):1865–77.
50. Glucksberg H, Storb R, Fefer A, Buckner CD, Neiman PE, Clift RA, et al. Clinical manifestations of graft-versus-host disease in human recipients of marrow from HL-A-matched sibling donors. Transplantation. 1974;18(4):295–304.
51. Jagasia MH, Greinix HT, Arora M, Williams KM, Wolff D, Cowen EW, et al. National Institutes of Health consensus development project on criteria for clinical trials in chronic graft-versus-host disease: I. the 2014 diagnosis and staging working group report. Biol Blood Marrow Transplant. 2015;21(3):389–401. e1
52. Tomblyn M, Chiller T, Einsele H, Gress R, Sepkowitz K, Storek J, et al. Guidelines for preventing infectious complications among hematopoietic cell transplant recipients: a global perspective. Preface. Bone Marrow Transplant. 2009;44(8):453–5.
53. Marty FM, Ljungman P, Chemaly RF, Maertens J, Dadwal SS, Duarte RF, et al. Letermovir prophylaxis for cytomegalovirus in hematopoietic-cell transplantation. N Engl J Med. 2017;377(25):2433–44.
54. Bhatt V, Vendrell N, Nau K, Crumb D, Roy V. Implementation of a standardized protocol for prevention and management of oral mucositis in patients undergoing hematopoietic cell transplantation. J Oncol Pharm Pract. 2010;16(3):195–204.
55. Filicko J, Lazarus HM, Flomenberg N. Mucosal injury in patients undergoing hematopoietic progenitor cell transplantation: new approaches to prophylaxis and treatment. Bone Marrow Transplant. 2003;31(1):1–10.
56. Worthington HV, Clarkson JE, Bryan G, Furness S, Glenny AM, Littlewood A, et al. Interventions for preventing oral mucositis for patients with cancer receiving treatment. Cochrane Database Syst Rev. 2010;(12):CD000978.
57. Spielberger R, Stiff P, Bensinger W, Gentile T, Weisdorf D, Kewalramani T, et al. Palifermin for oral mucositis after intensive therapy for hematologic cancers. N Engl J Med. 2004;351(25):2590–8.
58. Lunde LE, Dasaraju S, Cao Q, Cohn CS, Reding M, Bejanyan N, et al. Hemorrhagic cystitis after allogeneic hematopoietic cell transplantation: risk factors, graft source and survival. Bone Marrow Transplant. 2015;50(11):1432–7.
59. Coppell JA, Richardson PG, Soiffer R, Martin PL, Kernan NA, Chen A, et al. Hepatic veno-occlusive disease following stem cell transplantation: incidence, clinical course, and outcome. Biol Blood Marrow Transplant. 2010;16(2):157–68.
60. McDonald GB, Sharma P, Matthews DE, Shulman HM, Thomas ED. Venocclusive disease of the liver after bone marrow transplantation: diagnosis, incidence, and predisposing factors. Hepatology. 1984;4(1):116–22.
61. Jones RJ, Lee KS, Beschorner WE, Vogel VG, Grochow LB, Braine HG, et al. Venoocclusive disease of the liver following bone marrow transplantation. Transplantation. 1987;44(6):778–83.
62. Cheuk DK, Chiang AK, Ha SY, Chan GC. Interventions for prophylaxis of hepatic veno-occlusive disease in people undergoing haematopoietic stem cell transplantation. Cochrane Database Syst Rev. 2015;(5):CD009311.
63. Richardson P, Aggarwal S, Topaloglu O, Villa KF, Corbacioglu S. Systematic review of defibrotide studies in the treatment of veno-occlusive disease/sinusoidal obstruction syndrome (VOD/SOS). Bone Marrow Transplant. 2019;54(12):1951–62.
64. Richardson PG, Riches ML, Kernan NA, Brochstein JA, Mineishi S, Termuhlen AM, et al. Phase 3 trial of defibrotide for the treatment of severe veno-occlusive disease and multi-organ failure. Blood. 2016;127(13):1656–65.
65. Epperla N, Li A, Logan B, Fretham C, Chhabra S, Aljurf M, et al. Incidence, risk factors for and outcomes of transplant-associated thrombotic microangiopathy. Br J Haematol. 2020;189(6):1171–81.
66. Khera N, Storer B, Flowers ME, Carpenter PA, Inamoto Y, Sandmaier BM, et al. Nonmalignant late effects and compromised functional status in survivors of hematopoietic cell transplantation. J Clin Oncol. 2012;30(1):71–7.
67. Chow EJ, Cushing-Haugen KL, Cheng GS, Boeckh M, Khera N, Lee SJ, et al. Morbidity and mortality differences between hematopoietic cell transplantation survivors and other cancer survivors. J Clin Oncol. 2017;35(3):306–13.
68. Armenian SH, Sun CL, Shannon T, Mills G, Francisco L, Venkataraman K, et al. Incidence and predictors of congestive heart failure after autologous hematopoietic cell transplantation. Blood. 2011;118(23):6023–9.
69. Majhail NS, Challa TR, Mulrooney DA, Baker KS, Burns LJ. Hypertension and diabetes mellitus in adult and pediatric survivors of allogeneic hematopoietic

cell transplantation. Biol Blood Marrow Transplant. 2009;15(9):1100–7.
70. Tichelli A, Passweg J, Wojcik D, Rovo A, Harousseau JL, Masszi T, et al. Late cardiovascular events after allogeneic hematopoietic stem cell transplantation: a retrospective multicenter study of the late effects working party of the European Group for blood and marrow transplantation. Haematologica. 2008;93(8):1203–10.
71. Chow EJ, Wong K, Lee SJ, Cushing-Haugen KL, Flowers ME, Friedman DL, et al. Late cardiovascular complications after hematopoietic cell transplantation. Biol Blood Marrow Transplant. 2014;20(6):794–800.
72. Majhail NS, DeFor T, Lazarus HM, Burns LJ. High prevalence of iron overload in adult allogeneic hematopoietic cell transplant survivors. Biol Blood Marrow Transplant. 2008;14(7):790–4.
73. Majhail NS, DeFor TE, Lazarus HM, Burns LJ. Iron-overload after autologous hematopoietic cell transplantation. Leuk Res. 2009;33(4):578–9.
74. Rose C, Ernst O, Hecquet B, Maboudou P, Renom P, Noel MP, et al. Quantification by magnetic resonance imaging and liver consequences of post-transfusional iron overload alone in long term survivors after allogeneic hematopoietic stem cell transplantation (HSCT). Haematologica. 2007;92(6):850–3.
75. Baker KS, Ness KK, Steinberger J, Carter A, Francisco L, Burns LJ, et al. Diabetes, hypertension, and cardiovascular events in survivors of hematopoietic cell transplantation: a report from the bone marrow transplantation survivor study. Blood. 2007;109(4):1765–72.
76. Sanders JE, Hoffmeister PA, Woolfrey AE, Carpenter PA, Storer BE, Storb RF, et al. Thyroid function following hematopoietic cell transplantation in children: 30 years' experience. Blood. 2009;113(2):306–8.
77. Anserini P, Chiodi S, Spinelli S, Costa M, Conte N, Copello F, et al. Semen analysis following allogeneic bone marrow transplantation. Additional data for evidence-based counselling. Bone Marrow Transplant. 2002;30(7):447–51.
78. Chatterjee R, Andrews HO, McGarrigle HH, Kottaridis PD, Lees WR, Mackinnon S, et al. Cavernosal arterial insufficiency is a major component of erectile dysfunction in some recipients of high-dose chemotherapy/chemo-radiotherapy for haematological malignancies. Bone Marrow Transplant. 2000;25(11):1185–9.
79. Molassiotis A, van den Akker OB, Milligan DW, Boughton BJ. Gonadal function and psychosexual adjustment in male long-term survivors of bone marrow transplantation. Bone Marrow Transplant. 1995;16(2):253–9.
80. Phelan R, Mann E, Napurski C, DeFor TE, Petryk A, Miller WP, et al. Ovarian function after hematopoietic cell transplantation: a descriptive study following the use of GnRH agonists for myeloablative conditioning and observation only for reduced-intensity conditioning. Bone Marrow Transplant. 2016;51(10):1369–75.
81. Sanders JE, Buckner CD, Amos D, Levy W, Appelbaum FR, Doney K, et al. Ovarian function following marrow transplantation for aplastic anemia or leukemia. J Clin Oncol. 1988;6(5):813–8.
82. Le Meignen M, Auquier P, Barlogis V, Sirvent N, Contet A, Simeoni MC, et al. Bone mineral density in adult survivors of childhood acute leukemia: impact of hematopoietic stem cell transplantation and other treatment modalities. Blood. 2011;118(6):1481–9.
83. Savani BN, Donohue T, Kozanas E, Shenoy A, Singh AK, Childs RW, et al. Increased risk of bone loss without fracture risk in long-term survivors after allogeneic stem cell transplantation. Biol Blood Marrow Transplant. 2007;13(5):517–20.
84. Yao S, McCarthy PL, Dunford LM, Roy DM, Brown K, Paplham P, et al. High prevalence of early-onset osteopenia/osteoporosis after allogeneic stem cell transplantation and improvement after bisphosphonate therapy. Bone Marrow Transplant. 2008;41(4):393–8.
85. Campbell S, Sun CL, Kurian S, Francisco L, Carter A, Kulkarni S, et al. Predictors of avascular necrosis of bone in long-term survivors of hematopoietic cell transplantation. Cancer. 2009;115(18):4127–35.
86. Enright H, Haake R, Weisdorf D. Avascular necrosis of bone: a common serious complication of allogeneic bone marrow transplantation. Am J Med. 1990;89(6):733–8.
87. Majhail NS, Rizzo JD, Lee SJ, Aljurf M, Atsuta Y, Bonfim C, et al. Recommended screening and preventive practices for long-term survivors after hematopoietic cell transplantation. Biol Blood Marrow Transplant. 2012;18(3):348–71.
88. Rizzo JD, Wingard JR, Tichelli A, Lee SJ, Van Lint MT, Burns LJ, et al. Recommended screening and preventive practices for long-term survivors after hematopoietic cell transplantation: joint recommendations of the European Group for Blood and Marrow Transplantation, the Center for International Blood and Marrow Transplant Research, and the American Society of Blood and Marrow Transplantation. Biol Blood Marrow Transplant. 2006;12(2):138–51.
89. Inamoto Y, Petricek I, Burns L, Chhabra S, DeFilipp Z, Hematti P, et al. Non-graft-versus-host disease ocular complications after hematopoietic cell transplantation: expert review from the late effects and quality of life working Committee of the Center for international blood and marrow transplant research and the transplant complications working Party of the European Society for blood and marrow transplantation. Biol Blood Marrow Transplant. 2019;25(5):e145–e54.
90. Cohen A, Rovelli A, Merlo DF, van Lint MT, Lanino E, Bresters D, et al. Risk for secondary thyroid carcinoma after hematopoietic stem-cell transplantation: an EBMT late effects working party study. J Clin Oncol. 2007;25(17):2449–54.
91. Curtis RE, Rowlings PA, Deeg HJ, Shriner DA, Socie G, Travis LB, et al. Solid cancers after bone marrow transplantation. N Engl J Med. 1997;336(13):897–904.
92. Danner-Koptik KE, Majhail NS, Brazauskas R, Wang Z, Buchbinder D, Cahn JY, et al. Second malignancies

after autologous hematopoietic cell transplantation in children. Bone Marrow Transplant. 2013;48(3):363–8.
93. Rizzo JD, Curtis RE, Socie G, Sobocinski KA, Gilbert E, Landgren O, et al. Solid cancers after allogeneic hematopoietic cell transplantation. Blood. 2009;113(5):1175–83.
94. Leisenring W, Friedman DL, Flowers ME, Schwartz JL, Deeg HJ. Nonmelanoma skin and mucosal cancers after hematopoietic cell transplantation. J Clin Oncol. 2006;24(7):1119–26.
95. Friedman DL, Rovo A, Leisenring W, Locasciulli A, Flowers ME, Tichelli A, et al. Increased risk of breast cancer among survivors of allogeneic hematopoietic cell transplantation: a report from the FHCRC and the EBMT-late effect working party. Blood. 2008;111(2):939–44.
96. Metayer C, Curtis RE, Vose J, Sobocinski KA, Horowitz MM, Bhatia S, et al. Myelodysplastic syndrome and acute myeloid leukemia after autotransplantation for lymphoma: a multicenter case-control study. Blood. 2003;101(5):2015–23.
97. Tarella C, Passera R, Magni M, Benedetti F, Rossi A, Gueli A, et al. Risk factors for the development of secondary malignancy after high-dose chemotherapy and autograft, with or without rituximab: a 20-year retrospective follow-up study in patients with lymphoma. J Clin Oncol. 2011;29(7):814–24.
98. Straathof KC, Savoldo B, Heslop HE, Rooney CM. Immunotherapy for post-transplant lymphoproliferative disease. Br J Haematol. 2002;118(3):728–40.

# An Overview of Graft-Versus-Host Disease

2

Rohtesh Mehta, Ajay Sheshadri, and Amin M. Alousi

## Introduction

It is essential for consultants who provide care for allogeneic hematopoietic cell transplant (AHCT) recipients to have an understanding of the procedure and the main determinants of morbidity and mortality. Accordingly, an understanding of graft-versus-host disease (GVHD) is required to provide thoughtful care. For pulmonologists, intensivists, and other providers, this requires the ability to recognize the diverse manifestations of the disease, predictors of outcomes, and familiarity with the therapies used for prevention and treatment along with their potential for toxicity and infectious risks. This chapter is meant to provide such an overview.

GVHD is a multisystem disorder that occurs when immune cells transplanted from a nonidentical donor (the graft) recognize the recipient (host) as foreign resulting in an immunologic process causing tissue injury. Two forms of GVHD are distinguished, *acute* and *chronic*. Historically, the arbitrary time point of day 100 was used to distinguish acute from chronic. More recently, the limitations of this artificial time point has been recognized, and instead clinical manifestation and histologic findings are now the sole factors used in defining these entities. Inherent in this distinction is the belief that acute and chronic GVHD have distinct, albeit interrelated, pathophysiology for which our understanding is unfolding and driving the development of novel therapies.

## Pathophysiology of GVHD

The pathophysiology of acute GVHD can be conceptualized as occurring in three phases, which proposes a central role of the gastrointestinal (GI) tract in the initiation and propagation of the cytokine storm characteristic of this disease [1]. The priming phase occurs as a result of tissue damage, especially the intestinal mucosa, caused by the conditioning chemoradiotherapy leading to the release of inflammatory cytokines (e.g., interleukin-6 [IL-6], tissue necrosis factor [TNF]), alarmins (IL-1α and IL-33), damage-associated molecular patterns (DAMPs), and pathogen-associated molecular pattern (PAMP) molecules [2], which could be bacterial (e.g., lipopolysac-

R. Mehta
Stem Cell Transplant and Cellular Therapy, The University of Texas MD Anderson Cancer Center, Houston, TX, USA

Clinical Research Division, Fred Hutch and the University of Washington School of Medicine, Seattle, USA

A. Sheshadri · A. M. Alousi (✉)
Stem Cell Transplant and Cellular Therapy, The University of Texas MD Anderson Cancer Center, Houston, TX, USA
e-mail: asheshadri@mdanderson.org; aalousi@mdanderson.org



A. O. Soubani (ed.), *Pulmonary and Critical Care Considerations of Hematopoietic Stem Cell Transplantation*, https://doi.org/10.1007/978-3-031-28797-8_2

charides, lipoproteins, peptidoglycan, and flagellin), fungal components (e.g., β-glucans, α-mannans), or viral nucleic acids. These tissue- and microbiota-derived molecules further stimulate the production of other inflammatory cytokines (e.g., TNF, IL-1, IL-6, IL-33, IL-12, IL-23, type1 interferon [IFN]) and chemokines (e.g., CCL5), which enhance the expression of MHC antigens and augment alloantigen presentation by the recipient antigen-presenting cells (APCs) [3]. The second phase is characterized by the activation and expansion of donor T cells. The infused mature donor CD4 and CD8 T cells activate, expand, and differentiate into effector T cells upon the recognition of alloantigens on the recipient. In the final phase, effector T cells secrete cytokines (e.g., IFN-γ, TNF, IL-2, IL-17), which render monocytes and macrophages extremely sensitive to endogenous LPS leading to target tissue apoptosis [1].

The pathophysiology of chronic GVHD is more complex and less understood. Similar to acute, chronic GVHD pathophysiology can also be conceptualized into three phases: phase 1: tissue injury causing acute inflammation; phase 2: chronic inflammation, thymic injury, and dysregulated B-cell and T-cell immunity; and phase 3: tissue repair and subsequent fibrosis [4, 5]. Similar to acute, the first phase of chronic GVHD also starts with the tissue damage caused by the conditioning regimen, which in addition to the activation of T cells also leads to the activation of innate immune cells and non-hematopoietic cells such as endothelial cells and fibroblasts. Additional stimuli such as infections and acute GVHD further increase the DAMPs and the PAMPs. The second phase is characterized by adaptive immune responses leading to the activation of alloreactive effector cells, particularly T cells and B cells, autoreactive CD4 T cells that escape thymic selection and produce IL-17A, and activated follicular helper T cells (Tfh) that produce IL-21. This immune dysregulation is further intensified with the loss of regulatory cell populations, including regulatory T cells (Tregs), regulatory type 1 T cells, regulatory B cells, regulatory natural killer (NK) cells, and invariant natural killer (iNK) T cells, in part due to conditioning regimen-related thymic injury causing loss of thymic epithelial cells. In the third phase, activated macrophages secrete platelet-derived growth factor-α (PDGF-α) and transforming growth factor-β (TGF-β), which cause activation of fibroblasts resulting in the sclerotic manifestations of chronic GVHD. In addition, differentiated B cells/plasma cells, in the presence of B-cell activating factor (BAFF), produce isotype-switched immunoglobulins which are deposited in various organs leading to fibrosis [4].

## GVHD: Incidence and Impact on Non-relapse Mortality (NRM)

Despite GVHD prophylaxis, a significant proportion of transplant recipients develop acute and/or chronic GVHD. Variability in identifying, measuring, and documenting GVHD across centers makes reliable estimates for its true incidence challenging. Nonetheless, estimates for grades II–IV and grades III/IV acute GVHD range from 25 to 50% and 5 to 20%, while incidences for chronic and extensive chronic range from 15 to 65% and 10 to 50%, respectively, after myeloablative conditioning (MAC) [6–10]. Incidences are lower after reduced-intensity conditioning (RIC) and can vary widely based on the presence of risk factors reviewed below. Despite challenges in estimating incidences of GVHD, its impact on transplant outcomes is clear as a leading cause of non-relapse mortality (NRM) beyond day 100 in human leukocyte antigen (HLA) matched sibling donor (MSD) and the second leading cause of NRM in HLA matched unrelated donor (MUD) recipients [11]. At the same time, outcomes are improving for patients who develop acute GVHD. A recent Center for International Blood and Marrow Transplant Research (CIBMTR) analysis showed a significant decrease over time in the proportion of grades III–IV disease among patients who develop grades II–IV acute GVHD and corresponding improvements in overall survival and NRM [12]. Similarly, a recent retrospective review demonstrated significant improvement in survival through reduction in NRM for patients who developed grades III/IV acute GVHD in more recent time periods [13]. In contrast to the declining rates for acute GVHD,

CIBMTR has shown an increased incidence of chronic GVHD, which could be partly attributed to growing recognition and diagnosis or increased use of peripheral blood (PB) graft, with no improvement in the 5-year NRM among those who develop the disease [14].

Among patients with acute GVHD, the risk of NRM ranges from <10% to 30–35% at 6 months [15] and up to 50% at 2 years [16], depending upon the risk stratification. Organ involvement and clinical GVHD stage and overall grade are key factors predictive of NRM in those who develop acute GVHD. Additional factors include recipient age, refractory disease (cancer) at the time of transplant, shorter time to acute GVHD onset, and donor type [13, 17].

Survivors of acute GVHD are at higher risk of developing chronic GVHD, which is a major contributor of late morbidity and impaired quality of life [18, 19] either related to GVHD itself or due to its prolonged treatment, which could be lifelong in some patients. Studies have shown that about 15% of transplant recipients were still on immunosuppressive treatment (IST) at 7 years' follow-up [20]. The cumulative incidence of discontinuation of IST after the resolution of chronic GVHD has been shown to be 50%, with a median duration of roughly 2 years. Beyond chronic GVHD's impact on the need for prolonged IST, it is a major contributor to late NRM with one recent study reporting a cumulative incidence of NRM at 5 years of 22% which increased to 40% at 12 years [21]. In this analysis, predictors for NRM included having any degree of lung GVHD, advanced skin involvement, and an impaired distance walk test (among others). Thus, minimizing chronic GVHD is deemed essential for reducing late mortality and impaired QOL.

## Risk Factors of GVHD

HLA matching between the donor and recipient is the single most important determinant of GVHD [22–25]. However, even with HLA matching between a patient and donor, substantial numbers of patients still develop acute and/or chronic GVHD due to differences in minor histocompatibility antigens (MiHA) that lie outside the HLA loci. The major histocompatibility complex (MHC) in humans, also known as the HLA, comprises more than 220 genes and over 29,000 allele sequences and is the most polymorphic region of the human genome. In addition to numerous classical and nonclassical HLA genes, more than 100 MiHA have been identified and sequenced. Unrelated donors are expected to harbor greater differences in MiHA than the HLA genotypically identical sibling donors, and data suggest that more than half of the acute and chronic GVHD cases are attributed to MiHA mismatching [26].

Other risk factors for GVHD include older age of recipient or donor, female donor for a male, parity of the female donor causing allosensitization, granulocyte colony-stimulating factor (G-CSF) mobilized PB versus bone marrow (BM) graft, conditioning intensity, use of donor lymphocyte infusion (DLI), receipt of total body irradiation (TBI)-based regimens, and the absence of serotherapy for GVHD prevention, to name a few [27–30].

## Classification of GVHD

The 2005 National Institutes of Health (NIH) Consensus Criteria established definitions for acute and chronic GVHD based on clinical features. According to these criteria, acute GVHD occurring within 100 days is "classic acute" and that occurring after 100 days is "late acute." Further, a new category of "overlap syndrome" was coined to include patients with concurrent features of acute and chronic GVHD. Patients with overlap GVHD have significantly greater functional impairment and poorer prognosis than classical chronic GVHD [31, 32]. The median time of development of chronic GVHD is approximately 5 months, and about 90% of chronic GVHD develops within 1 year of HCT [14].

### Staging and Grading of Acute GVHD

The diagnosis, staging, and grading of acute GVHD are purely clinical. Biopsy confirmation is helpful; however, pathological grading is not part of staging or grading. Acute GVHD is instead graded using a standardized system which takes into account the clinical stages in the primarily affected organs: skin, liver, and GI tract. The skin is the most commonly affected organ of acute GVHD and typically manifests as an morbilliform (macular-papular) eruption; however, less common manifestations may include pruritus alone, dysesthesias, or erythema. The gastrointestinal tract is the second most commonly involved organ and can present as "upper" GI (defined by clinical manifestations of nausea, vomiting, and anorexia) or "lower" GI involvement manifesting as a secretory diarrhea. In the modern era, the liver is the least common affected organ by acute GVHD with its hallmark being a cholestatic jaundice associated with elevated alkaline phosphatase and bilirubin.

Recently, a simplified and updated staging/grading system for acute GVHD staging/grading was proposed by the Mount Sinai Acute GVHD International Consortium (MAGIC) [33]. Based on this, each organ is staged as 0–4, with 0 being no GVHD and 4 being the worst stage (Table 2.1). Skin stage is based on the body surface area (BSA) involvement using the "rules of nines" with stage 1: <25%; stage 2: 25- <50%; and stage 3: ≥50% BSA. The development of bullae or a positive Nikolsky sign heralds the onset of more severe disease (stage 4) characterized by epidermal denudation often with involvement of other mucosal surfaces including the eye and mucus membranes. The presence of upper GI GVHD symptoms (anorexia, nausea, vomiting, and dyspepsia) is called stage 1 GI GVHD; and biopsy confirmation, although encouraged, is not mandated. As the symptoms of upper GI GVHD can be caused by several non-GVHD etiologies, it is suggested that in patients with milder symptoms, a diagnosis other than GVHD should be considered. Lower GI GVHD staging relies on stool volume and the presence of hematochezia or severe abdominal pain. Adults with stool volume of 500–999 mL/day are classified as stage 1, 1000–1500 mL/day as stage 2, and >1500 mL/day as stage 3. Patients with severe abdominal pain (requiring intravenous narcotic pain medication) with or without ileus or grossly bloody stool are classified as stage 4 regardless of the stool volume. As formal measurement of stool volume can be challenging, the number of diarrhea episodes can be used for staging (Table 2.2). Formed or mostly formed stools are not included in this assessment. Liver GVHD is categorized based on total bilirubin, and values 2–3 mg/dL, 3.1–6 mg/dL, 6.1–15 mg/dL, and >15 mg/dL represent stages 1, 2, 3, and 4, respectively. An overall grade is calculated based on the combination of individual stages. Patients with stage 2–3 liver and/or GI GVHD are categorized as grade III, and higher stages make them grade IV.

**Table 2.1** Acute GVHD grading systems

| Overall grade | Original Glucksberg criteria | "Modified Glucksberg" or "Keystone" criteria | MAGIC criteria |
|---|---|---|---|
| 0 | No organ involvement (skin = 0; and liver = 0; and GI = 0) corresponds to the absence of aGvHD | | |
| I | Skin = 1 or 2, without liver/GI involvement or decrease in performance status/fever | Skin = 1 or 2, without liver/GI involvement | Stage 1–2 skin without liver, upper GI, or lower GI involvement |
| II | Skin = 1 or 2 and (liver and/or GI involvement = 1 or 2) with mild decrease in performance status | Skin = 3, and/or liver = 1, and/or GI = 1 | Stage 3 rash and/or stage 1 liver and/or stage 1 upper GI and/or stage 1 lower GI |
| III | (Skin and/or liver and/or GI = 2, 3, or 4) with marked decrease in performance status | Liver = 2 or 3; and/or GI = 2–4 | Stage 2–3 liver and/or stage 2–3 lower GI, with stage 0–3 skin and/or stage 0–1 upper GI |
| IV | (Skin and/or liver and/or GI = 2, 3, or 4) with Karnofsky <30% | Skin = 4; and/or liver = 4 | Stage 4 skin, liver, or lower GI involvement, with stage 0–1 upper GI |

The overall aGvHD grade typically corresponds to the highest grade conferred by the individual staging of each organ. *GI* gastrointestinal tract, *GvHD* graft-versus-host disease, *IBMTR* International Bone Marrow Transplantation Registry, *MAGIC* Mount Sinai Acute GvHD International Consortium

**Table 2.2** Acute GVHD staging systems

| Organ severity stage | Original Glucksberg criteria | "Modified Glucksberg" or "Keystone" criteria | MAGIC criteria |
|---|---|---|---|
| *Skin* | | | |
| 0 | No rash | No rash | No rash |
| 1 | Rash <25% of BSA | Rash <25% of BSA | Rash <25% of BSA |
| 2 | Rash 25% to 50% of BSA | Rash 25% to 50% of BSA | Rash 25% to 50% of BSA |
| 3 | Rash >50% of BSA | Rash >50% of BSA | Rash >50% of BSA |
| 4 | Generalized erythroderma with bullous formation | Generalized erythroderma with bullous formation | Generalized erythroderma (> 50% BSA) plus bullous formation and desquamation **>5% of BSA** |
| *Liver* | | | |
| 0 | Total serum bilirubin <34 µmol/L (<2 mg/dL) or AST/SGOT 150–750 IU | Total serum bilirubin <34 µmol/L (<2 mg/dL) | Total serum bilirubin <34 µmol/L (<2 mg/dL) |
| 1 | Total serum bilirubin 34–50 µmol/L (2 to 3 mg/dL) | Total serum bilirubin 34–50 µmol/L (2 to 3 mg/dL) | Total serum bilirubin 34–50 µmol/L (2 to 3 mg/dL) |
| 2 | Total serum bilirubin 51–102 µmol/L (3.1 to 6 mg/dL) | Total serum bilirubin 51–102 µmol/L (3.1 to 6 mg/dL) | Total serum bilirubin 51–102 µmol/L (3.1 to 6 mg/dL) |
| 3 | Total serum bilirubin 103–255 µmol/L (6.1 to 15 mg/dL) | Total serum bilirubin 103–255 µmol/L (6.1 to 15 mg/dL) | Total serum bilirubin 103–255 µmol/L (6.1 to 15 mg/dL) |
| 4 | Total serum bilirubin >255 µmol/L (>15 mg/dL) | Total serum bilirubin >255 µmol/L (> 15 mg/dL) | Total serum bilirubin >255 µmol/L (> 15 mg/dL) |
| *Upper GI* | | | |
| 0 | NA | No persistent nausea and no histologic evidence of GvHD in the stomach or duodenum | **No or intermittent** anorexia or nausea or vomiting |
| 1 | NA | **Persistent** nausea **with histologic evidence of GvHD** in the stomach or duodenum | **Persistent** anorexia *accompanied by* ***weight loss*** or nausea or vomiting (*should last* ***at least 3 days*** *or be accompanied by* ***at least two vomiting episodes per day*** *for* ***at least 2 days***) |
| *Lower GI* | | | |
| 0 | Diarrhea <500 mL/day | Diarrhea <500 mL/day | Diarrhea <500 mL/day or <3 episodes/day for adults[a,b] |
| 1 | Diarrhea >500 mL/day | Diarrhea >500 mL/day | Diarrhea 500–999 mL/day or three to four episodes/day for adults[a,c] |
| 2 | Diarrhea >1000 mL/day | Diarrhea >1000 mL/day | Diarrhea 1000–1500 mL/day or five to seven episodes/day for adults[a,d] |
| 3 | Diarrhea >1500 mL/day | Diarrhea >1500 mL/day | Diarrhea >1500 mL/day or >7 episodes/day for adults[a,e] |
| 4 | Diarrhea >2000 mL/day | Severe abdominal pain with or without ileus | Severe abdominal pain **with or without ileus or grossly bloody stools (regardless of stool volume)** |

*AST* aspartate transaminase, *BSA* body surface area, *GI* gastrointestinal tract, *GvHD* graft-versus-host disease, *IBMTR* International Bone Marrow Transplantation Registry, *IU* international units, *MAGIC* Mount Sinai Acute GvHD International Consortium, *NA* not applicable, *SGOT* serum glutamic oxaloacetic acid transaminase

[a]One episode of diarrhea is considered to be about 200 mL for an adult and 3 mL/kg for a child (<50 kg) [16]

[b]Diarrhea <10 mL/kg/day or <4 episodes/day for children

[c]Diarrhea 10–19.9 mL/kg/day or four to six episodes/day for children

[d]Diarrhea 20–30 mL/kg/day or seven to ten episodes/day for children

[e]Diarrhea >30 mL/kg/day or >10 episodes/day for children

## Staging/Grading of Chronic GVHD

Historically, chronic GVHD was classified as limited or extensive. Limited chronic GVHD included localized skin involvement or hepatic dysfunction due to chronic GVHD, and all others were classified as extensive [34, 35]. As this classification system was based on a small retrospective study and was not shown predictive of NRM, the NIH convened a working group in 2004 to standardize the criteria for diagnosis and scoring of chronic GVHD. The first NIH consensus criteria were published in 2005 [36] and updated in 2014 [37].

Based on these criteria, signs and symptoms of chronic GVHD are categorized as either "diagnostic" (manifestations that are sufficient to establish the diagnosis of chronic GVHD without need for further testing) or "distinctive" (manifestations that are usually not seen in acute GVHD, and are commonly seen in chronic GVHD, but are insufficient alone to establish an unequivocal diagnosis of chronic GVHD). *Distinctive* features require additional testing to establish the diagnosis of chronic GVHD, which could include a biopsy, other tests (e.g., pulmonary function test (PFT), Schirmer's test), or evaluation by a specialist (e.g., ophthalmologist, gynecologist). For the diagnosis of chronic GVHD, the NIH consensus criteria require at least one *diagnostic* manifestation or at least one *distinctive* manifestation plus additional testing.

Chronic GVHD commonly involves eight organs—the skin (and appendages such as hair and nails), mouth, eyes, GI tract, liver, lungs, joints/musculoskeletal system, and genitalia. *Diagnostic* features in the skin are poikiloderma, lichen planus, lichen sclerosus-like eruptions, deep sclerotic features, or morphea-like superficial sclerotic features. Lichen planus-like changes in the mouth are *diagnostic* of oral GVHD, and lichen planus- or lichen sclerosus-like features in the genitalia are *diagnostic* of genital GVHD. Other *diagnostic* criteria for genital GVHD include vaginal scarring or clitoral/labial agglutination in females and phimosis or urethral/meatus scarring or stenosis in males. Esophageal webs, strictures, and stenosis in the upper to mid-third of the esophagus are *diagnostic* features of chronic GI GVHD. *Diagnostic* findings of the musculoskeletal system GVHD include fasciitis, joint stiffness, or contractures secondary to fasciitis or sclerosis. Bronchiolitis obliterans syndrome (BOS) is *diagnostic* of lung GVHD. Cryptogenic organizing pneumonia (COP) and restrictive lung disease are neither diagnostic nor distinctive of lung GVHD. There are no *diagnostic* features for ocular, hair, or nail, and there is no *diagnostic* or *distinctive* feature of liver GVHD. *Diagnostic*, *distinctive*, and other features of chronic GVHD are elaborated in Table 2.3.

Each of the common eight organs/sites (skin, mouth, eyes, GI tract, liver, lungs, joints/fascia,

**Table 2.3** Signs and symptoms of chronic GVHD

| Organ or site | Diagnostic (sufficient to establish the diagnosis of chronic GVHD) | Distinctive[a] (seen in chronic GVHD, but insufficient alone to establish a diagnosis) | Other features or unclassified entities[b] | Common[c] (seen with both acute and chronic GVHD) |
|---|---|---|---|---|
| Skin | Poikiloderma | Depigmentation | Sweat impairment | Erythema |
| | Lichen planus–like features | Papulosquamous lesions | Ichthyosis | Maculopapular rash |
| | | | Keratosis pilaris | Pruritus |
| | Sclerotic features Morphea-like features | | Hypopigmentation | |
| | | | Hyperpigmentation | |
| | Lichen sclerosus–like features | | | |

**Table 2.3** (continued)

| | | | | |
|---|---|---|---|---|
| Nails | | Dystrophy | | |
| | | Longitudinal ridging, splitting or brittle features | | |
| | | Onycholysis | | |
| | | Pterygium unguis | | |
| | | Nail loss (usually symmetric, affects most nails) | | |
| Scalp and body hair | | New onset of scarring or nonscarring scalp alopecia (after recovery from chemoradiotherapy) | Thinning scalp hair, typically patchy, coarse or dull (not explained by endocrine or other causes) | |
| | | Loss of body hair Sealing | Premature gray hair | |
| Mouth | Lichen planus–like changes | Xerostomia | | Gingivitis |
| | | Mucoceles | | Mucositis |
| | | Mucosal astrophy | | Erythema |
| | | Ulcers | | Pain |
| | | Pseudomembranes | | |
| Eyes | | New onset dry, gritty, or painful eyes | Photophobia | |
| | | | Periorbital hyperpigmentation | |
| | | Cicatricial conjunctivitis | Blepharitis (erythema of the eyelids with edema) | |
| | | KCS | | |
| | | Confluent areas of punctate keratopathy | | |
| Genitalia | Lichen planus–like features | Erosions | | |
| | Lichen sclerosus–like features | Fissures | | |
| Female | Vaginal scarring or clitoral/labial agglutination | Ulcers | | |
| Males | Phimosis or urethral/meatus scarring or stenosis | | | |
| CI Tract | Esophageal web | | Exocrine pancreatic insufficiency | Anorexia |
| | Strictures or stenosis in the upper to mid third of the esophagus | | | Nausea |
| | | | | Vomiting |
| | | | | Diarrhea |
| | | | | Weight loss |
| | | | | Failure to thrive (infants and children |

(continued)

**Table 2.3** (continued)

| | | | | |
|---|---|---|---|---|
| Liver | | | | Total bilirubin, alkaline phosphatase > 2 × upper limit of normal |
| | | | | ALT > 2 × upper limit of normal |
| Lung | Bronchiolitis obliterans diagnosed with lung biopsy | Air trapping and bronchiectasis on chest CT | Cryptogenic organizing pneumonia | |
| | BOS[d, f] | | Restrictive lung disease[c] | |
| Muscles, fascia, joints | Fasciitis | Myositis or polymyositis[e, f] | Edema | |
| | Joint stiffness or contractures secondary to fasciitis or sclerosis | | Muscle cramps | |
| | | | Arthralgia or arthritis | |
| Hematopoietic and immune | | Thrombocytopenia | | |
| | | | Eosinophilia | |
| | | | Lymphopenia | |
| | | | Hypo- or hyper-gammaglobulinemia | |
| | | | Autoantibodies (AIHA, ITP) | |
| | | | Raynaud's phenomenon | |
| Other | | | Pericardial or pleural effusions | |
| | | | Ascites | |
| | | | Peripheral neuropathy | |
| | | | Nephrotic syndrome | |
| | | | Myasthenia gravis | |
| | | | Cardiac conduction abnormality or cardiomyopathy | |

*Ref: Biol Blood Marrow Transplant. 2015 Mar; 21(3): 389–401.e1*
*ALT* alanine aminotransferase, *AIHA* autoimmune hemolytic anemia, *ITP* idiopathic thrombocytopenic purpura
[a]In all cases, infection, drug effect, malignancy, or other causes must be excluded
[b]Can be acknowledged as part of the chronic GVHD manifestations if diagnosis is confirmed
[c]Common refers to shared features by both acute and chronic GVHD
[d]BOS can be diagnostic for lung chronic GVHD only if distinctive sign or symptom present in another organ (see text)
[e]Pulmonary entities under investigation or unclassified
[f]Diagnosis of chronic GVHD requires biopsy

and genital tract) is staged from 0–3, with 0 being normal and 3 being the worst score. Based on the number and severity of organs/sites involved, a global score is calculated, based on which chronic GVHD is categorized as mild, moderate, or severe. Mild chronic GVHD includes one or two organs/site(s) with no more than score 1 and a lung score of 0. Moderate chronic GVHD includes more than two organs/sites involved with no more than score 1 or one organ/site (not lung) with a score of 2 or lung score 1. Severe chronic GVHD includes at least one organ/site with a score of 3 or a lung score of >1. The degree to which the presence of even mild lung GVHD

(BOS) impacts scoring is reflective of the increased mortality associated with this organ involvement (Table 2.4). At the time of chronic GVHD onset, a majority have mild (45–55%) or moderate (35–40%) chronic GVHD, while severe (5–15%) is relatively uncommon [31, 32].

**Table 2.4** Organ scoring of chronic GVHD

| | SCORE 0 | SCORE 1 | SCORE 2 | SCORE 3 |
|---|---|---|---|---|
| **PERFORMANCE SCORE:**<br>[ ]<br>**KPS ECOG LPS** | ☐ Asymptomatic and fully active (ECOG 0; KPS or LPS 100%) | ☐ Symptomatic, fully ambulatory, restricted only in physically strenuous activity (ECOG 1, KPS or LPS 80-90%) | ☐ Symptomatic, ambulatory, capabl of self-care, >50% of waking hours ou of bed (ECOG 2, KPS or LPS 60-70%) | ☐ Symptomatic, limited self-care, >50% of waking hours in bed (ECOG 3-4, KPS or LPS <60%) |
| **SKIN†**<br>**SCORE % BSA** [ ]<br>*GVHD features to be scored by BSA:*<br>**Check all that apply:**<br>☐ Maculopapular rash/erythema<br>☐ Lichen planus-like features<br>☐ Sclerotic features<br>☐ Papulosquamous lesions or ichthyosis<br>☐ Keratosis pilaris-like GVHD | ☐ No BSA involved | ☐ 1-18% BSA | ☐ 19-50% BSA | ☐ >50% BSA |
| **SKIN FEATURES SCORE:** | ☐ No sclerotic features | | ☐ Superficial sclerotic features "not hidebound" (able to pinch) | **Check all that apply:**<br>☐ Deep sclerotic features<br>☐ "Hidebound" (unable to pinch)<br>☐ Impaired mobility<br>☐ Ulceration |
| *Other skin GVHD features (NOT scored by BSA)*<br>**Check all that apply:**<br>☐ Hyperpigmentation<br>☐ Hypopigmentation<br>☐ Poikiloderma<br>☐ Severe or generalized pruritus<br>☐ Hair involvement<br>☐ Nail involvement<br>☐ *Abnormality present but explained entirely by non-GVHD documented cause (specify):*____ | | | | |
| **MOUTH**<br>*Lichen planus-like features present:*<br>☐ **Yes**<br>☐ **No** | ☐ No symptoms | ☐ Mild symptoms **with** disease signs but not limiting oral intake significantly | ☐ Moderate symptoms with disease signs **with** partial limitation of oral intake | ☐ Severe symptoms with disease signs on examination **with** major limitation of oral intake |
| ☐ *Abnormality present but explained entirely by non-GVHD documented cause (specify):*____ | | | | |

**Figure 1.** Organ scoring of chronic GVHD. ECOG indicates Eastern Cooperative Oncology Group; KPS, Karnofsky Performance Status; LPS, Lansky Performance Status; BSA, body surface area; ADL, activities of daily living; LFTs, liver function tests; AP, alkaline phosphatase; ALT, alanine aminotransferase; ULN, normal upper limit. *Weight loss within 3 months. †Skin scoring should use both percentage of BSA involved by disease signs and the cutaneous features scales. When a discrepancy exists between the percentage of total body surface (BSA) score and the skin feature score, OR if superficial sclerotic features are present (Score 2), but there is impaired mobility or ulceration (Score 3), the higher level should be used for the final skin scoring. ‡To be completed by specialist or trained medical providers (see Supplemental Figure). **Lung scoring should be performed using both the symptoms and FEV1 scores whenever possible. FEV1 should be used in the final lung scoring where there is discrepancy between symptoms and FEV1 scores.

*Ref: Biol Blood Marrow Transplant. 2015 Mar; 21(3): 389–401.e1*

(continued)

**Table 2.4** (continued)

| | SCORE 0 | SCORE 1 | SCORE 2 | SCORE 3 |
|---|---|---|---|---|
| **EYES**<br><br>*Keratoconjunctivitis sicca (KCS) confirmed by ophthalmologist:*<br>☐ **Yes**<br>☐ **No**<br>☐ **Not examined** | ☐ No symptoms | ☐ Mild dry eye symptoms not affecting ADL (requirement of lubricant eye drops ≤ 3 x per day) | ☐ Moderate dry eye symptoms partially affecting ADL (requiring lubricant eye drops > 3 x per day or punctal plugs), **WITHOUT** new vision impairment due to KCS | ☐ Severe dry eye symptoms significantly affecting ADL (special eyeware to relieve pain) **OR** unable to work because of ocular symptoms **OR** loss of vision due to KCS |
| ☐ *Abnormality present but explained entirely by non-GVHD documented cause (specify):* ________ | | | | |
| **GI Tract**<br>***Check all that apply:***<br>☐ Esophageal web/ proximal stricture or ring<br>☐ Dysphagia<br>☐ Anorexia<br>☐ Nausea<br>☐ Vomiting<br>☐ Diarrhea<br>☐ Weight loss ≥5%*<br>☐ Failure to thrive | ☐ No symptoms | ☐ Symptoms without significant weight loss* (<5%) | ☐ Symptoms associated with mild to moderate weight loss* (5-15%) **OR** moderate diarrhea without significant interference with daily living | ☐ Symptoms associated with significant weight loss* >15%, requires nutritional supplement for most calorie needs **OR** esophageal dilation **OR** severe diarrhea with significant interference with daily living |
| ☐ *Abnormality present but explained entirely by non-GVHD documented cause (specify):* ________ | | | | |
| **LIVER** | ☐ Normal total bilirubin and ALT or AP < 3 x ULN | ☐ Normal total bilirubin with ALT ≥3 to 5 x ULN or AP ≥ 3 x ULN | ☐ Elevated total bilirubin but ≤3 mg/dL or ALT > 5 ULN | ☐ Elevated total bilirubin > 3 mg/dL |
| ☐ *Abnormality present but explained entirely by non-GVHD documented cause (specify):* | | | | |
| **LUNGS****<br><u>**Symptom score**</u>: | ☐ No symptoms | ☐ Mild symptoms (shortness of breath after climbing one flight of steps) | ☐ Moderate symptoms (shortness of breath after walking on flat ground) | ☐ Severe symptoms (shortness of breath at rest; requiring $0_2$) |
| <u>**Lung score**</u>:<br>**% FEV1** ☐<br><br>*Pulmonary function tests*<br>☐ Not performed | ☐ FEV1≥80% | ☐ FEV1 60-79% | ☐ FEV1 40-59% | ☐ FEV1 ≤39% |
| ☐ *Abnormality present but explained entirely by non-GVHD documented cause (specify):* ________ | | | | |

**Table 2.4** (continued)

| | SCORE 0 | SCORE 1 | SCORE 2 | SCORE 3 |
|---|---|---|---|---|
| JOINTS AND FASCIA<br><br>P-ROM score<br>*(see below)*<br>Shoulder (1-7):___<br>Elbow (1-7): ____<br>Wrist/finger (1-7):___<br>Ankle (1-4):___ | ☐ No symptoms | ☐ Mild tightness of arms or legs, normal or mild decreased range of motion (ROM) **AND** not affecting ADL | ☐ Tightness of arms or legs **OR** joint contractures, erythema thought due to fasciitis, moderate decrease ROM **AND** mild to moderate limitation of ADL | ☐ Contractures **WITH** significant decrease of ROM ***AND*** significant limitation of ADL (unable to tie shoes, button shirts, dress self etc.) |
| ☐ *Abnormality present but explained entirely by non-GVHD documented cause (specify):*_________________ | | | | |
| GENITAL TRACT<br>(*See Supplemental figure*[‡])<br>☐ Not examined<br>*Currently sexually active*<br>☐ Yes<br>☐ No | ☐ No signs | ☐ Mild signs[‡] and females with or without discomfort on exam | ☐ Moderate signs[‡] and may have symptoms with discomfort on exam | ☐ Severe signs[‡] with or without symptoms |
| ☐ *Abnormality present but explained entirely by non-GVHD documented cause (specify):* | | | | |

**Other indicators, clinical features or complications related to chronic GVHD (check all that apply and assign a score to severity (0-3) based on functional impact where applicable none – 0,mild -1, moderate -2, severe – 3)**

| | | |
|---|---|---|
| ☐ Ascites (serositis)___ | ☐ Myasthenia Gravis___ | |
| ☐ Pericardial Effusion___ | ☐ Peripheral Neuropathy___ | ☐ Eosinophilia > 500/µl___ |
| ☐ Pleural Effusion(s)___ | ☐ Polymyositis___ | ☐ Platelets <100,000/µl ___ |
| ☐ Nephrotic syndrome___ | ☐ Weight loss>5%* without GI symptoms ___ | ☐ Others (specify):_____________ |

| | | | | |
|---|---|---|---|---|
| **Overall GVHD Severity**<br>*(Opinion of the evaluator)* | ❑ **No GVHD** | ❑ **Mild** | ❑ **Moderate** | ❑ **Severe** |

**Photographic Range of Motion (P-ROM)**

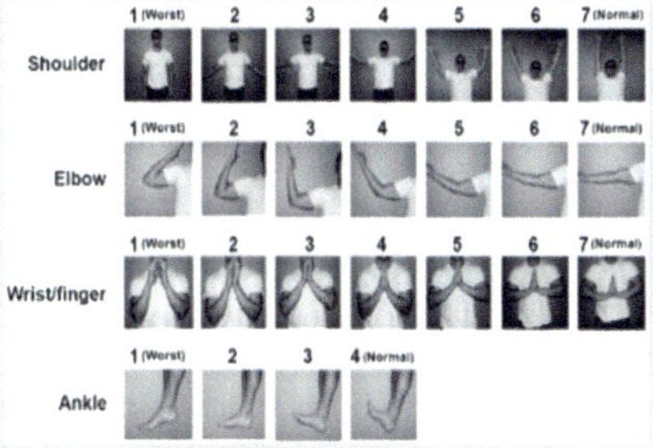


***Ref:*** *Biol Blood Marrow Transplant. 2015 Mar; 21(3): 389–401.e1.*

## Introduction of the Concept of GVHD Prophylaxis

The first evidence that interventions could be used to prevent GVHD came with the recognition that treating animals with antimetabolites (such as methotrexate (MTX)) improved engraftment as well as survival by limiting "secondary syndrome" which was later recognized as GVHD [38–46]. Simultaneously, several other antimetabolites (6-mercaptopurine, azathioprine, procarbazine, and cytosine arabinoside, cyclophosphamide (Cy), 6-mercaptopurine, azathioprine) and other drugs (cyclosporine A (CsA), prednisone, and antithymocyte globulin (ATG)) either alone or in combination were tested in animal models. Among antimetabolites, both MTX and Cy were found to be effective for GVHD prevention in preclinical models leading to human trials examining MTX for GVHD prophylaxis [35, 47]. These trials determined a shorter course of MTX to be as effective as longer course therapy [48]. Accordingly, MTX is administered on days +1, +3, +6, and +11 posttransplant, with some omitting the day +11, especially in the recipients of low-intensity conditioning.

## Introduction of Cyclosporine A for GVHD Prophylaxis

In the late 1970s, a novel antilymphocytic agent—CsA—was described by Jean Borel and colleagues [49]. It is a calcineurin inhibitor (CNI) that exerts its immunosuppressive effects by blocking transcription of cytokine genes, including interleukin-2 (IL-2) and IL-4 [50]. After entering T lymphocytes, it binds to an intracellular protein—cyclophilin A forming a cyclophilin-CsA complex which inhibits calcineurin, a Ca+/calmodulin-dependent serine/threonine phosphatase required for early T-cell activation. Calcineurin normally dephosphorylates the nuclear factor of activated T cells (NFAT), allowing it to translocate into the nucleus and activate expression of genes involved in the transcription of cytokines. Therefore, by preventing calcineurin-mediated dephosphorylation, CsA inhibits the nuclear translocation of NFAT and subsequent cytokine gene expression in activated T cells [50].

After the discovery of CsA, controlled studies were done in animals and subsequently in humans demonstrating efficacy with a reduction in acute GVHD and improved survival [51–54]. While effective as GVHD prophylaxis, CSA has significant toxicities including hypertension, nephrotoxicity, hypomagnesemia, risks for seizures, hypertrichosis, gingival hyperplasia, tremors, and anorexia [55]. Typically CSA is initiated intravenously 1–2 days prior to stem cell infusion and converted to oral dosing when possible. The risk of acute GVHD increases when cyclosporine trough concentrations drop below a target level [56].

## Use of Combination Drugs for GVHD Prophylaxis

Preclinical models examining the addition of CSA to MTX for GVHD prophylaxis demonstrated synergism between these agents and improved survival [51]. From these experiments, it was learned that CsA has to be present early after HCT to prevent sensitization between donor and recipient cells, and when delayed, lymphocytes could proliferate into cytotoxic effector cells. Subsequently, two prospective randomized clinical trials in humans showed a significant reduction in acute GVHD and improved overall survival (OS) with the combination of CSA to MTX when compared to MTX alone [57, 58].

## Trials Assessing Tacrolimus Versus CsA

Tacrolimus (FK506), another CNI, is a macrolide lactone that was first isolated from the fermentation broth of *Streptomyces tsukubaensis* in 1984 and was noted to have more potent in vitro and in vivo immunosuppressive effects in mice than CsA [59–61]. Tacrolimus and CsA both bind to immunophilins but belong to distinct families, called FK506-binding proteins (FKBPs) and cyclophilins, respectively, which form distinct drug: immunophilin complexes - CsA-cyclophilin and FK506-FKBP-12, respectively [62]. These complexes bind to and inhibit the activity of calcineurin.

After its introduction, studies in dogs [63] and four prospective randomized trials in humans compared the safety and efficacy of tacrolimus to CsA in combination with MTX [64–67] for GVHD prophylaxis. These trials differed significantly by donor type, patient population, and target calcineurin inhibitor (CNI) levels, in addition to other factors. These differences led to conflicting conclusions regarding the benefit of tacrolimus vs. CSA with respect to a number of key transplant outcomes including reduction in (severe) acute and chronic GVHD, mortality and relapse. The implications of these studies and their oftentimes divergent findings are unclear, and generally CSA and tacrolimus are viewed as equivalent agents.

## Mycophenolate Mofetil (MMF)

Another antimetabolite often used for GVHD prophylaxis is MMF. MMF is rapidly hydrolyzed to an active metabolite—mycophenolic acid (MPA), which is a potent, selective, and reversible inhibitor of inosine 5′-monophosphate dehydrogenase (IMPDH), a key enzyme in the de novo synthesis of guanine nucleotides, and is expressed in activated human T and B lymphocytes [68]. MMF has a more potent cytostatic effect on lymphocytes than other cells [69]. Canine models demonstrated synergy between MMF and CsA [68]. In practice, MMF is often used as an alternative to MTX, mostly in older-aged or frail patients receiving NMA or RIC [70]. The most common side effects attributed to MMF are cytopenia and GI side effects. A few prospective trials compared MMF to MTX, both in combination with a CNI [71–73]. One study in MUD and MSD recipients who received either MAC or RIC showed a higher risk of severe acute GVHD with MMF vs. MTX, 19% vs. 4%, respectively, $P = 0.03$, with no differences in other outcomes [71]. Two other smaller studies showed no differences in GVHD or survival for MMF vs. MTX arms in MSD recipients receiving MAC [72, 74].

## Antithymocyte Globulin (ATG) for In Vivo T-Cell Depletion

Several preclinical studies in the late 1960s and early 1970s showed that pretreatment of donor cells with horse or rabbit anti*lymphocyte* serum (ALS) or anti*thymocyte* serum (ATS) was effective in preventing acute GVHD [75–79]. Several formulations of these polyclonal sera have been tested in humans, and it is important to recognize the differences in these formulations. They are broadly classified as anti*thymocyte* globulin (ATG) or anti-T-*lymphocyte* globulin (ATLG). Both of these can be derived from either horse or rabbit source [80, 81] and rarely from pigs [82] by inoculation of human thymocytes (generating anti*thymocyte* globulin, ATG) or human cell lines, such as Jurkat T-lymphoblastoid cell line, which resembles human activated T lymphocytes (thus, generating anti-T-*lymphocyte* globulin, ATLG). Rabbit ATG more efficiently depletes lymphocytes in vivo and is more cytotoxic on a weight basis in vitro as compared to horse ATG [81]. Also, rabbit ATG but not horse ATG induces the development of regulatory T cells (Tregs) [83, 84]. Anti*thymocyte* polyclonal sera derived from horses is known as "**ATGAM®**" (hATG, Pfizer Inc. NY, US) or **lymphoglobulin/hATG** (Lymphoglobulin, Genzyme, Cambridge, MA, USA), which was later withdrawn from the market and replaced by the one derived from rabbits, known as **thymoglobulin** or simply **ATG** (Sanofi Genzyme, Cambridge, MA) [80]. Anti-*T-lymphocyte* polyclonal sera are available only from rabbit source and is known as **ATLG (formerly ATG Fresenius®,** Neovii Biotech, Lexington, MA) [80]. Since polyclonal serum reacts against both host and donor lymphocytes, the expected effects are the reduction of the risk of GVHD and the prevention of graft failure.

Several large phase III prospective clinical trials assessed the safety and efficacy of ATG/ATLG in the MAC setting with either MSD [9] or MUD [7, 85, 86] using different formulations and doses. One prospective randomized trial was conducted in the MSD setting, where patients with acute leukemia received MAC and PB graft and CsA/MTX for GVHD prophylaxis with or without ATLG/ATG Fresenius (30 mg/kg over 3 days—days −3, −2, and −1). There was no difference in the risk of grades II–IV or grades III–IV (2% vs. 8%, $p = 0.10$) acute GVHD with ATLG vs. no ATLG, respectively; however, the risk of chronic GVHD (32% vs 69%; $P < 0.001$) and moderate-severe chronic GVHD (11% vs.

47%, $P < 0.001$) were significantly lower with ATLG. There were no differences in relapse, infectious complications, adverse events, or OS between the groups [9].

Three prospective phase III randomized trials were conducted in the MUD setting. A European trial included acute leukemia patients who received MAC, and a majority received PB graft (82%). GVHD prophylaxis included CsA/MTX with or without ATLG (60 mg/kg over 3 days; days −3, −2, −1). The use of ATLG was associated with a significantly lower risk of grades II–IV acute GVHD (33% vs. 51% [HR 0.56; $p = 0.011$]), grades III–IV acute GVHD (12% vs. 25% [HR 0.50; $p = 0.054$]), chronic GVHD (31% vs. 59% [HR 0.34; $p < 0.0001$]), and extensive chronic GVHD (12% vs. 43% [HR 0.22; $p < 0.0001$]). There were no differences in relapse, NRM, OS, or mortality from infectious causes [86]. A Canadian trial included patients with various hematologic malignancies, most of whom were treated with MAC, and a majority received PB (88%). GVHD prophylaxis included CNI plus either MTX or MMF, with or without rabbit ATG. The rates of grades II–IV acute GVHD (50% vs. 65%; $p = 0.012$) and moderate-severe chronic GVHD (13% vs. 29%; $p = 0.0083$) were significantly lower with ATG. Again, there was no difference in relapse, NRM, and OS, but more Epstein-Barr virus (EBV) reactivations occurred in the ATG arm [85]. The most recent addition to these trials was a double-blind placebo-controlled trial conducted in the USA. This study included patients with acute leukemia or myelodysplastic syndrome, all treated with MAC, and a majority received PB (~ 75%) grafts. GVHD prophylaxis included Tac/MTX with or without ATLG (ATG Fresenius). The rates of grades II–IV acute GVHD (23% vs. 40%; $p = 0.004$), grades III–IV acute GVHD (4.3% vs. 11%; $p = 0.09$), chronic GVHD (16% vs. 38%; $p < 0.001$), and moderate-severe chronic GVHD (12% vs. 33%; $p < 0.001$) all favored the ATLG arm. There was no difference in relapse or NRM. However, DFS (65% vs. 47%; $p = 0.04$) and OS (74% vs. 59%; $p = 0.034$) were significantly worse in the ATLG arm (predominantly seen in patients who received TBI), and CMV reactivation was higher with ATG [7].

Although ATG/ATLG is effective in reducing the risk of graft rejection and GVHD, it depletes T cells nonselectively, resulting in global immunodeficiency. Moreover, the mean elimination half-life of ATG in humans ranges from about 6 days (equine source) to as long as 30 days (rabbit source) [87] and increases the risk of viral [7, 85, 88] and fungal infections [89] and posttransplant lymphoproliferative disorders (PTLD) [90].

Another agent used for in vivo T-cell depletion is alemtuzumab (Campath-1H or "Cambridge Pathology 1"), which is a monoclonal antibody directed against CD52 [91]. As CD52 is expressed on the surface of B and T lymphocytes, natural killer (NK) cells, monocytes, macrophages, and some dendritic cells, alemtuzumab is broadly immunosuppressive. One study assessing pharmacokinetics of alemtuzumab showed potentially lympholytic levels (>0.1 μg/mL) of alemtuzumab for approximately 56 days post-HCT in the RIC group, which was 26 days longer than in the MAC group [92]. This results in significantly prolonged lymphopenia and delayed CD4 reconstitution [92]. A subsequent study conducted at the MD Anderson Cancer Center only included patients with CD52 expressing malignancies and used a lower dose of alemtuzumab (10 mg/day, days −7 to −3) with Cy/TBI MAC. Alemtuzumab level was undetectable in all serum samples tested between days −1 and +21 post-HCT; all patients engrafted and all patients attained 100% donor chimerism by 3 months post-HCT [93]. Several other studies evaluated the role of alemtuzumab for GVHD prevention (reviewed in [94]), but there are no large-scale prospective randomized trials with or without alemtuzumab or comparing its efficacy against ATG/ATLG.

## Posttransplantation Cyclophosphamide (PTCy)

Hematopoietic stem cells express high levels of cytosolic aldehyde dehydrogenase (ALDH), an enzyme responsible for Cy metabolism, thus making HSCs resistant to Cy, whereas B and T lymphocytes and NK cells express low levels of the enzyme and are extremely sensitive to the cytotoxic properties of Cy [95, 96]. Post-HCT Cy is hypothesized to induce tolerance by three mechanisms: (a) clonal destruction of antigen-stimulated rapidly proliferating peripheral T cells while sparing T cells that do not react to either host or donor alloantigens, (b) depletion of intrathymic clonal donor-reactive T cells, and (c) generation of tolerogen-specific suppressor T cells [97].

The use of Cy for GVHD prophylaxis dates back over five decades where preclinical models demonstrated a reduction GVHD in a dose dependent fashion [98–100]. The interest in Cy prophylaxis reemerged after further studies from Johns Hopkins in the late 1990s and early 2000s demonstrated its efficacy in HLA-mismatched models [101]. The use of posttransplantation Cy (PTCy) 200 mg/kg on day +3 in preclinical models led to the induction of stable, mixed chimerism after MHC-mismatched BMT and NMA conditioning. Survival was prolonged in the recipients of PTCy compared with animals that received alloBMT without PTCy [101]. Subsequently, a prospective phase I/II trial evaluated PTCy in recipients of T cell-replete BM graft from HLA-haploidentical donors [102]. The study included 13 patients who received NMA conditioning and PTCy 50 mg/kg on day +3 along with MMF and tacrolimus starting from day +4. The cumulative incidence of graft failure and severe GVHD was about 60% at 6 months. The conditioning regimen was then modified, and PTCy 50 mg/kg was given on either day +3 alone or days +3 and +4 in two different cohorts [103]. All patients also received MMF and tacrolimus starting a day following the completion of Cy. With this regimen, graft rejection occurred in 13%, and grades II–IV and III–IV acute GVHD by day 200 were 34% and 6%, respectively, with no statistically significant differences between patients who received one versus two doses of PTCy. However, most impressively, the incidence of extensive chronic GVHD at 1 year was 5% in those who received two doses of PTCy versus 25% in those who received one dose (hazard ratio [HR] 0.21; 95% confidence interval [CI] 0.04–1.01; $P = 0.05$). The cumulative incidence of relapse, NRM, and survival did not differ between the groups [103].

Since then, the use of PTCy has been extended to the HLA-matched/HLA-mismatched related/unrelated donor setting after either MAC or RIC HCT. In the setting of MAC, when used as the sole prophylactic agent in patients undergoing HLA-matched related or MUD HCT with BM graft, the incidence of grades II–IV acute GVHD was 51%, grades III–IV was 15%, and chronic GVHD at 2 years was 14% [104]. The incidence of GVHD can be reduced further when additional prophylaxis is added with PTCy. In a prospective phase II clinical trial at MDACC [105], patients with HLA-matched or HLA-mismatched related or unrelated donors received IV Bu/Flu+/−thiotepa MAC and GVHD prophylaxis with PTCy/Tac/MMF. The rates of grades II–IV and III–IV acute GVHD were 38% and 9%, respectively; 1-year chronic GVHD and extensive chronic GVHD rates were 10% and 8%, respectively [105].

In the setting of RIC, a prospective phase III clinical trial conducted by the Blood and Marrow Transplant Clinical Trials Network (BMT CTN) compared PTCy/Tac/MMF prophylaxis with two other novel GVHD prophylaxis regimens including bortezomib (with Tac/MTX) and maraviroc (with Tac/MTX). Each of these arms was compared separately to a contemporary nonrandomized prospective control group who received Tac/MTX prophylaxis. The best GVHD-free relapse-free survival (GRFS) was noted in the PTCy arm (HR 0·72; $p = 0{\cdot}044$), while bortezomib (HR 0·98; $p = 0{\cdot}92$) and maraviroc arms (HR 1·10; $p = 0{\cdot}49$) were not different as compared to the control group. The rates of grades II–IV acute GVHD and overall chronic GVHD were not statistically different across the three investigational arms when compared to contemporary controls. However, the rates of grades III–IV acute GVHD and immunosuppression-requiring chronic GVHD were both significantly lower in the PTCy arm (2% and 22%) than bortezomib (8% and 29%), maraviroc (9% and 33%), and the controls (13% and 37%) [6]. The BMT CTN is now conducting a randomized prospective phase III clinical trial comparing PTCy/Tac/MMF to the Tac/MTX regimen.

## Sirolimus

Sirolimus is produced by the bacterium *Streptomyces hygroscopicus*, which was first isolated from a soil sample collected from Rapa Nui commonly known as Easter Island in 1972 by Surendra Nath Sehgal and colleagues [106]. The compound was named rapamycin after the native name of the island. It was developed as an antifungal, given its potent anti-candida activity, but was also found to possess antitumor, antiproliferative, and immunosuppressive properties in subsequent studies [106]. Sirolimus shares structural similarity with tacrolimus in the binding domains, and they both bind to FKBP, but sirolimus exerts different biological activities than tacrolimus, and it neither affects calcineurin activity, nor does it interfere with T-cell receptor-induced NFAT nuclear translocation. The target of the sirolimus-FKBP complex is the mammalian target of rapamycin (mTOR), the inhibition of which blocks IL-2 mediated signal transduction pathways that prevent cell cycle progression from G1 to S phase in T cells [107]. Sirolimus is also postulated to facilitate the expansion of regulatory T cells (CD4 + CD25 + FoxP3+; Tregs) which have a protective effect against GVHD [108, 109], making it a particularly appealing drug for use as GVHD prophylaxis.

A Blood and Marrow Transplant Clinical Trials Network (BMT CTN) phase III randomized prospective clinical trial compared the use of Tac/MTX to Tac/Siro after MSD HCT and Cy/TBI or TBI/Etoposide MAC. The trial initially allowed myeloablative busulfan-based conditioning; however, it was later removed due to excess toxicity and veno-occlusive disease (VOD)/sinusoidal obstruction syndrome (SOS) of the liver observed in the sirolimus arm. The study showed no difference in acute or chronic GVHD; however, sirolimus was associated with faster engraftment of neutrophils and platelets and less severe mucositis than MTX [110].

Sirolimus-based CNI-free GVHD regimens were also demonstrated to be safe in the setting of haploidentical [111] and MMUD [112] HCT after either NMA or MAC and in the setting of double-unit umbilical cord blood transplantation (UCBT) after RIC [113]. A recent phase II prospective clinical trial by the National Marrow Donor Program/Be The Match (NMDP) enrolled 80 patients across 11 US centers and assessed the role of PTCy/sirolimus/MMF prophylaxis in patients undergoing mismatched unrelated donor (MMUD) HCT with BM graft after myeloablative ($n = 40$) or non-myeloablative ($n = 40$) conditioning. In the MAC and the RIC groups, the cumulative incidence of grades II–IV acute GVHD at day 100 was 43% and 33%, grades III–IV was 18% and 0%, 1-year chronic GVHD was 36% and 18%, and 1-year OS was 72% and 79%, respectively. Only one case of VOD/SOS was noted, and there was no case of thrombotic microangiopathy (TMA) [112]. Another prospective phase II trial assessed the role of PTCy/sirolimus/MMF prophylaxis in patients undergoing PB haploidentical HCT demonstrating low rates of acute and comparable rates of chronic GVHD as other forms of prophylaxis [111].

The addition of sirolimus to standard CNI/MMF prophylaxis enhanced the outcomes after NMA MUD HCT, with a lower risk of GVHD, lower NRM, and improved survival. This was shown in a multicenter, randomized, phase III trial comparing sirolimus/CsA/MMF to CsA/MMF prophylaxis in patients undergoing MUD HCT after NMA conditioning. The sirolimus-based regimen was associated with a significantly lower risk of grades II–IV acute GVHD (26% vs. 52%), 1-year NRM (4% vs. 16%), and better PFS (77% vs. 64%) as well as OS at 1 year (86% vs. 70%) than CsA/MMF regimen. There was no difference in grades III–IV acute GVHD (2% vs. 8%) or chronic GVHD (49% vs. 50%) between the arms [114].

## Ex Vivo T-Cell Depletion for GVHD Prophylaxis

In the early 1980s, multiple studies were conducted using ex vivo T cell-deplete (TCD) grafts without the need for post-grafting immunosuppression. These studies indeed showed a significant reduction in the risk of both acute and chronic GVHD but also showed higher risks of graft rejection, delayed immune reconstitution, increased PTLD, and disease relapse. The degree of T-cell depletion needed to prevent GVHD was also studied; some studies showed that reducing the T-cell content in the BM graft from $1 \times 10^6$ cells/kg to $0.5 \times 10^6$ cells/kg can reduce the risk of acute GVHD by half from 45% to 22% [115, 116], and others showed that even a lower CD3 dose ($0.03 \times 10^6$ cells/kg) was sufficient for successful engraftment and resulted in no GVHD in recipients of haploidentical HCT, although the risk of relapse and NRM remained high [117]. Then several prospective and retrospective studies independently assessed the role of TCD (reviewed [118]), but prospective randomized trials comparing its safety and efficacy to other techniques remained unanswered until recently.

In a recent prospective phase III randomized trial (BMT CTN 1301) [119], patients aged 65 years or younger with acute leukemia or myelodysplasia with MSD (about 40%) or MUD (about 60%) were randomized to one of three CNI-free GVHD approaches. Group 1 received a CD34+ selected PB graft without any post-HCT immune suppression, group 2 received BM graft and PTCy alone for GVHD prophylaxis, and group 3 (control) received BM graft and standard Tac/MTX prophylaxis. Of note, only 85% of patients in group 1 received the planned CD34+ selected graft. The primary endpoint was chronic GVHD-free relapse-free survival at 1 year, which was not statistically different between the groups. The CD34+ selected arm was associated with impressive reductions in the rates of acute and chronic GVHD (including severe manifestations); however, despite reducing GVHD, this arm was associated with the worst NRM, DFS, and OS of all groups. The DFS was 76% for CD34+ group (HR 1.74, $p = 0.02$; HR for CD34 vs. PTCy was 1.77, $p = 0.02$) versus 85% in the PTCy (HR 1.02, $p = 0.95$) and 84.2% in the controls. Rates of NRM at 1 year were 16.5% (HR 2.76 vs. control, $p = 0.01$), 12% (HR 2.01 vs. control, $p = 0.09$), and 7% for CD34, PTCy, and control, respectively. The rates of grades II–III infections at 2 year were high in both CD34+ and PTCy groups, with a significantly higher risk of EBV reactivation by day 180.

## Targeting T-Cell Co-stimulatory Receptors

CD28 and **cytotoxic T-cell lymphocyte-4 (CTLA-4)** are two of the opposing costimulatory receptors on T cells that bind to the same ligands (CD80 and CD86) on APCs and provide positive and negative feedback, respectively, for T-cell activation. **Abatacept** is a fusion protein composed of the Fc region of the immunoglobulin IgG1 fused to the extracellular domain of CTLA-4. In a randomized double-blind placebo-controlled phase II trial [120], patients with 8/8-HLA-matched donors were randomized to receive either abatacept (10 mg/kg/dose, on days −1, +5, +14, and +28) or placebo. In addition, all patients received a CNI (Tac or CsA) and MTX. Patients in the abatacept arm had a reduced risk of grades III–IV acute GVHD at day 100 (6.8%) as compared to placebo (14.8%), but it did not reach statistical significance (HR, 0.45; 80% CI, 0.22 to 0.9, $p = 0.13$). Day 180 severe acute GVHD-free survival was significantly better in the abatacept arm (93.2%) than in placebo (82.0%): HR, 0.37; 80% CI, 0.19 to 0.73, $p = 0.05$. The rates of chronic GVHD were not different nor were differences in the risk of relapse, NRM, OS, or viral reactivations. In addition to the 8/8-HLA group, the study also had a 7/8-HLA cohort which was treated with open-label abatacept along with CNI/MTX. This cohort was compared to a CIBMTR control group that received no ATG. In this 7/8-MUD group, patients treated with abatacept had a substantial decrease in the risk of grades III–IV acute GVHD at day 100 (2.3% vs. 30.2% in controls; HR, 0.0, $P < 0.001$) and significantly improved severe acute GVHD-free survival at day 180 (97.7% vs. 58.7%; HR: 0.00, $P < 0.001$). The rates of grades II–IV acute GVHD and chronic GVHD at 1 year were not different. Based on these results, the US Food and Drug Administration (FDA) granted it breakthrough therapy designation for the prevention of moderate to severe acute GVHD in patients undergoing HCT from unrelated donors.

## Treatment of GVHD

The detailed management of acute and chronic GVHD is beyond the scope of the chapter and is reviewed elsewhere [121–125]. Briefly, the standard first-line therapy for acute GVHD is high-dose corticosteroids. The addition of immunosuppressants to steroid therapy, including mycophenolate mofetil [126, 127], pentostatin [127], denileukin diftitox [127], etanercept [127], daclizumab [128], anti-interleukin-2 receptor monoclonal antibody [129], infliximab [130], or antithymocyte globulin [131], has not shown additional benefits in multiple randomized trials. Response to first-line treatment varies from about 40% to 70% based on the stage and organs involved [17, 121, 124], and only 25–40% of patients achieve durable responses [132]. Failure to respond to corticosteroids (steroid-refractory (SR)-acute GVHD, defined as progression of GVHD after 3 days or no response by 7–10 of treatment) is a marker of poor prognosis, with an overall response rate (ORR) of generally less than 50% and complete response (CR) rate of <30% to subsequent therapies [133]. Although day 28 overall response to treatment is a well-validated surrogate marker of NRM [15, 17, 134–136], physicians generally do not have time to wait for a month before starting second-line treatment, and decisions are often made early based on the response within the first 7–10 days of treatment. Patients who do not respond to steroids early (within a week) generally remain treatment-resistant by day 28. However, about 40% of the patients who are deemed treatment-refractory at 1 week subsequently respond to treatment by day 28 [135], suggesting that these patients are delayed responders rather than truly steroid-refractory. Ruxolitinib is the only Food and Drug Administration (FDA)-approved therapy for SR-acute GVHD, as it showed promising efficacy in a phase III clinical trial leading to an ORR of 62% at day 28 and 40% at day 56 and a median overall survival (OS) of about 11 months [137].

Similar to acute GVHD, corticosteroids are the standard first-line therapy for patients with moderate to severe chronic GVHD. As in acute GVHD, roughly half of the patients with chronic GVHD require treatment with a second-line agent, and until recently, ibrutinib was the only FDA-approved in this setting [138]. Ibrutinib inhibits Bruton tyrosine kinase (BTK) in B cells and interleukin-2-inducible T-cell kinase (ITK) in T cells. Approval of ibrutinib was based on an open-label, multicenter, single-arm study of 42 patients with chronic GVHD who had failed at least 1 prior treatment and were treated with ibrutinib 420 mg orally once daily. At a median follow-up of about 14 months, the best overall response was 67%. The median time-to-response was about 3 months, and the responses were seen across all organs evaluated (skin, mouth, gastrointestinal tract, and liver). Responses lasting 5 months or longer were observed in less than half of the patients (48%). Also, about one-third (31%) of patients needed dose reductions due to an adverse event (AE)—the most common being fatigue—and AEs led to treatment discontinuation in another one-third of patients: the most common being fatigue and pneumonia [138]. Other drugs that have been tested in the treatment of SR-chronic GVHD are ruxolitinib [139] and belumosudil [140].

Belumosudil is a novel oral selective rho-associated coiled-coil kinase 2 (ROCK2) inhibitor. In a phase II, open-label, randomized, multicenter study, patients with cGVHD who had received two to five prior lines of therapy were treated with belumosudil 200 mg once a day ($n$ = 66) or twice a day ($n$ = 66) [141]. Most (67%) patients had severe cGVHD and over half (52%) had ≥4 organs involved, and 72% had received 3 or more previous lines of treatment. In this highly advanced population, with a median follow-up of 8 months, the overall response rate (ORR) was 73% (once daily arm) and 74% (twice daily arm). The ORR was 65% and 72%, respectively, in patients who previously received ruxolitinib and 73% and 71%, respectively, in patients who previously received ibrutinib. The median time-to-response was 4 weeks, and about half of the patients (49%) maintained the response for ≥20 weeks. The drug was very well tolerated, and only 10% of patients discontinued therapy due to possible drug-related AE leading to recent

FDA approval in patients 12 years and older with chronic GVHD that has failed at least two prior lines of systemic therapy.

Ruxolitinib was evaluated in a phase III, open-label, randomized study in patients with SR- or steroid-dependent chronic GVHD [139]. Of note, patients treated with ≥2 prior lines of systemic therapy for chronic GVHD in addition to corticosteroids ± CNI were excluded. Patients were randomized (1:1) to ruxolitinib 10 mg orally twice daily ($n$ = 165) versus investigator-selected best available therapy (BAT; $n$ = 164) for six cycles of 28 days each, along with the continuation of corticosteroids +/− CNI. At data cutoff, 50% in the ruxolitinib arm and 74% in the BAT arm had discontinued the treatment (reason: lack of efficacy (15% vs. 43%), adverse events (17% vs. 5%), and relapse (5% vs. 4%), respectively). After six cycles, the ORR was significantly higher in the ruxolitinib arm (50%) versus the BAT arm (26%): odds ratio, 2.99, $P < 0.0001$. The rates of grade ≥3 AEs were similar in both arms (57% vs. 58%). The most common AEs were anemia (29% vs. 13%), hypertension (16% vs. 13%), pyrexia (16% vs. 9%), and ALT increase (15% vs. 4%), respectively, and infections of any type occurred in 64% vs. 56%, respectively [139].

## Pulmonary Perspectives

A significant proportion of allogeneic HCT recipients will develop pulmonary complications, whether infectious or noninfectious [142]. In the setting of GVHD, these complications can occur as a result of immunosuppression, increasing the chance for opportunistic and routine infections, or as direct alloimmune injury to the lung, resulting in GVHD. As a result, when a pulmonary complication is suspected, a thorough knowledge of the range of pulmonary diseases that can affect HCT recipients, as well as a knowledge of the appropriate and timely workup for these conditions (discussed in Chap. 6), is crucial. HCT recipients can be immunocompromised for numerous reasons, including incomplete or partial graft recovery, pharmacological immunosuppression, or other mechanisms. Therefore, the evaluation of new pulmonary disease requires a broad evaluation for infectious pathologies, often necessitating bronchoscopy, as recommended for immunocompromised hosts [143]. These infections, considered in detail in Chaps. 8–14, require close communication and collaboration between pulmonary, transplant, and infectious diseases experts in order to achieve prompt diagnosis and initiation of treatment.

Noninfectious pulmonary complications (NIPCs) occur in about 20% of allogeneic HCT recipients and are linked to higher mortality [144]. NIPCs are discussed in detail in Chaps. 15–20. Some entities, such as cryptogenic organizing pneumonia and idiopathic pneumonia syndrome, may be indistinguishable from infectious pneumonia without a prompt pulmonary evaluation. The pathophysiology underpinning these conditions has become clearer over time, requiring pulmonary consultants to remain engaged with these scientific advances. For example, the advent of widespread nucleic acid amplification testing led to the insight that occult viral infections were often found in cases of presumed "idiopathic" pneumonia [145]. Finally, the knowledge of the mechanisms of disease in the general population helps guide us when seeing similar entities in HCT recipients, particularly when crucial differences are evident. For example, while diffuse alveolar hemorrhage in the general population is often due to autoimmune vasculitis and requires prompt, aggressive immunosuppression, support for aggressive immunosuppression to treat alveolar hemorrhage in the setting of HCT is less convincing [146].

One of the most common NIPCs that affect allogeneic HCT recipients is lung GVHD, almost always in the form of bronchiolitis obliterans syndrome (BOS), an obstructive airways disorder that is discussed in detail in Chap. 18. BOS is rare, occurring in 3–5% of HCT recipients, and the median onset is often during a time period where lung function monitoring is less frequent [147]. Because the symptoms of BOS occur insidiously, new-onset BOS is often detected by pulmonary function testing [148]. A thorough pulmonary consultation must not only distinguish BOS from mimicking conditions, like asthma or viral bronchiolitis, but also distinguish BOS from other conditions that cause lung impairment. For example, BOS may occur in the setting of truncal sclerosis, which may hinder the detection of an obstructive disorder when in the background of significant lung restriction. Furthermore, BOS often occurs in the context of GVHD of other organs and must occasionally be detected against the background of muscle weakness caused by corticosteroids [149] or pleural disease due to serositis [150]. Furthermore, diaphragmatic weakness can cause breathlessness and can occur even in the absence of overt peripheral muscle weakness. It should be considered as a possible cause of dyspnea in any patient who has received extensive corticosteroid therapy and can often worsen breathlessness already present in patients with BOS. Diagnostic evaluations for BOS and other pulmonary complications are discussed in detail in Chap. 6. Finally, pulmonary rehabilitation is beneficial for patients with BOS [151] but is likely to be underutilized [152], particularly when considering the pleiotropic benefits of exercise against the minimal drawbacks. Pulmonary rehabilitation is discussed in detail in Chap. 21.

Finally, pulmonary consultants must be aware of the dire prognosis of patients with GVHD who are admitted to intensive care units [153]. In part due to necessary immunosuppression and coexisting frailty, the care of patients with GVHD with critical illness requires a detailed, multidisciplinary approach, outlined in the second half of this book. Even in modern cohorts, the in-hospital mortality of GVHD patients with respiratory failure who require intensive care unit admission is often well over 50% [154].

In short, a broad understanding of GVHD and its treatments as outlined in this chapter will benefit all pulmonary consultants who care for these patients.

## References


1. Hill GR, Ferrara JL. The primacy of the gastrointestinal tract as a target organ of acute graft-versus-host disease: rationale for the use of cytokine shields in allogeneic bone marrow transplantation. Blood. 2000;95(9):2754–9. e-pub ahead of print 2000/04/26.
2. Brubaker SW, Bonham KS, Zanoni I, Kagan JC. Innate immune pattern recognition: a cell biological perspective. Annu Rev Immunol. 2015;33:257–90. e-pub ahead of print 2015/01/13. https://doi.org/10.1146/annurev-immunol-032414-112240.
3. Hill GR, Koyama M. Cytokines and costimulation in acute graft-versus-host disease. Blood. 2020;136(4):418–28. e-pub ahead of print 2020/06/12. https://doi.org/10.1182/blood.2019000952.
4. Zeiser R, Blazar BR. Pathophysiology of chronic graft-versus-host disease and therapeutic targets. N Engl J Med. 2017;377(26):2565–79. e-pub ahead of print 2017/12/28. https://doi.org/10.1056/NEJMra1703472.
5. Cooke KR, Luznik L, Sarantopoulos S, Hakim FT, Jagasia M, Fowler DH, et al. The biology of chronic graft-versus-host disease: a task force report from the National Institutes of Health consensus development project on criteria for clinical trials in chronic graft-versus-host disease. Biol Blood Marrow Transplant. 2017;23(2):211–34. e-pub ahead of print 2016/10/08. https://doi.org/10.1016/j.bbmt.2016.09.023.
6. Bolanos-Meade J, Reshef R, Fraser R, Fei M, Abhyankar S, Al-Kadhimi Z, et al. Three prophylaxis regimens (tacrolimus, mycophenolate mofetil, and cyclophosphamide; tacrolimus, methotrexate, and bortezomib; or tacrolimus, methotrexate, and maraviroc) versus tacrolimus and methotrexate for prevention of graft-versus-host disease with haemopoietic cell transplantation with reduced-intensity conditioning: a randomised phase 2 trial with a non-randomised contemporaneous control group (BMT CTN 1203). Lancet Haematol. 2019;6(3):e132–43. e-pub ahead of print 2019/03/03. https://doi.org/10.1016/S2352-3026(18)30221-7.
7. Soiffer RJ, Kim HT, McGuirk J, Horwitz ME, Johnston L, Patnaik MM, et al. Prospective, randomized, double-blind, phase III clinical trial of anti-T-lymphocyte globulin to assess impact on chronic graft-versus-host disease-free survival in patients undergoing HLA-matched unrelated myeloablative hematopoietic cell transplantation. J Clin Oncol. 2017;35(36):4003–11. e-pub ahead of print 2017/10/19. https://doi.org/10.1200/JCO.2017.75.8177.
8. Scott BL, Pasquini MC, Logan BR, Wu J, Devine SM, Porter DL, et al. Myeloablative versus reduced-intensity hematopoietic cell transplantation for acute myeloid Leukemia and myelodysplastic syndromes. J Clin Oncol. 2017;35(11):1154–61. e-pub ahead of print 2017/04/06. https://doi.org/10.1200/JCO.2016.70.7091.
9. Kroger N, Solano C, Wolschke C, Bandini G, Patriarca F, Pini M, et al. Antilymphocyte globulin for prevention of chronic graft-versus-host disease. N Engl J Med. 2016;374(1):43–53. e-pub

ahead of print 2016/01/07. https://doi.org/10.1056/NEJMoa1506002.
10. Anasetti C, Logan BR, Lee SJ, Waller EK, Weisdorf DJ, Wingard JR, et al. Peripheral-blood stem cells versus bone marrow from unrelated donors. N Engl J Med. 2012;367(16):1487–96. e-pub ahead of print 2012/10/19. https://doi.org/10.1056/NEJMoa1203517.
11. D'Souza A, Fretham C, Lee SJ, Arora M, Brunner J, Chhabra S, et al. Current use of and trends in hematopoietic cell transplantation in the United States. Biol Blood Marrow Transplant. 2020;26(8):e177–82. e-pub ahead of print 2020/05/22. https://doi.org/10.1016/j.bbmt.2020.04.013.
12. Khoury HJ, Wang T, Hemmer MT, Couriel D, Alousi A, Cutler C, et al. Improved survival after acute graft-versus-host disease diagnosis in the modern era. Haematologica. 2017;102(5):958–66. e-pub ahead of print 2017/03/18. https://doi.org/10.3324/haematol.2016.156356.
13. El-Jawahri A, Li S, Antin JH, Spitzer TR, Armand PA, Koreth J, et al. Improved treatment-related mortality and overall survival of patients with grade IV acute GVHD in the modern years. Biol Blood Marrow Transplant. 2016;22(5):910–8. e-pub ahead of print 2016/01/10. https://doi.org/10.1016/j.bbmt.2015.12.024.
14. Arai S, Arora M, Wang T, Spellman SR, He W, Couriel DR, et al. Increasing incidence of chronic graft-versus-host disease in allogeneic transplantation: a report from the Center for International Blood and Marrow Transplant Research. Biol Blood Marrow Transplant. 2015;21(2):266–74. e-pub ahead of print 2014/12/03. https://doi.org/10.1016/j.bbmt.2014.10.021.
15. Hartwell MJ, Ozbek U, Holler E, Renteria AS, Major-Monfried H, Reddy P, et al. An early-biomarker algorithm predicts lethal graft-versus-host disease and survival. JCI Insight. 2017;2(3):e89798. e-pub ahead of print 2017/02/15. https://doi.org/10.1172/jci.insight.89798.
16. MacMillan ML, DeFor TE, Weisdorf DJ. What predicts high risk acute graft-versus-host disease (GVHD) at onset?: identification of those at highest risk by a novel acute GVHD risk score. Br J Haematol. 2012;157(6):732–41. e-pub ahead of print 2012/04/11. https://doi.org/10.1111/j.1365-2141.2012.09114.x.
17. MacMillan ML, Robin M, Harris AC, DeFor TE, Martin PJ, Alousi A, et al. A refined risk score for acute graft-versus-host disease that predicts response to initial therapy, survival, and transplant-related mortality. Biol Blood Marrow Transplant. 2015;21(4):761–7. e-pub ahead of print 2015/01/15. https://doi.org/10.1016/j.bbmt.2015.01.001.
18. Pidala J, Anasetti C, Jim H. Quality of life after allogeneic hematopoietic cell transplantation. Blood. 2009;114(1):7–19. e-pub ahead of print 2009/04/02. https://doi.org/10.1182/blood-2008-10-182592.
19. Lee SJ, Kim HT, Ho VT, Cutler C, Alyea EP, Soiffer RJ, et al. Quality of life associated with acute and chronic graft-versus-host disease. Bone Marrow Transplant. 2006;38(4):305–10. e-pub ahead of print 2006/07/05. https://doi.org/10.1038/sj.bmt.1705434.
20. Stewart BL, Storer B, Storek J, Deeg HJ, Storb R, Hansen JA, et al. Duration of immunosuppressive treatment for chronic graft-versus-host disease. Blood. 2004;104(12):3501–6. e-pub ahead of print 2004/08/05. https://doi.org/10.1182/blood-2004-01-0200.
21. DeFilipp Z, Alousi AM, Pidala JA, Carpenter PA, Onstad LE, Arai S, et al. Nonrelapse mortality among patients diagnosed with chronic GVHD: an updated analysis from the chronic GVHD consortium. Blood Adv. 2021;5(20):4278–84. e-pub ahead of print 2021/09/15. https://doi.org/10.1182/bloodadvances.2021004941.
22. Petersdorf EW. Which factors influence the development of GVHD in HLA-matched or mismatched transplants? Best Pract Res Clin Haematol. 2017;30(4):333–5. e-pub ahead of print 2017/11/21. https://doi.org/10.1016/j.beha.2017.09.003.
23. Kollman C, Spellman SR, Zhang MJ, Hassebroek A, Anasetti C, Antin JH, et al. The effect of donor characteristics on survival after unrelated donor transplantation for hematologic malignancy. Blood. 2016;127(2):260–7. e-pub ahead of print 2015/11/04. https://doi.org/10.1182/blood-2015-08-663823.
24. Morishima Y, Kashiwase K, Matsuo K, Azuma F, Morishima S, Onizuka M, et al. Biological significance of HLA locus matching in unrelated donor bone marrow transplantation. Blood. 2015;125(7):1189–97. e-pub ahead of print 2014/12/19. https://doi.org/10.1182/blood-2014-10-604785.
25. Fernandez-Vina MA, Klein JP, Haagenson M, Spellman SR, Anasetti C, Noreen H, et al. Multiple mismatches at the low expression HLA loci DP, DQ, and DRB3/4/5 associate with adverse outcomes in hematopoietic stem cell transplantation. Blood. 2013;121(22):4603–10. e-pub ahead of print 2013/04/19. https://doi.org/10.1182/blood-2013-02-481945.
26. Martin PJ, Levine DM, Storer BE, Warren EH, Zheng X, Nelson SC, et al. Genome-wide minor histocompatibility matching as related to the risk of graft-versus-host disease. Blood. 2017;129(6):791–8. e-pub ahead of print 2016/11/23. https://doi.org/10.1182/blood-2016-09-737700.
27. Flowers ME, Inamoto Y, Carpenter PA, Lee SJ, Kiem HP, Petersdorf EW, et al. Comparative analysis of risk factors for acute graft-versus-host disease and for chronic graft-versus-host disease according to National Institutes of Health consensus criteria. Blood. 2011;117(11):3214–9. e-pub ahead of print 2011/01/26. https://doi.org/10.1182/blood-2010-08-302109.
28. Jagasia M, Arora M, Flowers ME, Chao NJ, McCarthy PL, Cutler CS, et al. Risk factors for acute GVHD and survival after hematopoietic cell

transplantation. Blood. 2012;119(1):296–307. e-pub ahead of print 2011/10/20. https://doi.org/10.1182/blood-2011-06-364265.
29. Gupta V, Tallman MS, He W, Logan BR, Copelan E, Gale RP, et al. Comparable survival after HLA-well-matched unrelated or matched sibling donor transplantation for acute myeloid leukemia in first remission with unfavorable cytogenetics at diagnosis. Blood. 2010;116(11):1839–48. e-pub ahead of print 2010/06/12. https://doi.org/10.1182/blood-2010-04-278317.
30. Yakoub-Agha I, Mesnil F, Kuentz M, Boiron JM, Ifrah N, Milpied N, et al. Allogeneic marrow stem-cell transplantation from human leukocyte antigen-identical siblings versus human leukocyte antigen-allelic-matched unrelated donors (10/10) in patients with standard-risk hematologic malignancy: a prospective study from the French Society of Bone Marrow Transplantation and Cell Therapy. J Clin Oncol. 2006;24(36):5695–702. e-pub ahead of print 2006/11/23. https://doi.org/10.1200/JCO.2006.08.0952.
31. Moon JH, Sohn SK, Lambie A, Ellis L, Hamad N, Uhm J, et al. Validation of National Institutes of Health global scoring system for chronic graft-versus-host disease (GVHD) according to overall and GVHD-specific survival. Biol Blood Marrow Transplant. 2014;20(4):556–63. e-pub ahead of print 2014/01/23. https://doi.org/10.1016/j.bbmt.2014.01.010.
32. Pidala J, Vogelsang G, Martin P, Chai X, Storer B, Pavletic S, et al. Overlap subtype of chronic graft-versus-host disease is associated with an adverse prognosis, functional impairment, and inferior patient-reported outcomes: a chronic graft-versus-host disease consortium study. Haematologica. 2012;97(3):451–8. e-pub ahead of print 2011/11/08. https://doi.org/10.3324/haematol.2011.055186.
33. Harris AC, Young R, Devine S, Hogan WJ, Ayuk F, Bunworasate U, et al. International, Multicenter standardization of acute graft-versus-host disease clinical data collection: a report from the Mount Sinai acute GVHD international consortium. Biol Blood Marrow Transplant. 2016;22(1):4–10. e-pub ahead of print 2015/09/20. https://doi.org/10.1016/j.bbmt.2015.09.001.
34. Sullivan KM, Shulman HM, Storb R, Weiden PL, Witherspoon RP, McDonald GB, et al. Chronic graft-versus-host disease in 52 patients: adverse natural course and successful treatment with combination immunosuppression. Blood. 1981;57(2):267–76. e-pub ahead of print 1981/02/01.
35. Shulman HM, Sullivan KM, Weiden PL, McDonald GB, Striker GE, Sale GE, et al. Chronic graft-versus-host syndrome in man. A long-term clinicopathologic study of 20 Seattle patients. Am J Med. 1980;69(2):204–17. e-pub ahead of print 1980/08/01. https://doi.org/10.1016/0002-9343(80)90380-0.
36. Filipovich AH, Weisdorf D, Pavletic S, Socie G, Wingard JR, Lee SJ, et al. National Institutes of Health consensus development project on criteria for clinical trials in chronic graft-versus-host disease: I. diagnosis and staging working group report. Biol Blood Marrow Transplant. 2005;11(12):945–56. e-pub ahead of print 2005/12/13. https://doi.org/10.1016/j.bbmt.2005.09.004.
37. Jagasia MH, Greinix HT, Arora M, Williams KM, Wolff D, Cowen EW, et al. National Institutes of Health Consensus Development Project on Criteria for Clinical Trials in Chronic Graft-versus-Host Disease: I. The 2014 Diagnosis and staging working group report. Biol Blood Marrow Transplant. 2015;21(3)):389–401e381. e-pub ahead of print 2014/12/23. https://doi.org/10.1016/j.bbmt.2014.12.001.
38. Storb R, Rudolph RH, Thomas ED. Marrow grafts between canine siblings matched by serotyping and mixed leukocyte culture. J Clin Invest. 1971;50(6):1272–5. https://doi.org/10.1172/JCI106605.
39. Storb R, Epstein RB, Graham TC, Thomas ED. Methotrexate regimens for control of graft-versus-host disease in dogs with allogeneic marrow grafts. Transplantation. 1970;9(3):240–6.
40. Storb R, Epstein RB, Bryant J, Ragde H, Thomas ED. Marrow grafts by combined marrow and leukocyte infusions in unrelated dogs selected by histocompatibility typing. Transplantation. 1968;6(4):587–93.
41. Thomas ED, Kasakura S, Cavins JA, Ferrebee JW. Marrow transplants in lethally irradiated dogs: the effect of methotrexate on survival of the host and the homograft. Transplantation. 1963;1:571–4.
42. Lochte HL Jr, Levy AS, Guenther DM, Thomas ED, Ferrebee JW. Prevention of delayed foreign marrow reaction in lethally irradiated mice by early administration of methotrexate. Nature. 1962;196:1110–1.
43. Thomas ED, Collins JA, Herman EC Jr, Ferrebee JW. Marrow transplants in lethally irradiated dogs given methotrexate. Blood. 1962;19:217–28.
44. Uphoff DE. Drug-induced immunological "tolerance" for homotransplantation. Plast Reconstr Surg. 1961;28:12–6.
45. Hager EB, Mannick JA, Thomas ED, Ferrebee JW. Dogs that survive "lethal" exposures to radiation. Radiat Res. 1961;14:192–205.
46. Uphoff DE. Alteration of homograft reaction by A-methopterin in lethally irradiated mice treated with homologous marrow. Proc Soc Exp Biol Med. 1958;99(3):651–3.
47. Thomas E, Storb R, Clift RA, Fefer A, Johnson FL, Neiman PE, et al. Bone-marrow transplantation (first of two parts). N Engl J Med. 1975;292(16):832–43. e-pub ahead of print 1975/04/17. https://doi.org/10.1056/NEJM197504172921605.
48. Smith BR, Parkman R, Lipton J, Nathan DG, Rappeport JM. Efficacy of a short course (four doses) of methotrexate following bone marrow transplantation for prevention of graft-versus-host disease. Transplantation. 1985;39(3):326–9.

e-pub ahead of print 1985/03/01. https://doi.org/10.1097/00007890-198503000-00028.
49. Borel JF, Feurer C, Magnee C, Stahelin H. Effects of the new anti-lymphocytic peptide cyclosporin a in animals. Immunology. 1977;32(6):1017–25. e-pub ahead of print 1977/06/01.
50. Matsuda S, Koyasu S. Mechanisms of action of cyclosporine. Immunopharmacology. 2000;47(2–3):119–25. e-pub ahead of print 2000/07/06. https://doi.org/10.1016/s0162-3109(00)00192-2.
51. Deeg HJ, Storb R, Weiden PL, Raff RF, Sale GE, Atkinson K, et al. Cyclosporin a and methotrexate in canine marrow transplantation: engraftment, graft-versus-host disease, and induction of intolerance. Transplantation. 1982;34(1):30–5. e-pub ahead of print 1982/07/01. https://doi.org/10.1097/00007890-198207000-00006.
52. Hows JM, Palmer S, Gordon-Smith EC. Use of cyclosporin a in allogeneic bone marrow transplantation for severe aplastic anemia. Transplantation. 1982;33(4):382–6. e-pub ahead of print 1982/04/01. https://doi.org/10.1097/00007890-198204000-00008.
53. Speck B, Gratwohl A, Nissen C, Osterwalder B, Muller M, Luthy A, et al. New development in clinical bone marrow transplantation in leukemia. Schweiz Med Wochenschr. 1981;111(50):1975–7. e-pub ahead of print 1981/12/12.
54. Powles RL, Clink HM, Spence D, Morgenstern G, Watson JG, Selby PJ, et al. Cyclosporin a to prevent graft-versus-host disease in man after allogeneic bone-marrow transplantation. Lancet. 1980;1(8164):327–9. e-pub ahead of print 1980/02/16. https://doi.org/10.1016/s0140-6736(80)90881-8.
55. Rossi SJ, Schroeder TJ, Hariharan S, First MR. Prevention and management of the adverse effects associated with immunosuppressive therapy. Drug Saf. 1993;9(2):104–31. e-pub ahead of print 1993/08/01. https://doi.org/10.2165/00002018-199309020-00004.
56. Przepiorka D, Shapiro S, Schwinghammer TL, Bloom EJ, Rosenfeld CS, Shadduck RK, et al. Cyclosporine and methylprednisolone after allogeneic marrow transplantation: association between low cyclosporine concentration and risk of acute graft-versus-host disease. Bone Marrow Transplant. 1991;7(6):461–5. e-pub ahead of print 1991/06/01.
57. Storb R, Deeg HJ, Farewell V, Doney K, Appelbaum F, Beatty P, et al. Marrow transplantation for severe aplastic anemia: methotrexate alone compared with a combination of methotrexate and cyclosporine for prevention of acute graft-versus-host disease. Blood. 1986;68(1):119–25. e-pub ahead of print 1986/07/01.
58. Storb R, Deeg HJ, Whitehead J, Appelbaum F, Beatty P, Bensinger W, et al. Methotrexate and cyclosporine compared with cyclosporine alone for prophylaxis of acute graft versus host disease after marrow transplantation for leukemia. N Engl J Med. 1986;314(12):729–35. e-pub ahead of print 1986/03/20. https://doi.org/10.1056/NEJM198603203141201.
59. Goto T, Kino T, Hatanaka H, Nishiyama M, Okuhara M, Kohsaka M, et al. Discovery of FK-506, a novel immunosuppressant isolated from Streptomyces tsukubaensis. Transplant Proc. 1987;19(5 Suppl 6):4–8. e-pub ahead of print 1987/10/01.
60. Kino T, Inamura N, Sakai F, Nakahara K, Goto T, Okuhara M, et al. Effect of FK-506 on human mixed lymphocyte reaction in vitro. Transplant Proc. 1987;19(5 Suppl 6):36–9. e-pub ahead of print 1987/10/01.
61. Kino T, Hatanaka H, Hashimoto M, Nishiyama M, Goto T, Okuhara M, et al. FK-506, a novel immunosuppressant isolated from a streptomyces. I. Fermentation, isolation, and physicochemical and biological characteristics. J Antibiot (Tokyo). 1987;40(9):1249–55. e-pub ahead of print 1987/09/01. https://doi.org/10.7164/antibiotics.40.1249.
62. Fruman DA, Klee CB, Bierer BE, Burakoff SJ. Calcineurin phosphatase activity in T lymphocytes is inhibited by FK 506 and cyclosporin a. Proc Natl Acad Sci U S A. 1992;89(9):3686–90. e-pub ahead of print 1992/05/01. https://doi.org/10.1073/pnas.89.9.3686.
63. Storb R, Raff RF, Appelbaum FR, Deeg HJ, Fitzsimmons W, Graham TC, et al. FK-506 and methotrexate prevent graft-versus-host disease in dogs given 9.2 Gy total body irradiation and marrow grafts from unrelated dog leukocyte antigen-nonidentical donors. Transplantation. 1993;56(4):800–7. e-pub ahead of print 1993/10/01. https://doi.org/10.1097/00007890-199310000-00005.
64. Nash RA, Antin JH, Karanes C, Fay JW, Avalos BR, Yeager AM, et al. Phase 3 study comparing methotrexate and tacrolimus with methotrexate and cyclosporine for prophylaxis of acute graft-versus-host disease after marrow transplantation from unrelated donors. Blood. 2000;96(6):2062–8. e-pub ahead of print 2000/09/09.
65. Kanda Y, Kobayashi T, Mori T, Tanaka M, Nakaseko C, Yokota A, et al. A randomized controlled trial of cyclosporine and tacrolimus with strict control of blood concentrations after unrelated bone marrow transplantation. Bone Marrow Transplant. 2016;51(1):103–9. e-pub ahead of print 2015/10/06. https://doi.org/10.1038/bmt.2015.222.
66. Ratanatharathorn V, Nash RA, Przepiorka D, Devine SM, Klein JL, Weisdorf D, et al. Phase III study comparing methotrexate and tacrolimus (prograf, FK506) with methotrexate and cyclosporine for graft-versus-host disease prophylaxis after HLA-identical sibling bone marrow transplantation. Blood. 1998;92(7):2303–14. e-pub ahead of print 1998/09/25.
67. Hiraoka A, Ohashi Y, Okamoto S, Moriyama Y, Nagao T, Kodera Y, et al. Phase III study comparing tacrolimus (FK506) with cyclosporine for graft-

versus-host disease prophylaxis after allogeneic bone marrow transplantation. Bone Marrow Transplant. 2001;28(2):181–5. e-pub ahead of print 2001/08/18. https://doi.org/10.1038/sj.bmt.1703097.
68. Yu C, Seidel K, Nash RA, Deeg HJ, Sandmaier BM, Barsoukov A, et al. Synergism between mycophenolate mofetil and cyclosporine in preventing graft-versus-host disease among lethally irradiated dogs given DLA-nonidentical unrelated marrow grafts. Blood. 1998;91(7):2581–7. e-pub ahead of print 1998/04/18.
69. Allison AC, Eugui EM. Purine metabolism and immunosuppressive effects of mycophenolate mofetil (MMF). Clin Transpl. 1996;10(1 Pt 2):77–84. e-pub ahead of print 1996/02/01.
70. McSweeney PA, Niederwieser D, Shizuru JA, Sandmaier BM, Molina AJ, Maloney DG, et al. Hematopoietic cell transplantation in older patients with hematologic malignancies: replacing high-dose cytotoxic therapy with graft-versus-tumor effects. Blood. 2001;97(11):3390–400. e-pub ahead of print 2001/05/23. https://doi.org/10.1182/blood.v97.11.3390.
71. Perkins J, Field T, Kim J, Kharfan-Dabaja MA, Fernandez H, Ayala E, et al. A randomized phase II trial comparing tacrolimus and mycophenolate mofetil to tacrolimus and methotrexate for acute graft-versus-host disease prophylaxis. Biol Blood Marrow Transplant. 2010;16(7):937–47. e-pub ahead of print 2010/01/28. https://doi.org/10.1016/j.bbmt.2010.01.010.
72. Bolwell B, Sobecks R, Pohlman B, Andresen S, Rybicki L, Kuczkowski E, et al. A prospective randomized trial comparing cyclosporine and short course methotrexate with cyclosporine and mycophenolate mofetil for GVHD prophylaxis in myeloablative allogeneic bone marrow transplantation. Bone Marrow Transplant. 2004;34(7):621–5. e-pub ahead of print 2004/08/10. https://doi.org/10.1038/sj.bmt.1704647.
73. Kiehl MG, Schafer-Eckart K, Kroger M, Bornhauser M, Basara N, Blau IW, et al. Mycophenolate mofetil for the prophylaxis of acute graft-versus-host disease in stem cell transplant recipients. Transplant Proc. 2002;34(7):2922–4. e-pub ahead of print 2002/11/15. https://doi.org/10.1016/s0041-1345(02)03489-9.
74. Bornhauser M, Schuler U, Porksen G, Naumann R, Geissler G, Thiede C, et al. Mycophenolate mofetil and cyclosporine as graft-versus-host disease prophylaxis after allogeneic blood stem cell transplantation. Transplantation. 1999;67(4):499–504. e-pub ahead of print 1999/03/10. https://doi.org/10.1097/00007890-199902270-00001.
75. Storb R, Kolb HJ, Graham TC, Kolb H, Weiden PL, Thomas ED. Treatment of established graft-versus-host disease in dogs by antithymocyte serum or prednisone. Blood. 1973;42(4):601–9. e-pub ahead of print 1973/10/01.
76. Kolb HJ, Storb R, Graham TC, Kolb H, Thomas ED. Antithymocyte serum and methotrexate for control of graft-versus-host disease in dogs. Transplantation. 1973;16(1):17–23. e-pub ahead of print 1973/07/01. https://doi.org/10.1097/00007890-197307000-00004.
77. van Bekkum DW, Balner H, Dicke KA, van den Berg FG, Prinsen GH, Hollander CF. The effect of pretreatment of allogeneic bone marrow graft recipients with antilymphocytic serum on the acute graft-versus-host reaction in monkeys. Transplantation. 1972;13(4):400–7. e-pub ahead of print 1972/04/01. https://doi.org/10.1097/00007890-197204000-00007.
78. Haskovcova H, Nouza K. Treatment and pretreatment of graft-versus-host reaction by antilymphocyte serum. Folia Biol (Praha). 1970;16(6):397–406. e-pub ahead of print 1970/01/01.
79. Boak JL, Dagher RK, Corson JM, Wilson RE. Modification of the graft-versus-host syndrome by anti-lymphocyte serum treatment of the host. Clin Exp Immunol. 1968;3(8):801–8. e-pub ahead of print 1968/10/01.
80. Mohty M. Mechanisms of action of antithymocyte globulin: T-cell depletion and beyond. Leukemia. 2007;21(7):1387–94. e-pub ahead of print 2007/04/06. https://doi.org/10.1038/sj.leu.2404683.
81. Scheinberg P, Fischer SH, Li L, Nunez O, Wu CO, Sloand EM, et al. Distinct EBV and CMV reactivation patterns following antibody-based immunosuppressive regimens in patients with severe aplastic anemia. Blood. 2007;109(8):3219–24. e-pub ahead of print 2006/12/07. https://doi.org/10.1182/blood-2006-09-045625.
82. Chen M, Liu C, Zhuang J, Zou N, Xu Y, Zhang W, et al. Long-term follow-up study of porcine anti-human thymocyte immunoglobulin therapy combined with cyclosporine for severe aplastic anemia. Eur J Haematol. 2016;96(3):291–6. e-pub ahead of print 2015/05/23. https://doi.org/10.1111/ejh.12590.
83. Feng X, Kajigaya S, Solomou EE, Keyvanfar K, Xu X, Raghavachari N, et al. Rabbit ATG but not horse ATG promotes expansion of functional CD4+CD25highFOXP3+ regulatory T cells in vitro. Blood. 2008;111(7):3675–83. e-pub ahead of print 2008/02/06. https://doi.org/10.1182/blood-2008-01-130146.
84. Lopez M, Clarkson MR, Albin M, Sayegh MH, Najafian N. A novel mechanism of action for anti-thymocyte globulin: induction of CD4+CD25+Foxp3+ regulatory T cells. J Am Soc Nephrol. 2006;17(10):2844–53. e-pub ahead of print 2006/08/18. https://doi.org/10.1681/ASN.2006050422.
85. Walker I, Panzarella T, Couban S, Couture F, Devins G, Elemary M, et al. Pretreatment with anti-thymocyte globulin versus no anti-thymocyte globulin in patients with haematological malignancies undergoing haemopoietic cell transplantation from unrelated donors: a randomised, controlled, open-label, phase 3, multicentre trial. Lancet Oncol.

2016;17(2):164–73. e-pub ahead of print 2016/01/03. https://doi.org/10.1016/S1470-2045(15)00462-3.
86. Finke J, Bethge WA, Schmoor C, Ottinger HD, Stelljes M, Zander AR, et al. Standard graft-versus-host disease prophylaxis with or without anti-T-cell globulin in haematopoietic cell transplantation from matched unrelated donors: a randomised, open-label, multicentre phase 3 trial. Lancet Oncol. 2009;10(9):855–64. e-pub ahead of print 2009/08/22. https://doi.org/10.1016/S1470-2045(09)70225-6.
87. Bunn D, Lea CK, Bevan DJ, Higgins RM, Hendry BM. The pharmacokinetics of anti-thymocyte globulin (ATG) following intravenous infusion in man. Clin Nephrol. 1996;45(1):29–32. e-pub ahead of print 1996/01/01.
88. Enright H, Haake R, Weisdorf D, Ramsay N, McGlave P, Kersey J, et al. Cytomegalovirus pneumonia after bone marrow transplantation. Risk factors and response to therapy. Transplantation. 1993;55(6):1339–46. e-pub ahead of print 1993/06/01. https://doi.org/10.1097/00007890-199306000-00024.
89. Tollemar J, Ringden O, Bostrom L, Nilsson B, Sundberg B. Variables predicting deep fungal infections in bone marrow transplant recipients. Bone Marrow Transplant. 1989;4(6):635–41. e-pub ahead of print 1989/11/01.
90. Curtis RE, Travis LB, Rowlings PA, Socie G, Kingma DW, Banks PM, et al. Risk of lymphoproliferative disorders after bone marrow transplantation: a multi-institutional study. Blood. 1999;94(7):2208–16. e-pub ahead of print 1999/09/25.
91. Waldmann H. A personal history of the CAMPATH-1H antibody. Med Oncol. 2002;19(Suppl):S3–9. e-pub ahead of print 2002/08/16. https://doi.org/10.1385/mo:19:2s:s03.
92. Morris EC, Rebello P, Thomson KJ, Peggs KS, Kyriakou C, Goldstone AH, et al. Pharmacokinetics of alemtuzumab used for in vivo and in vitro T-cell depletion in allogeneic transplantations: relevance for early adoptive immunotherapy and infectious complications. Blood. 2003;102(1):404–6. e-pub ahead of print 2003/03/08. https://doi.org/10.1182/blood-2002-09-2687.
93. Khouri IF, Albitar M, Saliba RM, Ippoliti C, Ma YC, Keating MJ, et al. Low-dose alemtuzumab (Campath) in myeloablative allogeneic stem cell transplantation for CD52-positive malignancies: decreased incidence of acute graft-versus-host-disease with unique pharmacokinetics. Bone Marrow Transplant. 2004;33(8):833–7. e-pub ahead of print 2004/02/03. https://doi.org/10.1038/sj.bmt.1704435.
94. Kanda J, Lopez RD, Rizzieri DA. Alemtuzumab for the prevention and treatment of graft-versus-host disease. Int J Hematol. 2011;93(5):586–93. e-pub ahead of print 2011/03/04. https://doi.org/10.1007/s12185-011-0802-2.
95. Wachsmuth LP, Patterson MT, Eckhaus MA, Venzon DJ, Gress RE, Kanakry CG. Post-transplantation cyclophosphamide prevents graft-versus-host disease by inducing alloreactive T cell dysfunction and suppression. J Clin Invest. 2019;129(6):2357–73. e-pub ahead of print 2019/03/27. https://doi.org/10.1172/JCI124218.
96. Kanakry CG, Ganguly S, Zahurak M, Bolanos-Meade J, Thoburn C, Perkins B, et al. Aldehyde dehydrogenase expression drives human regulatory T cell resistance to posttransplantation cyclophosphamide. Sci Transl Med. 2013;5(211):211ra157. e-pub ahead of print 2013/11/15. https://doi.org/10.1126/scitranslmed.3006960.
97. Mayumi H, Umesue M, Nomoto K. Cyclophosphamide-induced immunological tolerance: an overview. Immunobiology. 1996;195(2):129–39. e-pub ahead of print 1996/07/01. https://doi.org/10.1016/S0171-2985(96)80033-7.
98. Owens AH Jr, Santos GW. The effect of cytotoxic drugs on graft-versus-host disease in mice. Transplantation. 1971;11(4):378–82. e-pub ahead of print 1971/04/01. https://doi.org/10.1097/00007890-197104000-00004.
99. Santos GW, Owens AH. Production of graft-versus-host disease in the rat and its treatment with cytotoxic agents. Nature. 1966;210(5032):139–40. e-pub ahead of print 1966/04/09. https://doi.org/10.1038/210139a0.
100. Storb R, Graham TC, Shiurba R, Thomas ED. Treatment of canine graft-versus-host disease with methotrexate and cyclo-phosphamide following bone marrow transplantation from histoincompatible donors. Transplantation. 1970;10(2):165–72. e-pub ahead of print 1970/08/01. https://doi.org/10.1097/00007890-197008000-00003.
101. Luznik L, Jalla S, Engstrom LW, Iannone R, Fuchs EJ. Durable engraftment of major histocompatibility complex-incompatible cells after nonmyeloablative conditioning with fludarabine, low-dose total body irradiation, and posttransplantation cyclophosphamide. Blood. 2001;98(12):3456–64. e-pub ahead of print 2001/11/24. https://doi.org/10.1182/blood.v98.12.3456.
102. O'Donnell PV, Luznik L, Jones RJ, Vogelsang GB, Leffell MS, Phelps M, et al. Nonmyeloablative bone marrow transplantation from partially HLA-mismatched related donors using posttransplantation cyclophosphamide. Biol Blood Marrow Transplant. 2002;8(7):377–86. e-pub ahead of print 2002/08/13. https://doi.org/10.1053/bbmt.2002.v8.pm12171484.
103. Luznik L, O'Donnell PV, Symons HJ, Chen AR, Leffell MS, Zahurak M, et al. HLA-haploidentical bone marrow transplantation for hematologic malignancies using nonmyeloablative conditioning and high-dose, posttransplantation cyclophosphamide. Biol Blood Marrow Transplant. 2008;14(6):641–50. e-pub ahead of print 2008/05/21. https://doi.org/10.1016/j.bbmt.2008.03.005.
104. Kanakry CG, O'Donnell PV, Furlong T, de Lima MJ, Wei W, Medeot M, et al. Multi-institutional study of post-transplantation cyclophosphamide as

single-agent graft-versus-host disease prophylaxis after allogeneic bone marrow transplantation using myeloablative busulfan and fludarabine conditioning. J Clin Oncol. 2014;32(31):3497–505. e-pub ahead of print 2014/10/01. https://doi.org/10.1200/JCO.2013.54.0625.
105. Popat UR, Mehta RS, Bassett R, Olson AL, Alousi AM, Anderlini P, et al. Post-transplant cyclophosphamide in matched and haploidentical transplant recipients receiving myeloablative timed sequential busulfan conditioning regimen: results of a phase II study. J Clin Oncol. 2019;37(15_suppl):7007.
106. Sehgal SN. Sirolimus: its discovery, biological properties, and mechanism of action. Transplant Proc. 2003;35(3 Suppl):7S–14S. e-pub ahead of print 2003/05/14. https://doi.org/10.1016/s0041-1345(03)00211-2.
107. Sehgal SN. Rapamune (RAPA, rapamycin, Sirolimus): mechanism of action immunosuppressive effect results from blockade of signal transduction and inhibition of cell cycle progression. Clin Biochem. 1998;31(5):335–40. e-pub ahead of print 1998/08/29. https://doi.org/10.1016/s0009-9120(98)00045-9.
108. Li Z, Li D, Tsun A, Li B. FOXP3+ regulatory T cells and their functional regulation. Cell Mol Immunol. 2015;12(5):558–65. e-pub ahead of print 2015/02/17. https://doi.org/10.1038/cmi.2015.10.
109. Peccatori J, Forcina A, Clerici D, Crocchiolo R, Vago L, Stanghellini MT, et al. Sirolimus-based graft-versus-host disease prophylaxis promotes the in vivo expansion of regulatory T cells and permits peripheral blood stem cell transplantation from haploidentical donors. Leukemia. 2015;29(2):396–405. e-pub ahead of print 2014/06/05. https://doi.org/10.1038/leu.2014.180.
110. Cutler C, Logan B, Nakamura R, Johnston L, Choi S, Porter D, et al. Tacrolimus/sirolimus vs tacrolimus/methotrexate as GVHD prophylaxis after matched, related donor allogeneic HCT. Blood. 2014;124(8):1372–7. e-pub ahead of print 2014/07/02. https://doi.org/10.1182/blood-2014-04-567164.
111. Bejanyan N, Pidala JA, Wang X, Thapa R, Nishihori T, Elmariah H, et al. A phase 2 trial of GVHD prophylaxis with PTCy, sirolimus, and MMF after peripheral blood haploidentical transplantation. Blood Adv. 2021;5(5):1154–63. e-pub ahead of print 2021/02/27. https://doi.org/10.1182/bloodadvances.2020003779.
112. Shaw BE, Jimenez-Jimenez AM, Burns LJ, Logan BR, Khimani F, Shaffer BC, et al. National Marrow Donor Program-Sponsored Multicenter, phase II trial of HLA-mismatched unrelated donor bone marrow transplantation using post-transplant cyclophosphamide. J Clin Oncol. 2021;39:1971. e-pub ahead of print 2021/04/28. https://doi.org/10.1200/JCO.20.03502.
113. Bejanyan N, Rogosheske J, DeFor TE, Lazaryan A, Arora M, Holtan SG, et al. Sirolimus and mycophenolate mofetil as calcineurin inhibitor-free graft-versus-host disease prophylaxis for reduced-intensity conditioning umbilical cord blood transplantation. Biol Blood Marrow Transplant. 2016;22(11):2025–30. e-pub ahead of print 2016/08/16. https://doi.org/10.1016/j.bbmt.2016.08.005.
114. Sandmaier BM, Kornblit B, Storer BE, Olesen G, Maris MB, Langston AA, et al. Addition of sirolimus to standard cyclosporine plus mycophenolate mofetil-based graft-versus-host disease prophylaxis for patients after unrelated non-myeloablative haemopoietic stem cell transplantation: a multicentre, randomised, phase 3 trial. Lancet Haematol. 2019;6(8):e409–18. e-pub ahead of print 2019/06/30. https://doi.org/10.1016/S2352-3026(19)30088-2.
115. Wagner JE, Santos GW, Noga SJ, Rowley SD, Davis J, Vogelsang GB, et al. Bone marrow graft engineering by counterflow centrifugal elutriation: results of a phase I-II clinical trial. Blood. 1990;75(6):1370–7. e-pub ahead of print 1990/03/15.
116. Wagner JE, Donnenberg AD, Noga SJ, Cremo CA, Gao IK, Yin HJ, et al. Lymphocyte depletion of donor bone marrow by counterflow centrifugal elutriation: results of a phase I clinical trial. Blood. 1988;72(4):1168–76. e-pub ahead of print 1988/10/01.
117. Aversa F, Tabilio A, Velardi A, Cunningham I, Terenzi A, Falzetti F, et al. Treatment of high-risk acute leukemia with T-cell-depleted stem cells from related donors with one fully mismatched HLA haplotype. N Engl J Med. 1998;339(17):1186–93. e-pub ahead of print 1998/10/22. https://doi.org/10.1056/NEJM199810223391702.
118. Ho VT, Soiffer RJ. The history and future of T-cell depletion as graft-versus-host disease prophylaxis for allogeneic hematopoietic stem cell transplantation. Blood. 2001;98(12):3192–204. e-pub ahead of print 2001/11/24. https://doi.org/10.1182/blood.v98.12.3192.
119. Calcineurin Inhibitor-Free Graft-Versus-Host Disease (GVHD) prophylaxis in hematopoietic cell transplantation (HCT) with myeloablative conditioning regimens (MAC) and HLA-matched donors: results of the BMT CTN 1301 Progress II trial. TCT Annual Meeting, Feb 2021; 2021.
120. Watkins B, Qayed M, McCracken C, Bratrude B, Betz K, Suessmuth Y, et al. Phase II trial of Costimulation blockade with abatacept for prevention of acute GVHD. J Clin Oncol. 2021;39(17):1865–77. e-pub ahead of print 2021/01/16. https://doi.org/10.1200/JCO.20.01086.
121. Martin PJ. How I treat steroid-refractory acute graft-versus-host disease. Blood. 2020;135(19):1630–8. e-pub ahead of print 2020/03/24. https://doi.org/10.1182/blood.2019000960.
122. Sarantopoulos S, Cardones AR, Sullivan KM. How I treat refractory chronic graft-versus-host disease. Blood. 2019;133(11):1191–200. e-pub ahead of print 2019/01/25. https://doi.org/10.1182/blood-2018-04-785899.

123. Hill L, Alousi A, Kebriaei P, Mehta R, Rezvani K, Shpall E. New and emerging therapies for acute and chronic graft versus host disease. Ther Adv Hematol. 2018;9(1):21–46. e-pub ahead of print 2018/01/11. https://doi.org/10.1177/2040620717741860.
124. McDonald GB. How I treat acute graft-versus-host disease of the gastrointestinal tract and the liver. Blood. 2016;127(12):1544–50. e-pub ahead of print 2016/01/06. https://doi.org/10.1182/blood-2015-10-612747.
125. Flowers ME, Martin PJ. How we treat chronic graft-versus-host disease. Blood. 2015;125(4):606–15. e-pub ahead of print 2014/11/16. https://doi.org/10.1182/blood-2014-08-551994.
126. Bolanos-Meade J, Logan BR, Alousi AM, Antin JH, Barowski K, Carter SL, et al. Phase 3 clinical trial of steroids/mycophenolate mofetil vs steroids/placebo as therapy for acute GVHD: BMT CTN 0802. Blood. 2014;124(22):3221–7; quiz 3335. https://doi.org/10.1182/blood-2014-06-577023.
127. Alousi AM, Weisdorf DJ, Logan BR, Bolanos-Meade J, Carter S, Difronzo N, et al. Etanercept, mycophenolate, denileukin, or pentostatin plus corticosteroids for acute graft-versus-host disease: a randomized phase 2 trial from the blood and marrow transplant clinical trials network. Blood. 2009;114(3):511–7. https://doi.org/10.1182/blood-2009-03-212290.
128. Lee SJ, Zahrieh D, Agura E, MacMillan ML, Maziarz RT, McCarthy PL Jr, et al. Effect of up-front daclizumab when combined with steroids for the treatment of acute graft-versus-host disease: results of a randomized trial. Blood. 2004;104(5):1559–64. https://doi.org/10.1182/blood-2004-03-0854.
129. Cahn JY, Bordigoni P, Tiberghien P, Milpied N, Brion A, Widjenes J, et al. Treatment of acute graft-versus-host disease with methylprednisolone and cyclosporine with or without an anti-interleukin-2 receptor monoclonal antibody. A multicenter phase III study. Transplantation. 1995;60(9):939–42.
130. Couriel DR, Saliba R, de Lima M, Giralt S, Andersson B, Khouri I, et al. A phase III study of infliximab and corticosteroids for the initial treatment of acute graft-versus-host disease. Biol Blood Marrow Transplant. 2009;15(12):1555–62. https://doi.org/10.1016/j.bbmt.2009.08.003.
131. Cragg L, Blazar BR, Defor T, Kolatker N, Miller W, Kersey J, et al. A randomized trial comparing prednisone with antithymocyte globulin/prednisone as an initial systemic therapy for moderately severe acute graft-versus-host disease. Biol Blood Marrow Transplant. 2000;6(4A):441–7.
132. Antin JH, Chen AR, Couriel DR, Ho VT, Nash RA, Weisdorf D. Novel approaches to the therapy of steroid-resistant acute graft-versus-host disease. Biol Blood Marrow Transplant. 2004;10(10):655–68. https://doi.org/10.1016/j.bbmt.2004.07.007.
133. Pidala J, Anasetti C. Glucocorticoid-refractory acute graft-versus-host disease. Biol Blood Marrow Transplant. 2010;16(11):1504–18. e-pub ahead of print 2010/01/26. https://doi.org/10.1016/j.bbmt.2010.01.007.
134. MacMillan ML, Weisdorf DJ, Wagner JE, DeFor TE, Burns LJ, Ramsay NK, et al. Response of 443 patients to steroids as primary therapy for acute graft-versus-host disease: comparison of grading systems. Biol Blood Marrow Transplant. 2002;8(7):387–94. e-pub ahead of print 2002/08/13. https://doi.org/10.1053/bbmt.2002.v8.pm12171485.
135. Major-Monfried H, Renteria AS, Pawarode A, Reddy P, Ayuk F, Holler E, et al. MAGIC biomarkers predict long-term outcomes for steroid-resistant acute GVHD. Blood. 2018;131(25):2846–55. e-pub ahead of print 2018/03/17. https://doi.org/10.1182/blood-2018-01-822957.
136. Levine JE, Braun TM, Harris AC, Holler E, Taylor A, Miller H, et al. A prognostic score for acute graft-versus-host disease based on biomarkers: a multicentre study. Lancet Haematol. 2015;2(1):e21–9. e-pub ahead of print 2015/12/22. https://doi.org/10.1016/S2352-3026(14)00035-0.
137. Zeiser R, von Bubnoff N, Butler J, Mohty M, Niederwieser D, Or R, et al. Ruxolitinib for glucocorticoid-refractory acute graft-versus-host disease. N Engl J Med. 2020;382(19):1800–10. e-pub ahead of print 2020/04/23. https://doi.org/10.1056/NEJMoa1917635.
138. Miklos D, Cutler CS, Arora M, Waller EK, Jagasia M, Pusic I, et al. Ibrutinib for chronic graft-versus-host disease after failure of prior therapy. Blood. 2017;130(21):2243–50. e-pub ahead of print 2017/09/20. https://doi.org/10.1182/blood-2017-07-793786.
139. Zeiser R, Polverelli N, Ram R, Hashmi SK, Chakraverty R, Flowers MED, et al. Ruxolitinib (RUX) vs best available therapy (BAT) in patients with steroid-refractory/steroid-dependent chronic graft-vs-host disease (cGVHD): primary findings from the phase 3, Randomized REACH 3 study. In: Presented at the ASH 2020 annual meeting, session: 732. Clinical allogeneic transplantation: results I; 2020.
140. Cutler C, Lee SJ, Arai S, Rotta M, Zoghi B, Ramakrishnan A, et al. Belumosudil for chronic graft-versus-host disease (cGVHD) after 2 or more prior lines of therapy: the rockstar study (KD025-213). Blood. 2020;136(Supplement 1):45–6.
141. Cutler C, Lee SJ, Arai S, Rotta M, Zoghi B, Lazaryan A, et al. Belumosudil for chronic graft-versus-host disease after 2 or more prior lines of therapy: the ROCKstar study. Blood. 2021;138(22):2278–89. e-pub ahead of print 2021/07/16. https://doi.org/10.1182/blood.2021012021.
142. Diab KJ, Yu Z, Wood KL, Shmalo JA, Sheski FD, Farber MO, et al. Comparison of pulmonary complications after nonmyeloablative and conventional allogeneic hematopoietic cell transplant. Biol Blood Marrow Transplant. 2012;18(12):1827–34. e-pub

ahead of print 2012/07/07. https://doi.org/10.1016/j.bbmt.2012.06.013.

143. Dela Cruz CS, Evans SE, Restrepo MI, Dean N, Torres A, Amara-Elori I, et al. Understanding the host in the management of pneumonia. an official American Thoracic Society workshop report. Ann Am Thorac Soc. 2021;18(7):1087–97. e-pub ahead of print 2021/07/10. https://doi.org/10.1513/AnnalsATS.202102-209ST.

144. Bergeron A, Chevret S, Peffault de Latour R, Chagnon K, de Margerie-Mellon C, Riviere F, et al. Noninfectious lung complications after allogeneic haematopoietic stem cell transplantation. Eur Respir J. 2018;51(5):1702617. e-pub ahead of print 2018/04/14. https://doi.org/10.1183/13993003.02617-2017.

145. Seo S, Renaud C, Kuypers JM, Chiu CY, Huang ML, Samayoa E, et al. Idiopathic pneumonia syndrome after hematopoietic cell transplantation: evidence of occult infectious etiologies. Blood. 2015;125(24):3789–97. e-pub ahead of print 2015/04/29. https://doi.org/10.1182/blood-2014-12-617035.

146. Rathi NK, Tanner AR, Dinh A, Dong W, Feng L, Ensor J, et al. Low-, medium- and high-dose steroids with or without aminocaproic acid in adult hematopoietic SCT patients with diffuse alveolar hemorrhage. Bone Marrow Transplant. 2015;50(3):420–6. e-pub ahead of print 2014/12/23. https://doi.org/10.1038/bmt.2014.287.

147. Clark JG, Crawford SW, Madtes DK, Sullivan KM. Obstructive lung disease after allogeneic marrow transplantation. Clinical presentation and course. Ann Intern Med. 1989;111(5):368–76.

148. Palmer J, Williams K, Inamoto Y, Chai X, Martin PJ, Tomas LS, et al. Pulmonary symptoms measured by the national institutes of health lung score predict overall survival, nonrelapse mortality, and patient-reported outcomes in chronic graft-versus-host disease. Biol Blood Marrow Transplant. 2014;20(3):337–44. e-pub ahead of print 2013/12/10. https://doi.org/10.1016/j.bbmt.2013.11.025.

149. Ngo-Huang A, Yadav R, Bansal S, Williams J, Wu J, Fu JB, et al. An exploratory study on physical function in stem cell transplant patients undergoing corticosteroid treatment for acute graft-versus-host-disease. Am J Phys Med Rehabil. 2021;100(4):402–6. e-pub ahead of print 2020/12/06. https://doi.org/10.1097/PHM.0000000000001660.

150. Leonard JT, Newell LF, Meyers G, Hayes-Lattin B, Gajewski J, Heitner S, et al. Chronic GvHD-associated serositis and pericarditis. Bone Marrow Transplant. 2015;50(8):1098–104. e-pub ahead of print 2015/05/12. https://doi.org/10.1038/bmt.2015.105.

151. Tran J, Norder EE, Diaz PT, Phillips GS, Elder P, Devine SM, et al. Pulmonary rehabilitation for bronchiolitis obliterans syndrome after hematopoietic stem cell transplantation. Biol Blood Marrow Transplant. 2012;18(8):1250–4. https://doi.org/10.1016/j.bbmt.2012.01.017.

152. Spitzer KA, Stefan MS, Priya A, Pack QR, Pekow PS, Lagu T, et al. Participation in pulmonary rehabilitation after hospitalization for chronic obstructive pulmonary disease among Medicare beneficiaries. Ann Am Thorac Soc. 2019;16(1):99–106. e-pub ahead of print 2018/11/13. https://doi.org/10.1513/AnnalsATS.201805-332OC.

153. Bach PB, Schrag D, Nierman DM, Horak D, White P Jr, Young JW, et al. Identification of poor prognostic features among patients requiring mechanical ventilation after hematopoietic stem cell transplantation. Blood. 2001;98(12):3234–40. e-pub ahead of print 2001/11/24. https://doi.org/10.1182/blood.v98.12.3234.

154. Saillard C, Blaise D, Mokart D. Critically ill allogeneic hematopoietic stem cell transplantation patients in the intensive care unit: reappraisal of actual prognosis. Bone Marrow Transplant. 2016;51(8):1050–61. e-pub ahead of print 2016/04/05. https://doi.org/10.1038/bmt.2016.72.

# Pulmonary Complications Following Hematopoietic Stem Cell Transplantation: Spectrum, Incidence, Risk Factors, and Outcomes

3

Naser Mahmoud, Cassondra Cramer-Bour, and Ayman O. Soubani

## Introduction

Since the first successful HSCT done by Edward Donnall Thomas in 1957 [1], HSCT has been a very important treatment modality in the management of a variety of benign and malignant conditions with more than one and a half million transplants done worldwide [2]. It is useful to consider the pulmonary diseases post-HSCT separated by infectious and noninfectious etiologies (Fig. 3.1) which span a time frame segmented by the immunologic status of the patient. The timeline and immunologic status posttransplantation can be divided into three phases: phase I or the pre-engraftment phase from days 0 to 30 post-HSCT associated with severe neutropenia, phase II or the early post-engraftment phase from days 30 to 100 post-HSCT associated with cellular dysfunction, and phase III or the late post-engraftment phase after 100 days associated with cellular and humoral dysfunction (see Chap. 1). For each phase, it is important to consider not only the immunologic status of the patient but also the prophylactic medications the patient is receiving, as well as any graft-versus-host disease (GVHD) that may be contributing as well (see Chap. 2).

During the last few decades, tremendous improvements in critical care management, infection prophylaxis, and supportive care have resulted in decreased morbidity and mortality for these patients [3, 4] and thereby emphasize the need to develop a survivorship model of care (outlined in Chap. 37). Despite these advances, the incidence of pulmonary complications is still relatively high with about one-third of recipients developing at least one respiratory concern during the first year after transplant [5, 6]. Respiratory diseases remain one of the common causes of non-relapse mortality in HSCT recipients [7, 8]. Particularly in the subset of patients who develop critical illness, the need for an optimal approach for respiratory support (see Chap. 25) and a multidisciplinary team (see Chap. 36) is paramount to achieving the best outcomes for the critically ill HSCT patient (see Chap. 24).

Understanding the risk factors which make patients more susceptible to developing these

N. Mahmoud
Section of Pulmonary Medicine, Department of Internal Medicine, King Hussein Cancer Center, Amman, Jordan

C. Cramer-Bour · A. O. Soubani (✉)
Division of Pulmonary, Critical Care and Sleep Medicine, Wayne State University School of Medicine, Detroit, MI, USA
e-mail: asoubani@med.wayne.edu


A. O. Soubani (ed.), *Pulmonary and Critical Care Considerations of Hematopoietic Stem Cell Transplantation*, https://doi.org/10.1007/978-3-031-28797-8_3

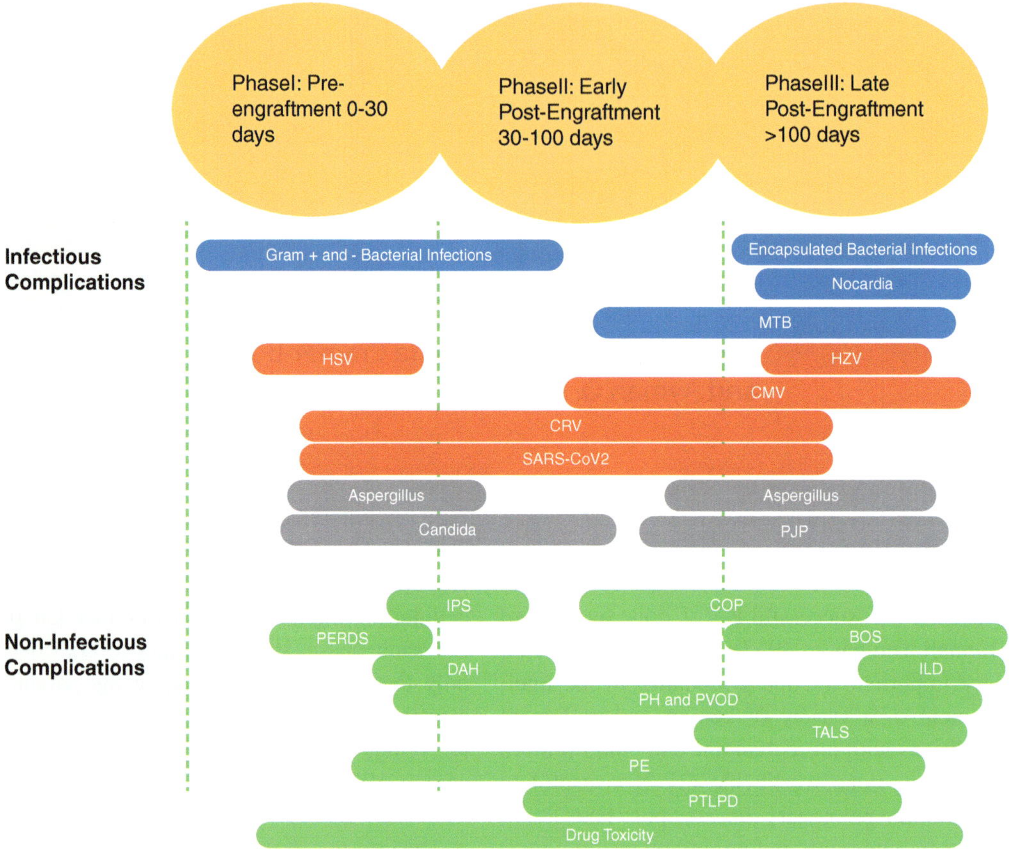


**Fig. 3.1** The spectrum and time course of pulmonary complications post-HSCT. *BOS* bronchiolitis obliterans syndrome, *COP* cryptogenic organizing pneumonia, *CRV* common respiratory viruses, *CMV* cytomegalovirus, *DAH* diffuse alveolar hemorrhage, *HSV* herpes simplex virus, *HZV* herpes zoster virus, *ILD* interstitial lung disease, *IPS* idiopathic pneumonia syndrome, *MTB Mycobacterium tuberculosis*, *PE* pleural effusion, *PERDS* peri-engraftment respiratory distress syndrome, *PH* pulmonary hypertension, *PJP* pneumocystis jirovecii pneumonia, *PTLPD* posttransplant lymphoproliferative disorder, *PVOD* pulmonary veno-occlusive disease, *SARS-CoV-2* severe acute respiratory syndrome coronavirus 2, *TALS* thoracic air leak syndrome

complications is critical. Older age and a history of preexisting lung disease are examples of baseline risk factors, which are discussed in the pretransplant evaluation in Chap. 4. Other important risk factors include gender, conditioning regimen, indication for transplant, modality of transplant harvest, and history of previous pulmonary infections [6, 9–12]. In this chapter, important hazards will be highlighted in the context of the pulmonary condition described, with references to the appropriate chapter for more information (Table 3.1). Given the complex and wide variety of infectious and noninfectious pulmonary complications, it is necessary to have a framework in mind when approaching the HSCT patient – Chap. 5 delves into this topic in more detail (Table 3.2). As a part of this workup, radiographic findings are extremely important and will be discussed in Chap. 6. The following sections provide a brief overview of the bulk of the respiratory conditions outlined in this text.

**Table 3.1** Potential risk factors for pulmonary complications post-HSCT

| | |
|---|---|
| Consistent | Allogeneic HSCT |
| | Chronic GVHD |
| | Myeloablative therapy (compared to reduced intensity regimens) |
| | Serostatus of the recipient and donor (for viral infections and PTLPD) |
| | Seasonal outbreaks (RVI and SARS-CoV-2) |
| | Longer duration of neutropenia (for fungal infections) |
| Probable | HLA mismatch |
| | Unrelated donor HSCT |
| | Smoking |
| | Abnormal pretransplant PFT |
| | Transplant for hematologic malignancy |
| | Low performance scores |
| | Total body irradiation |
| | Older age of recipient |
| | Severe acute GVHD |
| | Mucositis (for bacterial infections) |
| | Indwelling catheters (for bacterial infections and thrombosis) |
| | Corticosteroid use |
| | Conditioning regimen |
| | Lung-gut microbiome |
| Possible | CMV infection |
| | Source of HSCT (cord blood or peripheral blood) |
| | Bacterial colonization with MRSA and VRE (for bacterial infections) |
| | Use of granulocyte macrophage colony stimulating factor (PERDS) |
| | Fluoroquinolone prophylaxis |
| | Younger age |
| | Female to male HSCT |
| | Use of antithymocyte globulin |
| | Toll-like receptor polymorphisms |
| | Iron overload |

**Table 3.2** Relative frequencies of infectious and noninfectious complications based on type of transplant

| Disease | Autologous | Allogeneic |
|---|---|---|
| *Infectious* | | |
| Bacterial (gram + and −) | + + | + + + |
| *Nocardia* | ± | + |
| MTB and NTM | ± | + |
| Fungal | + + | + + + |
| *PJP* | + | + + |
| CMV | ± | + + |
| Other viruses | ++ | + + + |
| *Noninfectious* | | |
| PERDS | + + | ++ |
| DAH | + | ++ |
| IPS | + | ++ |
| BOS | ± | + + |
| COP | + + | + + |
| ILD | + | + + |
| PH and PVOD | ± | + + |
| TALS | ± | + |
| Pleural effusion | + + | + + |
| VTE | + + | + + |
| PCT | ± | ± |
| PTLPD | ± | + |
| PAP | ± | ± |

+ + +: common; + +: less common; +: rare; ±: very rare

*BOS* bronchiolitis obliterans syndrome, *COP* cryptogenic organizing pneumonia, *CRV* common respiratory viruses, *CMV* cytomegalovirus, *DAH* diffuse alveolar hemorrhage, *HSV* herpes simplex virus, *HZV* herpes zoster virus, *ILD* interstitial lung disease, *IPS* idiopathic pneumonia syndrome, *MTB Mycobacterium tuberculosis*, *NTM* nontuberculous mycobacterium, *PAP* pulmonary alveolar proteinosis, *PCT* pulmonary cytolytic thrombi, *PERDS* peri-engraftment respiratory distress syndrome, *PH* pulmonary hypertension, *PJP Pneumocystis jirovecii* pneumonia, *PTLPD* posttransplant lymphoproliferative disorder, *PVOD* pulmonary veno-occlusive disease, *SARS-CoV-2* severe acute respiratory syndrome coronavirus 2, *TALS* thoracic air leak syndrome, *VTE* venous thromboembolism

## Infectious Complications

It is not surprising given the severity of the immune compromise patients undergoing HSCT therapy experience those infectious complications are not only more common than noninfectious complications but also are responsible for a large percentage of non-relapse mortality among HSCT recipients. Given the more intense conditioning regimen necessary for allogeneic HSCT and the ongoing concerns for GVHD, infectious complications are usually more common in allogeneic HSCT.

## Bacterial Complications

### Pneumonia

It is a common infection with a reported incidence of 15–25% of post-HSCT patients meeting a clinical diagnosis of pneumonia, making it the predominant infection in the early-stage post-HSCT [13, 14]. Bacterial pneumonia usually develops during phase I and II. Risk factors such as mucositis, neutropenia, prolonged use of central venous catheters, low performance status, GVHD, prior use of fluoroquinolones, and colonization of bacteria may predispose patients to these infections [15]. Gram negative bacteria like *E. coli*, *Pseudomonas* (including multidrug resistant organisms), and *Klebsiella pneumoniae*, as well as gram positive bacteria such as pneumococcus, streptococcus species, and staphylococci, are the most common causes of pneumonia [13, 14, 16, 17]. Early recognition is important, and early initiation of antibiotics is of paramount importance as mortality can be high, particularly in phase I prior to engraftment. Please refer to Chap. 7 for more details about bacterial infections.

### Nocardia

Infection is less common than other bacterial infections with an incidence of less than 2% [18, 19] and usually occurs late during phase III post-HSCT. Risk factors for *Nocardia* infections include use of corticosteroids, chronic GVHD, CMV reactivation, high calcineurin inhibitors' levels, and trimethoprim sulfamethoxazole free periods. The presence of pulmonary nodules, cavities, masses, and consolidations or failure to respond to beta-lactam antibiotic therapy should raise the suspicion for *Nocardia* infections [20]. Treatment should be started with trimethoprim sulfamethoxazole. Outcome is usually good with most patients responsive to treatment.

### *Mycobacterium tuberculosis* (MTB)

Infections are rare in non-endemic areas with incidence less than 0.1% compared to 16% in endemic areas [21–23]. Risk factors include allogeneic HSCT, older age, chronic GVHD, prolonged immunosuppression, use of tyrosine kinase inhibitors, total body irradiation, and corticosteroid use [22, 24–26]. It usually occurs during the second and third phase post-HSCT. Fever is very common [27] and cough, dyspnea, and extra pulmonary involvement are also common. The outcomes for MTB disease are favorable if it is localized with no resistant organisms but less favorable in allogeneic HSCT, multidrug resistant or extensively drug resistant tuberculosis, or disseminated disease [22, 24, 28].

### Nontuberculous Mycobacterial Infections

The incidence of nontuberculous mycobacterial infections in HSCT is about 1–3% [29, 30] and, overall, much more common in the USA compared to MTB. In a retrospective review of 1047 allogeneic HSCT patients, important risk factors included CMV viremia and the presence of severe chronic GVHD [29]. Patients present with diffuse lymphadenopathy, skin and soft tissue infections, pneumonia, or a disseminated bloodstream infection [31]. Treatment can be complex in the setting of multiple drug interactions and concomitant GVHD; in this same retrospective study, the median survival after diagnosis was 398 days, with a survival of 40.8% at 2 years [29].

## Viral Complications

As depicted in Fig. 3.1, viral infections post-HSCT can happen at any stage: cytomegalovirus (CMV) and respiratory virus infections (RVI) typically occur during phase II and III, while herpes simplex virus (HSV) reactivation pneumonitis is typically diagnosed early in phase I.

### Cytomegalovirus

Although the use of prophylactic and preemptive treatment of patients at risk resulted in decrease in the incidence of CMV pneumonitis, it is still one of the common viral infections posttransplant. The rate of reactivation has dropped from around 60 to 70% to a little over a third of patients with improved treatment regimens [32–34]. The most important risk factor is the serostatus of the recipient and donor (highest risk if seropositive recipient and seronegative donor), total body irradiation, myeloablative conditioning, acute or chronic GVHD, unrelated or mismatched donor, use of alemtuzumab or fludarabine in seropositive patients, and high doses of corticosteroids [35–37]. CMV infection can present with a wide range of presentations from asymptomatic viremia to tissue invasive disease of the lung, gut, eye, liver, or brain, and it can – through immunomodulation – increase the risk of other infections. Tissue biopsy is the gold standard of diagnosis, but this is rarely performed in HSCT patients, and the diagnosis can still be made clinically using blood or bronchoalveolar lavage (BAL) PCR. Treatments used for CMV infections include valganciclovir, foscarnet, and cidofovir [33]. CMV viremia is associated with increased mortality, but it is infrequently linked as the cause of death for these patients [33, 34]. In a retrospective cohort study of 926 post-HSCT patients, 346 patients (37%) had reported plasma viral load greater than 150 IU/mL, but CMV disease was listed as a cause of death in only three patients (1%) during the first year after transplant [33]. For more information regarding CMV disease, see Chap. 10.

**Herpesviruses** (including HSV, VZV, and other herpesviruses) involvement in the course of the HSCT is an exciting area of future study. Previously herpes simplex virus 1 or 2 (HSV-1, HSV-2) were felt to be rare causes of pneumonitis in this population [38]. Prophylaxis with acyclovir is commonly administered in antibody + HSV + VZV HSCT recipients to reduce the risk of reactivation, which is most common in phase I of the time frame [39, 40]. An emerging area of study is the identification of latent human herpesviruses (commonly HHV-6, but HSV and EBV also described) in the BAL fluid of patients later diagnosed to have idiopathic pneumonia syndrome and bronchiolitis obliterans syndrome, two important noninfectious causes of non-relapse mortality [41]. There is ongoing work regarding the association of diagnosed respiratory infections within the first 100 days post-transplant (phases I and II) as an important identified risk factor for later noninfectious pulmonary diseases.

## Respiratory Virus Infections (RVI)

This category includes influenza, parainfluenza, respiratory syncytial virus (RSV), human metapneumovirus, rhino viruses, corona viruses (other than SARS-CoV-2), and adenoviruses. They collectively infect a high percentage of HSCT recipients. The reported incidence has increased with the use of more advanced techniques such as nasopharyngeal multiplex PCR with ranges of 11%–40% [42, 43]. Risk factors include seasonal outbreaks, exposure to household infected contacts, GVHD, immunosuppressive therapy, and unvaccinated status. Risk factors for progression to pneumonia include age greater than 65 years, lymphopenia, neutropenia, use of high dose corticosteroids, and GVHD [44]. Fever, cough, shortness of breath, sneezing, fatigue, and sore throat are common. Acute respiratory distress syndrome can develop in severe cases. Initiating appropriate antiviral therapy may help decrease mortality in some infections. The overall mortality of RVI pneumonias is about 12%–15% [43, 45]. Treatment with oseltamivir can decrease morbidity and mortality in influenza virus infections [46], and use of ribavirin is proven to decrease mortality in RSV pneumonias [44]. Mortality of different viruses may vary and can be high in some viruses like influenza A/H1N1 strains and reach up to 29.6% [47]. For more information, please refer to Chap. 11.

## SARS-CoV-2

It is still an ongoing pandemic. Its incidence is variable across many studies and reflects the changing pandemic status in different areas of the world. SARS-CoV-2 infection may range from asymptomatic infection to a life-threatening acute respiratory distress syndrome and multi-organ failure. Fever, myalgia, cough, shortness of breath, and upper respiratory tract symptoms are common. Diagnosis is confirmed with PCR testing of swabs from the throat and nasopharynx or samples from BAL. Treatment is evolving, but use of dexamethasone in severe cases has shown a mortality benefit in the non-HSCT population, as well as immunomodulatory medications such as IL-6 inhibitors (tocilizumab, sarilumab) or Janus kinase (JAK) inhibitors (baricitinib) [48]. Older age, developing SARS-CoV 2 during the first year, allogeneic HSCT, and transplantation for lymphomas may have a higher risk for severe disease and mortality [49]. The outcomes in HSCT recipients appear to be worse than the general population with a mortality of about 22%–36% [49–51] 30 days after infection. Mounting an appropriate immune response to vaccines may be suboptimal [52] depending on when the vaccine is given in the post-HSCT timeline. The European Conference on Infections in Leukemia, along with the American Society for Transplantation and Cellular Therapy and the CDC, has endorsed COVID-19 vaccines for use in HSCT recipients. The current guidance is to initiate the vaccine series (with preference for m-RNA vaccines) at least 6 months after HSCT but can be considered as soon as 3 months post-HSCT if community transmission is high, though the efficacy is felt to be less optimal. For further reading on this emerging pathogen, please refer to Chap. 12.

## Invasive Fungal Infections

Invasive fungal infections (IFI) may occur at any phase posttransplant but peak during the early neutropenic phase which is associated with profound cellular immunodeficiency or late phase secondary to the immunosuppressive effects of medications used to treat chronic GVHD. Commonly encountered invasive fungi include aspergillus species, candida species, zygomycetes species, fusarium, scedosporium, and others.

The incidence of invasive fungal infections in HSCT recipients has decreased due to the use of antifungal prophylaxis [53, 54]. The annual incidence of IFI is 1.3%–10% with *Aspergillus* species being the most common IFI [55]. Risk factors for IFI include neutropenia, use of antithymocyte globulin, radiation, use of corticosteroids and other immunosuppressive therapy that affect T cells, severe GVHD, HLA-mismatched donors, use of cord blood as graft, CMV reactivation, toll-like receptor polymorphisms, and iron overload [56, 57]. Patients with IFI and HSCT are often critically ill and are admitted to an ICU more often [55, 56] compared to other types of infections. Mortality of different types of IFI continues to be high despite treatment and can reach 12%–65% [55, 58].

**Invasive pulmonary aspergillosis** is the most common invasive fungal infection and carries a high mortality. Imaging may show nodules, masses, cavities, peribronchial infiltration, halo sign, tree-in-bud appearance, air crescent sign, and pulmonary hemorrhage [59]. A proven diagnosis requires tissue biopsy demonstrating angioinvasion which is rarely performed. A probable diagnosis may be made with culture of *Aspergillus* spp. or by indirect tests such as elevated β-D-glucan and galactomannan (in serum or BAL) in a patient with appropriate host features. Finally, a possible diagnosis may be made with appropriate clinical features and imaging findings but absence of positive mycologic data [60]. Treatment with voriconazole should be started in confirmed or suspected cases. For more information, please see Chap. 8.

**Mucormycosis** is a cause of invasive sinusitis and pneumonia and usually requires surgical treatment in addition to antifungals with a high mortality. For more information on this life-threatening infection, please see Chap. 9.

**Pneumocystis jiroveci pneumonia** (PJP) usually occurs in the second or third phase post-HSCT. The incidence rate of PJP decreased dramatically with the use of trimethoprim sulfamethoxazole (TMP-SMX) prophylaxis. The incidence is about 2.5% in one retrospective study of 519 allogeneic stem cell transplanted patients, and prophylaxis had been discontinued in all but three [58]. Patients present with fever, dry cough, dyspnea, and acute respiratory failure. Microscopic examination of respiratory samples, as well as PCR and β-d-glucan, is used in diagnosis. First line treatment is with TMP-SMX. See Chap. 9 for more information.

**Fusarium infections** (incidence is 5.97 per 1000 transplants [58]) and **scedosporium** are rare examples of IFI which can involve the lungs and may be rising in incidence given widespread mold-active prophylaxis and selection pressure. See Chap. 9 for more information on these infections.

## Noninfectious Complications

Modern HSCT medicine has shown a decline in the incidence and severity of the infectious pulmonary complications with the use of prophylactic antibiotics and preemptive diagnosis and treatment. This trend has placed greater emphasis and recognition for the noninfectious pulmonary complications, which continue to be a very important cause of morbidity and mortality following HSCT in both the near and long term.

## Idiopathic Pneumonia Syndrome (IPS)

IPS is defined as idiopathic syndrome of pneumopathy following HSCT and characterized by respiratory symptoms with deranged lung physiology and multilobar lung infiltrates on imaging and requires the exclusion of infectious causes, cardiac dysfunction, acute renal failure, or fluid overload [61]. The incidence of IPS is about 3%–21% and usually develops a median of 25 days post-HSCT [62, 63]. Risk factors for IPS include allogeneic HSCT, full-intensity conditioning, total body irradiation >12 Gy, acute GVHD, older age, and pretransplant poor lung function [61, 63, 64]. More recent investigations have identified HHV-6 infection as an important risk factor for later development of IPS [41].

Treatment is usually supportive; many patients will be on empiric antibiotics while undergoing simultaneous infectious disease evaluation. There may be benefits from adding corticosteroids with or without etanercept [65]. The outcome for IPS is poor with high mortality that can reach more than 75%. Many patients will progress to fulminant respiratory failure and die within a few days. The need for mechanical ventilation and the presence of renal insufficiency were associated with higher mortality [62, 64]. For more information on IPS, please see Chap. 16.

## Peri-Engraftment Respiratory Distress Syndrome (PERDS)

PERDS is defined as new-onset acute lung injury requiring oxygen supplementation with radiographic abnormalities that happen within 5 days of neutrophil engraftment in the absence of cardiac or infectious etiologies. It reflects the pulmonary subtype of the engraftment syndrome (ES). It is more frequent in autologous HSCT compared to allogeneic HSCT. The incidence of PERDS varies widely in the literature due to the heterogeneity of ES definitions, but in a retrospective study of 3473 patients undergoing an autologous transplant, the reported incidence was 4.8% [66]. Risk factors for PERDS include autologous HSCT, female sex, use of granulocyte macrophage colony stimulating factor, non-myeloablative conditioning, and peripheral blood versus bone marrow source of HSCT [67–71]. The clinical presentation of PERDS is nonspecific and may mimic other diagnoses. Treatment is largely supportive with a portion of patients improving without therapy; however, corticosteroids are efficacious in those requiring treatment with excellent outcomes and only 3.6% in-hospital mortality [66] but may increase the non-relapse mortality at 2 years [70, 72]. For more information on PERDS, please see Chap. 15.

## Diffuse Alveolar Hemorrhage (DAH)

DAH is characterized by acute respiratory failure with bilateral lung infiltrates resulting from bleeding into the alveolar surfaces. It can progress rapidly to respiratory failure and result in death. In addition to the diffuse alveolar infiltrates and new oxygen requirement, the diagnosis is made by progressively bloody return from consecutive bronchoalveolar lavages. A cutoff of "20% hemosiderin laden macrophages" is also used to obtain a cytologic definition of hemorrhage. The incidence of DAH is 2%–16% [73–75] based on variable applications of the definition. Risk factors include allogeneic HSCT, delayed platelet engraftment, myeloablative therapy, and older age [74, 76, 77].

Treatment is with supportive care, corticosteroids, and correction of platelet and coagulation abnormalities. The outcome is poor with high mortality and the need for mechanical ventilation in many patients [78, 79]. Early DAH in the first month carries a better prognosis and outcome compared to late DAH [75]. For more information regarding DAH, please see Chap. 14.

## Cryptogenic Organizing Pneumonia (COP)

COP is a pneumonia-like syndrome characterized by fever, cough, and shortness of breath with alveolar and interstitial changes on imaging. Pulmonary function testing will show a restrictive physiology. The incidence is between 2% and 11% and usually occurs between 2- and

15-month post-HSCT [79, 80]. Risk factors include HLA disparity, female sex, and peripheral blood HSCT. On the other hand, busulfan based myeloablative conditioning and fludarabine based reduced intensity conditioning have lower risk [81, 82]. COP usually has a favorable prognosis with good response to corticosteroids, but up to 30% may relapse [79, 82].

## Bronchiolitis Obliterans Syndrome (BOS)

BOS is a new-onset obstructive lung disease that develops after allogeneic HSCT secondary to bronchiolar wall fibrosis and narrowing. The incidence rate of BOS is 3.4%–10% [83] and is considered the most common late presenting noninfectious pulmonary complication. It is most often diagnosed well into phase III, typically around the 1-year mark post-HSCT. The typical presentation will include new cough, dyspnea, and exercise limitation, which may be progressive in nature or slowly stabilizes. Important risk factors include myeloablative conditioning regimen, chronic GVHD, multiparous female donors, unrelated donors, and a lower respiratory tract infection prior to day 100. Antithymocyte globulin administration and reduced intensity regimen were associated with reduced risk [84–88].

After ruling out infectious etiologies, BOS can be diagnosed based on PFT showing irreversible obstruction, a decline of FEV1 < 75% of predicted with ≥10% decline over less than 2 years and either HRCT findings of air trapping and bronchiectasis, or PFT findings of air trapping [89]. Treatment is difficult with no curative therapy known. Corticosteroids, azithromycin, inhaled budesonide/formoterol, and montelukast can be used [90–92] with variable reports of stabilizing lung function decline. Lung transplant is an option in advanced disease [93]. BOS is a significant source of mortality in the phase III HSCT patient, and estimates of mortality range from approximately 50% in 5 years, with early onset BOS as an independent risk factor for poor survival [86, 94, 95]. For more information on BOS, please see Chap. 17.

## Interstitial Lung Disease (ILD)

ILD is a late complication of HSCT with a low incidence of 2.4%–2.6% [96, 97]. The median duration from transplantation to diagnosis in one cohort was 44 months [96]. Risk factors include peripheral blood allogeneic HSCT and extra-thoracic GVHD [97]. ILD pathology varies and includes pleuroparenchymal fibroelastosis, diffuse alveolar damage, nonspecific interstitial pneumonia, organizing pneumonia, or lymphoid interstitial pneumonia [97, 98]. The outcome for ILD is poor especially in pleuroparenchymal fibroelastosis with no clear guidelines on treatment. The median survival at 2 years is 61% [97]. Please refer to Chap. 18 for more details.

## Pulmonary Hypertension and Pulmonary Veno-Occlusive Disease (PVOD)

Pulmonary hypertension after HSCT is likely an underreported condition with most cases reported in children. It is common in patients with BOS with an incidence of 32.5% [99]. PVOD is a rare form of pulmonary hypertension defined by post-capillary intimal fibrosis of the pulmonary venules seen via a surgical lung biopsy. Clinically it can mimic heart failure on imaging – making the syndrome difficult to recognize. There is a suggestion that PVOD may be a result of endothelial injury from cytotoxic treatment or radiation [100]. Patients with PVOD often do worse if treated with pulmonary vasodilator therapy that is typically used for pulmonary arterial hypertension, at the time of diagnosis; it is recommended to refer such patients to lung transplant as the effective 1-year mortality approaches 70% [101]. For more information on pulmonary hypertension and PVOD, please see Chap. 19.

## Thoracic Air Leak Syndrome (TALS)

It refers to the presence of extra-alveolar air known as the development of pneumothorax, pneumomediastinum, pneumopericardium, and/

or subcutaneous emphysema following allogeneic HSCT. The reported incidence is 0.83%–3.1% [102–104]. Risk factors include chronic GVHD, history of invasive fungal infection, male sex, younger age, and tacrolimus based GVHD prophylaxis with BOS being the main risk factor for this condition [105]. It is typically a late presenting condition; in one retrospective review of 18 patients with TALS, the onset was on average day 425 after HSCT, and the mean duration of air leak was long at 16 days [104]. Treatment is largely supportive, focused on oxygen therapy and chest tube placement when appropriate. TALS—especially if associated with severe GVHD—reflects a poor overall condition with high mortality that can reach 88.9% [102, 104]. For more information on TALS, please see Chap. 19.

## Pleural Effusions

Pleural effusions are frequent after HSCT with an incidence of 9.9% at 1 year posttransplant. They can result from infectious processes, fluid overload, GVHD related serositis, ES, or malignancy. Treatment is directed toward correcting the underlying condition. The development of pleural effusions is associated with decrease in overall survival [106] regardless of underlying etiology. More information on pleural effusions is available in Chap. 19.

## Venous Thromboembolic Disease (VTE) and Pulmonary Cytolytic Thrombi (PCT)

Following a stem cell transplant, patients are at an above average risk of VTE; in one meta-analysis, this risk has been estimated to be as high as 5% for the post-HSCT population at day 180 [107]. The most prevalent and strongest risk factors are identified as prior VTE, indwelling catheter devices, and GVHD [107–111]. Somewhat counterintuitively, VTE can be seen even in patients with profound thrombocytopenia, in one series up to 13% of patients with platelet counts of less than $20 \times 10^9$/L [108]. As expected, treatment can be challenging in the face of significant thrombocytopenia as this population is at risk for significant bleeding complications as well. Mechanical thromboprophylaxis is widely recommended in those who cannot tolerate chemical thromboprophylaxis. Lower extremity deep vein thrombosis and pulmonary embolism are associated with an increased risk of non-relapse mortality [111].

Pulmonary cytolytic thrombi (PCT) are a rare and unusual complication following HSCT. Patients present with fever and pulmonary nodules. After ruling out infectious etiologies, the diagnosis is made following a surgical biopsy. Pathology will show necrotic occlusive basophilic thromboemboli on the small pulmonary arteries. PCT can be reversible with treatment with immunosuppressive therapy [112, 113].

For more information on VTE and PCT, please see Chap. 19.

## Other Noninfectious Complications

**Posttransplant lymphoproliferative disorder** (PTLD) is an Epstein-Barr virus (EBV) related lymphoid proliferation that results from significant immunosuppression of T-cell immunity. It is a rare condition with an incidence of 1–17% and usually occurs during the first 6 months post-HSCT [114] when the degree of immunosuppression is the greatest. Risk factors include allogeneic HSCT, T-cell depletion of the donor marrow, antithymocyte globulin use, unrelated or HLA-mismatched grafts, acute and chronic graft-versus-host disease, second transplantation, and EBV sero-mismatch (recipient-negative/donor-positive) [114–116]. Patients may develop fever, thoracic lymphadenopathy, and lung parenchymal involvement—though lymph node enlargement can be identified throughout the body [117]. Treatment includes decreasing the immunosuppressive therapy, rituximab, and chemotherapy. The disease is fatal without treatment, and the 3-year overall survival with treatment is 37.3% [118]. For more information on PTLD, please see Chap. 19.

**Pulmonary alveolar proteinosis** (PAP) is a rare condition related to a dysfunction in surfactant clearance by alveolar macrophages that can develop post-HSCT. Pathology will show abnormal periodic acid-Schiff lipo-proteinaceous material accumulation inside the airways. The outcome is good, and it can be reversible with appropriate management [119]; severe respiratory failure and death may result without treatment. Please see Chap. 19.

**Acute radiation pneumonitis** (ARP): ARP is directly related to the dose and field that the radiation therapy is applied to. It happens less commonly after whole-body irradiation, but it is more common in mediastinal lymphomas given the proximity to the lung fields. Acute radiation pneumonitis is typically seen 4–12 weeks after therapy, and chronic radiation pneumonitis is seen 6–12 months following therapy and is also referred to as the fibrotic phase, associated with scar tissue and traction bronchiectasis [120]. Chapter 21 discusses further use of whole-body irradiation.

**Drug toxicity**: Many of the chemotherapeutic and immunosuppressive medications used in patients with HSCT can potentially affect the lung and cause a wide range of diseases (e.g., cyclophosphamide, busulfan, sirolimus etc.). For a detailed discussion of pulmonary complications following these therapies, please see Chap. 21.

## Acute Respiratory Failure and Mechanical Ventilation

It is estimated that 15.7%–20% of patients with HSCT will be admitted to the ICU [121, 122] within their first year. Acute respiratory failure is one of the most common causes for admission to the ICU in the HSCT population. Many of the infectious and noninfectious conditions discussed in this chapter can result in acute respiratory failure and the need to use mechanical ventilation or noninvasive ventilation. Infectious complications are the most common cause of respiratory failure among HSCT recipients. Despite the tremendous improvement in supportive intensive care, advancement in technology, and prophylactic measures, the mortality for allogeneic HSCT in respiratory failure did not improve significantly with overall mortality of 51.7% but is higher if requiring mechanical ventilation and may reach up to 80% [123]. Risk factors for increased ICU mortality include the need for mechanical ventilation, use of vasopressors, renal replacement therapy, acute respiratory failure, acute kidney injury, acute GVHD, and allogeneic HSCT [123, 124]. The long-term survival of more than 6 months is 40%–86% [125]. Autologous HSCT patients in the ICU have a much better prognosis. For more information on use of respiratory support in the ICU, see Chap. 25, and for critical care outcomes, please see Chap. 24.

## Diagnostic Considerations of Noninfectious Pulmonary Complications Following HSCT

It is important for the management of pulmonary complications following HSCT that these patients are evaluated pretransplant by thorough history, physical examination, pulmonary function testing, and chest radiograph. Chest CT scan may be indicated especially in older patients, smokers, or those who have an abnormal initial evaluation. These investigations should serve as a baseline for any posttransplant changes.

Respiratory symptoms in the early posttransplant period (generally in the first 100 days following transplant) should be evaluated in the context of acuity of symptoms and patient's immune status (neutrophil count, immunosuppressive medications, presence of acute GVHD, and antimicrobial prophylactic measures). Infectious conditions should be considered first during this period. HRCT of the chest is more sensitive in detecting pulmonary opacities and may provide useful information on the etiology of the patient's symptoms [126]. Bronchoscopy with BAL is well tolerated and provides a diagnosis in around half of the patients [127]. Recent advances in noninvasive diagnostic methods have reduced the need for bronchoscopy in this patient population. These include viral PCR studies of nasal washing and serological tests such as galactomannan and CMV PCR [120]. Surgical lung

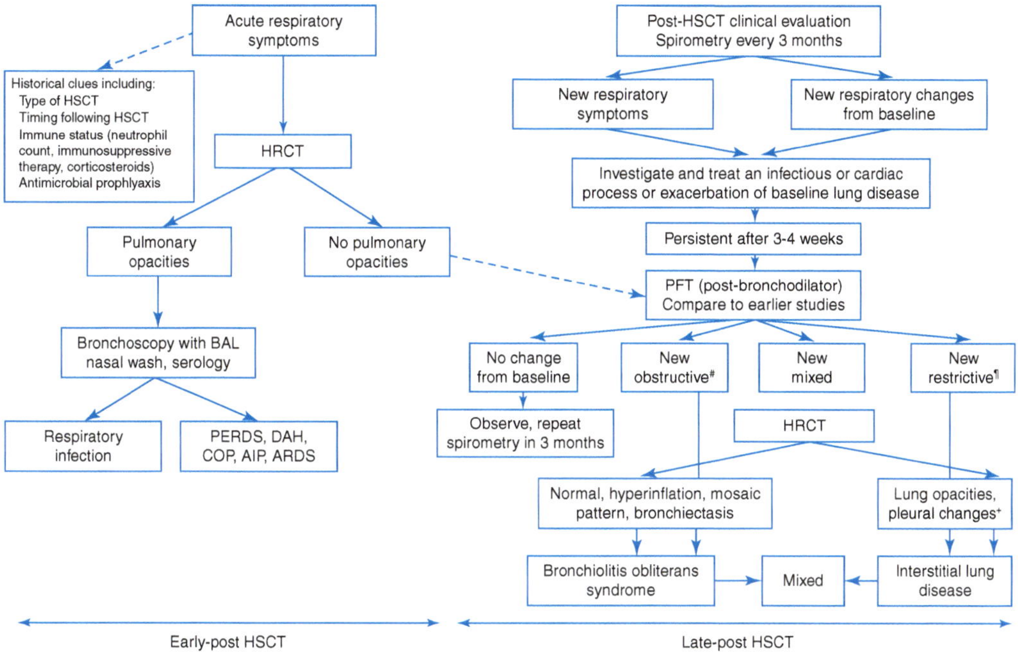


**Fig. 3.2** Suggested diagnostic approach to pulmonary complications post-HSCT. *HRCT* high resolution CT, *BAL* bronchoalveolar lavage, *PERDS* peri-engraftment respiratory distress syndrome, *DAH* diffuse alveolar hemorrhage, *COP* cryptogenic organizing pneumonia, *AIP* acute interstitial pneumonia, *ARDS* acute respiratory distress syndrome, *PFT* pulmonary function test

biopsies are rarely needed nowadays following HSCT, and the decision to proceed with this procedure should be made in a multidisciplinary approach and on a case-by-case basis [128].

In the late post-HSCT period, chronic noninfectious pulmonary complications including BOS, ILD, or mixed changes gain more significance. Given the limited treatment options once the damage associated with these conditions has been established, it is recommended to monitor patients carefully following HSCT by regular outpatient visits and review of the patient's respiratory symptoms. Screening spirometry every 3 months after the initial 100 days and for the first 2 years following allogeneic HSCT is recommended by the National Institutes of Health 2014 Consensus Conference on chronic GVHD and Consensus Conference on Clinical Practice in chronic GVHD [129]. The presence of a new obstructive pattern as compared to baseline values is consistent with BOS, while a new restrictive finding is suggestive of ILD. Occasionally, patients may have combined new obstructive and restrictive changes that reflect a mixed pattern of BOS and ILD. If there are persistent new changes on PFT, HRCT is helpful in delineating the pulmonary disease. The findings of nonhomogeneous air trapping by expiratory CT (mosaic pattern) or small airway thickening or bronchiectasis are consistent with BOS, while ILD associated with GVHD usually manifests radiologically with persistent multilobar opacities (ground glass, consolidation, small linear and reticular changes) with or without pleural changes. An approach to the evaluation of late noninfectious pulmonary complications following HSCT is summarized in Fig. 3.2. More details about the diagnosis of pulmonary complications following HSCT are offered in Chap. 5.

## Conclusion

The pulmonary complications following HSCT are significant and are a major cause of morbidity and mortality. Knowledge of the spectrum of conditions that are seen in this patient population and developing an organized framework to approach the HSCT patient are pivotal to timely diagnosis and management. An important theme in this regard is considering the type of transplant, the immune status of the patient, and the timing following transplant. The best outcome in the care of these patients is when there is systematic communication and collaboration by a multidisciplinary team of experts that include the transplant specialist, pulmonologist and intensivist, infectious disease specialist, radiologist, bedside nurse, pharmacist, and other providers as needed.

## References


1. Thomas E, Lochte H, Lu W, Ferrebee J. Intravenous infusion of bone marrow in patients receiving radiation and chemotherapy. N Engl J Med. 1957;257(11):491–6.
2. Niederwieser D, Baldomero H, Atsuta Y, Aljurf M, Seber A, Greinix H, et al. One and half million hematopoietic stem cell transplants (HSCT). Dissemination, trends and potential to improve activity by telemedicine from the worldwide network for blood and marrow transplantation (WBMT). Blood. 2019;134(Supplement_1):2035.
3. McDonald G, Sandmaier B, Mielcarek M, Sorror M, Pergam S, Mokoto G, et al. Survival, nonrelapse mortality, and relapse-related mortality after allogeneic hematopoietic cell transplantation: comparing 2003–2007 versus 2013–2017 cohorts. Ann Intern Med. 2020;172(4):229.
4. Gooley T, Chien J, Pergam S, Hingorani S, Sorror M, Boeckh M, et al. Reduced mortality after allogeneic hematopoietic-cell transplantation. N Engl J Med. 2010;363(22):2091–101.
5. Lucena C, Torres A, Rovira M, Marcos M, de la Bellacasa J, Sánchez M, et al. Pulmonary complications in hematopoietic SCT: a prospective study. Bone Marrow Transplant. 2014;49(10):1293–9.
6. Afessa B, Abdulai R, Kremers W, Hogan W, Litzow M, Peters S. Risk factors and outcome of pulmonary complications after autologous hematopoietic stem cell transplant. Chest. 2012;141(2):442–50.
7. Martin P, Counts G, Appelbaum F, Lee S, Sanders J, Deeg H, et al. Life expectancy in patients surviving more than 5 years after hematopoietic cell transplantation. J Clin Oncol. 2010;28(6):1011–6.
8. Bhatia S, Francisco L, Carter A, Sun C, Baker K, Gurney J, et al. Late mortality after allogeneic hematopoietic cell transplantation and functional status of long-term survivors: report from the bone marrow transplant survivor study. Blood. 2007;110(10):3784–92.
9. Junghanss C, Marr K, Carter R, Sandmaier B, Maris M, Maloney D, et al. Incidence and outcome of bacterial and fungal infections following nonmyeloablative compared with myeloablative allogeneic hematopoietic stem cell transplantation: a matched control study. Biol Blood Marrow Transplant. 2002;8(9):512–20.
10. Tran B, Halperin A, Chien J. Cigarette smoking and outcomes after allogeneic hematopoietic stem cell transplantation. Biol Blood Marrow Transplant. 2011;17(7):1004–11.
11. Onizuka M, Fujii N, Nakasone H, Ogata M, Atsuta Y, Suzuki R, Uchida N, Ohashi K, Ozawa Y, Eto T, Ikegame K, Nakamae H, Inoue M, Fukuda T. Transplant complications working Group of the Japan Society for hematopoietic cell transplantation. Risk factors and prognosis of non-infectious pulmonary complications after allogeneic hematopoietic stem cell transplantation. Int J Hematol. 2022;115(4):534–44.
12. Cheng GS. Pulmonary function and pretransplant evaluation of the hematopoietic cell transplant candidate. Clin Chest Med. 2017;38:307–16.
13. Aguilar-Guisado M, Jiménez-Jambrina M, Espigado I, Rovira M, Martino R, Oriol A, et al. Pneumonia in allogeneic stem cell transplantation recipients: a multicenter prospective study. Clin Transpl. 2011;25(6):E629–38.
14. Dettenkofer M, Wenzler-Rottele S, Babikir R, Bertz H, Ebner W, Meyer E, et al. Surveillance of nosocomial sepsis and pneumonia in patients with a bone marrow or peripheral blood stem cell transplant: a multicenter project. Clin Infect Dis. 2005;40(7):926–31.
15. Balletto E, Mikulska M. Bacterial infections in hematopoietic stem cell transplant recipients. Mediterr J Hematol Infect Dis. 2015;7:e2015045.
16. Kumar D, Humar A, Plevneshi A, Siegal D, Franke N, Green K, et al. Invasive pneumococcal disease in adult hematopoietic stem cell transplant recipients: a decade of prospective population-based surveillance. Bone Marrow Transplant. 2008;41(8):743–7.
17. Torda A, Chong Q, Lee A, Chen S, Dodds A, Greenwood M, et al. Invasive pneumococcal disease following adult allogeneic hematopoietic stem cell transplantation. Transpl Infect Dis. 2014;16(5):751–9.
18. Coussement J, Lebeaux D, Rouzaud C, Lortholary O. Nocardia infections in solid organ and hematopoietic stem cell transplant recipients. Curr Opin Infect Dis. 2017;30(6):545–51.
19. Molina A, Winston D, Pan D, Schiller G. Increased incidence of nocardial infections in an era of atovaquone prophylaxis in allogeneic hematopoietic stem cell transplant recipients. Biol Blood Marrow Transplant. 2018;24(8):1715–20.
20. Kanne J, Yandow D, Mohammed T, Meyer C. CT findings of pulmonary nocardiosis. Am J Roentgenol. 2011;197(2):W266–72.

21. Abad C, Razonable R. An update on mycobacterium tuberculosis infection after hematopoietic stem cell transplantation in adults. Clin Transpl. 2018;32(12):e13430.
22. Al-Anazi K, Al-Jasser A, Alsaleh K. Infections caused by mycobacterium tuberculosis in recipients of hematopoietic stem cell transplantation. Front Oncol. 2014;4:231.
23. Russo R, Dulley F, Suganuma L, França I, Yasuda M, Costa S. Tuberculosis in hematopoietic stem cell transplant patients: case report and review of the literature. Int J Infect Dis. 2010;14:e187–91.
24. Kapoor J, Mirgh S, Khushoo V, Mehta P, Ahmed R, Bansal N, et al. Study of clinical characteristics, risk factors and outcomes for tuberculosis post allogeneic stem cell transplant: never count it out. Therapeut Adv Infect Dis. 2021;8:204993612110086.
25. Yang A, Shi J, Luo Y, Ye Y, Tan Y, Huang H, et al. Allo-HSCT recipients with invasive fungal disease and ongoing immunosuppression have a high risk for developing tuberculosis. Sci Rep. 2019;9(1):20402.
26. Ip MS, Yuen KY, Woo PC, Luk WK, Tsang KW, Lam WK, Liang RH. Risk factors for pulmonary tuberculosis in bone marrow transplant recipients. Am J Respir Crit Care Med. 1998;158(4):1173–7.
27. Costa S, Ramos J, Batista M. Tuberculosis in hematopoietic stem cell transplant recipients. Mediterr J Hematol Infect Dis. 2013;5(1):e2013061.
28. de la Cámara R, Martino R, Granados E, Rodriguez-Salvanés F, Rovira M, Cabrera R, et al. Tuberculosis after hematopoietic stem cell transplantation: incidence, clinical characteristics and outcome. Bone Marrow Transplant. 2000;26(3):291–8.
29. Beswick J, Shin E, Michelis F, Thyagu S, Viswabandya A, Lipton J, et al. Incidence and risk factors for nontuberculous mycobacterial infection after allogeneic hematopoietic cell transplantation. Biol Blood Marrow Transplant. 2018;24(2):366–72.
30. Al-Anazi K, Al-Jasser A, Al-Anazi W. Infections caused by non-tuberculous mycobacteria in recipients of hematopoietic stem cell transplantation. Front Oncol. 2014;4:311.
31. Brissot E, Gomez A, Aline-Fardin A, Lalande V, Lapusan S, Isnard F, et al. Report of disseminated mycobacterium haemophilum infection after double cord blood Allo-SCT. Bone Marrow Transplant. 2014;49(10):1347–8.
32. Cho S, Lee D, Kim H. Cytomegalovirus infections after hematopoietic stem cell transplantation: current status and future immunotherapy. Int J Mol Sci. 2019;20(11):2666.
33. Green M, Leisenring W, Xie H, Mast T, Cui Y, Sandmaier B, et al. Cytomegalovirus viral load and mortality after haemopoietic stem cell transplantation in the era of pre-emptive therapy: a retrospective cohort study. Lancet Haematol. 2016;3(3):e119–27.
34. Avery R, Silveira F, Benedict K, Cleveland A, Kauffman C, Schuster M, et al. Cytomegalovirus infections in lung and hematopoietic cell transplant recipients in the organ transplant infection prevention and detection study: a multi-year, multicenter prospective cohort study. Transpl Infect Dis. 2018;20(3):e12877.
35. Dziedzic M, Sadowska-Krawczenko I, Styczynski J. Risk factors for cytomegalovirus infection after allogeneic hematopoietic cell transplantation in malignancies: proposal for classification. Anticancer Res. 2017;37(12):6551–6.
36. Styczynski J. Who is the patient at risk of CMV recurrence: a review of the current scientific evidence with a focus on hematopoietic cell transplantation. Infect Dis Ther. 2017;7(1):1–16.
37. Montesinos P, Sanz J, Cantero S, Lorenzo I, Martín G, Saavedra S, et al. Incidence, risk factors, and outcome of cytomegalovirus infection and disease in patients receiving prophylaxis with Oral valganciclovir or intravenous ganciclovir after umbilical cord blood transplantation. Biol Blood Marrow Transplant. 2009;15(6):730–40.
38. Kitabayashi A, Hirokawa M, Horiuchi T, Kawabata Y, Miura A. Late-onset herpes simplex virus-associated interstitial pneumonia after allogeneic bone marrow transplantation. Bone Marrow Transplant. 2000;25(2):225–6.
39. Kim D, Messner H, Minden M, Gupta V, Kuruvilla J, Wright J, et al. Factors influencing varicella zoster virus infection after allogeneic peripheral blood stem cell transplantation: low-dose acyclovir prophylaxis and pre-transplant diagnosis of lymphoproliferative disorders. Transpl Infect Dis. 2008;10(2):90–8.
40. Gasparetto E, Escuissato D, Inoue C, Marchiori E, Muller N. Herpes simplex virus type 2 pneumonia after bone marrow transplantation. J Thorac Imaging. 2005;20(2):71–3.
41. Zhou X, O'Dwyer DN, Xia M, Miller HK, Chan PR, Trulik K, Chadwick MM, Hoffman TC, Bulte C, Sekerak K, Wilke CA, Patel SJ, Yokoyama WM, Murray S, Yanik GA, Moore BB. First-onset Herpesviral infection and lung injury in allogeneic hematopoietic cell transplantation. Am J Respir Crit Care Med. 2019;200(1):63–74.
42. Schuster M, Cleveland A, Dubberke E, Kauffman C, Avery R, Husain S, et al. Infections in hematopoietic cell transplant recipients: results from the organ transplant infection project, a multicenter, prospective, cohort study. Open forum. Infect Dis. 2017;4(2):ofx050.
43. Wolfromm A, Porcher R, Legoff J, de Latour R, Xhaard A, de Fontbrune F, et al. Viral respiratory infections diagnosed by multiplex PCR after allogeneic hematopoietic stem cell transplantation: long-term incidence and outcome. Biol Blood Marrow Transplant. 2014;20(8):1238–41.
44. Paulsen G, Danziger-Isakov L. Respiratory viral infections in solid organ and hematopoietic stem cell transplantation. Clin Chest Med. 2017;38(4):707–26.
45. Chemaly R, Ghosh S, Bodey G, Rohatgi N, Safdar A, Keating M, et al. Respiratory viral infections in adults with hematologic malignancies and human

stem cell transplantation recipients. Medicine. 2006;85(5):278–87.
46. Khanna N, Steffen I, Studt J, Schreiber A, Lehmann T, Weisser M, et al. Outcome of influenza infections in outpatients after allogeneic hematopoietic stem cell transplantation. Transpl Infect Dis. 2009;11(2):100–5.
47. Reid G, Huprikar S, Patel G, Razonable R, Mossad S, Levi M, et al. A multicenter evaluation of pandemic influenza a/H1N1 in hematopoietic stem cell transplant recipients. Transpl Infect Dis. 2013;15(5):487–92.
48. https://www.covid19treatmentguidelines.nih.gov/. Accessed 24 Feb 2022.
49. Sharma A, Bhatt N, St Martin A, Abid M, Bloomquist J, Chemaly R, et al. Clinical characteristics and outcomes of COVID-19 in haematopoietic stem-cell transplantation recipients: an observational cohort study. Lancet Haematol. 2021;8(3):e185–93.
50. Shahzad M, Chaudhary S, Zafar M, Hassan M, Hussain A, Ali F, et al. Impact of COVID-19 in hematopoietic stem cell transplant recipients: a systematic review and meta-analysis. Transpl Infect Dis. 2022;24(2):e13792.
51. Kanellopoulos A, Ahmed M, Kishore B, Lovell R, Horgan C, Paneesha S, et al. COVID-19 in bone marrow transplant recipients: reflecting on a single Centre experience. Br J Haematol. 2020;190(2):e67–70.
52. Dhakal B, Abedin S, Fenske T, Chhabra S, Ledeboer N, Hari P, et al. Response to SARS-CoV-2 vaccination in patients after hematopoietic cell transplantation and CAR T-cell therapy. Blood. 2021;138(14):1278–81.
53. Cordonnier C, Rovira M, Maertens J, Olavarria E, Faucher C, Bilger K, et al. Voriconazole for secondary prophylaxis of invasive fungal infections in allogeneic stem cell transplant recipients: results of the VOSIFI study. Haematologica. 2010;95(10):1762–8.
54. Robenshtok E, Gafter-Gvili A, Goldberg E, Weinberger M, Yeshurun M, Leibovici L, et al. Antifungal prophylaxis in cancer patients after chemotherapy or hematopoietic stem-cell transplantation: systematic review and meta-analysis. J Clin Oncol. 2007;25(34):5471–89.
55. Young A, Leiva Juarez M, Evans S. Fungal pneumonia in patients with hematologic malignancy and hematopoietic stem cell transplantation. Clin Chest Med. 2017;38(3):479–91.
56. Harrison N, Mitterbauer M, Tobudic S, Kalhs P, Rabitsch W, Greinix H, et al. Incidence and characteristics of invasive fungal diseases in allogeneic hematopoietic stem cell transplant recipients: a retrospective cohort study. BMC Infect Dis. 2015;15(1):584.
57. Marr K, Carter R, Crippa F, Wald A, Corey L. Epidemiology and outcome of mould infections in hematopoietic stem cell transplant recipients. Clin Infect Dis. 2002;34(7):909–17.
58. De Castro N, Neuville S, Sarfati C, Ribaud P, Derouin F, Gluckman E, et al. Occurrence of pneumocystis jiroveci pneumonia after allogeneic stem cell transplantation: a 6-year retrospective study. Bone Marrow Transplant. 2005;36(10):879–83.
59. Raveendran S, Lu Z. CT findings and differential diagnosis in adults with invasive pulmonary aspergillosis. Radiol Infect Dis. 2018;5(1):14–25.
60. Blot SI, Taccone FS, Van den Abeele AM, Bulpa P, Meersseman W, Brusselaers N, Dimopoulos G, Paiva JA, Misset B, Rello J, Vandewoude K, Vogelaers D, AspICU Study Investigators. A clinical algorithm to diagnose invasive pulmonary aspergillosis in critically ill patients. Am J Respir Crit Care Med. 2012;186(1):56–64.
61. Panoskaltsis-Mortari A, Griese M, Madtes D, Belperio J, Haddad I, Folz R, et al. An official American Thoracic Society research statement: noninfectious lung injury after hematopoietic stem cell transplantation: idiopathic pneumonia syndrome. Am J Respir Crit Care Med. 2011;183(9):1262–79.
62. Wenger D, Triplette M, Crothers K, Cheng G, Hill J, Milano F, et al. Incidence, risk factors, and outcomes of idiopathic pneumonia syndrome after allogeneic hematopoietic cell transplantation. Biol Blood Marrow Transplant. 2020;26(2):413–20.
63. Zhu K, Hu J, Zhang T, Chen J, Zhong J, Lu Y. Incidence, risks, and outcome of idiopathic pneumonia syndrome early after allogeneic hematopoietic stem cell transplantation. Eur J Haematol. 2008;81(6):461–6.
64. Fukuda T, Hackman R, Guthrie K, Sandmaier B, Boeckh M, Maris M, et al. Risks and outcomes of idiopathic pneumonia syndrome after nonmyeloablative and conventional conditioning regimens for allogeneic hematopoietic stem cell transplantation. Blood. 2003;102(8):2777–85.
65. Thompson J, Yin Z, D'Souza A, Fenske T, Hamadani M, Hari P, et al. Etanercept and corticosteroid therapy for the treatment of late-onset idiopathic pneumonia syndrome. Biol Blood Marrow Transplant. 2017;23(11):1955–60.
66. Wieruszewski P, May H, Peters S, Gajic O, Hogan W, Dierkhising R, et al. Characteristics and outcome of periengraftment respiratory distress syndrome after autologous hematopoietic cell transplant. Ann Am Thorac Soc. 2021;18(6):1013–9.
67. Akasheh M, Eastwood D, Vesole D. Engraftment syndrome after autologous hematopoietic stem cell transplant supported by granulocyte-colony-stimulating factor (G-CSF) versus granulocyte-macrophage colony-stimulating factor (GM-CSF). Bone Marrow Transplant. 2003;31(2):113–6.
68. Martínez-Cibrian N, Magnano L, Gutiérrez-García G, Andrade X, Correa J, Suárez-Lledó M, et al. At-home autologous stem cell transplantation in multiple myeloma with and without G-CSF administration: a comparative study. Bone Marrow Transplant. 2015;51(4):593–5.

69. Carreras E, Fernández-Avilés F, Silva L, Guerrero M, de Larrea C, Martínez C, et al. Engraftment syndrome after auto-SCT: analysis of diagnostic criteria and risk factors in a large series from a single center. Bone Marrow Transplant. 2010;45(9):1417–22.
70. Cornell R, Hari P, Drobyski W. Engraftment syndrome after autologous stem cell transplantation: an update unifying the definition and management approach. Biol Blood Marrow Transplant. 2015;21(12):2061–8.
71. Gorak E, Geller N, Srinivasan R, Espinoza-Delgado I, Donohue T, Barrett A, et al. Engraftment syndrome after nonmyeloablative allogeneic hematopoietic stem cell transplantation: incidence and effects on survival. Biol Blood Marrow Transplant. 2005;11(7):542–50.
72. Chang L, Frame D, Braun T, Gatza E, Hanauer D, Zhao S, et al. Engraftment syndrome after allogeneic hematopoietic cell transplantation predicts poor outcomes. Biol Blood Marrow Transplant. 2014;20(9):1407–17.
73. Zhang Z, Wang C, Peters S, Hogan W, Hashmi S, Litzow M, et al. Epidemiology, risk factors, and outcomes of diffuse alveolar Hemorrhage after hematopoietic stem cell transplantation. Chest. 2021;159(6):2325–33.
74. Afessa B, Tefferi A, Litzow M, Peters S. Outcome of diffuse alveolar hemorrhage in hematopoietic stem cell transplant recipients. Am J Respir Crit Care Med. 2002;166(10):1364–8.
75. Abdulai R, Cartin-Ceba R. Diffuse alveolar hemorrhage in hematopoietic stem cell transplant recipients: 10-year experience in a single center. Chest. 2013;144(4):1019A.
76. Majhail N, Parks K, Defor T, Weisdorf D. Diffuse alveolar Hemorrhage and infection-associated alveolar hemorrhage following hematopoietic stem cell transplantation: related and high-risk clinical syndromes. Biol Blood Marrow Transplant. 2006;12(10):1038–46.
77. Lewis I, DeFor T, Weisdorf D. Increasing incidence of diffuse alveolar hemorrhage following allogeneic bone marrow transplantation: cryptic etiology and uncertain therapy. Bone Marrow Transplant. 2000;26(5):539–43.
78. Keklik F, Alrawi E, Cao Q, Bejanyan N, Rashidi A, Lazaryan A, et al. Diffuse alveolar hemorrhage is most often fatal and is affected by graft source, conditioning regimen toxicity, and engraftment kinetics. Haematologica. 2018;103(12):2109–15.
79. Adachi Y, Ozeki K, Ukai S, Sagou K, Fukushima N, Kohno A. Patterns of onset and outcome of cryptogenic organizing pneumonia after allogeneic hematopoietic stem cell transplantation. Int J Hematol. 2019;109(6):700–10.
80. Nakasone H, Onizuka M, Suzuki N, Fujii N, Taniguchi S, Kakihana K, et al. Pre-transplant risk factors for cryptogenic organizing pneumonia/bronchiolitis obliterans organizing pneumonia after hematopoietic cell transplantation. Bone Marrow Transplant. 2013;48(10):1317–23.
81. Freudenberger T, Madtes D, Curtis J, Cummings P, Storer B, Hackman R. Association between acute and chronic graft-versus-host disease and bronchiolitis obliterans organizing pneumonia in recipients of hematopoietic stem cell transplants. Blood. 2003;102(10):3822–8.
82. Kim M, Cha S, Seo H, Shin K, Lim J, Kim H, et al. Predictors of relapse in patients with organizing pneumonia. Tuberc Respir Dis. 2015;78(3):190.
83. Hofstetter E, Henig N, Kappeler D. Prevalence of bronchiolitis obliterans syndrome (BOS) following allogeneic hematopoietic stem cell transplant (alloHSCT) in the USA, Europe and Japan. Blood. 2019;134(Supplement_1):5678.
84. Pham J, Rangaswamy J, Avery S, Borg B, Martin C, Munsif M, et al. Updated prevalence, predictors and treatment outcomes for bronchiolitis obliterans syndrome after allogeneic stem cell transplantation. Respir Med. 2021;177:106286.
85. Yoshihara S, Tateishi U, Ando T, Kunitoh H, Suyama H, Onishi Y, et al. Lower incidence of bronchiolitis obliterans in allogeneic hematopoietic stem cell transplantation with reduced-intensity conditioning compared with myeloablative conditioning. Bone Marrow Transplant. 2005;35(12):1195–200.
86. Chen Y, Xu J, Fan Z, Xu N, Huang F, Shi P, et al. Retrospective analysis of bronchiolitis obliterans syndrome after allogeneic hematopoietic stem cell transplantation. Blood. 2021;138(Supplement 1):4877.
87. Gazourian L, Rogers A, Ibanga R, Weinhouse G, Pinto-Plata V, Ritz J, et al. Factors associated with bronchiolitis obliterans syndrome and chronic graft-versus-host disease after allogeneic hematopoietic cell transplantation. Am J Hematol. 2014;89(4):404–9.
88. Duque-Afonso J, Ihorst G, Wäsch R, Bertz H, Müller-Quernheim J, Finke J, et al. Identification of risk factors for bronchiolitis obliterans syndrome after reduced toxicity conditioning before hematopoietic cell transplantation. Bone Marrow Transplant. 2013;48(8):1098–103.
89. Jagasia M, Greinix H, Arora M, Williams K, Wolff D, Cowen E, et al. National Institutes of Health Consensus Development Project on Criteria for Clinical Trials in Chronic Graft-versus-Host Disease: I. The 2014 Diagnosis and Staging Working Group Report. Biol Blood Marrow Transplant. 2015;21(3):389–401.e1.
90. Williams K. How I treat bronchiolitis obliterans syndrome after hematopoietic stem cell transplantation. Blood. 2017;129(4):448–55.
91. Bergeron A, Chevret S, Chagnon K, Godet C, Bergot E, Peffault de Latour R, et al. Budesonide/formoterol for bronchiolitis obliterans after hematopoietic stem cell transplantation. Am J Respir Crit Care Med. 2015;191(11):1242–9.

92. Yadav H, Peters S, Keogh K, Hogan W, Erwin P, West C, et al. Azithromycin for the treatment of obliterative bronchiolitis after hematopoietic stem cell transplantation: a systematic review and meta-analysis. Biol Blood Marrow Transplant. 2016;22(12):2264–9.
93. Soubani A, Kingah P, Alshabani K, Muma G, Haq A. Lung transplantation following hematopoietic stem cell transplantation: report of two cases and systematic review of literature. Clin Transpl. 2014;28(7):776–82.
94. Au B, Au M, Chien J. Bronchiolitis obliterans syndrome epidemiology after allogeneic hematopoietic cell transplantation. Biol Blood Marrow Transplant. 2011;17(7):1072–8.
95. Rhee C, Ha J, Yoon J, Cho B, Min W, Yoon H, et al. Risk factor and clinical outcome of bronchiolitis obliterans syndrome after allogeneic hematopoietic stem cell transplantation. Yonsei Med J. 2016;57(2):365.
96. Namkoong H, Ishii M, Mori T, Sugiura H, Tasaka S, Sakurai M, et al. Clinical and radiological characteristics of patients with late-onset severe restrictive lung defect after hematopoietic stem cell transplantation. BMC Pulm Med. 2017;17(1):123.
97. Schlemmer F, Chevret S, Lorillon G, De Bazelaire C, Peffault de Latour R, Meignin V, et al. Late-onset noninfectious interstitial lung disease after allogeneic hematopoietic stem cell transplantation. Respir Med. 2014;108(10):1525–33.
98. Bondeelle L, Gras J, Michonneau D, Houdouin V, Hermet E, Blin N, et al. Pleuroparenchymal fibroelastosis after allogeneic hematopoietic stem cell transplantation. Bone Marrow Transplant. 2019;55(5):982–6.
99. Nathan S, Shlobin O, Ahmad S, Barnett S, Burton N, Gladwin M, et al. Pulmonary hypertension in patients with bronchiolitis obliterans syndrome listed for retransplantation. Am J Transplant. 2008;8(7):1506–11.
100. Bunte M, Patnaik M, Pritzker M, Burns L. Pulmonary veno-occlusive disease following hematopoietic stem cell transplantation: a rare model of endothelial dysfunction. Bone Marrow Transplant. 2008;41(8):677–86.
101. Dandoy C, Hirsch R, Chima R, Davies S, Jodele S. Pulmonary hypertension after hematopoietic stem cell transplantation. Biol Blood Marrow Transplant. 2013;19(11):1546–56.
102. Liu Y, Chou Y, Ko P, Wang H, Fan N, Liu C, et al. Risk factors and clinical features for post-transplant thoracic air-leak syndrome in adult patients receiving allogeneic haematopoietic stem cell transplantation. Sci Rep. 2019;9(1):11795.
103. Franquet T, Rodríguez S, Hernández J, Martino R, Giménez A, Hidalgo A, et al. Air-leak syndromes in hematopoietic stem cell transplant recipients with chronic GVHD. J Thorac Imaging. 2007;22(4):335–40.
104. Moon M, Sa Y, Cho K, Jo K, Lee S, Sim S. Thoracic air-leak syndromes in hematopoietic stem cell transplant recipients with graft-versus-host disease: a possible sign for poor response to treatment and poor prognosis. J Korean Med Sci. 2010;25(5):658.
105. Sakai R, Kanamori H, Nakaseko C, Yoshiba F, Fujimaki K, Sakura T, et al. Air-leak syndrome following Allo-SCT in adult patients: report from the Kanto study Group for Cell Therapy in Japan. Bone Marrow Transplant. 2010;46(3):379–84.
106. Modi D, Jang H, Kim S, Deol A, Ayash L, Bhutani D, et al. Incidence, etiology, and outcome of pleural effusions in allogeneic hematopoietic stem cell transplantation. Am J Hematol. 2016;91(9):E341–7.
107. Zahid M, Murad M, Litzow M, Hogan W, Patnaik M, Khorana A, et al. Venous thromboembolism following hematopoietic stem cell transplantation—a systematic review and meta-analysis. Ann Hematol. 2016;95(9):1457–64.
108. Gerber D, Segal J, Levy M, Kane J, Jones R, Streiff M. The incidence of and risk factors for venous thromboembolism (VTE) and bleeding among 1514 patients undergoing hematopoietic stem cell transplantation: implications for VTE prevention. Blood. 2008;112(3):504–10.
109. Labrador J, Lopez-Anglada L, Perez-Lopez E, Lozano F, Lopez-Corral L, Sanchez-Guijo F, et al. Analysis of incidence, risk factors and clinical outcome of thromboembolic and bleeding events in 431 allogeneic hematopoietic stem cell transplantation recipients. Haematologica. 2012;98(3):437–43.
110. Kekre N, Connors J. Venous thromboembolism incidence in hematologic malignancies. Blood Rev. 2019;33:24–32.
111. Kekre N, Kim HT, Ho VT, et al. Venous thromboembolism is associated with graft-*versus*-host disease and increased non-relapse mortality after allogeneic hematopoietic stem cell transplantation. Haematologica. 2017;102:1185–91.
112. Morales I, Anderson P, Tazelaar H, Wylam M. Pulmonary cytolytic thrombi: unusual complication of hematopoietic stem cell transplantation. J Pediatr Hematol Oncol. 2003;25(1):89–92.
113. Woodard J, Gulbahce E, Shreve M, Steiner M, Peters C, Hite S, et al. Pulmonary cytolytic thrombi: a newly recognized complication of stem cell transplantation. Bone Marrow Transplant. 2000;25(3):293–300.
114. Barlev A, Xu H, Fulcher N, Watson C, Sruti I, Sudhindra A. Risk of patients developing post-transplant lymphoproliferative disorder within the first year after an allogeneic hemopoietic stem cell transplant, 2011 to 2016: a US claims database analysis. Blood. 2018;132(Supplement 1):5840.
115. Landgren O, Gilbert E, Rizzo J, Socié G, Banks P, Sobocinski K, et al. Risk factors for lymphoproliferative disorders after allogeneic hematopoietic cell transplantation. Blood. 2009;113(20):4992–5001.
116. Liu L, Zhang X, Feng S. Epstein-Barr virus-related post-transplantation lymphoproliferative disorders after allogeneic hematopoietic stem cell

transplantation. Biol Blood Marrow Transplant. 2018;24(7):1341–9.
117. Halkos M, Miller J, Mann K, Miller D, Gal A. Thoracic presentations of posttransplant lymphoproliferative disorders. Chest. 2004;126(6):2013–20.
118. Xuan L, Jiang X, Sun J, Zhang Y, Huang F, Fan Z, et al. Spectrum of Epstein-Barr virus–associated diseases in recipients of allogeneic hematopoietic stem cell transplantation. Transplantation. 2013;96(6):560–6.
119. Salvator H, Tcherakian C, Maillard N, Milin S, Bergeron A, Bondeelle L, et al. Pulmonary alveolar proteinosis after allogeneic hematopoietic stem-cell transplantation in adults. Chest. 2021;160(5):1783–8.
120. Legoff J, Zucman N, Lemiale V, et al. Clinical significance of upper airway virus detection in critically ill hematology patients. Am J Respir Crit Care Med. 2019;199(4):518–28.
121. Pène F, Salluh J, Staudinger T. Has survival increased in cancer patients admitted to the ICU? No. Intensive Care Med. 2014;40(10):1573–5.
122. Afessa B, Azoulay E. Critical care of the hematopoietic stem cell transplant recipient. Crit Care Clin. 2010;26(1):133–50.
123. Saillard C, Darmon M, Bisbal M, Sannini A, Chow-Chine L, Faucher M, et al. Critically ill allogenic HSCT patients in the intensive care unit: a systematic review and meta-analysis of prognostic factors of mortality. Bone Marrow Transplant. 2018;53(10):1233–41.
124. Al-Zubaidi N, Shehada E, Alshabani K, ZazaDitYafawi J, Kingah P, Soubani A. Predictors of outcome in patients with hematologic malignancies admitted to the intensive care unit. Hematol Oncol Stem Cell Ther. 2018;11(4):206–18.
125. Soubani A. Critical care prognosis and outcomes in patients with cancer. Clin Chest Med. 2017;38(2):333–53.
126. Caillot D, Casasnovas O, Bernard A, et al. Improved management of invasive pulmonary aspergillosis in neutropenic patients using early thoracic computed tomographic scan and surgery. J Clin Oncol. 1997;15(1):139–47.
127. Bauer PR, Chevret S, Yadav H, et al. Diagnosis and outcome of acute respiratory failure in immunocompromised patients after bronchoscopy. Eur Respir J. 2019;54(1):1802442.
128. Cheng GS, Stednick ZJ, Madtes DK, Boeckh M, McDonald GB, Pergam SA. Decline in the use of surgical biopsy for diagnosis of pulmonary disease in hematopoietic cell transplantation recipients in an era of improved diagnostics and empirical therapy. Biol Blood Marrow Transplant. 2016;22(12):2243–9.
129. Hildebrandt GC, Fazekas T, Lawitschka A, et al. Diagnosis and treatment of pulmonary chronic GVHD: report from the consensus conference on clinical practice in chronic GVHD. Bone Marrow Transplant. 2011;46(10):1283–95.

# Pretransplant Pulmonary Evaluation

4

Mansour Alkhunaizi, Ricardo José, and Ajay Sheshadri

## Introduction

Since its introduction more than 50 years ago, hematopoietic stem cell transplant (HSCT) has remained integral for the treatment of many benign and malignant hematological conditions. More than 50,000 HSCT cases are performed annually, and advancements in pre- and post-HSCT care have led to a significant reduction in transplant-related mortality [1, 2]. However, pulmonary complications, both infectious and non-infectious, continue to affect a significant number of HSCT recipients and contribute greatly to early post-HSCT mortality [3, 4]. Despite improvements in outcomes after infections, non-infectious pulmonary complications (NIPC) continue to pose a significant challenge [5–7], accounting for two-thirds of all pulmonary transplant-related mortalities [8]. Finally, impairments in pulmonary function in the general population are well known to be associated with decreased survival [9]; forced spirometric measurements (FEV1 and FVC) are independent risk factors for cardiovascular [10, 11] and all-cause mortality [12–14]. By providing objective and quantifiable measures of lung function to gain insight on post-HSCT outcomes, pulmonary function tests represent the cornerstone of the pre-HSCT pulmonary evaluation and can help shape HSCT strategies to mitigate post-HSCT risk.

In this chapter, we explore the pre-HSCT pulmonary evaluation, which gives crucial information to the transplant team for determining who is at the greatest risk of respiratory complications and non-relapse mortality. We have organized this chapter by focusing on the purpose of the pre-HSCT pulmonary evaluation, the evidence for different components of pulmonary function testing (PFT), special considerations regarding the use of specific cutoffs, the role of other pulmonary tests, smoking cessation, and future directions regarding cardiopulmonary fitness.

## Pulmonary Function Tests Overview

Pulmonary function testing consists of a suite of distinct measurements that help clinicians with a diverse array of scenarios, including the diagnosis and evaluation of pulmonary and non-pulmonary diseases, monitoring disease progression and

M. Alkhunaizi
Department of Medicine, Baylor College of Medicine, Houston, TX, USA
e-mail: Mansour.alkhunaizi@bcm.edu

R. José
Department of Respiratory Medicine (Host Defence), Royal Brompton Hospital, Chelsea, London, UK
e-mail: r.jose@rbht.nhs.uk

A. Sheshadri (✉)
Department of Pulmonary Medicine, The University of Texas MD Anderson Cancer Center, Houston, TX, USA
e-mail: asheshadri@mdanderson.org



A. O. Soubani (ed.), *Pulmonary and Critical Care Considerations of Hematopoietic Stem Cell Transplantation*, https://doi.org/10.1007/978-3-031-28797-8_4

response to therapy, screening for specific diseases or exposures, and preoperative assessment [15]. Measurements from certain pulmonary function tests, such as forced vital capacity, have far-reaching implications regarding the future risk for cardiopulmonary complications and death [16, 17]. It is critical to minimize variability in PFTs in order to eliminate technical variability and isolate changes in lung function parameters that are related to disease processes. Therefore, PFT laboratories put substantial effort into maintaining and calibrating equipment and have standard operating procedures for lung function physiologists and clear instructions coupled with encouragement for patients to give their best performance during tests and maximize reproducibility.

General considerations when conducting pulmonary function tests include asking individuals not to smoke on the day of the test, not to drink alcohol for at least 4 h before the test, avoid eating a large meal within 2 h of the test, and avoid vigorous activity 30 min before the test. For specific tests, such as assessment of bronchodilator reversibility or bronchial provocation testing, bronchodilators should be withheld before the test. In certain cases, it is inappropriate to conduct lung function tests due to the potential for harm during testing where forceful maneuvers may aggravate underlying conditions. Relative contraindications to spirometry include hemoptysis of unknown origin; pneumothorax; recent myocardial infarction; unstable cardiovascular status or pulmonary embolism; thoracic, abdominal, or cerebral aneurysms; recent eye, thoracic, or abdominal surgery; or the presence of an acute illness that may affect the performance of the test [18]. More information about the technical aspects of performing pulmonary function testing are available elsewhere [19].

When conducting PFTs, it is important to obtain the individual's age, birth sex, standing height (to the nearest 0.5 cm without shoes), and weight (to the nearest 0.5 kg wearing light clothes without shoes) as these indices are used to estimate predictive values. Predicted normal values for an individual are based on equations derived from the testing of large, healthy populations [20]. Two approaches have been used to determine whether a given PFT result is normal or abnormal. Historically, values below a given threshold (e.g., 80% of predictive values) were used as a cutoff to distinguish normal and abnormal PFTs, but more recent data suggest that using values below a percentile (e.g., fifth percentile or less) may result in better classification of health and disease [21], particularly when considering the diversity of height measurements and age in populations of interest [22–24]. Therefore, we recommend the use of the lower limit of normal (LLN), calculated as the mean parameter − 1.645 × standard deviation (SD)—and present this as a standardized residual (also known as *z*-score). While the most recent recommendations from the European Respiratory Society and American Thoracic Society endorse this approach [25], fixed cutoffs have shown to classify disease better than LLN in certain populations [26], such as patients with smoking-related obstructive lung disease [27]. A similar study should be conducted in HSCT recipients to better understand which definition of impairment has better predictive and diagnostic value.

While it is commonplace to measure self-identified race in order to use race-specific equations, with the intent to give additional normative context to pulmonary function data, this practice may change in the coming years with the growing realization that self-identified race is not an immutable biological characteristic [28] and that in certain contexts, race-neutral interpretation of lung function may offer a superior estimate of pulmonary health [29]. Race adjustment has a long history based upon observations that certain races or social classes have had historically lower values for pulmonary function after adjusting for age, sex, and height. This practice has seeped into the medical dogma but has recently come under scrutiny. Most studies examining the role of race in spirometry have failed to report structural or social determinants of health or environmental exposures, all of which can affect maximally attained lung function [30–34]. Furthermore, race correction may result in the underdiagnosis of lung disease in black individuals, which can further contribute to biased medical care and health disparities [30–35]. However, in the context of HSCT, one crucial concern is that race-neutral interpretation may result in patients with pulmonary impairment being deemed ineligible for transplantation due to the use of a race-neutral interpretative approach as opposed to a race-specific equation. It is not clear whether race-neutral interpretation is superior to race-specific interpretation in the context of determining post-HSCT complications, which we will discuss in detail in a subsequent section. Further detail regarding the interpretation of spirometry is available elsewhere [25]. The following section describes specific PFT measurements and their attendant considerations from a pulmonary perspective.

## Spirometry

Spirometry is a useful noninvasive technique to detect airflow limitation. It measures the amount of airflow over time (L/s). During the procedure, the patient is asked by a trained technician to take a deep breath in until they have reached maximal lung capacity. Within 2 s, the individual forcefully and rapidly exhales, with ongoing exhalation for at least 6 s or until they reach their residual volume and can no longer further exhale. This allows determination of the forced expiratory volume in 1 s (FEV1) and the forced vital capacity (FVC), two of the most important PFT measures that are used to determine if a pulmonary impairment is present and if it is due to airflow obstruction (Fig. 4.1a, b). To ensure that the test results are reproducible and accurate, for FEV1 and FVC, the difference between the two largest values must be ≤0.150 L [19]. Obstructive airway disease is determined on spirometry by an FEV1/FVC ratio of <70% predicted or to be more accurate by a FEV1/FVC ratio lower than the LLN determined by the *z*-score [36]. While a

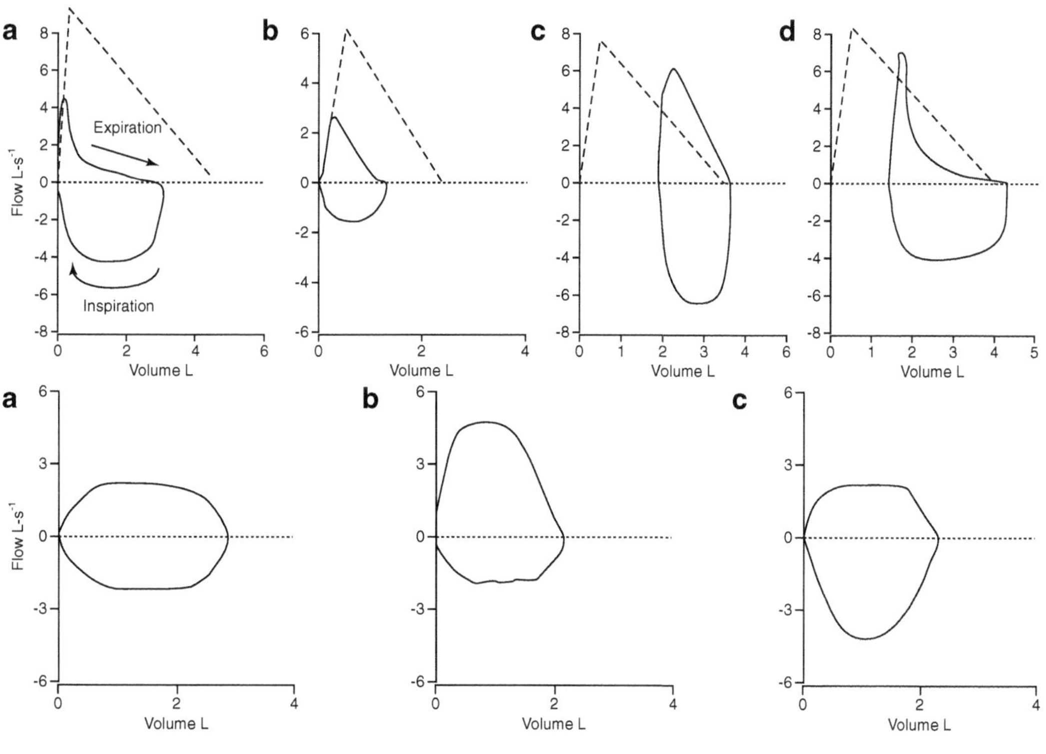


**Fig. 4.1** (**a**) Flow-volume loops. (**a, b**) Examples of obstructive pulmonary defects with a low (**a**; forced expiratory volume in 1 s (FEV1) 38%; FEV1/vital capacity (VC) 46%; peak expiratory flow (PEF) 48%; total lung capacity (TLC) 101%) or normal (**b**; FEV1 57%; FEV1/VC 73%; PEF 43%; TLC 96%) ratio of FEV1/VC. In both cases, TLC is normal, and flows are less than expected over the entire volume range. (**c**) Example of a typical restrictive defect (FEV1 66%; FEV1/VC 80%; PEF 79%; TLC 62%). The TLC is low and flow is higher than expected at a given lung volume. (**d**) Example of a typical mixed defect characterized by a low TLC and a low FEV1/VC ratio (FEV1 64%; FEV1/VC 64%; PEF 82%; TLC 72%). (**b**) Patterns of airway obstruction: (**a**) fixed, (**b**) variable extra-thoracic, and (**c**) variable intrathoracic airway obstruction

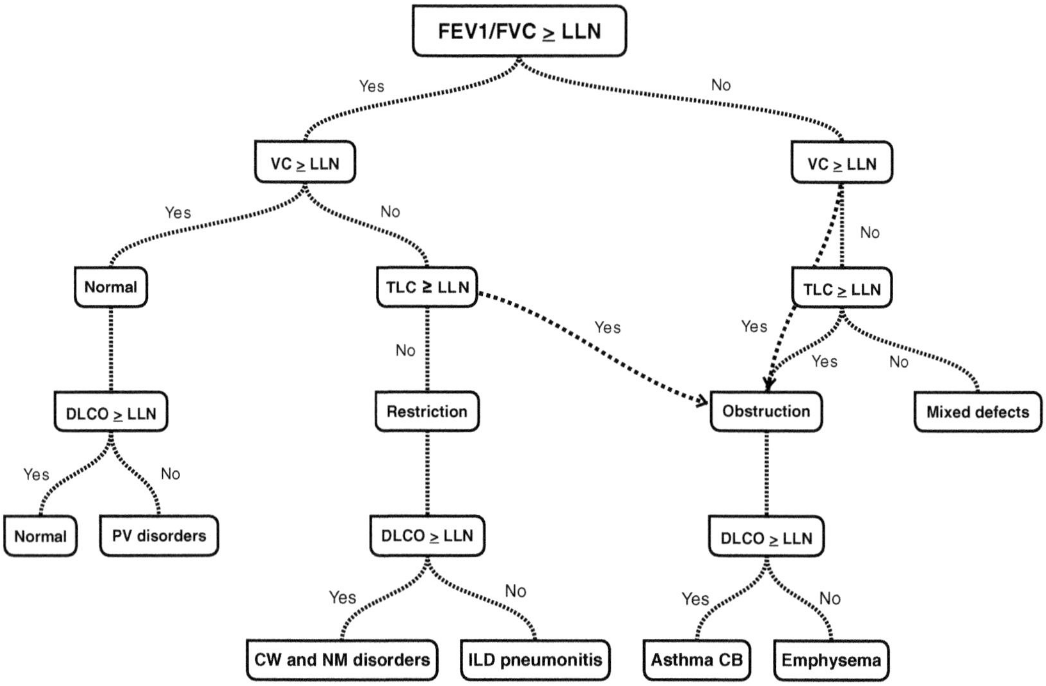


**Fig. 4.2** PFT interpretation algorithm. (Reproduced with permission from ERS: Interpretative strategies for lung function tests. R. Pellegrino, G. Viegi, V. Brusasco, R. O. Crapo, F. Burgos, R. Casaburi, A. Coates, C. P. M. van der Grinten, P. Gustafsson, J. Hankinson, R. Jensen, D. C. Johnson, N. MacIntyre, R. McKay, M. R. Miller, D. Navajas, O. F. Pedersen, J. Wanger. European Respiratory Journal 26 (5) 948-968; DOI: 10.1183/09031936.05.00035205 Published 1 November 2005. Acknowledgement Wording: Reproduced with permission of the © ERS 2022: European Respiratory Journal 53 (1) 1801889; DOI: 10.1183/13993003.01889-2018 Published 24 January 2019)

symmetric reduction in FEV1 and FVC may indicate the presence of a restrictive lung disease, lung volumes are necessary to distinguish symmetric reductions due to air trapping (e.g., pseudorestriction) [37], which indicates small airflow obstruction, from true lung restriction. In cases of mixed obstructive and restrictive disorders, expert interpretation is needed, and determining the relative contribution of airflow obstruction and lung restriction toward the degree of pulmonary impairment may not be possible. In these cases, the overall severity of impairment will likely suffice when determining the risk for post-HSCT complications. In cases of airflow obstruction, it may be helpful to measure FEV1 before and after bronchodilation in order to determine whether there is reversible airflow limitation, as can be seen in asthma. However, in general, pre-bronchodilator spirometry has been used in most studies examining how pre-HSCT pulmonary function impacts post-HSCT health [38]. Figure 4.2 demonstrates a general approach to interpreting PFTs.

## Lung Volumes

The measurement of static lung volumes, which include the residual volume (RV), functional residual capacity (FRC), and total lung capacity (TLC), provides valuable information regarding the presence of restrictive lung diseases as well as air trapping (Fig. 4.3). The most common method to measure static lung volumes is body plethysmography. Helium dilution or nitrogen washout methods can also be used but tend to underestimate the FRC in people with obstructive airway disease. However, plethysmography may overestimate FRC in obstructive lung disease [39]. Generally speaking, either method is acceptable and the agreement between the two methods is reasonably high [40], but plethysmography is

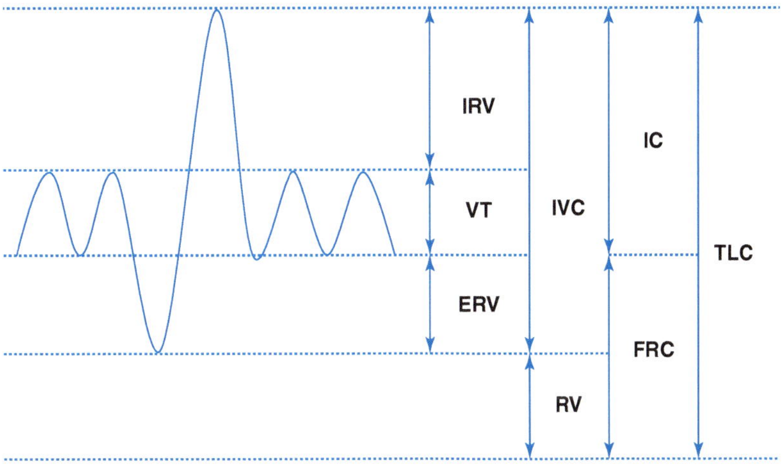


**Fig. 4.3** Lung volumes. *IRV* inspiratory reserve volume, *Vt* tidal volume, *ERV* expiratory reserve volume, *IVC* inspiratory vital capacity, *RV* residual volume, *IC* inspiratory capacity, *FRC* functional residual capacity, *TLC* total lung capacity

more commonly used in PFT labs. Gas dilution techniques may further be useful in the diagnosis of lung graft-versus-host disease [41, 42], but unlike plethysmography [43], it is not known whether pre-HSCT gas dilution measurements can predict post-HSCT risk.

During plethysmography, the patient sits upright in a hermetically sealed body box with their head in a neutral position (Fig. 4.4). A nose clip closes the nostrils and the patient breathes normally through a mouthpiece. At the end of normal tidal expiration, when a stable end-expiratory volume has been achieved, the shutter at the end of the mouthpiece is closed and the patient pants against the shutter at a rate of approximately one breath per second. After 2–3 s the shutter is opened and the patient breathes normally to obtain a baseline of the FRC. Once this is established, the patient inhales maximally to reach their total lung capacity and then exhales fully with a steady flow until no further air can be exhaled, reaching their residual volume. The test is repeated until three acceptable measurements are obtained. Measurement of lung volumes is achieved by the principles outlined in Boyle's law – $\text{Pressure}_1 \times \text{Volume}_1 = \text{Pressure}_2 \times \text{Volume}_2$—with the lung volumes being estimated based upon the change in pressure during the panting maneuver. A detailed list of assumptions and calculations involved with plethysmography is available elsewhere [44]. In general, a reduction in the VC, FRC, and RV is seen in restrictive lung disease, while in obstructive airway disease, there is an increase in the RV due to air trapping.

## Diffusing Capacity

The ability of the lungs to exchange gases between the atmosphere and the pulmonary capillaries is proportional to the lung volume available for gas exchange, the solubility of the gas, and the concentration of the gas on either side of the alveolar-capillary membrane while being inversely proportional to the thickness of the alveolar-capillary membrane. Other factors that influence gas exchange include the hemoglobin concentration and the blood transit time (i.e., cardiac output). Carbon monoxide (CO) is used to measure gas exchange because it is safe at low concentrations and has similar solubility as oxygen, but because of its high affinity for hemoglobin, the rate of uptake of CO is almost completely limited by diffusing capacity and not by other factors, such as lung perfusion. Furthermore, the affinity of CO to hemoglobin is not affected by the numerous factors that affect oxygen-hemoglobin binding, including temperature, PH, the partial pressure of carbon dioxide, and other considerations. The resulting measurement, the diffusing lung capacity for carbon monoxide (DLCO), gives a global estimate of the ability of the lung to exchange gases.

With the advent of rapid gas analyzers, DLCO is generally measured with a single 10-s breath-hold. If possible, the maneuver should be performed with a patient breathing room air; supplemental oxygen should be withheld for at least 10 min if feasible. Cigarette smoking should be noted, since this can reduce DLCO acutely, but this reduction typically resolves after several hours. Patients should be instructed not to smoke cigarettes on the day of DLCO testing. The patient is asked to breathe normally through a mouthpiece with the nose clipped. They then are asked to exhale maximally to RV, and at this point, they inhale a gas mixture consisting of 0.3% CO, 21% $O_2$, and tracer gas (typically 10% helium or 0.3% methane) and the remainder consisting of nitrogen. This inspired volume should be within 90% of known vital capacity measurements. Patients then inhale maximally to reach their TLC and, after a 10-s breath-hold, exhale maximally again. During exhalation, the total dead-space volume (equipment and anatomic) is discarded, and the rest of the exhaled air is collected for gas analysis [45]. A minimum VC of 1.5 L is usually necessary to calculate DLCO accurately, in part due to this need to discard dead-space gas. Correcting DLCO values for hemoglobin is particularly important in patients undergoing HSCT because hemoglobin levels can vary significantly from PFT to PFT. The DLCO is then corrected for alveolar volume (KCO) and for hemoglobin concentration (Fig. 4.5). More detailed information regarding the measurement of DLCO is available elsewhere [46].

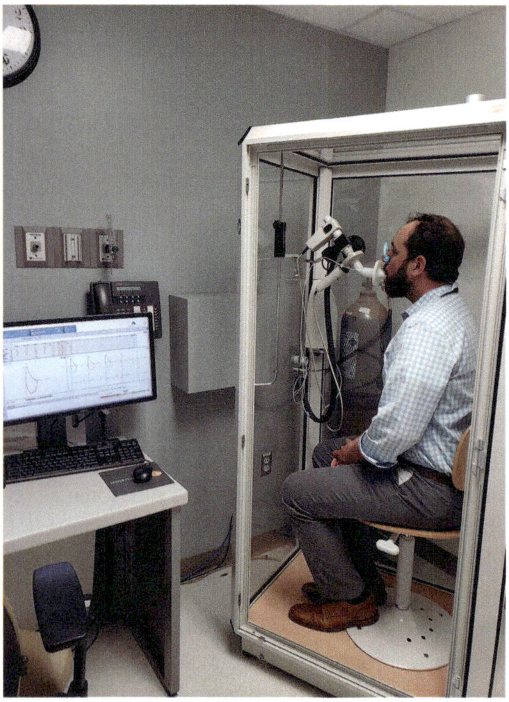

**Fig. 4.4** Plethysmography

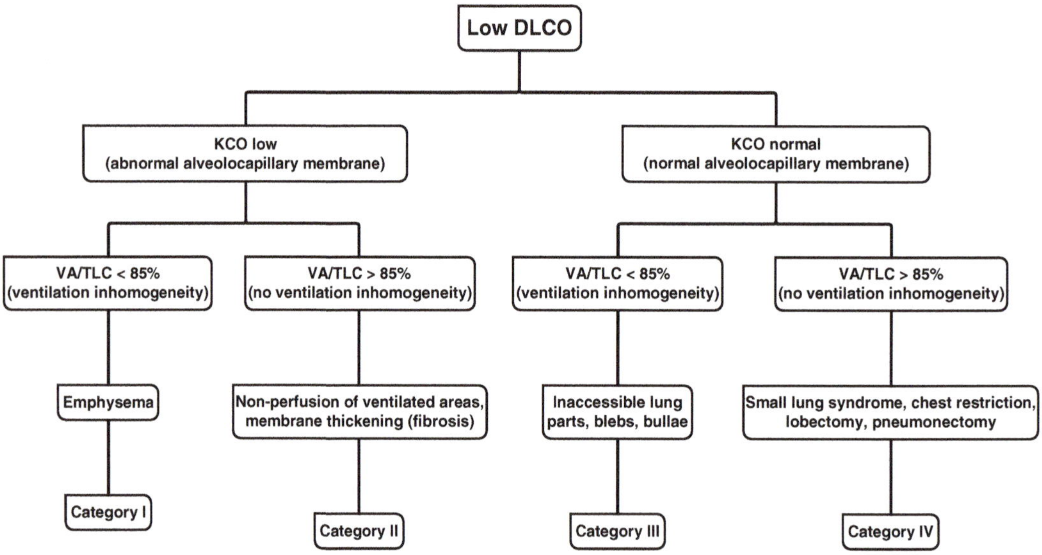


**Fig. 4.5** Low DLCO algorithm. *DLCO* diffusion capacity of carbon monoxide, *KCO* carbon monoxide transfer coefficient, *TLC* total lung capacity, *VA* alveolar volume. (Adapted from: van der Lee I, Zanen P, van den Bosch JMM, Lammers J-WJ. Pattern of diffusion disturbance related to clinical diagnosis: The KCO has no diagnostic value next to the DLCO. Respiratory Medicine. 2006;100(1):101–109)

## Role of PFTs in the Pre-HSCT Pulmonary Evaluation

In the following section, we discuss some of the ways in which pre-HSCT PFTs can help inform the transplant team about the risk for complications following HSCT.

### Consideration of Type of Conditioning

Pre-HSCT pulmonary impairment imparts an increased risk for pulmonary complications and mortality after transplantation, especially with myeloablative conditioning, which is often used to lower relapse rates but is well known to increase the risk for pulmonary toxicity [47–49]. Identifying pre-HSCT pulmonary impairment may lead the transplant team to favor nonmyeloablative HSCT to mitigate the pulmonary risk. In a study of over 600 patients—with predominantly hematological malignancies—who underwent HSCT, the group of patients that received nonmyeloablative regimens experienced a significantly lower post-HSCT decline in FEV1 compared to patients that received myeloablative regimens, despite overall lower baseline pre-HSCT FEV1 values in the nonmyeloablative group. One study demonstrated that, despite the higher prevalence of pre-HSCT PFT abnormalities in patients undergoing nonmyeloablative regimens, those patients experienced a lesser decline in FEV1 than patients who received myeloablative regimens [47]. Idiopathic pulmonary syndrome (IPS), which is a major early post-HSCT complication with an incidence of about 4%, has been shown in studies to be two to four times more common with myeloablative conditioning [50, 51]. In a single-center large cohort of allogeneic HSCT recipients, a multivariable model of factors associated with IPS showed that myeloablative conditioning and greater pre-HSCT pulmonary impairment both increased the risk for IPS. Therefore, patients with significant pre-HSCT pulmonary impairment may have better outcomes after HSCT with nonmyeloablative conditioning regimens.

### Prediction of Respiratory Failure and Mortality

Crawford et al. were among the first to investigate the predictive value of pre-HSCT PFTs on post-HSCT mortality. Their study included 1297 patients aged 4 to 63 years, who had undergone HSCT for malignant neoplasms between 1986 and 1990. Patients received myeloablative conditioning regimens and had pre-HSCT PFTs performed within 2 weeks of transplant. FEV1/FVC ratio, predicted TLC, DLCO, and the alveolar-arterial gradient were the parameters used to assess pre-HSCT obstruction, restriction, and impairment in gas exchange as predictors of 1-year mortality. Patients with normal pre-HSCT PFTs had a 51% chance of survival at 1 year, as compared to 25% for those with moderate to severe restriction (TLC <60%), 34% for those with alveolar-arterial gradients >30 mmHg, and 26% for those with diffusion limitations (DLCO <60%). There was no significant association between airflow obstruction (FEV1/FVC <80%) and survival. Based on this univariate analysis, the authors concluded that impairments in pre-HSCT TLC, DLCO, and alveolar-arterial gradient, but not FEV1/FVC, were predictive of post-HSCT mortality [52].

Since then, several groups have examined the impact of pre-HSCT PFTs on post-HSCT outcomes [53–55]. They concordantly found that pre-HSCT lung impairment was associated with worse outcomes, be it airflow obstruction, respiratory failure requiring mechanical ventilation, or non-relapse mortality. A large retrospective cohort study in 2005 more definitively assessed this association. In 2800 adult patients who underwent a first autologous or allogeneic HSCT between 1990 and 2002, lower values of FEV1, FVC, TLC, and DLCO were associated with higher rates of respiratory failure at 120 days and long-term mortality. Because of the significant correlation found between FEV1, FVC, and TLC values but not DLCO, a study looked at FEV1 and DLCO collectively to develop the lung function score (LFS) (Table 4.1). Higher LFS categories were associated with a progressively higher risk of early respiratory failure and mortality, and

**Table 4.1** Pre-HSCT LFS categories

| Pre-HSCT LFS category | Description | Pre-HSCT LFS |
|---|---|---|
| I | Normal | 2 |
| II | Mildly decreased | 3–4 |
| III | Moderately decreased | 5–6 |
| IV | Severely decreased | 7–8 |

*LFS* lung function score
The pretransplant LFS represents the sum of the FEV1 and DLCO score. A value >80% = 1, 70–80% = 2, 60–70% = 3, and <60% = 4

LFS predicted these key outcomes better than FEV1 or DLCO alone. As a result, LFS is commonly used to assess post-HSCT risk for respiratory failure and death [38].

In a later study, the LFS was incorporated into a more comprehensive risk assessment tool: the Pretransplant Assessment of Mortality (PAM) score [56]. PAM incorporates eight variables (age, donor type, disease risk, conditioning regimen, FEV1, DLCO, ALT, and serum creatinine), all previously recognized as independent risk factors for mortality related to transplantation. Patients were classified into four different categories based on a cumulative score calculated from the individual values of those eight variables. The authors found that patients in the higher PAM score categories were associated with progressively worse 2-year mortality [56]. A major weakness of the PAM score is that it fails to integrate patients' functional status and other lung function parameters. In addition, given the evolution of transplant practices, PAM was recently revised to include donor/recipient CMV status and exclude clinical variables such as creatinine and liver function [57]. Risk models such as LFS and PAM periodically need to be revalidated, ideally with a sufficiently large external cohort, and properly calibrated to reflect current HSCT practices.

## Prediction of Airflow Obstruction and Bronchiolitis Obliterans Syndrome

Clark and colleagues were among the first to study the link of pre-HSCT lung function with post-HSCT airflow obstruction in 1987 [58]. In this single-center study, they included 281 patients with hematological malignancies who underwent HSCT between 1977 and 1985. In their bivariate analysis, they found that low pre-HSCT FEV1/FVC was among the factors associated with increased risk of post-HSCT obstructive lung disease (defined as FVC/FEV1 ratio < 70%) along with increased age, male gender, cigarette smoking, cGVHD, and the use of methotrexate. In 2003 Chein et al. studied this association on a larger cohort of patients [54]. 1131 patients who received HSCT between 1990 and 2000 were included. PFTs were measured according to ATS guidelines, similar to the studies described earlier. Airflow obstruction was defined as an annual decline in FEV1 of 5% or greater with an FEV1/FVC ratio of less than 0.8. Using multivariate analysis, the authors found that the following variables were significantly associated with the development of airflow obstruction: low pre-HSCT FEV1/FVC ratio (RR 2.4), advanced age (RR 2.5 for age > 60), chronic progressive GVHD (RR 1.9), and respiratory viral infection (RR 1.4) [54]. This suggests that post-HSCT airflow obstruction, which is a different definition than the NIH consensus criteria for lung graft-versus-host disease (also known as bronchiolitis obliterans syndrome, or BOS) [59], is more common among patients with pre-HSCT airflow obstruction, but does not necessarily inform the transplant team on how to mitigate this risk. For example, it is not known whether optimal treatment of pre-HSCT lung diseases can reduce the risk for post-HSCT airflow obstruction.

Additionally, pre-HSCT PFTs provide a baseline reference to interpret and detect clinically significant declines in post-HSCT lung function that might not be apparent otherwise [47]. An example of this is the diagnosis of BOS stage 0p (BOS 0p). BOS 0p is a spirometric parameter defined as a decline in the percent predicted FEV1 of 10% to 19% or a decrease in the percent predicted FEF25-75 of >25% (irrespective of the final percent predicted values) on two consecutive PFTs and not meeting criteria for BOS [60]. BOS 0p has been proposed as a tool to identify patients at risk of progression to BOS, arguably the most important late NIPC following allogeneic HSCT

[60, 61]. In a retrospective study of 442 patients who underwent HSCT, patients who met criteria of BOS 0p were three times more likely to develop BOS, which, in turn, was associated with a two-fold increase in mortality [60]. Furthermore, without knowledge of baseline lung function, many cases of BOS 0p may be misinterpreted as normal spirometry, resulting in delayed intervention and potentially worse outcomes. Reductions in pre-HSCT mid-flow expiratory rates are also associated with an increased risk for BOS. In a single-center study of 2941 HSCT recipients, low pre-HSCT forced expiratory flow between 25% and 75% of maximum (FEF25-75), as well as day 80 decline in post-HSCT FEV1 and FEF25-75, was found to have the strongest association with increased risk of BOS [62]. In summary, these studies show that a thorough pre-HSCT pulmonary evaluation may aid in the ability to predict early airflow obstruction or BOS after HSCT.

## Prediction of Non-pulmonary Complications

In addition to the post-HSCT pulmonary complications, pre-HSCT lung impairment can be associated with non-pulmonary complications. Based on the previously reported findings by Crawford and colleagues that the association between pre-HSCT DLCO impairment and mortality cannot be explained by an increased risk of respiratory failure alone [52], a subsequent study has investigated the association between reduced pre-HSCT DLCO and severe veno-occlusive disease (VOD) of the liver as an alternative explanation for the increased risk of mortality in these patients. It was a single-center study that included over 300 patients who received chemotherapy +/− irradiation in preparation for HSCT between 1987 and 1988 who had PFTs performed within 2 weeks of transplantation. They found that a DLCO of <70% of predicted values increased the risk for severe VOD by over twofold. The authors concluded that reduced DLCO could serve as an independent predictor for severe VOD, with a possible shared mechanism of systemic endothelial cell injury due to high-dose chemotherapy or radiation [63].

## Role of Other Tests in the Pre-HSCT Risk Assessment

Extrapolated from the preoperative data, pre-HSCT evaluation is similarly centered around detecting and addressing reversible causes of respiratory impairment. In the following section, we discuss non-PFT modalities that may provide useful information to the transplant team.

## Arterial Blood Gas (ABG)

ABGs are infrequently performed as part of routine PFTs, particularly given the significant overlap with ambulatory monitoring of oxygen saturation and the routine measurement of DLCO. In a retrospective multivariate analysis of 2852 patients, progressive decrease in all lung function parameters, including an A-a gradient of >20 mmHg, was associated with increased risk of early respiratory failure and mortality post-HSCT [38]; however, DLCO better captures the extent of diffusing capacity and is not painful to patients. Nonetheless, the PA-aO2 gradient could play a role in cases where DLCO values are borderline [3]. Because ABGs cause patient discomfort and have minimal additional informational value compared to complete PFTs, we do not recommend routinely performing them.

## Chest Imaging

The primary role of chest radiography (both plain films and computed tomography scans) in the pre-HSCT workup is to exclude infection when an infection is suspected on a clinical basis. While radiology can predict outcomes in obstructive and interstitial lung diseases [64–66], no studies have shown any value of chest imaging prior to HSCT beyond the exclusion of infections. In symptomatic individuals where there is a suspicion of bronchiectasis secondary to previous immunosuppression and infection, CT is useful to confirm the diagnosis, allowing the clinician to optimize the clinical condition and reduce posttransplant episodes of infection. In the absence of clinical symptoms suggesting pulmonary infection, CT is not routinely recommended because incidental findings in asymptomatic pre-HSCT patients may have indirect negative consequences, including additional costs or delay of HSCT [67]. On the other hand, CT may incidentally identify bronchiectasis, which may develop in malignancies like non-Hodgkin's lymphoma or chronic lymphocytic leukemia, but may be under-recognized and therefore not optimally treated [68]. While we do not recommend routine pre-HSCT chest imaging at this time, this recommendation may change if prospective studies show that routine CT screening decreases infectious complications or can identify radiomic markers that indicate a greater risk for post-HSCT complications. For example, 129-XeMRI is an emerging imaging modality that can capture true functional information about lung physiology, but the value of pre-HSCT XeMRI is unknown [69]. Parametric response mapping, a method that maps paired voxels on inspiratory and expiratory scans and can determine the volume of lung that is affected by small airway disease, is another modality that may add to lung function measurements when performed before HSCT, but prospective trial data is lacking [70, 71]. At this time, we do not recommend routine chest imaging in all pre-HSCT recipients, but chest imaging should be performed when there is a concern for active infection prior to HSCT.

## Assessment of Cardiopulmonary Fitness

NRM rates are exceptionally high in HSCT recipients with advanced age and those with low cardiopulmonary fitness [72, 73], the latter which can be measured via 6-min walk distance (6MWD) or cardiopulmonary exercise testing (CPET).

The 6-min walk test is a low-cost test that provides valuable information on respiratory function. A standard protocol is used where the patient rests in a chair for at least 10 min and then walks back and forth along a 30-to-60 m corridor while oxygen and heart rate are continuously assessed and total distance walked measured [74, 75]. A healthy person can walk at least 400 m in 6 min. A walking distance of less than 350 m during this time is associated with reduced survival in people with chronic lung disease [76], but a similar cutoff has not been validated for HSCT recipients.

CPET allows for the integrative assessment of the functional capacity of the heart, lungs, and skeletal muscles during submaximal and peak exercise. Protocols may differ from center to center, as well as the device used to measure fitness (e.g., stationary bicycle ergometers or treadmill). CPET allows for the analysis of heart rate, heart rhythm, blood pressure, airflow (flow-volume loops), gas ventilation ($CO_2$ and $O_2$), gas exchange, and blood lactate. The peak oxygen uptake ($VO_2$) is a measure of exercise capacity; low peak $VO_2$ during exercise suggests a problem with oxygen delivery or utilization. CPET is often used in the assessment of unexplained breathlessness when PFTs are normal but also in preoperative assessments for cardiac and noncardiac surgery, where an anaerobic threshold of less than 11 ml/min/Kg and peak $VO_2$ of less than 10 ml/min/Kg are associated with poor outcomes [77]. CPET has not been prospectively studied as a tool to assess cardiopulmonary fitness prior to HSCT.

While there is an abundance of solid evidence supporting exercise programs to improve the quality of life in patients post-HSCT [78–81], the prognostic value of improved cardiopulmonary fitness before HSCT ("pre-hab") has not been well studied in the HSCT population. In a small study on 32 patients before undergoing HSCT, functional capacity and cardiopulmonary fitness assessed through cycle ergometry and 6-min walk distance (6MWD) were linked to survival post-HSCT [72]. The 6 MW findings were replicated afterward by Jones and colleagues in a larger cohort of 407 patients [82], in which poor function capacity (6MWD <400 m) was associated with NRM, but there was no additional prognostic value to the 6MWD beyond markers such as pulmonary function testing, age, or conditioning, which makes the utility of routine pre-HSCT 6 MW testing unclear. Whether improving cardiopulmonary fitness prior to transplant improves survival remains unclear and is an area of active research.

## Risk Mitigation

After identifying patients at high risk of post-HSCT pulmonary complications, a key goal should be to maximally treat underlying lung disease within a reasonable time frame so that patients do not miss the window of transplantation. The following section offers a short overview on this subject, but is not exhaustive.

### Restrictive Impairment

Recent studies have shifted focus toward looking at the effect of pre-HSCT restriction, as evidenced by reduced percent predicted TLC, on post-HSCT outcomes [43, 83]. Although this association was reported in earlier studies [38, 84, 85], the work by Ramirez-Sarmiento and colleagues has shed more light on the strength of this association [43]. They found that a pre-HSCT TLC of less than 80% predicted was associated with a twofold increased risk of respiratory failure and non-relapse mortality (NRM) [43]. Additionally, they found that low TLC predicted values correlated with lower BMI and that most patients with restriction had normal chest radiographic findings [43]. This indicates that deconditioning and respiratory muscle weakness could be driving many cases of restrictive impairment, which suggests that these patients could potentially benefit from pre-habilitation to improve fitness prior to HSCT. However, the incidence of interstitial lung diseases prior to HSCT is low, except in certain unique circumstances (e.g., GATA2 mutations) [86]. It is not known whether anti-fibrotic therapies have similar utility in post-HSCT patients or whether they increase the rate of side effects or drug interactions with necessary post-HSCT immunosuppressive agents, making them intolerable. Overall, restrictive impairment should be managed according to the underlying etiology of restriction, but the optimal timing of treatment for newly diagnosed interstitial lung diseases remains unknown.

### Obstructive Lung Disease

Early studies failed to find an association between pre-HSCT airway obstruction, defined by a low FEV1/FVC ratio, and post-HSCT complications [38, 52, 84]. While it may be true that FEV1/FVC ratio is insensitive for the prediction of post-HSCT complications, other possible explanations include selection bias, in which patients with significant lung disease were not selected to undergo HSCT, or the inconsistent use of the lower limit of normal to define airflow obstruction, which is important in younger patients in whom a fixed FEV1/FVC cutoff of 0.7 would underdiagnose airflow obstruction, since normal FEV1/FVC ratios are higher in younger patients [3, 24]. For example, defining airflow obstruction using the LLN of the FEV1/FVC ratio instead of a fixed cutoff of 0.7 identified over twice the number of patients with airflow obstruction in a study of over 6000 people between 22 and 40 years of age [24]. This finding raises the question of whether the LLN should replace the fixed ratio cutoffs for pre-HSCT evaluation, especially since transplant recipients tend to be young on average [87]. However, using LLN as the marker for airflow obstruction may lead to missed cases of airflow obstruction in older patients. In fact, in a cohort of patients with COPD, the use of LLN was inferior to the use of a fixed ratio of 0.7 in terms of association with emphysema, gas trapping, and exacerbation rate [27]. Further work is necessary to determine which method is superior in HSCT recipients.

A recent study of 206 patients looked at the effects of different pre-HSCT PFT parameters including the ratio of the airflow rate at 50% of vital capacity to the airflow rate at 25% of vital capacity (V50/V25) as a marker of small airway disease. They found V50/V25 to be the most powerful predictor of survival post-HSCT, surpassing FEV1 and FVC, which mainly reflect central airway disease [83]. This provocative study suggests that pre-HSCT small airway disease is a strong predictor of post-HSCT mortality but also raises the question of how best to measure small airway disease. For example, high-quality studies of pre-HSCT impedance oscillometry (IOS) and 129-XeMRI are lacking [88]. While IOS is arguably easier to perform than forced spirometry, particularly for children, both IOS and XeMRI are more challenging to interpret than conventional PFTs. Future studies investigating the role of pre-HSCT small airway disease on post-HSCT outcomes are needed.

Putting aside the controversy regarding how best to measure and define obstruction, obstructive lung diseases, when clinically evident, should be treated to minimize their attendant symptoms. Our approach to obstructive airway disease centers around counseling on smoking cessation (discussed separately), ensuring the prescription of long-acting bronchodilators and inhaled corticosteroids as appropriate. It is essential when prescribing inhalers that correct inhaler technique is taught and observed on follow-up. A meta-analysis of 144 studies including 54,354 participants showed that only 31% of patients demonstrated correct inhaler technique, with the most common error in metered-dose inhalers (MDI) being incoordination [89]. This problem can be easily fixed with bedside education and spacer devices, which have been shown to significantly improve the delivery of inhaled particles significantly [90]. Furthermore, an array of new non-inhaler medications are available to treat obstructive lung diseases but are beyond the scope of this chapter.

## Smoking Cessation

The contribution of tobacco use to post-HSCT outcomes has long been a controversial topic [8, 53, 91]. The strong association between smoking and lung impairment has further confounded that data, since smoking is a causal factor for the development of obstructive lung diseases. However, more recent studies have shown smoking to be an independent predictor of long-term complications and death. In a retrospective single-center study of 286 patients with hematological disorders who underwent HSCT, smoking was associated with an increased incidence of post-HSCT pneumonia in a dose-dependent manner, with a cumulative incidence of 17% in the never smokers' group, 25% in the low-dose smokers' group, and 33% in the high-dose smokers' group, irrespective of baseline PFTs [92]. These findings were later supported by a study of 309 patients who underwent HSCT. Smoking was found to be independently associated with 5-year mortality compared to nonsmoking (45% vs. 26%, respectively) [93]. Smoking may worsen outcomes due to increased susceptibility to pulmonary infections secondary to the impaired mucociliary clearance, reduced phagocytosis, and lower secretion of cytokines by alveolar macrophages observed in smokers [92, 94], in addition to the numerous known consequences beyond the lungs. Smoking status must be assessed in all patients undergoing transplant evaluation. Patients should be offered necessary counseling, nicotine replacement therapies, and/or approved medications to aid with smoking cessation. Whether smoking cessation improves post-HSCT outcomes is unknown, but this intervention must be offered nonetheless due to the well-documented benefits outside of the lens of HSCT.

## Reducing the Risk of Respiratory Infection

Respiratory infection is a common pulmonary complication post-HSCT. The incidence has reduced over the years due to the implementation of antimicrobial protocols for at-risk individuals [95]. However, despite the success seen, it is still an important area resulting in morbidity, increased hospitalization, use of resources, and mortality. Individuals with hematological malignancy requiring HSCT may have immunodeficiency due to the underlying malignancy or due to treatments for their cancer resulting in secondary antibody deficiency or T-cell dysfunction [96]. The hematological malignancy may result in functional hypogammaglobulinemia and T-cell dysfunction due to alteration of immune checkpoint inhibitors, while those with chronic lymphocytic leukemia may have inadequate immunoglobulin production and inhibition of T-cell function. Furthermore, treatment with medication such as rituximab results in prolonged antibody deficiency. This predisposes patients to recurrent sinopulmonary infections that need to be treated prior to HSCT. As conditioning regimens and HSCT will further reduce immunity, a high index of pre-HSCT immunodeficiency is needed as the use of prophylactic antibiotics and intravenous immunoglobulin replacement can be useful to optimize these individuals' pretransplantation [97]. IVIG is often used in those who have a history of frequent infections, where antimicrobial prophylaxis is unsuccessful and total IgG is less than 4 g/L [96]. It is often continued until immune reconstitution is confirmed and the person has been infection-free for at least 6 months. In some instances, total IgG may be normal, but patients with hematological malignancy and a history of recurrent sinopulmonary infections may have polysaccharide antibody deficiency that may also benefit from IVIG. Immunoglobulin deficiency is a risk factor for the development of bronchiectasis in hematological malignancy [68], and these patients will need optimization of their treatment and ensure effective and regular airway clearance to mitigate their infection risk [98].

## Conclusions

In summary, PFT is an invaluable tool in the pre-HSCT pulmonary evaluation and should be performed routinely on all transplant candidates. Pulmonologists should endeavor to treat clinically evident lung diseases prior to HSCT and optimize the condition as much as possible within a reasonable time frame to not delay transplantation. Further work is needed to improve our ability to maximize our ability to provide useful information pre-HSCT, namely, (1) standardization of PFT interpretation in diverse pre-HSCT populations, particularly with regard to the definitions for obstructive and restrictive lung disease; (2) assessments of muscular strength and cardiopulmonary fitness that may provide valuable information beyond PFT, particularly in patients with pre-HSCT restrictive lung disease without interstitial lung disease; (3) prospective studies examining the role of pre-HSCT imaging; and (4) interventional studies that examine ways to mitigate the known risks associated with pulmonary impairment.

## References

1. Gratwohl A, Baldomero H, Aljurf M, et al. Hematopoietic stem cell transplantation: a global perspective. JAMA. 2010;303(16):1617–24. https://doi.org/10.1001/jama.2010.491.
2. Goldman JM, Horowitz MM. The international bone marrow transplant registry. Int J Hematol. 2002;76(Suppl 1):393–7. https://doi.org/10.1007/BF03165291.
3. Cheng G-S. Pulmonary function and pretransplant evaluation of the hematopoietic cell transplant candidate. Clin Chest Med. 2017;38(2):307–16. https://doi.org/10.1016/j.ccm.2016.12.014.
4. Soubani AO, Miller KB, Hassoun PM. Pulmonary complications of bone marrow transplantation. Chest. 1996;109(4):1066–77. https://doi.org/10.1378/chest.109.4.1066.
5. Haider S, Durairajan N, Soubani AO. Noninfectious pulmonary complications of haematopoietic stem cell transplantation. Eur Respir Rev. 2020;29(156):190119. https://doi.org/10.1183/16000617.0119-2019.
6. Henig I, Zuckerman T. Hematopoietic stem cell transplantation-50 years of evolution and future perspectives. Rambam Maimonides Med J. 2014;5(4):e0028. https://doi.org/10.5041/RMMJ.10162.
7. Dykewicz CA. Guidelines for preventing opportunistic infections among hematopoietic stem cell transplant recipients: focus on community respiratory virus infections. Biol Blood Marrow Transplant. 2001;7(Suppl):19S–22S. https://doi.org/10.1053/bbmt.2001.v7.pm11777100.
8. Savani BN, Montero A, Wu C, et al. Prediction and prevention of transplant-related mortality from pulmonary causes after total body irradiation and allogeneic stem cell transplantation. Biol Blood Marrow Transplant. 2005;11(3):223–30. https://doi.org/10.1016/j.bbmt.2004.12.328.
9. Hutchinson J. On the capacity of the lungs, and on the respiratory functions, with a view of establishing a precise and easy method of detecting disease by the spirometer. Med Chir Trans. 1846;29:137–252. https://doi.org/10.1177/095952874602900113.
10. Friedman GD, Klatsky AL, Siegelaub AB. Lung function and risk of myocardial infarction and sudden cardiac death. N Engl J Med. 1976;294(20):1071–5. https://doi.org/10.1056/NEJM197605132942001.
11. Kannel WB, Hubert H, Lew EA. Vital capacity as a predictor of cardiovascular disease: the Framingham study. Am Heart J. 1983;105(2):311–5. https://doi.org/10.1016/0002-8703(83)90532-x.

12. Ashley F, Kannel WB, Sorlie PD, Masson R. Pulmonary function: relation to aging, cigarette habit, and mortality. Ann Intern Med. 1975;82(6):739–45. https://doi.org/10.7326/0003-4819-82-6-739.
13. Lange P, Nyboe J, Appleyard M, Jensen G, Schnohr P. Spirometric findings and mortality in never-smokers. J Clin Epidemiol. 1990;43(9):867–73. https://doi.org/10.1016/0895-4356(90)90070-6.
14. Lee HM, Le H, Lee BT, Lopez VA, Wong ND. Forced vital capacity paired with Framingham risk score for prediction of all-cause mortality. Eur Respir J. 2010;36(5):1002–6. https://doi.org/10.1183/09031936.00042410.
15. Evans SE, Scanlon PD. Current practice in pulmonary function testing. Mayo Clin Proc. 2003;78(6):758–63; quiz 763. https://doi.org/10.4065/78.6.758.
16. Burney PGJ, Hooper RL. The use of ethnically specific norms for ventilatory function in African-American and white populations. Int J Epidemiol. 2012;41(3):782–90. https://doi.org/10.1093/ije/dys011.
17. Wan ES, Balte P, Schwartz JE, et al. Association between preserved ratio impaired spirometry and clinical outcomes in US adults. JAMA. 2021;326(22):2287–98. https://doi.org/10.1001/jama.2021.20939.
18. Cooper BG. An update on contraindications for lung function testing. Thorax. 2011;66(8):714–23. https://doi.org/10.1136/thx.2010.139881.
19. Graham BL, Steenbruggen I, Miller MR, et al. Standardization of spirometry 2019 update. An official American Thoracic Society and European Respiratory Society technical statement. Am J Respir Crit Care Med. 2019;200(8):e70–88. https://doi.org/10.1164/rccm.201908-1590ST.
20. Quanjer PH, Stanojevic S, Cole TJ, et al. Multi-ethnic reference values for spirometry for the 3-95-yr age range: the global lung function 2012 equations. Eur Respir J. 2012;40(6):1324–43. https://doi.org/10.1183/09031936.00080312.
21. Swanney MP, Ruppel G, Enright PL, et al. Using the lower limit of normal for the FEV1/FVC ratio reduces the misclassification of airway obstruction. Thorax. 2008;63(12):1046–51. https://doi.org/10.1136/thx.2008.098483.
22. Culver BH. How should the lower limit of the normal range be defined? Respir Care. 2012;57(1):135–6. https://doi.org/10.4187/respcare.01427.
23. Hansen JE, Sun X-G, Wasserman K. Spirometric criteria for airway obstruction: use percentage of FEV1/FVC ratio below the fifth percentile, not < 70%. Chest. 2007;131(2):349–55. https://doi.org/10.1378/chest.06-1349.
24. Cerveri I, Corsico AG, Accordini S, et al. Underestimation of airflow obstruction among young adults using FEV1/FVC <70% as a fixed cut-off: a longitudinal evaluation of clinical and functional outcomes. Thorax. 2008;63(12):1040–5. https://doi.org/10.1136/thx.2008.095554.
25. Stanojevic S, Kaminsky DA, Miller M, et al. ERS/ATS technical standard on interpretive strategies for routine lung function tests. Eur Respir J. 2021;60(1):2101499. https://doi.org/10.1183/13993003.01499-2021.
26. Mannino DM, Sonia Buist A, Vollmer WM. Chronic obstructive pulmonary disease in the older adult: what defines abnormal lung function? Thorax. 2007;62(3):237–41. https://doi.org/10.1136/thx.2006.068379.
27. Bhatt SP, Sieren JC, Dransfield MT, et al. Comparison of spirometric thresholds in diagnosing smoking-related airflow obstruction. Thorax. 2014;69(5):409–14. https://doi.org/10.1136/thoraxjnl-2012-202810.
28. Braun L. Race correction and spirometry: why history matters. Chest. 2021;159(4):1670–5. https://doi.org/10.1016/j.chest.2020.10.046.
29. Baugh AD, Shiboski S, Hansel NN, et al. Reconsidering the utility of race-specific lung function prediction equations. Am J Respir Crit Care Med. 2021;205:819. https://doi.org/10.1164/rccm.202105-1246OC.
30. Bhakta NR, Kaminsky DA, Bime C, et al. Addressing race in pulmonary function testing by aligning intent and evidence with practice and perception. Chest. 2022;161(1):288–97. https://doi.org/10.1016/j.chest.2021.08.053.
31. Hegewald MJ, Crapo RO. Socioeconomic status and lung function. Chest. 2007;132(5):1608–14. https://doi.org/10.1378/chest.07-1405.
32. Jones RL, Nzekwu M-MU. The effects of body mass index on lung volumes. Chest. 2006;130(3):827–33. https://doi.org/10.1378/chest.130.3.827.
33. Tennant PWG, Gibson GJ, Parker L, Pearce MS. Childhood respiratory illness and lung function at ages 14 and 50 years: childhood respiratory illness and lung function. Chest. 2010;137(1):146–55. https://doi.org/10.1378/chest.09-0352.
34. Rocha V, Fraga S, Moreira C, et al. Life-course socioeconomic disadvantage and lung function: a multicohort study of 70496 individuals. Eur Respir J. 2021;57(3):2001600. https://doi.org/10.1183/13993003.01600-2020.
35. Moffett AT, Eneanya ND, Halpern SD, Weissman GE. The impact of race correction on the interpretation of pulmonary function testing among black patients. In: A7. A007 impact of race, ethnicity, and social determinants on individuals with lung diseases. American Thoracic Society International conference abstracts. New York: American Thoracic Society; 2021. p. A1030. https://doi.org/10.1164/ajrccm--conference.2021.203.1_MeetingAbstracts.A1030.
36. Pellegrino R, Viegi G, Brusasco V, et al. Interpretative strategies for lung function tests. Eur Respir J. 2005;26(5):948–68. https://doi.org/10.1183/09031936.05.00035205.
37. Wanger J, Clausen JL, Coates A, et al. Standardisation of the measurement of lung volumes. Eur Respir J. 2005;26(3):511–22. https://doi.org/10.1183/09031936.05.00035005.
38. Parimon T, Madtes DK, Au DH, Clark JG, Chien JW. Pretransplant lung function, respiratory failure, and mortality after stem cell transplantation. Am J

Respir Crit Care Med. 2005;172(3):384–90. https://doi.org/10.1164/rccm.200502-212OC.
39. Sue DY. Measurement of lung volumes in patients with obstructive lung disease. A matter of time (constants). Ann Am Thorac Soc. 2013;10(5):525–30. https://doi.org/10.1513/AnnalsATS.201307-236OC.
40. Cliff IJ, Evans AH, Pantin CF, Baldwin DR. Comparison of two new methods for the measurement of lung volumes with two standard methods. Thorax. 1999;54(4):329–33. https://doi.org/10.1136/thx.54.4.329.
41. Rayment JH, Sandoval RA, Roden JP, Schultz KR. Multiple breath washout testing to identify pulmonary chronic graft versus host disease in children after hematopoietic stem cell transplantation. Transpl Cell Ther. 2022;28(6):328.e1–7. https://doi.org/10.1016/j.jtct.2022.02.002.
42. Nyilas S, Baumeler L, Tamm M, et al. Inert gas washout in bronchiolitis obliterans following hematopoietic cell transplantation. Chest. 2018;154(1):157–68. https://doi.org/10.1016/j.chest.2017.12.009.
43. Ramirez-Sarmiento A, Orozco-Levi M, Walter EC, Au MA, Chien JW. Influence of pretransplantation restrictive lung disease on allogeneic hematopoietic cell transplantation outcomes. Biol Blood Marrow Transplant. 2010;16(2):199–206. https://doi.org/10.1016/j.bbmt.2009.09.016.
44. Coates AL, Peslin R, Rodenstein D, Stocks J. Measurement of lung volumes by plethysmography. Eur Respir J. 1997;10(6):1415–27. https://doi.org/10.1183/09031936.97.10061415.
45. Fowler WS. Lung function studies; the respiratory dead space. Am J Physiol. 1948;154(3):405–16. https://doi.org/10.1152/ajplegacy.1948.154.3.405.
46. Graham BL, Brusasco V, Burgos F, et al. ERS/ATS standards for single-breath carbon monoxide uptake in the lung. Eur Respir J. 2017;49(1):1600016. https://doi.org/10.1183/13993003.00016-2016.
47. Chien JW, Maris MB, Sandmaier BM, Maloney DG, Storb RF, Clark JG. Comparison of lung function after myeloablative and 2 Gy of total body irradiation-based regimens for hematopoietic stem cell transplantation. Biol Blood Marrow Transplant. 2005;11(4):288–96. https://doi.org/10.1016/j.bbmt.2005.01.003.
48. Deeg HJ, Sandmaier BM. Who is fit for allogeneic transplantation? Blood. 2010;116(23):4762–70. https://doi.org/10.1182/blood-2010-07-259358.
49. Gyurkocza B, Sandmaier BM. Conditioning regimens for hematopoietic cell transplantation: one size does not fit all. Blood. 2014;124(3):344–53. https://doi.org/10.1182/blood-2014-02-514778.
50. Wenger DS, Triplette M, Crothers K, et al. Incidence, risk factors, and outcomes of idiopathic pneumonia syndrome after allogeneic hematopoietic cell transplantation. Biol Blood Marrow Transplant. 2020;26(2):413–20. https://doi.org/10.1016/j.bbmt.2019.09.034.
51. Fukuda T, Hackman RC, Guthrie KA, et al. Risks and outcomes of idiopathic pneumonia syndrome after nonmyeloablative and conventional conditioning regimens for allogeneic hematopoietic stem cell transplantation. Blood. 2003;102(8):2777–85. https://doi.org/10.1182/blood-2003-05-1597.
52. Crawford SW, Fisher L. Predictive value of pulmonary function tests before marrow transplantation. Chest. 1992;101(5):1257–64. https://doi.org/10.1378/chest.101.5.1257.
53. Ho VT, Weller E, Lee SJ, Alyea EP, Antin JH, Soiffer RJ. Prognostic factors for early severe pulmonary complications after hematopoietic stem cell transplantation. Biol Blood Marrow Transplant. 2001;7(4):223–9. https://doi.org/10.1053/bbmt.2001.v7.pm11349809.
54. Chien JW, Martin PJ, Gooley TA, et al. Airflow obstruction after myeloablative allogeneic hematopoietic stem cell transplantation. Am J Respir Crit Care Med. 2003;168(2):208–14. https://doi.org/10.1164/rccm.200212-1468OC.
55. Goldberg SL, Klumpp TR, Magdalinski AJ, Mangan KF. Value of the pretransplant evaluation in predicting toxic day-100 mortality among blood stem-cell and bone marrow transplant recipients. J Clin Oncol Off J Am Soc Clin Oncol. 1998;16(12):3796–802. https://doi.org/10.1200/JCO.1998.16.12.3796.
56. Parimon T, Au DH, Martin PJ, Chien JW. A risk score for mortality after allogeneic hematopoietic cell transplantation. Ann Intern Med. 2006;144(6):407–14. https://doi.org/10.7326/0003-4819-144-6-200603210-00007.
57. Au BKC, Gooley TA, Armand P, et al. Reevaluation of the pretransplant assessment of mortality score after allogeneic hematopoietic transplantation. Biol Blood Marrow Transplant. 2015;21(5):848–54. https://doi.org/10.1016/j.bbmt.2015.01.011.
58. Clark JG, Schwartz DA, Flournoy N, Sullivan KM, Crawford SW, Thomas ED. Risk factors for airflow obstruction in recipients of bone marrow transplants. Ann Intern Med. 1987;107(5):648–56. https://doi.org/10.7326/0003-4819-107-5-648.
59. Jagasia MH, Greinix HT, Arora M, et al. National Institutes of Health consensus development project on criteria for clinical trials in chronic graft-versus-host disease: I. the 2014 diagnosis and staging working group report. Biol Blood Marrow Transplant. 2015;21(3):389–401.e1. https://doi.org/10.1016/j.bbmt.2014.12.001.
60. Abedin S, Yanik GA, Braun T, et al. Predictive value of bronchiolitis obliterans syndrome stage 0p in chronic graft-versus-host disease of the lung. Biol Blood Marrow Transplant. 2015;21(6):1127–31. https://doi.org/10.1016/j.bbmt.2015.02.006.
61. Finlen Copeland CA, Snyder LD, Zaas DW, Turbyfill WJ, Davis WA, Palmer SM. Survival after bronchiolitis obliterans syndrome among bilateral lung transplant recipients. Am J Respir Crit Care Med. 2010;182(6):784–9. https://doi.org/10.1164/rccm.201002-0211OC.
62. Jamani K, He Q, Liu Y, et al. Early post-transplantation spirometry is associated with the development of bronchiolitis obliterans syndrome after alloge-

neic hematopoietic cell transplantation. Biol Blood Marrow Transplant. 2020;26(5):943–8. https://doi.org/10.1016/j.bbmt.2019.12.002.
63. Matute-Bello G, McDonald GD, Hinds MS, Schoch HG, Crawford SW. Association of pulmonary function testing abnormalities and severe veno-occlusive disease of the liver after marrow transplantation. Bone Marrow Transplant. 1998;21(11):1125–30. https://doi.org/10.1038/sj.bmt.1701225.
64. Krings JG, Goss CW, Lew D, et al. Quantitative CT metrics are associated with longitudinal lung function decline and future asthma exacerbations: results from SARP-3. J Allergy Clin Immunol. 2021;148(3):752–62. https://doi.org/10.1016/j.jaci.2021.01.029.
65. Witt CA, Sheshadri A, Carlstrom L, et al. Longitudinal changes in airway remodeling and air trapping in severe asthma. Acad Radiol. 2014;21(8):986–93. https://doi.org/10.1016/j.acra.2014.05.001.
66. Jacob J, Bartholmai BJ, Rajagopalan S, et al. Predicting outcomes in idiopathic pulmonary fibrosis using automated computed tomographic analysis. Am J Respir Crit Care Med. 2018;198(6):767–76. https://doi.org/10.1164/rccm.201711-2174OC.
67. El Boghdadly Z, Oran B, Jiang Y, Rondon G, Champlin R, Kontoyiannis DP. Pretransplant chest computed tomography screening in asymptomatic patients with leukemia and myelodysplastic syndrome. Bone Marrow Transplant. 2017;52(3):476–9. https://doi.org/10.1038/bmt.2016.309.
68. José RJ, Hall J, Brown JS. De novo bronchiectasis in haematological malignancies: patient characteristics, risk factors and survival. ERJ Open Res. 2019;5(4):00166. https://doi.org/10.1183/23120541.00166-2019.
69. Walkup LL, Myers K, El-Bietar J, et al. Xenon-129 MRI detects ventilation deficits in paediatric stem cell transplant patients unable to perform spirometry. Eur Respir J. 2019;53(5):1801779. https://doi.org/10.1183/13993003.01779-2018.
70. Cheng G-S, Selwa KE, Hatt C, et al. Multicenter evaluation of parametric response mapping as an indicator of bronchiolitis obliterans syndrome after hematopoietic stem cell transplantation. Am J Transplant. 2020;20(8):2198–205. https://doi.org/10.1111/ajt.15814.
71. Galbán CJ, Boes JL, Bule M, et al. Parametric response mapping as an indicator of bronchiolitis obliterans syndrome after hematopoietic stem cell transplantation. Biol Blood Marrow Transplant. 2014;20(10):1592–8. https://doi.org/10.1016/j.bbmt.2014.06.014.
72. Wood WA, Deal AM, Reeve BB, et al. Cardiopulmonary fitness in patients undergoing hematopoietic SCT: a pilot study. Bone Marrow Transplant. 2013;48(10):1342–9. https://doi.org/10.1038/bmt.2013.58.
73. Kelsey CR, Scott JM, Lane A, et al. Cardiopulmonary exercise testing prior to myeloablative Allo-SCT: a feasibility study. Bone Marrow Transplant. 2014;49(10):1330–6. https://doi.org/10.1038/bmt.2014.159.
74. ATS Committee. ATS statement: guidelines for the six-minute walk test. Am J Respir Crit Care Med. 2002;166(1):111–7. https://doi.org/10.1164/ajrccm.166.1.at1102.
75. Holland AE, Spruit MA, Troosters T, et al. An official European Respiratory Society/American Thoracic Society technical standard: field walking tests in chronic respiratory disease. Eur Respir J. 2014;44(6):1428–46. https://doi.org/10.1183/09031936.00150314.
76. Sánchez-Martínez MP, Bernabeu-Mora R, Martínez-González M, Gacto-Sánchez M, Martín San Agustín R, Medina-Mirapeix F. Stability and predictors of poor 6-min walking test performance over 2 years in patients with COPD. J Clin Med. 2020;9(4):1155. https://doi.org/10.3390/jcm9041155.
77. Older PO, Levett DZH. Cardiopulmonary exercise testing and surgery. Ann Am Thorac Soc. 2017;14(Supplement_1):S74–83. https://doi.org/10.1513/AnnalsATS.201610-780FR.
78. Wilson RW, Jacobsen PB, Fields KK. Pilot study of a home-based aerobic exercise program for sedentary cancer survivors treated with hematopoietic stem cell transplantation. Bone Marrow Transplant. 2005;35(7):721–7. https://doi.org/10.1038/sj.bmt.1704815.
79. Jarden M, Baadsgaard MT, Hovgaard DJ, Boesen E, Adamsen L. A randomized trial on the effect of a multimodal intervention on physical capacity, functional performance and quality of life in adult patients undergoing allogeneic SCT. Bone Marrow Transplant. 2009;43(9):725–37. https://doi.org/10.1038/bmt.2009.27.
80. DeFor TE, Burns LJ, Gold E-MA, Weisdorf DJ. A randomized trial of the effect of a walking regimen on the functional status of 100 adult allogeneic donor hematopoietic cell transplant patients. Biol Blood Marrow Transplant. 2007;13(8):948–55. https://doi.org/10.1016/j.bbmt.2007.04.008.
81. Dimeo F, Fetscher S, Lange W, Mertelsmann R, Keul J. Effects of aerobic exercise on the physical performance and incidence of treatment-related complications after high-dose chemotherapy. Blood. 1997;90(9):3390–4.
82. Jones LW, Devlin SM, Maloy MA, et al. Prognostic importance of pretransplant functional capacity after allogeneic hematopoietic cell transplantation. Oncologist. 2015;20(11):1290–7. https://doi.org/10.1634/theoncologist.2015-0200.
83. Nakamae M, Yamashita M, Koh H, et al. Lung function score including a parameter of small airway disease as a highly predictive indicator of survival after allogeneic hematopoietic cell transplantation. Transpl Int. 2016;29(6):707–14. https://doi.org/10.1111/tri.12779.
84. Ghalie R, Szidon JP, Thompson L, Nawas YN, Dolce A, Kaizer H. Evaluation of pulmonary complications after bone marrow transplantation: the role of pretransplant pulmonary function tests. Bone Marrow Transplant. 1992;10(4):359–65.

85. Piñana JL, Martino R, Barba P, et al. Pulmonary function testing prior to reduced intensity conditioning allogeneic stem cell transplantation in an unselected patient cohort predicts posttransplantation pulmonary complications and outcome. Am J Hematol. 2012;87(1):9–14. https://doi.org/10.1002/ajh.22183.
86. Cuellar-Rodriguez J, Gea-Banacloche J, Freeman AF, et al. Successful allogeneic hematopoietic stem cell transplantation for GATA2 deficiency. Blood. 2011;118(13):3715–20. https://doi.org/10.1182/blood-2011-06-365049.
87. Popplewell LL, Forman SJ. Is there an upper age limit for bone marrow transplantation? Bone Marrow Transplant. 2002;29(4):277–84. https://doi.org/10.1038/sj.bmt.1703382.
88. Rutting S, Badal T, Wallis R, et al. Long-term variability of oscillatory impedance in stable obstructive airways disease. Eur Respir J. 2021;58(1):2004318. https://doi.org/10.1183/13993003.04318-2020.
89. Sanchis J, Gich I, Pedersen S. Systematic review of errors in inhaler use: has patient technique improved over time? Chest. 2016;150(2):394–406. https://doi.org/10.1016/j.chest.2016.03.041.
90. O'Callaghan C, Lynch J, Cant M, Robertson C. Improvement in sodium cromoglycate delivery from a spacer device by use of an antistatic lining, immediate inhalation, and avoiding multiple actuations of drug. Thorax. 1993;48(6):603–6. https://doi.org/10.1136/thx.48.6.603.
91. Tran BT, Halperin A, Chien JW. Cigarette smoking and outcomes after allogeneic hematopoietic stem cell transplantation. Biol Blood Marrow Transplant. 2011;17(7):1004–11. https://doi.org/10.1016/j.bbmt.2010.10.032.
92. Hanajiri R, Kakihana K, Kobayashi T, Doki N, Sakamaki H, Ohashi K. Tobacco smoking is associated with infectious pulmonary complications after allogeneic hematopoietic stem cell transplantation. Bone Marrow Transplant. 2015;50(8):1141–3. https://doi.org/10.1038/bmt.2015.116.
93. Scheidl S, Zinke-Cerwenka W, Flick H, et al. Whole-body lung function test-derived outcome predictors in allogenic stem cell transplantation. Biol Blood Marrow Transplant. 2019;25(1):129–36. https://doi.org/10.1016/j.bbmt.2018.07.036.
94. Feldman C, Anderson R. Cigarette smoking and mechanisms of susceptibility to infections of the respiratory tract and other organ systems. J Infect. 2013;67(3):169–84. https://doi.org/10.1016/j.jinf.2013.05.004.
95. Jose RJ, Dickey BF, Brown JS. Infectious respiratory disease in non-HIV immunocompromised patients. Br J Hosp Med (Lond). 2014;75(12):685–90. https://doi.org/10.12968/hmed.2014.75.12.685.
96. Allegra A, Tonacci A, Musolino C, Pioggia G, Gangemi S. Secondary immunodeficiency in hematological malignancies: focus on multiple myeloma and chronic lymphocytic leukemia. Front Immunol. 2021;12:738915. https://doi.org/10.3389/fimmu.2021.738915.
97. Foster JH, Cheng WS, Nguyen N-Y, Krance R, Martinez C. Immunoglobulin prophylaxis in pediatric hematopoietic stem cell transplant. Pediatr Blood Cancer. 2018;65(12):e27348. https://doi.org/10.1002/pbc.27348.
98. José RJ, Brown JS. Bronchiectasis. Br J Hosp Med (Lond). 2014;75(Suppl 10):C146–51. https://doi.org/10.12968/hmed.2014.75.Sup10.C146.

# 5 Diagnostic Evaluation of Pulmonary Disease Following Hematopoietic Stem Cell Transplantation

Philippe R. Bauer

## Diagnosis Evaluation: Overview

Pulmonary diseases are frequent complications following hematopoietic stem cell transplantation (HSCT) and represent a major cause of mortality and a hindrance to the overall success of HSCT [1, 2]. Up to 40% of HSCT recipients are admitted to the intensive care unit because of severe complications related to HSCT [3]. Pulmonary complications represent 30 to 60% of these complications [4]. In a 10-year retrospective review of autopsies, the major causes of death after allogeneic HSCT were pulmonary complications including diffuse alveolar damage, acute pneumonia, and invasive aspergillosis and after autologous HSCT relapse of malignancy, acute pneumonia, and diffuse alveolar damage [5]. Pulmonary complications can be infectious and noninfectious [6] and occur before and after engraftment or have a late onset [7]. They may involve the bronchi, alveoli, and capillary vessels (Fig. 5.1) [8] and are clinically under-recognized [9]. They can develop after autologous and allogeneic HSCT with similarities but also differences which depend on various factors such as age, underlying lung condition, and degree of immunosuppression. More than 25% of autologous HSCT recipients develop pulmonary complications within 1 year of transplant. Most of these complications are infectious and commonly occur while the patients are neutropenic. The most common noninfectious complications are acute pulmonary edema, diffuse alveolar hemorrhage, peri-engraftment syndrome, and idiopathic pneumonia syndrome [10]. In allogeneic HSCT, the most common noninfectious complications are bronchiolitis obliterans syndrome and interstitial lung disease [11]. Bronchiolitis obliterans syndrome remains the most challenging pulmonary complication after allogeneic HSCT [12]. New approaches with machine learning algorithms may offer a quantitative approach for the identification of bronchiolitis obliterans syndrome versus other lung diseases after HSCT [13]. Idiopathic pneumonia syndrome has less than 15% 1-year survival [14]. Clinical presentations are diverse, and an accurate and timely differential diagnosis is essential to limit their sometimes-disastrous consequences [15]. This presentation focuses on patients who are evaluated in the intensive care setting.

Infectious respiratory complications can be due to bacterial, viral, fungal, or parasitic organisms and can be affected by pretransplant status (e.g., cytomegalovirus), environmental exposure (e.g., histoplasmosis), type of immunosuppressive agents (e.g., corticosteroids), prophylaxis, and elapsed time since transplantation. Noninfectious complications may include radia-

P. R. Bauer (✉)
Division of Pulmonary and Critical Care Medicine, Department of Internal Medicine, Mayo Clinic, Rochester, MN, USA
e-mail: Bauer.Philippe@mayo.edu



A. O. Soubani (ed.), *Pulmonary and Critical Care Considerations of Hematopoietic Stem Cell Transplantation*, https://doi.org/10.1007/978-3-031-28797-8_5

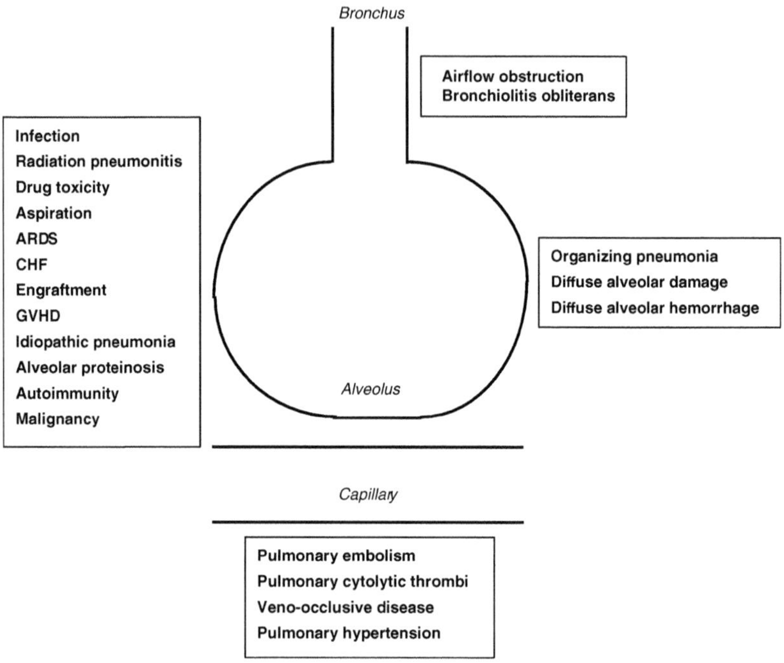


**Fig. 5.1** Overview of pulmonary diseases following HSCT (*ARDS* acute respiratory distress syndrome, *CHF* congestive heart failure, *GVHD* graft-versus-host disease)

tion- and drug-induced lung toxicity, aspiration pneumonitis (especially in case of mucositis), cardiogenic pulmonary edema, engraftment syndrome, idiopathic pneumonia syndrome, graft-versus-host disease, bronchiolitis obliterans, recurrence or secondary malignancy, connective tissue disease, vasculitis, pulmonary alveolar proteinosis, and pulmonary vascular disease including pulmonary veno-occlusive disease and pulmonary hypertension. Several complications can be combined. From a histopathological perspective, organizing pneumonia, diffuse alveolar damage, and diffuse alveolar hemorrhage are commonly encountered and can have different etiologies.

The approach to the diagnosis of pulmonary disease after HSCT must be systematic and progressive, from the least invasive to the most invasive, while considering pretest probability and the risk over benefit ratio of any given test or procedure (Table 5.1). In a secondary analysis of a prospective, multinational, observational study of 1611 immunocompromised patients with acute respiratory failure admitted to the intensive care unit, compared to noninvasive testing only, bronchoscopy achieved a 27% adjusted diagnostic yield and a 38% therapeutic yield but was associated with worsening of respiratory status in 11% of patients and higher ICU and hospital mortality (OR 1.41, 95% CI 1.08–1.81) [16]. Both noninvasive testing, including new molecular markers, and invasive procedures, such as bronchoscopy, should be complementary [17]. Managing pulmonary complications after HSCT remains challenging due to the lack of preventive strategies [18].

Chief complaints and clinical presentations that require transfer to the intensive care are usually dyspnea and increased oxygen requirement with or without frank respiratory distress. Other clinical features may include fever, cough, chest pain, and nonpulmonary signs (e.g., skin rash, diarrhea). After initial stabilization if clinically indicated (standard supplemental oxygen, high flow nasal cannula, noninvasive or invasive mechanical ventilation after intubation, vaso-

**Table 5.1** Pulmonary diseases after HSCT: diagnostic workup

| Diagnostics checklist | | Examples |
|---|---|---|
| Age | | |
| Comorbidities | Pulmonary disease | Previous PFT |
| | Cardiac disease | Previous echocardiogram |
| | Liver disease | Iron overload |
| | Renal disease | Nephrotoxic agents |
| Environmental exposure | Pets | Cats, birds |
| | Geographical location | TB, endemic fungi |
| Malignancy | Type | Leukemia, lymphoma, myeloma |
| | Chemotherapy | Cardiac toxicity |
| | Radiation therapy | Radiation toxicity |
| | Serostatus | CMV, HSV, HIV, EBV |
| | Prophylaxis | CMV, pneumocystis |
| HSCT | Type of HSCT | Autologous, allogeneic |
| | Preconditioning regimen | Myeloablative or not |
| | Time elapsed since HSCT | Pre-, post-engraftment |
| Physical examination | Signs and symptoms | Lungs, heart, skin, abdomen |
| | POCUS | Lungs, pleura, heart, abdomen |
| Labs | CBC with differential | Neutropenia |
| | Renal function | Acute kidney injury |
| | Liver function | Acute liver failure |
| Infectious workup | Blood culture | Bacterial, fungal |
| | Respiratory pathogens | Influenza, RSV, SARS-CoV-2 |
| | Sputum (induced) | Pneumocystis, TB |
| | Beta-D-glucan | *Candida*, *Aspergillus* |
| *Aspergillus galactomannan* | Galactomannan | *Aspergillus* |
| | Urine tests | *Streptococcus*, *Legionella* |
| Imaging | Chest radiograph | Focal, diffuse opacities |
| | Chest computed tomography | Focal, diffuse opacities, VTE |
| Bronchoscopy | BAL | Immunocompromised host |
| | Hemosiderin-laden macrophage | DAH if greater than 20% |
| | Transbronchial biopsy | Not if thrombocytopenia |
| Lung biopsy | VATS | Rarely done |
| | Open lung biopsy | Very rarely done |
| Skin biopsy | Skin rash | GVHD, engraftment |
| Cardiac workup | ECG | ACS, pericarditis |
| | Troponins | ACS |
| | Pro-BNP | Heart failure |
| | Echocardiogram | Heart failure, pericarditis |
| Autoimmunity | ANA | Scleroderma, Sjogren |
| | ENA | Scleroderma, Sjogren |
| | ANCAs | Vasculitis |

*PFT* pulmonary function test, *TB* tuberculosis, *CMV* cytomegalovirus, *HSV* herpes simplex virus, *HIV* human immunodeficiency virus, *EBV* Ebstein-Barr virus, *HSCT* hematopoietic stem cell transplant, *POCUS* point of care ultrasound, *CBC* complete blood count, *RSV* respiratory syncytial virus, *SARS-CoV-2* severe acute respiratory syndrome coronavirus 2, *VTE* venous thromboembolism, *BAL* bronchoalveolar lavage, *DAH* diffuse alveolar hemorrhage, *VATS* video-assisted thoracoscopic surgery, *GVHD* graft-versus-host disease, *ECG* electrocardiogram, *ACS* acute coronary syndrome, *BNP* brain natriuretic peptide, *ANA* antinuclear antibody, *ENA* extractable nuclear antigen antibody, *ANCAs* antineutrophil cytoplasmic antibodies

pressors, etc.), the diagnostic workup should focus on eliciting information regarding past medical history, type of malignancy, previous chemotherapy or radiation therapy, type of HSCT (autologous versus allogeneic), type of preparative conditioning regimen (e.g., myeloablative versus nonablative regimen), immunosuppression, cardiac toxicity, prophylaxis, pretransplant serostatus, environmental exposure, time since HSCT, engraftment, and graft-versus-host disease. Comorbidities are also important including age and preexisting pulmonary, cardiac, renal, and metabolic conditions [19, 20].

Physical examination should focus on assessing the presence of respiratory, circulatory, and neurological failure. Evidence for edema, jaundice, and maculopapular rash should be sought. A point of care ultrasound should be performed as an extension to the clinical examination, looking for evidence of B-lines attesting of interstitial process such as pulmonary edema or the presence of consolidation, atelectasis, pleural effusion, right or left ventricular failure, pericardial effusion, and ascites [21]. Usually, a chest radiograph is obtained first but may not be insufficient [22], and a chest computed tomography is obtained as soon as the patient is stable enough to be transported to the Radiology Department.

Diagnostic studies include the following: complete cell count with differential; blood culture for bacteria and fungi; sputum culture for bacteria, mycobacteria, and fungi including *Pneumocystis jirovecii*; nasal swab for polymerase chain reaction for severe acute respiratory syndrome coronavirus-2 (SARS-CoV-2), influenza and respiratory syncytial, or a more complete multiplex viral pathogen panel; and urine antigen for *Streptococcus pneumoniae*, *Legionella*, and, in the context of endemic fungi, histoplasma, or Blastomyces). Serum can be tested for CMV (viral load), beta-D-glucan, *Aspergillus galactomannan*, and cryptococcus antigen. Other blood tests may include antinuclear antibodies, extractable nuclear antigen antibodies, and vasculitis panel (antineutrophil cytoplasmic antibodies). Electrocardiogram, serial troponins, pro-brain natriuretic peptide, and formal echocardiogram may be useful if acute coronary syndrome, pericarditis, and congestive heart failure are suspected in case of preexisting heart failure, previous use of cardiotoxic drugs (e.g., anthracyclines), or weight gain with edema especially after large amount of intravenous fluid administration or in case of engraftment. A bronchoscopy should not be performed routinely unless noninvasive testing remains negative or cannot be obtained (e.g., induced sputum), or if there is a high clinical suspicion (e.g., diffuse alveolar hemorrhage), or if the patient requires immediate intubation. If the clinician feels that bronchoscopy is indicated, it should not be delayed until the patient's condition has worsened, since early bronchoscopy has a higher yield than delayed bronchoscopy [23, 24]. Bronchoalveolar lavage sent to the laboratory for an immunocompromised host panel should be obtained. Transbronchial biopsy is rarely useful in infectious complications but may contribute to the diagnostic management of noninfectious causes [25]. This procedure is often contraindicated because of the presence of thrombocytopenia. Lung biopsy (cryobiopsy, video-assisted thoracoscopic surgical biopsy, or open lung biopsy) has seldom any indication except in individualized cases of undetermined interstitial lung disease, concern for malignancy or idiopathic pulmonary syndrome [26]. Computed tomography-guided fine needle lung biopsy is an option in case of focal pulmonary lesions [27].

## Diagnosis Evaluation: Specifics

### Bacterial Pneumonias

Bacterial pneumonias (Gram-positive and Gram-negative bacteria) can occur during the pre-engraftment and post-engraftment period. At the late phase after allogeneic HSCT, encapsulated bacteria (*Streptococcus pneumoniae*, *Haemophilus influenzae*, *Neisseria meningitidis*) should also be considered. Workup includes imaging, blood cultures, sputum cultures, and urine antigens (e.g., *Streptococcus pneumoniae*, *Legionella*), and rarely bronchoalveolar lavage is necessary.

### Mycobacteria

Tuberculosis and atypical mycobacterial infections can be seen in the post-engraftment period. Tuberculosis is more common in patients from countries with high prevalence or in case of chronic graft-versus-host disease. Tuberculous skin test and interferon gamma-release assays are not reliable [28]. Imaging can show a miliary pattern. Induced sputum or bronchoalveolar lavage with acid-fast bacilli staining on smear and culture and the presence of caseating granuloma and/or acid-fast bacilli documented by histopathology are necessary for the diagnosis.

### Viral Pneumonias

Respiratory viruses (e.g., influenza, respiratory syncytial virus, adenovirus, SARS CoV-2) may be seasonal and can occur at any time during the pre-engraftment or post-engraftment period. Herpes simplex virus usually occurs during the pre-engraftment period, cytomegalovirus (CMV), human herpes virus-6, and varicella-zoster during the post-engraftment period [29]. Nasopharyngeal samples for viral cultures, viral antigen assays, and polymerase reaction assays are most useful. Chest imaging is often nonspecific [30]. For CMV, bronchoalveolar lavage and tissue sampling may be necessary when looking for intranuclear and intracytoplasmic inclusion bodies with confirmation by immunohistochemical staining. Serology may indicate prior exposure.

Epstein-Barr virus (EBV) is associated with posttransplant lymphoproliferative disorder [31]. It usually presents with B symptoms (fever, weight loss) and lung mass by chest computed tomography. Positron emission tomography scanning may be useful but not always feasible in critically ill patients. Opportunistic infections always need to be ruled out. Elevated lactate dehydrogenase may be a clue. Diagnosis is suspected by a markedly elevated EBV viral load by quantitative polymerase chain reaction and usually requires tissue diagnosis by lung biopsy.

### Fungal Pneumonias

Fungal infections are frequent and result from persistent immunosuppression caused by the underlying hematologic malignancy and its treatment with HSCT [32]. It may be less frequent in autologous HSCT than allogeneic HSCT. Infection due to *Candida* may occur in the pre-engraftment and *Pneumocystis* in the post-engraftment period. *Aspergillus* infection can occur at any time. On computed tomography, the classic halo sign is suggestive of invasive aspergillosis and the reverse halo sign of pulmonary mucormycosis. However, both are nonspecific and can also be seen with other infectious (e.g., *Candida* and other fungal infections) and noninfectious causes [33]. Aside from imaging, blood cultures and bronchoscopy with bronchoalveolar lavage are helpful. A common issue is how to make the distinction between colonization and invasive infection. The diagnosis of invasive aspergillosis relies on a positive culture in combination with histopathologic confirmation or the presence of *Aspergillus* in a culture from a normal sterile site (e.g., pleural space). Fungal markers (galactomannan, beta-D-glucan, and polymerase chain reaction) can be useful, particularly if measured in the bronchoalveolar lavage, but are not sufficient for a definite diagnosis. Beta-D-glucan can also suggest infection with *Candida* and *Pneumocystis*. Pneumocystis diagnosis relies on a positive identification by tinctorial staining, fluorescent antibody staining, or polymerase chain reaction on induced sputum or bronchoalveolar lavage.

Endemic fungi (histoplasmosis, blastomycosis, coccidioidomycosis) may be seen in endemic areas (e.g., the Mississippi basin, the southwest USA). Diagnosis relies on fungal cultures, antigen assay, serology, and histopathology.

### Parasitic Infections

Reactivation of toxoplasmosis and strongyloidiasis can rarely be observed. Polymerase chain reaction and serology testing are useful for toxoplasmosis. Rare cases of hyperinfection syndrome secondary to strongyloidiasis have been described after HSCT; the presence of eosinophilia and a history of travel, even remote, to endemic areas may be clues to the diagnosis [34]. Stool testing and serology confirm the diagnosis of strongyloidiasis.

### Radiation and Drug-Induced Toxicity

The clinical context usually is indicative of possible radiation- or drug-induced toxicity. A careful history of previous radiation therapy or pneumotoxic (e.g., cyclophosphamide) or cardiotoxic chemotherapy (e.g., anthracyclines) should raise concern for radiation therapy or chemotherapy as possible explanation for the pulmonary disease. Increased eosinophil in the bronchoalveolar lavage may suggest drug-induced toxicity. It remains a diagnosis of exclusion.

### Aspiration Pneumonitis

The clinical context is also indicative particularly when an aspiration event is witnessed. The presence of severe mucositis raises concern for aspiration which remains also a diagnosis of exclusion. The presence of atelectasis and intraluminal opacity on chest computed tomography is clue toward an aspiration event. In doubtful cases, bronchoscopy may be helpful.

### Cardiogenic Pulmonary Edema

Cardiogenic pulmonary edema can be seen in case of fluid overload, preexisting cardiac disease, drug cardiotoxicity, engraftment syndrome, and graft-versus-host disease. Diagnosis is made by clinical signs of heart failure, elevated pro-brain natriuretic peptide, abnormal chest radiograph and chest computed tomography with cardiomegaly, pulmonary edema, Kerley's B-lines, thickened interlobular septa, pleural effusion, and echocardiography showing evidence of left systolic or diastolic ventricular or right ventricular failure. Pericarditis and sometimes tamponade can be seen as well (e.g., post-irradiation or after sirolimus therapy).

### Diffuse Alveolar Hemorrhage

Diffuse alveolar hemorrhage can be seen in many circumstances. Hemoptysis is not always present. The diagnosis relies on bronchoalveolar lavage with progressively bloody return or greater than 20% of hemosiderin-laden macrophages. The clinical context and appropriate testing are necessary to account for its multiple causes [35].

### Acute Respiratory Distress Syndrome

Acute respiratory distress syndrome has many infectious and noninfectious causes. It follows the Berlin criteria to define its severity based on the presence of bilateral infiltrates with hypoxemia within 1 week of predisposal circumstances and not explained by heart failure [36]. Most cases of acute respiratory distress syndrome following HSCT do not meet criteria for a more specific posttransplantation pulmonary syndrome [37].

## Organizing Pneumonia

Organizing pneumonia is a histopathological diagnosis. It can be related to infectious and noninfectious causes or be idiopathic. Imaging shows patchy, nodular opacities and ground glass opacities with peripheral predominance. Bronchoalveolar lavage shows a mixed pattern with increased lymphocytes, neutrophils, and eosinophils. Lung biopsy is needed. Acute fibrinous and organizing pneumonia is a rare form of organizing pneumonia after allogeneic HSCT characterized by intra-alveolar fibrin deposition [38].

### Engraftment Syndrome

Engraftment syndrome is observed with both allogeneic and autologous HSCT, occurring at the time of neutrophil recovery and presenting with fever, skin rash, weight gain, and pulmonary edema [39]. Acute kidney injury, abnormal liver function, and encephalopathy can also be observed. Skin biopsy is sometimes helpful. Bronchoscopy may reveal the presence of diffuse alveolar hemorrhage. Infection needs to be ruled out. The use of a standard approach to diagnosis may be beneficial [40].

### Idiopathic Pneumonia Syndrome

Idiopathic pneumonia syndrome is a form of multifocal pneumonia with acute lung injury and increased oxygen requirement, diffuse alveolar damage, and no evidence of lower respiratory infection or noninfectious causes of pulmonary diseases after extensive evaluation. It is also more frequently observed with allogeneic than autologous HSCT. It occurs usually late (weeks or months) after HSCT [41]. It is a diagnosis of exclusion.

### Graft-Versus-Host Disease

Graft-versus-host disease is almost exclusively seen after allogeneic GSCT. It can be hyperacute, acute (classic acute, late acute), and chronic (classic chronic and overlap) [42]. Clinical manifestations include skin (maculopapular rash, erythroderma), gut (diarrhea), and liver (hyperbilirubinemia) involvement with other organ involvement such as eyes, kidney, lungs, and the hematopoietic system (e.g., thrombocytopenia, IgA deficiency). Pulmonary manifestations include diffuse alveolar damage, diffuse alveolar hemorrhage, and bronchiolitis obliterans with airflow obstruction at a later stage [43]. The diagnosis is clinical and can be reinforced by skin or intestinal biopsy and exclusion of other etiologies.

### Malignancy

Relapse of primary malignancy (e.g., lymphoma), secondary malignancy, and posttransplant lymphoproliferative disorders can occur. EBV status and tissue biopsy are necessary.

### Connective Tissue Disease, Vasculitis

Connective tissue disease (systemic lupus erythematosus, mixed connective tissue disease, Sjögren syndrome, polymyositis) associated interstitial lung diseases and antineutrophil cytoplasmic antibody vasculitis have been observed after allogeneic HSCT with three different histopathologic patterns of interstitial pneumonia (lymphocytic interstitial pneumonia, nonspecific interstitial pneumonia, and diffuse alveolar damage) [44]. Testing includes chest imaging and serological tests including antinuclear antibodies, extractable nuclear antigen antibodies, rheumatoid factor, and antineutrophil cytoplasmic antibodies.

### Pulmonary Alveolar Proteinosis

Pulmonary alveolar proteinosis is a reversible complication after allogeneic HSCT and a secondary cause of pulmonary disease affecting surfactant production and clearance [45]. On computed tomography, it shows patchy and diffuse bilateral ground glass opacities with sometimes crazy-paving pattern. The diagnosis is made by bronchoalveolar lavage showing a milky return with positive periodic acid-Schiff stain. When occurring after HSCT, there is no need to check for anti GM-CSF antibodies.

### Pulmonary Vascular Disease

Pulmonary veno-occlusive disease can be seen rarely after allogeneic HSCT [46]. Chest computed tomography may show ground glass opacities and increased interlobular septa. Echocardiogram shows increased right ventricular systolic pressure. Chest computed tomography angiography rules out pulmonary embolism. The diagnosis requires a right cardiac catheterization showing pulmonary hypertension.

Other pumonary vascular diseases include venous thromboembolic events, catheter-induced thrombosis diagnosed by Doppler ultrasound and computed tomography angiogram and transplant-associated thrombotic microangiopathy with microangiopathic hemolytic anemia with schistocytes, thrombocytopenia and acute renal failure [47].

Pulmonary cytolytic thrombi are a rare occurrence after allogeneic HSCT [48]. Chest computed tomography shows pulmonary nodules. Lung biopsy is necessary and shows necrotic basophilic cytolytic thromboemboli [49].

Preexisting pulmonary hypertension may be present, related to the underlying malignancy (e.g., myelofibrosis) or related to drug toxicity (e.g., dasatinib) [50].

In summary: Pulmonary complications after HSCT are frequent and associated with worse outcomes. Their occurrence is influenced by the degree of immunity of the host, the nature of the malignancy, and the therapies given. Several complications can come together, and a high index of suspicion should prevail. An early diagnosis is the key to a prompt and appropriate treatment. The diagnostic strategy should be structured, progressive, and individualized.

## References


1. Wieruszewski PM, Herasevich S, Gajic O, Yadav H. Respiratory failure in the hematopoietic stem cell transplant recipient. World J Crit Care Med. 2018;7(5):62–72.
2. Saunders IM, Tan M, Koura D, Young R. Long-term follow-up of hematopoietic stem cell transplant survivors: a focus on screening, monitoring, and therapeutics. Pharmacotherapy. 2020;40(8):808–41.
3. Soubani AO. Critical care considerations of hematopoietic stem cell transplantation. Crit Care Med. 2006;34(9 Suppl):S251–67.
4. Peters SG, Afessa B. Acute lung injury after hematopoietic stem cell transplantation. Clin Chest Med. 2005;26(4):561–9. vi
5. Khayyata S, Soubani AO, Bonnett M, Nassar H, Abidi MH, Al-Abbadi MA. The major autopsy findings in adult patients after hematopoietic stem cell transplantation. Ann Transplant. 2007;12(2):11–8.
6. Afessa B, Peters SG. Major complications following hematopoietic stem cell transplantation. Semin Respir Crit Care Med. 2006;27(3):297–309.
7. Schlemmer F, Chevret S, Lorillon G, De Bazelaire C, Peffault de Latour R, Meignin V, Michallet M, Hermet E, Wyplosz B, Houdouin V, Marchand-Adam S, Socié G, Tazi A, Bergeron A. Late-onset noninfectious interstitial lung disease after allogeneic hematopoietic stem cell transplantation. Respir Med. 2014;108(10):1525–33.
8. Meignin V, Thivolet-Bejui F, Kambouchner M, Hussenet C, Bondeelle L, Mitchell A, Chagnon K, Begueret H, Segers V, Cottin V, Tazi A, Chevret S, Danel C, Bergeron A. Lung histopathology of non-infectious pulmonary complications after allogeneic haematopoietic stem cell transplantation. Histopathology. 2018;73(5):832–42.
9. Gazourian L, Spring L, Meserve E, Hwang D, Diaz AA, Ash SY, Ho VT, Sholl LM, Washko GR. Pulmonary clinicopathological correlation after allogeneic hematopoietic stem cell transplantation: an autopsy series. Biol Blood Marrow Transplant. 2017;23(10):1767–72.
10. Afessa B, Abdulai RM, Kremers WK, Hogan WJ, Litzow MR, Peters SG. Risk factors and outcome of pulmonary complications after autologous hematopoietic stem cell transplant. Chest. 2012;141(2):442–50.
11. Bergeron A, Chevret S, Peffault de Latour R, Chagnon K, de Margerie-Mellon C, Rivière F, Robin M, Mani J, Lorillon G, Socié G, Tazi A. Noninfectious lung complications after allogeneic haematopoietic stem cell transplantation. Eur Respir J. 2018;51(5):1702617.
12. Haider S, Durairajan N, Soubani AO. Noninfectious pulmonary complications of haematopoietic stem cell transplantation. Eur Respir Rev. 2020;29(156):190119.
13. Sharifi H, Lai YK, Guo H, Hoppenfeld M, Guenther ZD, Johnston L, Brondstetter T, Chhatwani L, Nicolls MR, Hsu JL. Machine learning algorithms to differentiate among pulmonary complications after hematopoietic cell transplant. Chest. 2020;158(3):1090–103.
14. Afessa B, Litzow MR, Tefferi A. Bronchiolitis obliterans and other late onset non-infectious pulmonary complications in hematopoietic stem cell transplantation. Bone Marrow Transplant. 2001;28(5):425–34.
15. Shiari A, Nassar M, Soubani AO. Major pulmonary complications following hematopoietic stem cell transplantation: what the pulmonologist needs to know. Respir Med. 2021;185:106493.
16. Bauer PR, Chevret S, Yadav H, Mehta S, Pickkers P, Bukan RB, Rello J, van de Louw A, Klouche K, Meert AP, Martin-Loeches I, Marsh B, Socias Crespi L, Moreno-Gonzalez G, Buchtele N, Amrein K, Balik M, Antonelli M, Nyunga M, Barratt-Due A, Bergmans DCJJ, Spoelstra-de Man AME, Kuitunen A, Wallet F, Seguin A, Metaxa V, Lemiale V, Burghi G, Demoule A, Karvunidis T, Cotoia A, Klepstad P, Møller AM, Mokart D, Azoulay E, Efraim Investigators and the Nine-I Study Group. Diagnosis and outcome of acute respiratory failure in immunocompromised patients after bronchoscopy. Eur Respir J. 2019;54(1):1802442.
17. Feinstein MB, Habtes I, Giralt S, Stover DE. Utility of bronchoscopy with bronchoalveolar lavage among hematologic transplant recipients in the era of noninvasive testing. Respiration. 2021;100(4):339–46.
18. Bondeelle L, Bergeron A. Managing pulmonary complications in allogeneic hematopoietic stem cell transplantation. Expert Rev Respir Med. 2019;13(1):105–19.
19. Duque-Afonso J, Ewald S, Ihorst G, Waterhouse M, Struessmann T, Zeiser R, Wäsch R, Bertz H, Müller-Quernheim J, Duyster J, Finke J, Marks R, Engelhardt M. The impact of pulmonary function in patients undergoing autologous stem cell transplantation. Blood Adv. 2021;5(21):4327–37.
20. Diab KJ, Yu Z, Wood KL, Shmalo JA, Sheski FD, Farber MO, Wilkes DS, Nelson RP Jr. Comparison of pulmonary complications after nonmyeloablative and conventional allogeneic hematopoietic cell transplant. Biol Blood Marrow Transplant. 2012;18(12):1827–34.
21. Lichtenstein DA. BLUE-protocol and FALLS-protocol: two applications of lung ultrasound in the critically ill. Chest. 2015;147(6):1659–70.
22. Sirithanakul K, Salloum A, Klein JL, Soubani AO. Pulmonary complications following hematopoietic stem cell transplantation: diagnostic approaches. Am J Hematol. 2005;80(2):137–46.
23. Harris B, Geyer AI. Diagnostic evaluation of pulmonary abnormalities in patients with hematologic malignancies and hematopoietic cell transplantation. Clin Chest Med. 2017;38(2):317–31.

24. Lucena CM, Torres A, Rovira M, Marcos MA, de la Bellacasa JP, Sánchez M, Domingo R, Gabarrus A, Mensa J, Agustí C. Pulmonary complications in hematopoietic SCT: a prospective study. Bone Marrow Transplant. 2014;49(10):1293–9.
25. O'Dwyer DN, Duvall AS, Xia M, Hoffman TC, Bloye KS, Bulte CA, Zhou X, Murray S, Moore BB, Yanik GA. Transbronchial biopsy in the management of pulmonary complications of hematopoietic stem cell transplantation. Bone Marrow Transplant. 2018;53(2):193–8.
26. Dieffenbach BV, Madenci AL, Murphy AJ, Weldon CB, Weil BR, Lehmann LE. Therapeutic impact and complications associated with surgical lung biopsy after allogeneic hematopoietic stem cell transplantation in children. Biol Blood Marrow Transplant. 2019;25(11):2181–5.
27. Jantunen E, Piilonen A, Volin L, Ruutu P, Parkkali T, Koukila-Kähkölä P, Ruutu T. Radiologically guided fine needle lung biopsies in the evaluation of focal pulmonary lesions in allogeneic stem cell transplant recipients. Bone Marrow Transplant. 2002;29(4):353–6.
28. de Oliveira RM, de Almeida Testa LH, Dos Santos ACF, Zanetti LP, da Silva RL, de Souza MP, Colturato VR, Machado CM. Latent and active tuberculosis infection in allogeneic hematopoietic stem cell transplant recipients: a prospective cohort study. Bone Marrow Transplant. 2021;56(9):2241–7.
29. Jaskula E, Dlubek D, Sedzimirska M, Duda D, Tarnowska A, Lange A. Reactivations of cytomegalovirus, human herpes virus 6, and Epstein-Barr virus differ with respect to risk factors and clinical outcome after hematopoietic stem cell transplantation. Transplant Proc. 2010;42(8):3273–6.
30. Vakil E, Evans SE. Viral pneumonia in patients with hematologic malignancy or hematopoietic stem cell transplantation. Clin Chest Med. 2017;38(1):97–111.
31. Pegoraro F, Favre C. Post-transplantation lymphoproliferative disorder after haematopoietic stem cell transplantation. Ann Hematol. 2021;100(4):865–78.
32. Young AY, Leiva Juarez MM, Evans SE. Fungal pneumonia in patients with hematologic malignancy and hematopoietic stem cell transplantation. Clin Chest Med. 2017;38(3):479–91.
33. Georgiadou SP, Sipsas NV, Marom EM, Kontoyiannis DP. The diagnostic value of halo and reversed halo signs for invasive mold infections in compromised hosts. Clin Infect Dis. 2011;52(9):1144–55.
34. Wirk B, Wingard JR. Strongyloides stercoralis hyperinfection in hematopoietic stem cell transplantation. Transpl Infect Dis. 2009;11(2):143–8.
35. Zhang Z, Wang C, Peters SG, Hogan WJ, Hashmi SK, Litzow MR, Patnaik MS, Niven AS, Yadav H. Epidemiology, risk factors, and outcomes of diffuse alveolar Hemorrhage after hematopoietic stem cell transplantation. Chest. 2021;159(6):2325–33.
36. ARDS Definition Task Force, Ranieri VM, Rubenfeld GD, Thompson BT, Ferguson ND, Caldwell E, Fan E, Camporota L, Slutsky AS. Acute respiratory distress syndrome: the Berlin Definition. JAMA. 2012;307(23):2526–33.
37. Yadav H, Nolan ME, Bohman JK, Cartin-Ceba R, Peters SG, Hogan WJ, Gajic O, Kor DJ. Epidemiology of acute respiratory distress syndrome following hematopoietic stem cell transplantation. Crit Care Med. 2016;44(6):1082–90.
38. Nguyen LP, Ahdoot S, Sriratanaviriyakul N, Zhang Y, Stollenwerk N, Schivo M, Harper R. Acute fibrinous and organizing pneumonia associated with allogenic hematopoietic stem cell transplant successfully treated with corticosteroids: a two-patient case series. J Investig Med High Impact Case Rep. 2016;4(2):2324709616643990.
39. Chang L, Frame D, Braun T, Gatza E, Hanauer DA, Zhao S, Magenau JM, Schultz K, Tokala H, Ferrara JL, Levine JE, Reddy P, Paczesny S, Choi SW. Engraftment syndrome after allogeneic hematopoietic cell transplantation predicts poor outcomes. Biol Blood Marrow Transplant. 2014;20(9):1407–17.
40. Grant A, Chapman LRM, Mitchell R, O'Brien TA. Engraftment syndrome following hematopoietic stem cell transplant: a review of the literature. Clin Transpl. 2020;34(6):e13875.
41. Panoskaltsis-Mortari A, Griese M, Madtes DK, Belperio JA, Haddad IY, Folz RJ, Cooke KR, American Thoracic Society Committee on Idiopathic Pneumonia Syndrome. An official American Thoracic Society research statement: noninfectious lung injury after hematopoietic stem cell transplantation: idiopathic pneumonia syndrome. Am J Respir Crit Care Med. 2011;183(9):1262–79.
42. Jagasia MH, Greinix HT, Arora M, Williams KM, Wolff D, Cowen EW, Palmer J, Weisdorf D, Treister NS, Cheng GS, Kerr H, Stratton P, Duarte RF, McDonald GB, Inamoto Y, Vigorito A, Arai S, Datiles MB, Jacobsohn D, Heller T, Kitko CL, Mitchell SA, Martin PJ, Shulman H, Wu RS, Cutler CS, Vogelsang GB, Lee SJ, Pavletic SZ, Flowers ME. National Institutes of Health Consensus Development Project on Criteria for Clinical Trials in Chronic Graft-versus-Host Disease: I. The 2014 diagnosis and staging working group report. Biol Blood Marrow Transplant. 2015;21(3):389–401.e1.
43. Dudek AZ, Mahaseth H. Hematopoietic stem cell transplant-related airflow obstruction. Curr Opin Oncol. 2006;18(2):115–9.
44. Bergeron A, Bengoufa D, Feuillet S, Meignin V, de Latour RP, Rybojad M, Gossot D, Azoulay E, Socié G, Tazi A. The spectrum of lung involvement in collagen vascular-like diseases following allogeneic hematopoietic stem cell transplantation: report of 6 cases and review of the literature. Medicine (Baltimore). 2011;90(2):146–57.
45. Salvator H, Tcherakian C, Maillard N, Milin S, Bergeron A, Bondeelle L, Meignin V, Nguyen S, Souchet L, Guenounou S, Evrard SM, Rubio MT, Robin M, Sestili S, Brissot E, Fajac A, Catherinot E, Givel C, Chabrol A, Goyard C, Longchampt E, Chabi-Charvillat ML, Bernaudin JF, Couderc LJ. Pulmonary

alveolar proteinosis after allogeneic hematopoietic stem-cell transplantation in adults: a French Societe francophone de Greffe de Moelle et Therapie Cellulaire survey. Chest. 2021;160(5):1783–8.
46. Dandoy CE, Hirsch R, Chima R, Davies SM, Jodele S. Pulmonary hypertension after hematopoietic stem cell transplantation. Biol Blood Marrow Transplant. 2013;19(11):1546–56.
47. Sahin U, Ataca Atilla P, Atilla E, Toprak SK, Demirer T. An overview of hematopoietic stem cell transplantation related thrombotic complications. Crit Rev Oncol Hematol. 2016;107:149–55.
48. Peters A, Manivel JC, Dolan M, Gulbahce HE, Baker KS, Verneris MR. Pulmonary cytolytic thrombi after allogeneic hematopoietic cell transplantation: a further histologic description. Biol Blood Marrow Transplant. 2005;11(6):484–5.
49. Woodard JP, Gulbahce E, Shreve M, Steiner M, Peters C, Hite S, Ramsay NK, DeFor T, Baker KS. Pulmonary cytolytic thrombi: a newly recognized complication of stem cell transplantation. Bone Marrow Transplant. 2000;25(3):293–300.
50. Mattei D, Feola M, Orzan F, Mordini N, Rapezzi D, Gallamini A. Reversible dasatinib-induced pulmonary arterial hypertension and right ventricle failure in a previously allografted CML patient. Bone Marrow Transplant. 2009;43(12):967–8.

# 6 Pulmonary Complications Following Hematopoietic Stem Cell Transplantation: Radiological Considerations

Tomás Franquet, Ana Giménez, and Sandra Mazzini

Pulmonary complications are a common cause of morbidity and mortality after HSCT occurring in 40%–60% of recipients and accounting for more than 90% of mortality [1–3]. Specific pulmonary complications tend to occur during identifiable phases that correspond with the state of immune reconstitution after the marrow transplant [2, 4]. It is useful to divide the post-HSCT complications into three distinct phases after the procedure: (1) pre-engraftment (neutropenic) phase (the first 30 days), (2) early post-engraftment phase (days 31–100), and (3) late phase (beyond day 100) [3–7].

Imaging evaluation plays a crucial role in all phases of the HSCT process to identify the presence, location and extent of pulmonary abnormalities, and the course and evolution of complications [3, 8] and monitor the effect of therapy and detect recurrence if the transplant is unsuccessful [9].

Chest radiograph is the initial imaging tool in HSCT patients with fever, dyspnea, or cough and in most of these patients provides adequate imaging information [10]. However, a normal chest roentgenogram does not exclude pneumonia. It has limited sensitivity for the detection of early infection, being normal in up to 10% of patients with proven pulmonary disease. The low neutrophil counts may result in a poor inflammatory response, which may further decrease the sensitivity of the chest X-rays.

Although CT is not recommended for the initial evaluation of patients with pneumonia, it is useful in the detection, differential diagnosis, and management of the HSC transplanted recipient with acute pulmonary disease when chest radiographs show nonspecific abnormal findings or when the radiographic findings are normal with clinical findings of pulmonary disease [6, 11–13]. In addition, expiratory CT has established itself as an essential adjunct to conventional CT, in the demonstration of air-trapping in patients with suspected obstructive small airway disease [14–16]. Paired inspiratory and expiratory CT may help in the evaluation of air-trapping in HSCT recipients with bronchiolitis obliterans syndrome.

Pulmonary complications secondary to HSCT follow a predictable timeline that reflects the immunologic status of the patient in the peritransplant period [2, 7, 17, 18]. The combination of clinical factors and imaging findings favors an accurate differential diagnosis [19–21]. In the absence of clinical information, radiologists cannot reliably distinguish between pneumonia and other noninfectious pulmonary processes.

T. Franquet (✉)
Department of Radiology, Hospital de Sant Pau, Universidad Autónoma de Barcelona, Barcelona, Spain

Hospital de Sant Pau, Barcelona, Spain
e-mail: Tfranquet@santpau.cat

A. Giménez · S. Mazzini
Department of Radiology Hospital de Sant Pau, Universidad Autónoma de Barcelona, Barcelona, Spain



A. O. Soubani (ed.), *Pulmonary and Critical Care Considerations of Hematopoietic Stem Cell Transplantation*, https://doi.org/10.1007/978-3-031-28797-8_6

Diffuse parenchymal infiltrates are common radiographic findings in HSCT recipients. In the neutropenic phase, <30 days after transplantation, infectious causes of pulmonary infiltrates have been documented in fewer than 20% of recipients who underwent open lung biopsy [22]. However, between 30 and 180 days after transplantation, infections are the most common cause of diffuse parenchymal abnormalities [22, 23]. Pulmonary edema and the idiopathic pulmonary syndrome (IPS) are the most common conditions to be distinguished from bronchopneumonia when a generalized pulmonary abnormality is radiographically demonstrated [24–26].

Focal parenchymal infiltrates are frequently due to infection regardless of the time of presentation after transplant; however, distinction of localized pneumonia from other pulmonary processes cannot be made with certainty on radiologic grounds [11]. Localized pulmonary disease of a lobar or segmental distribution can also be produced by pulmonary edema and hemorrhage.

## Infectious Complications

Pneumonia remains to be a common life-threatening complication in HSC recipients occurring as a direct result of transplantation-induced immune suppression [27]. Pulmonary infection after HSCT occurs as a direct result of transplantation-induced immune suppression [24, 28].

During the initial posttransplant period, patients are profoundly neutropenic (absolute neutrophil count <500 cells/μL), and most microbiologically documented pneumonias are caused by fungi or bacteria [23]. If neutropenia is prolonged beyond 2 weeks, *Aspergillus* spp. as well as other opportunistic molds may cause life-threatening infections [29, 30]. While fungi are the most common cause of pulmonary infection in the early pre-engraftment phase, viruses most commonly occur in the post-engraftment phase [31, 32]. Conversely, in the late post-engraftment phase, from day 100 until the patient regains normal immunity usually 1–2 years later, there is no predominant pathogen, and most infections are usually bacterial [18, 33].

## Bacterial Infections

Nosocomial bacterial infections are responsible for approximately 90% of infections during the early phase of neutropenia [34, 35]. Gram-negative bacteria are the most virulent bacterial pathogens during neutropenia and the major causes of morbidity and mortality. Plain radiographs most commonly show focal alveolar infiltrates but may be normal in 30% of patients. On high-resolution CT, a focal air-space consolidation, which typically presents in either a segmental or lobar distribution, is identified (Fig. 6.1). Differentiation from atypical patterns of opportunistic infections is often impossible based on radiographic findings. Conversely, atypical patterns, including bilateral diffuse opacities, are not uncommon manifestations of bacterial pneumonia.

Bronchogenic dissemination of pyogenic bacteria can result in dilatation and thickening of bronchiolar walls. Chest radiography may have normal or nonspecific findings consisting of heterogeneous ill-defined opacities, especially visible in the lower lung regions. Other findings are peribronchial thickening occasionally observed as "tram tracking" images. Characteristic CT findings include (1) small ill-defined centrilobu-

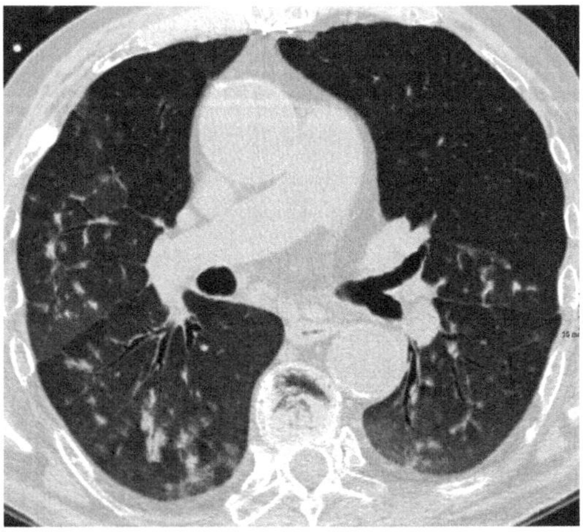

**Fig. 6.1** A 65-year-old man with multiple myeloma and *Pseudomonas aeruginosa* pneumonia. CT scan shows multiple centrilobular nodular and branching opacities

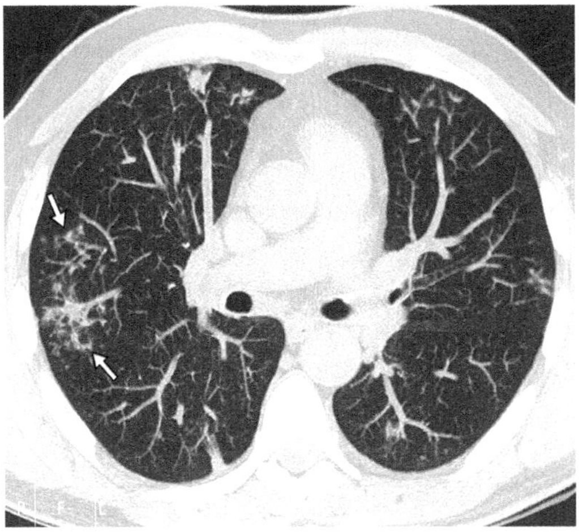

**Fig. 6.2** Endobronchial tuberculosis in a 54-year-old man with Hodgkin disease. CT scan shows multiple ill-defined nodules with a tree-in-bud appearance (arrows)

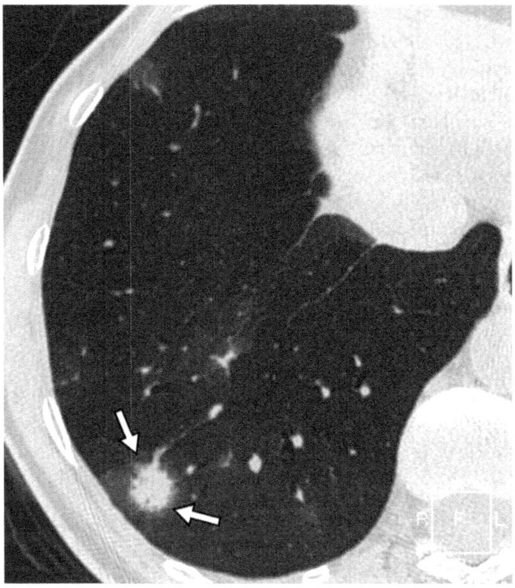

**Fig. 6.3** A 44-year-old woman with acute myeloblastic leukemia. Close-up view of a CT scan shows a right lower lobe nodular opacity with a surrounding halo of ground-glass attenuation (arrows)

lar densities representing bronchioles impacted with inflammatory material and peribronchiolar inflammation ("tree-in-bud"), (2) branching linear opacities due to airway inflammation, and (3) focal areas of consolidation due to bronchopneumonia [36].

Pulmonary tuberculosis in HSCT recipients can be difficult to diagnose due to simultaneous infection with other organisms [37]. *Mycobacterium tuberculosis* and a variety of nontuberculous mycobacteria have been reported to be between 0.4% and 4.9% of HSC transplant recipients [38–41]. Chest radiographic findings include nodules or air-space consolidation with a patchy multilobar distribution. Additional information from CT include tree-in-bud appearance with background areas of ill-defined nodules or consolidations (Fig. 6.2) [37].

## Fungal Infections

Invasive fungal infections are among the leading causes of infectious morbidity following HSCT in adults. *Aspergillus fumigatus* represents a common cause of life-threatening opportunistic infection in neutropenic patients [42, 43]. Beyond the first week after transplantation, 12%–50% of HSCT recipients are at increased risk of the angioinvasive or airway invasive forms of aspergillosis resulting in a variety of clinical, radiologic, and histologic manifestations [43–51].

Angioinvasive aspergillosis is characterized histologically by invasion and the occlusion of small to medium pulmonary arteries by fungal hyphae. This leads to the formation of necrotic hemorrhagic nodules or pleural-based wedge-shaped hemorrhagic infarcts. The characteristic CT findings consist of nodules surrounded by a halo of ground-glass attenuation (halo sign) or pleural-based wedge-shaped areas of consolidation (Fig. 6.3). In severely neutropenic patients, the halo sign is highly suggestive of angioinvasive aspergillosis [52, 53]. Separation of fragments of necrotic lung (pulmonary sequestra) from adjacent parenchyma results in air crescents like those seen in mycetomas (Fig. 6.4). The air-crescent sign in angioinvasive aspergillosis is usually seen during convalescence, i.e., 2–3 weeks after onset of treatment and concomitant with resolution of the neutropenia [54–56].

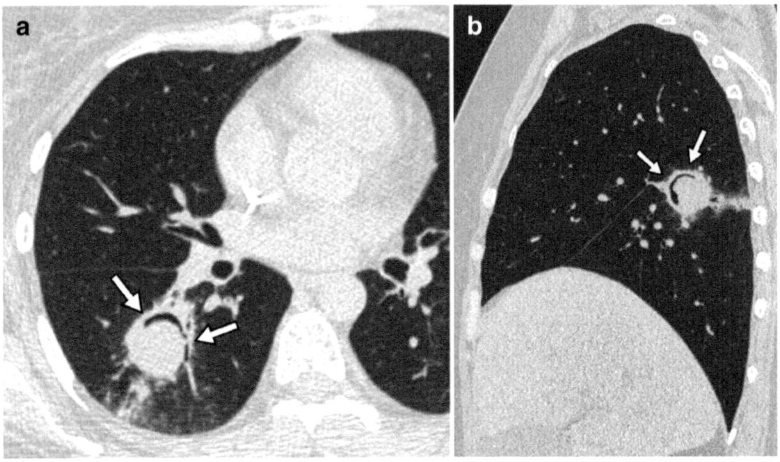


**Fig. 6.4** A 37-year-old woman with medullar aplasia and angioinvasive aspergillosis. (**a**) Axial and (**b**) sagittal CT scans show a nodular soft tissue opacity (necrotic sequestrum) separated from the surrounding parenchyma by a crescent of air (arrows). A characteristic air-crescent sign

Aspergillus bronchopneumonia, also known as airway invasive aspergillosis, occurs in up of 10% of cases of invasive pulmonary aspergillosis most commonly in neutropenic patients and in patients with acquired immunodeficiency syndrome (AIDS) [57]. The radiologic manifestations of *Aspergillus* bronchopneumonia are indistinguishable from those of bronchopneumonia caused by other microorganisms [36, 58]. CT findings of bronchiolitis are centrilobular nodules and branching linear or nodular opacities giving an appearance resembling a "tree-in-bud."

The *Mucor* species are ubiquitous, saprophytic molds, usually found in soil and in decaying food. Radiographic manifestations are nonspecific and include consolidation, cavitation, or abscess formation, nodules, and masses [59]. As occur in other angioinvasive fungal infections such as aspergillosis and candidiasis, the "air-crescent" sign and the "halo" sign may also be seen in patients with mucormycosis [60–62].

*Candida* sp. have been increasingly recognized as an important source of fungal pneumonia in patients with hematologic malignancies (acute leukemia and lymphoma) and allogeneic bone marrow transplant recipients [63, 64]. Chest radiographic and CT abnormalities consist of multifocal patchy areas of consolidation, focal cavitation, and multiple pulmonary nodules (Fig. 6.5) [64, 65].

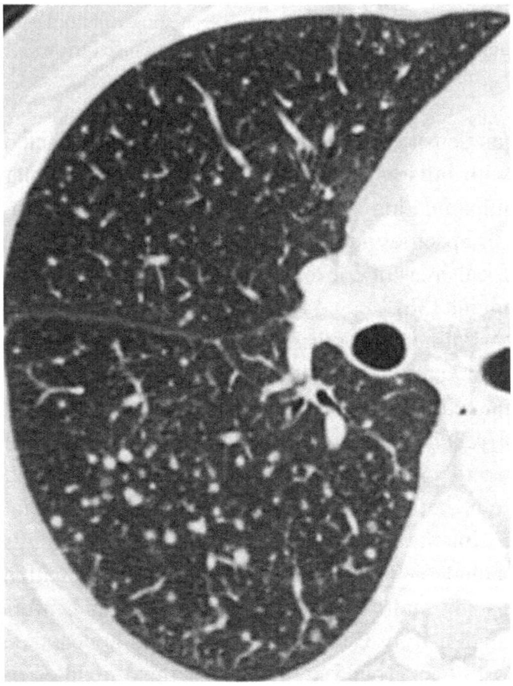

**Fig. 6.5** A 45-year-old man with acute myeloid leukemia and pulmonary candidiasis. CT scan demonstrates multiple well-defined tiny nodules in a random distribution

*Pneumocystis jiroveci* has been reported to be a rare cause of pulmonary infection in HSC transplant recipients [66]. Abnormal chest radiographs observed in up to 90% of patients with suspected pneumocystis pneumonia consist of diffuse bilateral interstitial infiltrates most marked in a perihilar distribution [3, 6]. Characteristic CT features are perihilar ground-glass opacity, often in a patchy or geographical distribution, with areas of affected lung interspersed by normal lung parenchyma (Fig. 6.6).

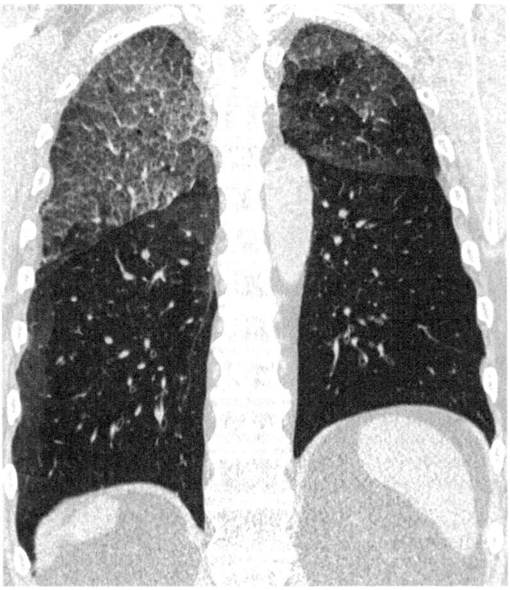

**Fig. 6.6** A 65-year-old man with *Pneumocystis* pneumonia (PJP) in angioimmunoblastic T-cell lymphoma. Coronal chest CT shows bilateral ground-glass opacities. Note interlobular and lobular septal thickening creating a "crazy-paving" pattern at the right upper lobe

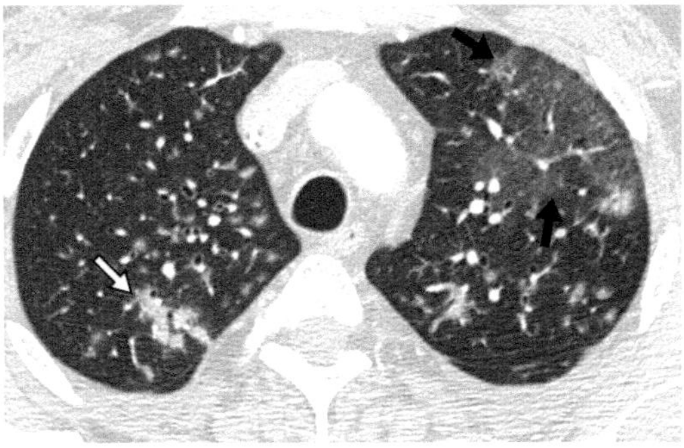

**Fig. 6.7** A 44-year-old man with respiratory syncytial virus (RSV) infection and peripheral T-cell lymphoma. CT scan shows multiple bilateral ill-defined nodular opacities. Note a ground-glass opacity in LUL (black arrows) and a focal consolidation in RUL (white arrow)

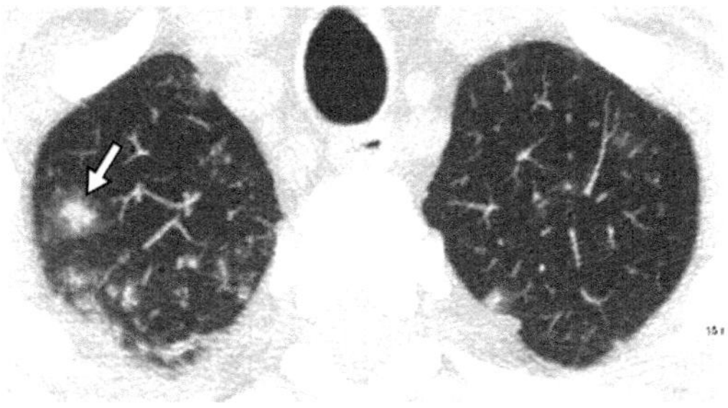

**Fig. 6.8** Cytomegalovirus (CMV) infection in a 63-year-old man with myeloblastic leukemia. CT scan shows multiple nodules with surrounding ground-glass halo (arrow)

Associated thickening of the interlobular septa with a "crazy-paving" appearance may also occur [67–69]. Less common patterns are parenchymal consolidation, mass lesions, nodules, cysts, spontaneous pneumothorax, pleural effusion, and lymph node enlargement [67].

## Viral Infection

Viruses have been increasingly recognized as important causes of serious respiratory illnesses in HSCT recipients. Viral infections may result from reactivation of a latent process or reflect newly acquired infection. Community respiratory viruses particularly respiratory syncytial virus (RSV), influenza, parainfluenza, adenovirus, and human metapneumovirus (HMPV) have been recognized as potential causes of severe pneumonia, accounting for the majority of non-CMV pulmonary infections in both autologous and allogeneic HSCT recipients [70–72]. The most common CT findings are similar and consist of small centrilobular nodules, multifocal areas of consolidation, and ground-glass opacities in a bilateral asymmetric distribution [73–77] (Fig. 6.7). Similar findings have also been described in patients with CMV, herpes simplex virus, and herpes varicella-zoster virus lung infections [74, 78–80].

CMV pneumonia remains one of the major complications in the post-engraftment phase, mostly within the first 4 months, being responsible for up to 50% of cases of pneumonia occurring in 50%–70% of HSCT recipients [18]. CT findings are diverse and consist of unilateral or bilateral interstitial infiltrates, alveolar consolidation, ground-glass opacities, and multiple small nodules with associated areas of ground-glass attenuation ("halo") (Fig. 6.8) [74, 80]. Nodule size is helpful in the differential diagnosis of infectious causes of nodules in immunocompromised patients [81].

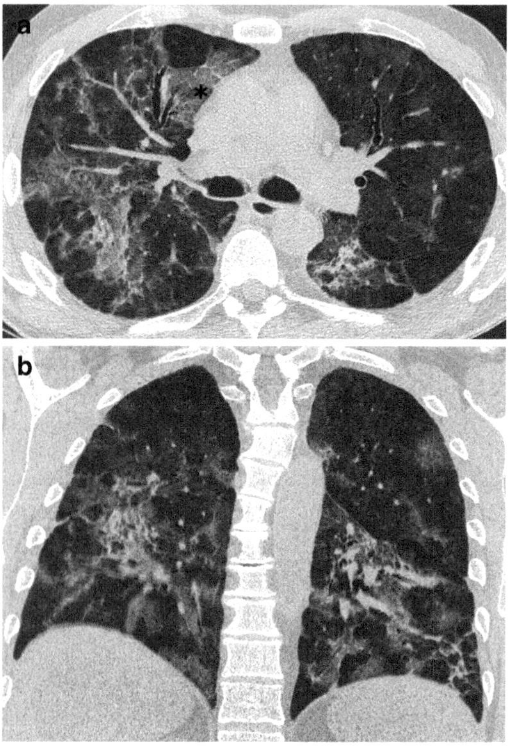


**Fig. 6.9** Hairy cell leukemia and COVID-19 pneumonia in a 55-year-old man. (**a**) Axial and (**b**) coronal CT scans show bilateral areas of ground-glass opacities in a peribronchovascular distribution

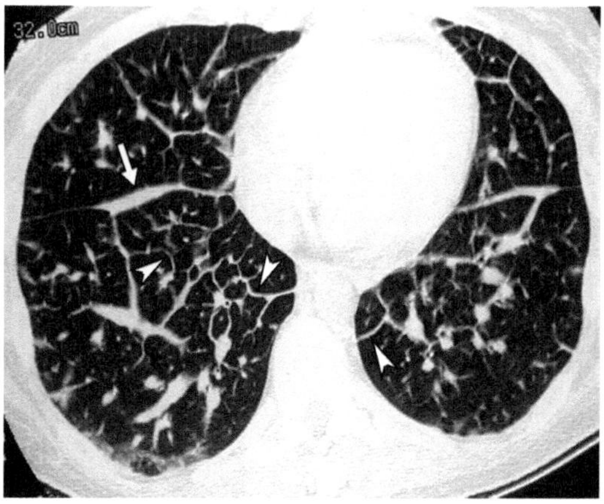

**Fig. 6.10** Pulmonary edema due to fluid overload in a 60-year-old woman with multiple myeloma. CT scan through lower lobes shows smooth septal thickening (arrowheads) in a gravity-dependent distribution. The right major fissure is also prominent due to subpleural edema (arrow)

Although the impact of COVID-19 infection on HSCT recipients has not yet been established, infected patients have a high mortality rate mainly in adults and patients with critical initial COVID-19 presentation (Fig. 6.9) [82].

## Noninfectious Complications

Noninfectious causes of lung injury after HSCT include a spectrum of syndromes: (a) pulmonary edema, (b) diffuse alveolar hemorrhage, (c) peri-engraftment respiratory distress syndrome, (d) drug-induced lung injury, (e) idiopathic pneumonia syndrome (IPS), (f) chronic graft-versus-host disease (cGVHD), (g) bronchiolitis obliterans syndrome (BOS), (h) air-leak syndrome, (i) organizing pneumonia (OP)/acute fibrinous organizing pneumonia (AFOP), and (j) posttransplant lymphoproliferative disorder (PTLD) [2, 6, 83].

Most of these causes are attributed to treatment-related toxicities and are influenced by the myeloablative conditioning regimens used before transplantation and tend to occur within specific time periods after transplantation [6].

Pulmonary edema is one of the earliest complications following HSCT and may occur even in those patients with normal cardiac function. It is usually secondary to the large volumes of fluids infused to minimize the toxicity of conditioning regimens and to transfusion of blood products [6]. Characteristic chest radiographic findings are diffuse interstitial lines such as Kerley A and Kerley B. The CT findings include enlarged pulmonary vessels, septal lines, peribronchial cuffing, ground-glass opacities, and small pleural effusions (Fig. 6.10) [10, 84].

Diffuse alveolar hemorrhage (DAH) is a life-threatening complication with a reported high mortality up to 70% [4, 85, 86]. It typically occurs as a diffuse process in the first month after transplant, often at the time of granulocyte recovery [8, 85, 87, 88]. The CT findings consist of extensive bilateral ground-glass opacities with or without superimposed intralobular linear opacities ("crazy-paving" pattern) (Fig. 6.11) [9, 10].

Peri-engraftment respiratory distress syndrome (PERDS), which is part of the engraft-

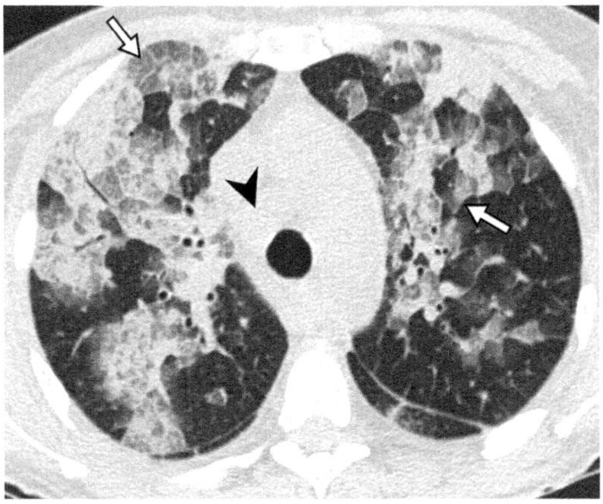

**Fig. 6.11** Diffuse alveolar hemorrhage in a 56-year-old man with non-Hodgkin lymphoma. CT scan demonstrates diffusely demarcated ground-glass opacities with some interstitial septal thickening (crazy-paving pattern) (arrows). Note paratracheal lymphadenopathy (arrowhead)

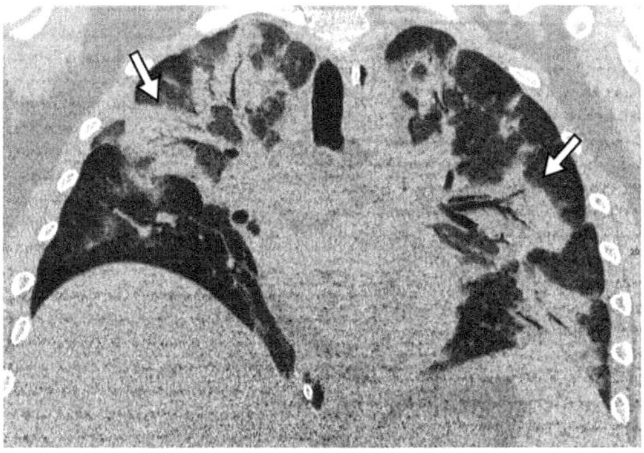

**Fig. 6.12** Peri-engraftment respiratory distress syndrome (PERDS) in a 25-year-old man with acute lymphoblastic leukemia. Coronal CT demonstrates bilateral areas of consolidation in a peribronchovascular distribution (arrows)

ment syndrome, represents a form of diffuse capillary leak associated with lung injury and pulmonary edema [4]. Chest radiograph findings are nonspecific and range from normality to bilateral air-space opacification, diffuse vascular redistribution, and pleural effusions. On CT, PERDS usually manifests as bilateral ground-glass opacification, air-space consolidation distributed at the hilar or peribronchial regions, and smooth thickening of interlobular septa (Fig. 6.12) [10, 84].

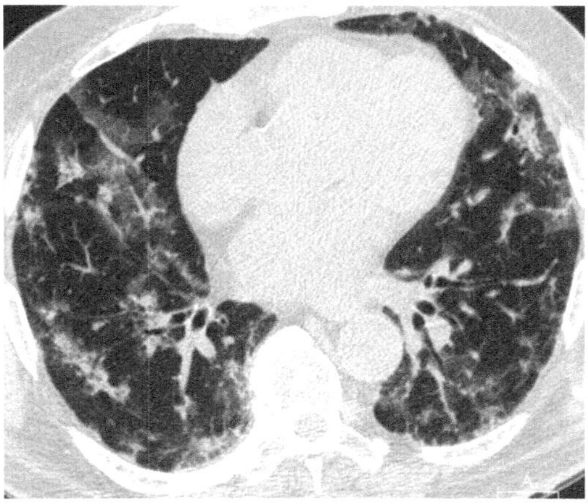

**Fig. 6.13** Bleomycin-induced lung injury in a 68-year-old man with Hodgkin disease. CT scan shows multiple areas of consolidation in a peripheral subpleural distribution

Drug-induced lung disease occurs in up to 10% of HSCT recipients and must always be considered in the differential diagnosis of pulmonary infiltrates. The CT findings have been divided into four categories according to their dominant pattern and distribution of disease: (1) fibrosis (irregular linear opacities with architectural distortion) with or without consolidation, (2) ground-glass opacities, (3) widespread bilateral consolidation (Fig. 6.13), and (4) bronchial wall thickening with areas of decreased attenuation [9, 10].

Idiopathic pneumonia syndrome (IPS) is defined by the American Thoracic Society as "an idiopathic syndrome of pneumopathy after HSCT, with evidence of widespread alveolar injury and in which an infectious etiology and cardiac dysfunction, acute renal failure or iatrogenic fluid overload have been excluded" [89]. The pathologic findings of IPS are like those found in acute interstitial pneumonia and acute respiratory distress syndrome (ARDS) and can be separated into acute exudative, subacute proliferative, and chronic fibrotic phases. Characteristic CT findings include focal or diffuse ground-glass opacity and air-space consolidation with a basilar predominance, a pattern consistent with non-cardiogenic pulmonary edema (Fig. 6.14) [90]. Architectural distortion, traction bronchiectasis, and the presence of honeycombing are indicative of the fibrotic phase of IPS [91].

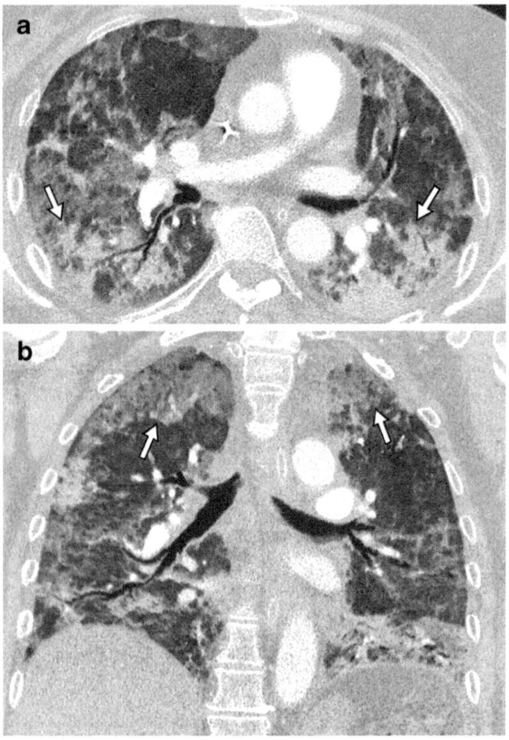


**Fig. 6.14** Idiopathic pneumonia syndrome in a 63-year-old woman with diffuse large B-cell lymphoma. (**a**) Axial and (**b**) coronal CT scans showing bilateral patchy areas of consolidation and ground-glass opacities (arrows)

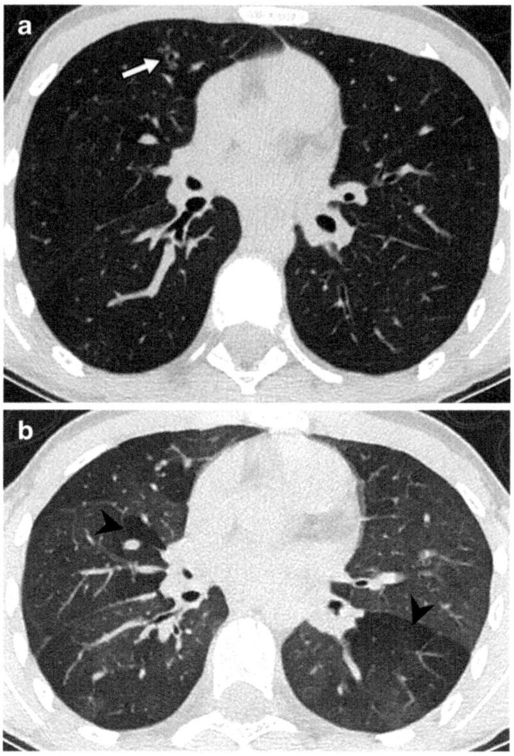


**Fig. 6.15** Bronchiolitis obliterans syndrome in an 18-year-old woman with acute lymphoblastic leukemia. (**a**) Inspiratory CT shows some dilatation of subsegmental airways in the right upper lobe (arrow). A tiny reduction in lung parenchymal density is also noted. (**b**) Expiratory CT performed at the same level demonstrates a significant reduction of parenchymal density representing air-trapping (arrows)

## Chronic Graft-Versus-Host Disease (cGVHD)

Chronic graft-versus-host disease is the most common non-relapse problem, occurring in approximately 60%–80% of long-term survivors of allogeneic HSC transplant, and is a major cause of late morbidity and mortality. Half of all patients who develop cGVHD are diagnosed between 100 days and 6 months after transplantation, although earlier and later developments are possible [92]. Pulmonary complications include bronchiolitis obliterans syndrome (BOS), organizing pneumonia (OP), and acute fibrinous and organizing pneumonia (AFOP).

Bronchiolitis obliterans syndrome (BOS), an obstructive pulmonary disorder that affects the small airways, has been reported in between 2% and 14% of allogeneic HSCT recipients who survive more than 3 months [93–95]. BOS is irreversible and associated with high mortality (up to 60%) at 3 years post-HSCT [96, 97]. Histologically, there is a predominantly constrictive bronchiolitis with destruction and narrowing of the bronchiolar lumen by fibrous tissue. Dynamic CT including paired inspiratory and expiratory scans may show patchy areas of decreased attenuation and vascularity (mosaic perfusion), air-trapping, and bronchial dilatation (Fig. 6.15) [98–100].

Air-leak syndromes have been recognized as a potentially fatal complication in HSCT recipients. Pneumothorax, pneumomediastinum, and subcutaneous emphysema are potential complications of patients with cGVHD and BOS (Fig. 6.16) [101]. Air in the peribronchial sheets (pulmonary interstitial emphysema) can be associated with impairment of respiratory function and/or chest pain, possibly resulting from compression of small vessels by the interstitial

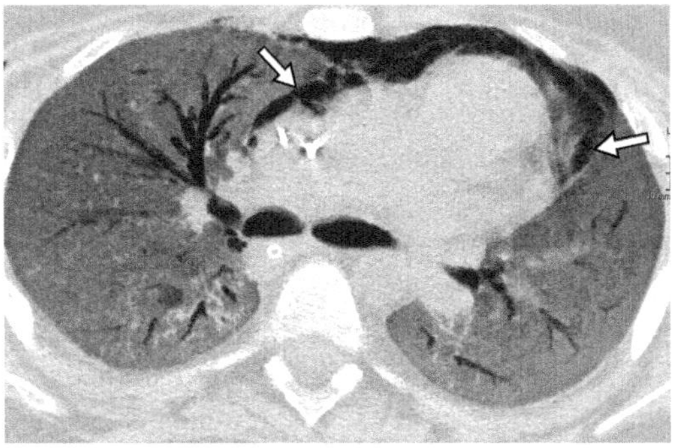

**Fig. 6.16** Air-leak syndrome in a 15-year-old boy with myelodysplastic syndrome and severe distress syndrome. CT scan shows diffuse ground-glass opacities associated with spontaneous pneumomediastinum (arrows)

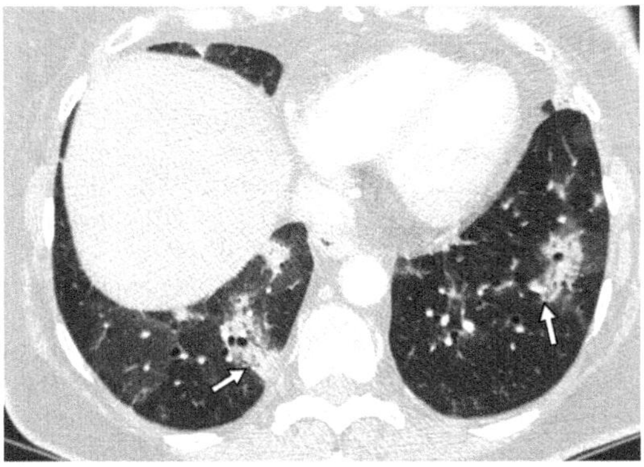

**Fig. 6.17** Organizing pneumonia in a 61-year-old woman. CT shows bilateral patchy areas of consolidation in lower lobes

air. Chest CT should be performed in any HSCT recipient with known or suspected cGVHD with acute clinical symptoms, especially chest pain, to rule out associated air-leak syndromes [101].

Organizing pneumonia (OP) is a well-known late manifestation of cGVHD occurring in up to 10% of HSCT [83, 93, 100]. CT findings consist of patchy or mass-like air-space consolidation, ground-glass opacities, reticular and linear opacities, and, occasionally, centrilobular nodules (Fig. 6.17) [21].

Acute fibrinous and organizing pneumonia (AFOP) is a recently described histologic pattern associated with acute lung injury in which the alveolar spaces are filled with organizing fibrin balls, in contrast to the true hyaline membranes found in diffuse alveolar damage [102, 103]. It has been described in the early and late post-HSCT period [104–106]. Imaging findings are

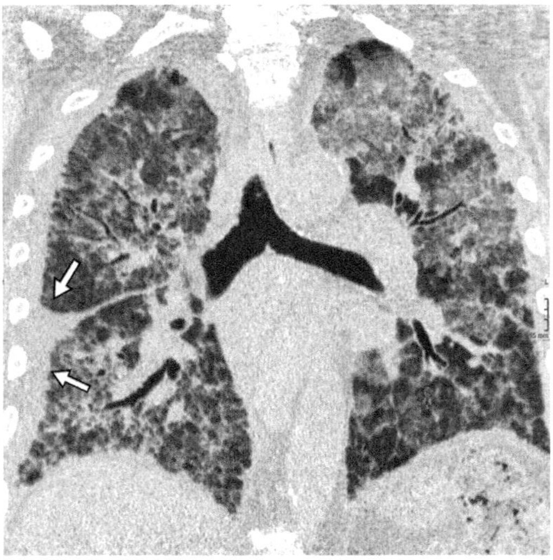

**Fig. 6.18** Acute fibrinous and organizing pneumonia (AFOP) in a 62-year-old man. Coronal CT shows diffuse bilateral ground-glass opacities and peribronchovascular consolidations. Note an associated right pleural effusion (arrows)

indistinguishable from OP and can encompass both focal and diffuse parenchymal abnormality (Fig. 6.18) [107].

## Other Noninfectious Pulmonary Complications

Pleuroparenchymal fibroelastosis (PPFE) is a rare entity characterized by an upper lobe pleural thickening with associated subpleural interstitial proliferation of predominantly elastic fibers [108–110]. The idiopathic form of PPF is categorized as a rare idiopathic interstitial pneumonia in the current classification [110, 111]. PPFE has been associated with chronic HP, connective tissue disease, drugs, and hematopoietic stem cell or lung transplantation. PPFE has been described in <0.5% of patients post-HSCT and typically presents many years posttransplantation [112–114]. Characteristic CT manifestations comprise nodular apical subpleural thickening, consolidation, and reticulation, associated with upper lobe volume loss, traction bronchiectasis, and superior retraction of the hila (Fig. 6.19) [109, 115, 116].

Posttransplant lymphoproliferative disorder (PTLD) represents a heterogeneous group of

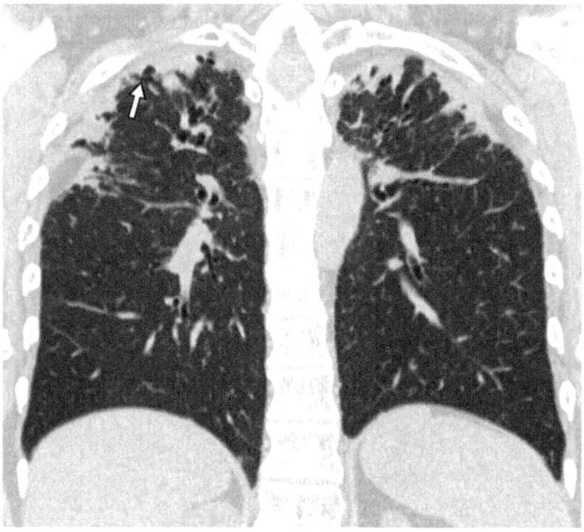

**Fig. 6.19** Pleuroparenchymal fibroelastosis in a 50-year-old woman with myeloblastic leukemia, 6 years after HSCT. Coronal CT shows biapical pleural thickening and subpleural fibrosis with traction bronchiectasis (arrow). Note associated upper lobes volume loss

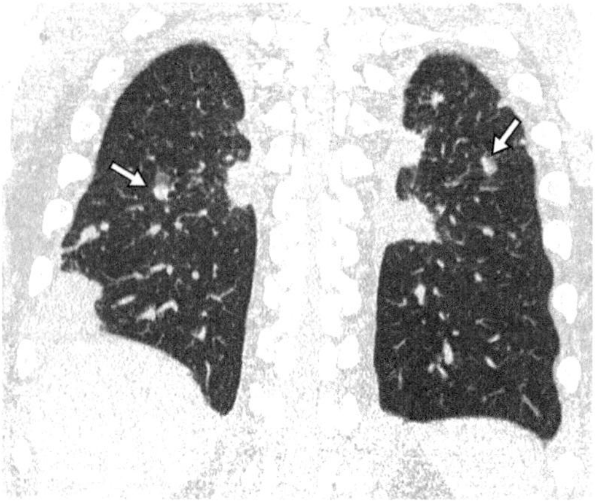

**Fig. 6.20** Posttransplantation lymphoproliferative disorder (PTLD) in a 54-year-old man with refractory anemia with excess blasts. Coronal CT shows bilateral ill-defined nodular opacities (arrows)

lymphoid/plasmacytic disorders that occurs by EBV reactivation after solid organ or HSCT [117–119]. The most common intrathoracic manifestations of PTLD are randomly distributed well-circumscribed pulmonary nodules (0.3–5 cm in diameter), mediastinal and hilar adenopathy, and patchy air-space consolidation (Fig. 6.20) [120–122].

## Conclusion

Imaging study plays an important role in the diagnosis and management of all phases of the HSCT recipients with suspected pulmonary complications. Although CT is not recommended for the initial evaluation, it is frequently appropriate in those cases with normal, equivocal, or nonspecific radiographic findings. A combination of the clinical information and CT findings, which are sometimes characteristic of several entities, may help the clinician and radiologist in forming a meaningful differential diagnosis of these disorders and improve the diagnosis and patient care.

## References


1. Yen KT, Lee AS, Krowka MJ, Burger CD. Pulmonary complications in bone marrow transplantation: a practical approach to diagnosis and treatment. Clin Chest Med. 2004;25(1):189–201. https://doi.org/10.1016/S0272-5231(03)00121-7.
2. Shiari A, Nassar M, Soubani AO. Major pulmonary complications following hematopoietic stem cell transplantation: what the pulmonologist needs to know. Respir Med. 2021;185:106493. https://doi.org/10.1016/j.rmed.2021.106493.
3. Soubani AO, Miller KB, Hassoun PM. Pulmonary complications of bone marrow transplantation. Chest. 1996;109(4):1066–77. https://doi.org/10.1378/chest.109.4.1066.
4. Chi AK, Soubani AO, White AC, Miller KB. An update on pulmonary complications of hematopoietic stem cell transplantation. Chest. 2013;144(6):1913–22. https://doi.org/10.1378/chest.12-1708.
5. Chan CK, Hyland RH, Hutcheon MA. Pulmonary complications following bone marrow transplantation. Clin Chest Med. 1990;11(2):323–32.
6. Worthy SA, Flint JD, Muller NL. Pulmonary complications after bone marrow transplantation: high-resolution CT and pathologic findings. Radiographics. 1997;17(6):1359–71. https://doi.org/10.1148/radiographics.17.6.9397451.
7. Ahya VN. Noninfectious acute lung injury syndromes early after hematopoietic stem cell transplantation. Clin Chest Med. 2017;38(4):595–606. https://doi.org/10.1016/j.ccm.2017.07.002.
8. Alam S, Chan KM. Noninfectious pulmonary complications after organ transplantation. Curr Opin Pulm Med. 1996;2(5):412–8. https://doi.org/10.1097/00063198-199609000-00011.
9. Evans A, Steward CG, Lyburn ID, Grier DJ. Imaging in haematopoietic stem cell transplantation. Clin

Radiol. 2003;58(3):201–14. https://doi.org/10.1016/s0009-9260(02)00475-0.
10. Wah TM, Moss HA, Robertson RJ, Barnard DL. Pulmonary complications following bone marrow transplantation. Br J Radiol. 2003;76(906):373–9. https://doi.org/10.1259/bjr/66835905.
11. Janzen DL, Padley SP, Adler BD, Muller NL. Acute pulmonary complications in immunocompromised non-AIDS patients: comparison of diagnostic accuracy of CT and chest radiography. Clin Radiol. 1993;47(3):159–65. https://doi.org/10.1016/s0009-9260(05)81153-5.
12. Tanaka N, Kunihiro Y, Yujiri T, Ando T, Gondo T, Kido S, et al. High-resolution computed tomography of chest complications in patients treated with hematopoietic stem cell transplantation. Jpn J Radiol. 2011;29(4):229–35. https://doi.org/10.1007/s11604-010-0544-8.
13. Tanaka N, Matsumoto T, Miura G, Emoto T, Matsunaga N. HRCT findings of chest complications in patients with leukemia. Eur Radiol. 2002;12(6):1512–22. https://doi.org/10.1007/s003300101112.
14. Arakawa H, Webb WR. Air trapping on expiratory high-resolution CT scans in the absence of inspiratory scan abnormalities: correlation with pulmonary function tests and differential diagnosis. AJR Am J Roentgenol. 1998;170(5):1349–53. https://doi.org/10.2214/ajr.170.5.9574614.
15. Franquet T, Gimenez A, Ketai L, Mazzini S, Rial A, Pomar V, et al. Air trapping in COVID-19 patients following hospital discharge: retrospective evaluation with paired inspiratory/expiratory thin-section CT. Eur Radiol. 2022;32:4427. https://doi.org/10.1007/s00330-022-08580-2.
16. Tanaka N, Matsumoto T, Miura G, Emoto T, Matsunaga N, Ueda K, et al. Air trapping at CT: high prevalence in asymptomatic subjects with normal pulmonary function. Radiology. 2003;227(3):776–85. https://doi.org/10.1148/radiol.2273020352.
17. Pena E, Souza CA, Escuissato DL, Gomes MM, Allan D, Tay J, et al. Noninfectious pulmonary complications after hematopoietic stem cell transplantation: practical approach to imaging diagnosis. Radiographics. 2014;34(3):663–83. https://doi.org/10.1148/rg.343135080.
18. Kotloff RM, Ahya VN, Crawford SW. Pulmonary complications of solid organ and hematopoietic stem cell transplantation. Am J Respir Crit Care Med. 2004;170(1):22–48. https://doi.org/10.1164/rccm.200309-1322SO.
19. Nusair S, Breuer R, Shapira MY, Berkman N, Or R. Low incidence of pulmonary complications following nonmyeloablative stem cell transplantation. Eur Respir J. 2004;23(3):440–5. https://doi.org/10.1183/09031936.04.00053004.
20. Coy DL, Ormazabal A, Godwin JD, Lalani T. Imaging evaluation of pulmonary and abdominal complications following hematopoietic stem cell transplantation. Radiographics. 2005;25(2):305–17; discussion 18. https://doi.org/10.1148/rg.252045037.
21. Franquet T, Muller NL, Lee KS, Gimenez A, Flint JD. High-resolution CT and pathologic findings of noninfectious pulmonary complications after hematopoietic stem cell transplantation. AJR Am J Roentgenol. 2005;184(2):629–37. https://doi.org/10.2214/ajr.184.2.01840629.
22. Crawford SW, Hackman RC, Clark JG. Open lung biopsy diagnosis of diffuse pulmonary infiltrates after marrow transplantation. Chest. 1988;94(5):949–53. https://doi.org/10.1378/chest.94.5.949.
23. Cunningham I. Pulmonary infections after bone marrow transplant. Semin Respir Infect. 1992;7(2):132–8.
24. Crawford SW. Noninfectious lung disease in the immunocompromised host. Respiration. 1999;66(5):385–95. https://doi.org/10.1159/000029418.
25. Cardozo BL, Hagenbeek A. Interstitial pneumonitis following bone marrow transplantation: pathogenesis and therapeutic considerations. Eur J Cancer Clin Oncol. 1985;21(1):43–51. https://doi.org/10.1016/0277-5379(85)90199-3.
26. Cardozo BL, Zoetelief H, van Bekkum DW, Zurcher C, Hagenbeek A. Lung damage following bone marrow transplantation: I. The contribution of irradiation. Int J Radiat Oncol Biol Phys. 1985;11(5):907–14. https://doi.org/10.1016/0360-3016(85)90112-9.
27. Aronchick JM. Pulmonary infections in cancer and bone marrow transplant patients. Semin Roentgenol. 2000;35(2):140–51. https://doi.org/10.1053/ro.2000.6152.
28. Choi YH, Leung AN. Radiologic findings: pulmonary infections after bone marrow transplantation. J Thorac Imaging. 1999;14(3):201–6.
29. Kaiser L, Huguenin T, Lew PD, Chapuis B, Pittet D. Invasive aspergillosis. Clinical features of 35 proven cases at a single institution. Medicine. 1998;77(3):188–94. https://doi.org/10.1097/00005792-199805000-00004.
30. Fukuda T, Boeckh M, Guthrie KA, Mattson DK, Owens S, Wald A, et al. Invasive aspergillosis before allogeneic hematopoietic stem cell transplantation: 10-year experience at a single transplant center. Biol Blood Marrow Transplant. 2004;10(7):494–503. https://doi.org/10.1016/j.bbmt.2004.02.006.
31. Kapoor N, Copelan EA, Tutschka PJ. Cytomegalovirus infection in bone marrow transplant recipients: use of intravenous gamma globulin as a prophylactic and therapeutic agent. Transplant Proc. 1989;21(1 Pt 3):3095–6.
32. Gosselin MV, Adams RH. Pulmonary complications in bone marrow transplantation. J Thorac Imaging. 2002;17(2):132–44. https://doi.org/10.1097/00005382-200204000-00005.
33. Paulin T, Ringden O, Nilsson B, Lonnqvist B, Gahrton G. Variables predicting bacterial and fungal infections after allogeneic marrow engraftment. Transplantation. 1987;43(3):393–8. https://doi.org/10.1097/00007890-198703000-00015.

34. Choi MH, Jung JI, Chung WD, Kim YJ, Lee SE, Han DH, et al. Acute pulmonary complications in patients with hematologic malignancies. Radiographics. 2014;34(6):1755–68. https://doi.org/10.1148/rg.346130107.
35. Maschmeyer G. Pneumonia in febrile neutropenic patients: radiologic diagnosis. Curr Opin Oncol. 2001;13(4):229–35. https://doi.org/10.1097/00001622-200107000-00004.
36. Aquino SL, Gamsu G, Webb WR, Kee ST. Tree-in-bud pattern: frequency and significance on thin section CT. J Comput Assist Tomogr. 1996;20(4):594–9. https://doi.org/10.1097/00004728-199607000-00018.
37. Jung JI, Lee DG, Kim YJ, Yoon HK, Kim CC, Park SH. Pulmonary tuberculosis after hematopoietic stem cell transplantation: radiologic findings. J Thorac Imaging. 2009;24(1):10–6. https://doi.org/10.1097/RTI.0b013e31818c6b97.
38. Navari RM, Sullivan KM, Springmeyer SC, Siegel MS, Meyers JD, Buckner CD, et al. Mycobacterial infections in marrow transplant patients. Transplantation. 1983;36(5):509–13. https://doi.org/10.1097/00007890-198311000-00008.
39. Mohite U, Das M, Saikia T, Parikh P, Gopal R, Kelkar R, et al. Mycobacterial pulmonary infection post allogeneic bone marrow transplantation. Leuk Lymphoma. 2001;40(5-6):675–8. https://doi.org/10.3109/10428190109097667.
40. Knoll BM. Update on nontuberculous mycobacterial infections in solid organ and hematopoietic stem cell transplant recipients. Curr Infect Dis Rep. 2014;16(9):421. https://doi.org/10.1007/s11908-014-0421-1.
41. Doucette K, Fishman JA. Nontuberculous mycobacterial infection in hematopoietic stem cell and solid organ transplant recipients. Clin Infect Dis. 2004;38(10):1428–39. https://doi.org/10.1086/420746.
42. Alangaden GJ, Wahiduzzaman M, Chandrasekar PH, Bone Marrow Transplant G. Aspergillosis: The most common community-acquired pneumonia with gram-negative Bacilli as copathogens in stem cell transplant recipients with graft-versus-host disease. Clin Infect Dis. 2002;35(6):659–64. https://doi.org/10.1086/342061.
43. Bag R. Fungal pneumonias in transplant recipients. Curr Opin Pulm Med. 2003;9(3):193–8. https://doi.org/10.1097/00063198-200305000-00007.
44. Aquino SL, Kee ST, Warnock ML, Gamsu G. Pulmonary aspergillosis: imaging findings with pathologic correlation. AJR Am J Roentgenol. 1994;163(4):811–5. https://doi.org/10.2214/ajr.163.4.8092014.
45. Gotway MB, Dawn SK, Caoili EM, Reddy GP, Araoz PA, Webb WR. The radiologic spectrum of pulmonary Aspergillus infections. J Comput Assist Tomogr. 2002;26(2):159–73. https://doi.org/10.1097/00004728-200203000-00001.
46. Franquet T, Gimenez A, Hidalgo A. Imaging of opportunistic fungal infections in immunocompromised patient. Eur J Radiol. 2004;51(2):130–8. https://doi.org/10.1016/j.ejrad.2004.03.007.
47. Mori M, Galvin JR, Barloon TJ, Gingrich RD, Stanford W. Fungal pulmonary infections after bone marrow transplantation: evaluation with radiography and CT. Radiology. 1991;178(3):721–6. https://doi.org/10.1148/radiology.178.3.1994408.
48. Young AY, Leiva Juarez MM, Evans SE. Fungal pneumonia in patients with hematologic malignancy and hematopoietic stem cell transplantation. Clin Chest Med. 2017;38(3):479–91. https://doi.org/10.1016/j.ccm.2017.04.009.
49. Harrison N, Mitterbauer M, Tobudic S, Kalhs P, Rabitsch W, Greinix H, et al. Incidence and characteristics of invasive fungal diseases in allogeneic hematopoietic stem cell transplant recipients: a retrospective cohort study. BMC Infect Dis. 2015;15:584. https://doi.org/10.1186/s12879-015-1329-6.
50. Gregg KS, Kauffman CA. Invasive aspergillosis: epidemiology, clinical aspects, and treatment. Semin Respir Crit Care Med. 2015;36(5):662–72. https://doi.org/10.1055/s-0035-1562893.
51. Denning DW. Early diagnosis of invasive aspergillosis. Lancet. 2000;355(9202):423–4. https://doi.org/10.1016/S0140-6736(00)82003-6.
52. Kuhlman JE, Fishman EK, Burch PA, Karp JE, Zerhouni EA, Siegelman SS. CT of invasive pulmonary aspergillosis. AJR Am J Roentgenol. 1988;150(5):1015–20. https://doi.org/10.2214/ajr.150.5.1015.
53. Kuhlman JE, Fishman EK, Siegelman SS. Invasive pulmonary aspergillosis in acute leukemia: characteristic findings on CT, the CT halo sign, and the role of CT in early diagnosis. Radiology. 1985;157(3):611–4. https://doi.org/10.1148/radiology.157.3.3864189.
54. Curtis AM, Smith GJ, Ravin CE. Air crescent sign of invasive aspergillosis. Radiology. 1979;133(1):17–21. https://doi.org/10.1148/133.1.17.
55. Gefter WB, Albelda SM, Talbot GH, Gerson SL, Cassileth PA, Miller WT. Invasive pulmonary aspergillosis and acute leukemia. Limitations in the diagnostic utility of the air crescent sign. Radiology. 1985;157(3):605–10. https://doi.org/10.1148/radiology.157.3.4059547.
56. Franquet T, Muller NL, Gimenez A, Guembe P, de La Torre J, Bague S. Spectrum of pulmonary aspergillosis: histologic, clinical, and radiologic findings. Radiographics. 2001;21(4):825–37. https://doi.org/10.1148/radiographics.21.4.g01jl03825.
57. Franquet T, Serrano F, Gimenez A, Rodriguez-Arias JM, Puzo C. Necrotizing Aspergillosis of large airways: CT findings in eight patients. J Comput Assist Tomogr. 2002;26(3):342–5. https://doi.org/10.1097/00004728-200205000-00004.
58. Franquet T, Muller NL, Oikonomou A, Flint JD. Aspergillus infection of the airways: computed tomography and pathologic findings. J Comput

Assist Tomogr. 2004;28(1):10–6. https://doi.org/10.1097/00004728-200401000-00002.
59. Georgiadou SP, Sipsas NV, Marom EM, Kontoyiannis DP. The diagnostic value of halo and reversed halo signs for invasive mold infections in compromised hosts. Clin Infect Dis. 2011;52(9):1144–55. https://doi.org/10.1093/cid/cir122.
60. McAdams HP, Rosado de Christenson M, Strollo DC, Patz EF Jr. Pulmonary mucormycosis: radiologic findings in 32 cases. AJR Am J Roentgenol. 1997;168(6):1541–8. https://doi.org/10.2214/ajr.168.6.9168721.
61. Connolly JE Jr, McAdams HP, Erasmus JJ, Rosado-de-Christenson ML. Opportunistic fungal pneumonia. J Thorac Imaging. 1999;14(1):51–62. https://doi.org/10.1097/00005382-199901000-00005.
62. Alexander BD, Lamoth F, Heussel CP, Prokop CS, Desai SR, Morrissey CO, et al. Guidance on imaging for invasive pulmonary Aspergillosis and Mucormycosis: from the Imaging Working Group for the Revision and Update of the Consensus Definitions of Fungal Disease from the EORTC/MSGERC. Clin Infect Dis. 2021;72(Suppl 2):S79–88. https://doi.org/10.1093/cid/ciaa1855.
63. Sharma S, Nadrous HF, Peters SG, Tefferi A, Litzow MR, Aubry MC, et al. Pulmonary complications in adult blood and marrow transplant recipients: autopsy findings. Chest. 2005;128(3):1385–92. https://doi.org/10.1378/chest.128.3.1385.
64. Buff SJ, McLelland R, Gallis HA, Matthay R, Putman CE. Candida albicans pneumonia: radiographic appearance. AJR Am J Roentgenol. 1982;138(4):645–8. https://doi.org/10.2214/ajr.138.4.645.
65. Franquet T, Muller NL, Lee KS, Oikonomou A, Flint JD. Pulmonary candidiasis after hematopoietic stem cell transplantation: thin-section CT findings. Radiology. 2005;236(1):332–7. https://doi.org/10.1148/radiol.2361031772.
66. Saito T, Seo S, Kanda Y, Shoji N, Ogasawara T, Murakami J, et al. Early onset Pneumocystis carinii pneumonia after allogeneic peripheral blood stem cell transplantation. Am J Hematol. 2001;67(3):206–9. https://doi.org/10.1002/ajh.1109.
67. Boiselle PM, Tocino I, Hooley RJ, Pumerantz AS, Selwyn PA, Neklesa VP, et al. Chest radiograph interpretation of Pneumocystis carinii pneumonia, bacterial pneumonia, and pulmonary tuberculosis in HIV-positive patients: accuracy, distinguishing features, and mimics. J Thorac Imaging. 1997;12(1):47–53. https://doi.org/10.1097/00005382-199701000-00007.
68. Gruden JF, Huang L, Turner J, Webb WR, Merrifield C, Stansell JD, et al. High-resolution CT in the evaluation of clinically suspected Pneumocystis carinii pneumonia in AIDS patients with normal, equivocal, or nonspecific radiographic findings. AJR Am J Roentgenol. 1997;169(4):967–75. https://doi.org/10.2214/ajr.169.4.9308446.
69. Kanne JP, Yandow DR, Meyer CA. Pneumocystis jiroveci pneumonia: high-resolution CT findings in patients with and without HIV infection. AJR Am J Roentgenol. 2012;198(6):W555–61. https://doi.org/10.2214/AJR.11.7329.
70. Krinzman S, Basgoz N, Kradin R, Shepard JA, Flieder DB, Wright CD, et al. Respiratory syncytial virus-associated infections in adult recipients of solid organ transplants. J Heart Lung Transplant. 1998;17(2):202–10.
71. Markovic SN, Adlakha A, Smith TF, Walker RC. Respiratory syncytial virus pneumonitis-induced diffuse alveolar damage in an autologous bone marrow transplant recipient. Mayo Clin Proc. 1998;73(2):153–6. https://doi.org/10.1016/S0025-6196(11)63648-3.
72. Nichols WG, Guthrie KA, Corey L, Boeckh M. Influenza infections after hematopoietic stem cell transplantation: risk factors, mortality, and the effect of antiviral therapy. Clin Infect Dis. 2004;39(9):1300–6. https://doi.org/10.1086/425004.
73. Franquet T. Imaging of pulmonary viral pneumonia. Radiology. 2011;260(1):18–39. https://doi.org/10.1148/radiol.11092149.
74. Franquet T, Lee KS, Muller NL. Thin-section CT findings in 32 immunocompromised patients with cytomegalovirus pneumonia who do not have AIDS. AJR Am J Roentgenol. 2003;181(4):1059–63. https://doi.org/10.2214/ajr.181.4.1811059.
75. Franquet T, Rodriguez S, Martino R, Salinas T, Gimenez A, Hidalgo A. Human metapneumovirus infection in hematopoietic stem cell transplant recipients: high-resolution computed tomography findings. J Comput Assist Tomogr. 2005;29(2):223–7. https://doi.org/10.1097/01.rct.0000157087.14838.4c.
76. Oikonomou A, Muller NL, Nantel S. Radiographic and high-resolution CT findings of influenza virus pneumonia in patients with hematologic malignancies. AJR Am J Roentgenol. 2003;181(2):507–11. https://doi.org/10.2214/ajr.181.2.1810507.
77. Gasparetto EL, Escuissato DL, Marchiori E, Ono S, Frare e Silva RL, Muller NL. High-resolution CT findings of respiratory syncytial virus pneumonia after bone marrow transplantation. AJR Am J Roentgenol. 2004;182(5):1133–7. https://doi.org/10.2214/ajr.182.5.1821133.
78. Foot AB, Caul EO, Roome AP, Darville JM, Oakhill A. Cytomegalovirus pneumonitis and bone marrow transplantation: identification of a specific high risk group. J Clin Pathol. 1993;46(5):415–9. https://doi.org/10.1136/jcp.46.5.415.
79. Gasparetto EL, Ono SE, Escuissato D, Marchiori E, Roldan L, Marques HL, et al. Cytomegalovirus pneumonia after bone marrow transplantation: high resolution CT findings. Br J Radiol. 2004;77(921):724–7. https://doi.org/10.1259/bjr/70800575.
80. Kang EY, Patz EF Jr, Muller NL. Cytomegalovirus pneumonia in transplant patients: CT findings. J

Comput Assist Tomogr. 1996;20(2):295–9. https://doi.org/10.1097/00004728-199603000-00024.
81. Franquet T, Muller NL, Gimenez A, Martinez S, Madrid M, Domingo P. Infectious pulmonary nodules in immunocompromised patients: usefulness of computed tomography in predicting their etiology. J Comput Assist Tomogr. 2003;27(4):461–8. https://doi.org/10.1097/00004728-200307000-00001.
82. Daudt LE, Corso MCM, Kerbauy MN, de Assis L, Rechenmacher C, Colturato I, et al. COVID-19 in HSCT recipients: a collaborative study of the Brazilian Society of Marrow Transplantation (SBTMO). Bone Marrow Transplant. 2022;57(3):453–9. https://doi.org/10.1038/s41409-021-01561-x.
83. Khurshid I, Anderson LC. Non-infectious pulmonary complications after bone marrow transplantation. Postgrad Med J. 2002;78(919):257–62. https://doi.org/10.1136/pmj.78.919.257.
84. Evans SE, Ost DE. Pneumonia in the neutropenic cancer patient. Curr Opin Pulm Med. 2015;21(3):260–71. https://doi.org/10.1097/MCP.0000000000000156.
85. Afessa B, Tefferi A, Litzow MR, Peters SG. Outcome of diffuse alveolar hemorrhage in hematopoietic stem cell transplant recipients. Am J Respir Crit Care Med. 2002;166(10):1364–8. https://doi.org/10.1164/rccm.200208-792OC.
86. Ben-Abraham R, Paret G, Cohen R, Szold O, Cividalli G, Toren A, et al. Diffuse alveolar hemorrhage following allogeneic bone marrow transplantation in children. Chest. 2003;124(2):660–4. https://doi.org/10.1378/chest.124.2.660.
87. Afessa B, Abdulai RM, Kremers WK, Hogan WJ, Litzow MR, Peters SG. Risk factors and outcome of pulmonary complications after autologous hematopoietic stem cell transplant. Chest. 2012;141(2):442–50. https://doi.org/10.1378/chest.10-2889.
88. Schmidt-Wolf I, Schwerdtfeger R, Schwella N, Gallardo J, Schmid HJ, Huhn D, et al. Diffuse pulmonary alveolar hemorrhage after allogeneic bone marrow transplantation. Ann Hematol. 1993;67(3):139–41. https://doi.org/10.1007/BF01701739.
89. Panoskaltsis-Mortari A, Griese M, Madtes DK, Belperio JA, Haddad IY, Folz RJ, et al. An official American Thoracic Society research statement: noninfectious lung injury after hematopoietic stem cell transplantation: idiopathic pneumonia syndrome. Am J Respir Crit Care Med. 2011;183(9):1262–79. https://doi.org/10.1164/rccm.2007-413ST.
90. Kantrow SP, Hackman RC, Boeckh M, Myerson D, Crawford SW. Idiopathic pneumonia syndrome: changing spectrum of lung injury after marrow transplantation. Transplantation. 1997;63(8):1079–86. https://doi.org/10.1097/00007890-199704270-00006.
91. Shankar G, Cohen DA. Idiopathic pneumonia syndrome after bone marrow transplantation: the role of pre-transplant radiation conditioning and local cytokine dysregulation in promoting lung inflammation and fibrosis. Int J Exp Pathol. 2001;82(2):101–13. https://doi.org/10.1111/j.1365-2613.2001.iep0082-0101-x.
92. Patriarca F, Skert C, Sperotto A, Damiani D, Cerno M, Geromin A, et al. Incidence, outcome, and risk factors of late-onset noninfectious pulmonary complications after unrelated donor stem cell transplantation. Bone Marrow Transplant. 2004;33(7):751–8. https://doi.org/10.1038/sj.bmt.1704426.
93. Pandya CM, Soubani AO. Bronchiolitis obliterans following hematopoietic stem cell transplantation: a clinical update. Clin Transplant. 2010;24(3):291–306. https://doi.org/10.1111/j.1399-0012.2009.01122.x.
94. Yoshihara S, Yanik G, Cooke KR, Mineishi S. Bronchiolitis obliterans syndrome (BOS), bronchiolitis obliterans organizing pneumonia (BOOP), and other late-onset noninfectious pulmonary complications following allogeneic hematopoietic stem cell transplantation. Biol Blood Marrow Transplant. 2007;13(7):749–59. https://doi.org/10.1016/j.bbmt.2007.05.001.
95. Bergeron A, Cheng GS. Bronchiolitis obliterans syndrome and other late pulmonary complications after allogeneic hematopoietic stem cell transplantation. Clin Chest Med. 2017;38(4):607–21. https://doi.org/10.1016/j.ccm.2017.07.003.
96. Freudenberger TD, Madtes DK, Curtis JR, Cummings P, Storer BE, Hackman RC. Association between acute and chronic graft-versus-host disease and bronchiolitis obliterans organizing pneumonia in recipients of hematopoietic stem cell transplants. Blood. 2003;102(10):3822–8. https://doi.org/10.1182/blood-2002-06-1813.
97. Kwok WC, Liang BM, Lui MMS, Tam TCC, Sim JPY, Tse EWC, et al. Rapid versus gradual lung function decline in bronchiolitis obliterans syndrome after haematopoietic stem cell transplantation is associated with survival outcome. Respirology. 2019;24(5):459–66. https://doi.org/10.1111/resp.13472.
98. Urbanski SJ, Kossakowska AE, Curtis J, Chan CK, Hutcheon MA, Hyland RH, et al. Idiopathic small airways pathology in patients with graft-versus-host disease following allogeneic bone marrow transplantation. Am J Surg Pathol. 1987;11(12):965–71. https://doi.org/10.1097/00000478-198712000-00007.
99. Ooi GC, Peh WC, Ip M. High-resolution computed tomography of bronchiolitis obliterans syndrome after bone marrow transplantation. Respiration. 1998;65(3):187–91. https://doi.org/10.1159/000029257.
100. Winer-Muram HT, Gurney JW, Bozeman PM, Krance RA. Pulmonary complications after bone marrow transplantation. Radiol Clin North Am. 1996;34(1):97–117.
101. Franquet T, Rodriguez S, Hernandez JM, Martino R, Gimenez A, Hidalgo A, et al. Air-leak syndromes in hematopoietic stem cell transplant recipients with chronic GVHD: high-resolution CT findings. J Thorac Imaging. 2007;22(4):335–40. https://doi.org/10.1097/RTI.0b013e3180cab6cf.

102. Beasley MB. The pathologist's approach to acute lung injury. Arch Pathol Lab Med. 2010;134(5):719–27. https://doi.org/10.1043/1543-2165-134.5.719.
103. Beasley MB, Franks TJ, Galvin JR, Gochuico B, Travis WD. Acute fibrinous and organizing pneumonia: a histological pattern of lung injury and possible variant of diffuse alveolar damage. Arch Pathol Lab Med. 2002;126(9):1064–70. https://doi.org/10.5858/2002-126-1064-AFAOP.
104. Nguyen LP, Ahdoot S, Sriratanaviriyakul N, Zhang Y, Stollenwerk N, Schivo M, et al. Acute fibrinous and organizing pneumonia associated with allogenic hematopoietic stem cell transplant successfully treated with corticosteroids: a two-patient case series. J Investig Med High Impact Case Rep. 2016;4(2):2324709616643990. https://doi.org/10.1177/2324709616643990.
105. Lee SM, Park JJ, Sung SH, Kim Y, Lee KE, Mun YC, et al. Acute fibrinous and organizing pneumonia following hematopoietic stem cell transplantation. Korean J Intern Med. 2009;24(2):156–9. https://doi.org/10.3904/kjim.2009.24.2.156.
106. Simmons GL, Chung HM, McCarty JM, Toor AA, Farkas D, Miller K, et al. Treatment of acute fibrinous organizing pneumonia following hematopoietic cell transplantation with etanercept. Bone Marrow Transplant. 2017;52(1):141–3. https://doi.org/10.1038/bmt.2016.197.
107. Kligerman SJ, Franks TJ, Galvin JR. From the radiologic pathology archives: organization and fibrosis as a response to lung injury in diffuse alveolar damage, organizing pneumonia, and acute fibrinous and organizing pneumonia. Radiographics. 2013;33(7):1951–75. https://doi.org/10.1148/rg.337130057.
108. Rosenbaum JN, Butt YM, Johnson KA, Meyer K, Batra K, Kanne JP, et al. Pleuroparenchymal fibroelastosis: a pattern of chronic lung injury. Hum Pathol. 2015;46(1):137–46. https://doi.org/10.1016/j.humpath.2014.10.007.
109. Reddy TL, Tominaga M, Hansell DM, von der Thusen J, Rassl D, Parfrey H, et al. Pleuroparenchymal fibroelastosis: a spectrum of histopathological and imaging phenotypes. Eur Respir J. 2012;40(2):377–85. https://doi.org/10.1183/09031936.00165111.
110. Travis WD, Costabel U, Hansell DM, King TE Jr, Lynch DA, Nicholson AG, et al. An official American Thoracic Society/European Respiratory Society statement: update of the international multidisciplinary classification of the idiopathic interstitial pneumonias. Am J Respir Crit Care Med. 2013;188(6):733–48. https://doi.org/10.1164/rccm.201308-1483ST.
111. Raghu G, Rochwerg B, Zhang Y, Garcia CA, Azuma A, Behr J, et al. An official ATS/ERS/JRS/ALAT clinical practice guideline: treatment of idiopathic pulmonary fibrosis. An update of the 2011 Clinical Practice Guideline. Am J Respir Crit Care Med. 2015;192(2):e3–19. https://doi.org/10.1164/rccm.201506-1063ST.
112. Astashchanka A, Ryan J, Lin E, Nokes B, Jamieson C, Kligerman S, et al. Pulmonary complications in hematopoietic stem cell transplant recipients—a clinician primer. J Clin Med. 2021;10(15):3227. https://doi.org/10.3390/jcm10153227.
113. Bondeelle L, Gras J, Michonneau D, Houdouin V, Hermet E, Blin N, et al. Pleuroparenchymal fibroelastosis after allogeneic hematopoietic stem cell transplantation. Bone Marrow Transplant. 2020;55(5):982–6. https://doi.org/10.1038/s41409-019-0636-8.
114. Mariani F, Gatti B, Rocca A, Bonifazi F, Cavazza A, Fanti S, et al. Pleuroparenchymal fibroelastosis: the prevalence of secondary forms in hematopoietic stem cell and lung transplantation recipients. Diagn Interv Radiol. 2016;22(5):400–6. https://doi.org/10.5152/dir.2016.15516.
115. Kusagaya H, Nakamura Y, Kono M, Kaida Y, Kuroishi S, Enomoto N, et al. Idiopathic pleuroparenchymal fibroelastosis: consideration of a clinicopathological entity in a series of Japanese patients. BMC Pulm Med. 2012;12:72. https://doi.org/10.1186/1471-2466-12-72.
116. Frankel SK, Cool CD, Lynch DA, Brown KK. Idiopathic pleuroparenchymal fibroelastosis: description of a novel clinicopathologic entity. Chest. 2004;126(6):2007–13. https://doi.org/10.1378/chest.126.6.2007.
117. Pegoraro F, Favre C. Post-transplantation lymphoproliferative disorder after haematopoietic stem cell transplantation. Ann Hematol. 2021;100(4):865–78. https://doi.org/10.1007/s00277-021-04433-y.
118. Ru Y, Zhang X, Song T, Ding Y, Zhu Z, Fan Y, et al. Epstein-Barr virus reactivation after allogeneic hematopoietic stem cell transplantation: multifactorial impact on transplant outcomes. Bone Marrow Transplant. 2020;55(9):1754–62. https://doi.org/10.1038/s41409-020-0831-7.
119. Halkos ME, Miller JI, Mann KP, Miller DL, Gal AA. Thoracic presentations of posttransplant lymphoproliferative disorders. Chest. 2004;126(6):2013–20. https://doi.org/10.1378/chest.126.6.2013.
120. Carignan S, Staples CA, Muller NL. Intrathoracic lymphoproliferative disorders in the immunocompromised patient: CT findings. Radiology. 1995;197(1):53–8. https://doi.org/10.1148/radiology.197.1.7568853.
121. Dodd GD 3rd, Ledesma-Medina J, Baron RL, Fuhrman CR. Posttransplant lymphoproliferative disorder: intrathoracic manifestations. Radiology. 1992;184(1):65–9. https://doi.org/10.1148/radiology.184.1.1609104.
122. Collins J, Muller NL, Leung AN, McGuinness G, Mergo PJ, Flint JD, et al. Epstein-Barr-virus-associated lymphoproliferative disease of the lung: CT and histologic findings. Radiology. 1998;208(3):749–59. https://doi.org/10.1148/radiology.208.3.9722856.

# Bacterial Pneumonia in Hematopoietic Stem Cell Transplant Recipients

7

D. Martin Ashley and Scott E. Evans

## Overview

Despite advances in both conditioning and prophylactic antimicrobial regimens in recent decades, infectious pulmonary complications remain a substantial cause of morbidity and mortality in patients who have undergone hematopoietic stem cell transplantation (HSCT) [1–3]. As many as 80% HSCT recipients will experience one or more episode of pneumonia, which is the most frequent lethal complication of HSCT and is identified as the proximate cause of death in up to 20% of HSCT patients [2, 4, 5]. HSCT patients' susceptibility to bacterial infections derives from such disparate, concurrent mechanisms of immune impairment as systemic leukocytopenias, lung architectural derangements due to prior treatments, and nutritional deficiencies [3, 6–9]. Even among those HSCT recipients who survive an episode of pneumonia, a diagnosis of pneumonia often portends poorer transplant outcomes with increased frequency and complexity of hospitalizations in the posttransplant period, making understanding of this complication important in the care of these patients [10–13].

The complex and often prolonged host immunity derangements associated with HSCT result in susceptibility to a wide range of opportunistic pneumonia-causing bacterial pathogens [14]. Further, repeated encounters with the healthcare system predispose HSCT patients to uncommon or antibiotic-resistant organisms [15]. Nonetheless, the most frequently detected bacterial pathogens in this population remain those that commonly cause community- or hospital-acquired pneumonia in the general population [4, 7, 8, 16].

HSCT recipients require thoughtful and thorough evaluation of suspected infection to facilitate the prompt pathogen identification and effective initial treatment that are associated with improved clinical outcomes of bacterial pneumonia [17]. The diagnosis of bacterial pneumonia may be particularly challenging in this population, as the clinical presentation of post-HSCT pneumonia is often nonspecific and may overlap with syndromes associated with other aspects of the disease or treatment (e.g., treatment toxicities, peri-engraftment syndromes, leukemic infiltration, etc.). Further, due to transplant-related attenuation of host response elements, typical clinical clues to the presence of bacterial pneumonia, such as cough with sputum production, fever, elevated leukocyte counts, or suggestive

D. M. Ashley
Division of Pulmonary and Critical Care Medicine, University of Texas McGovern Medical School, Houston, TX, USA
e-mail: Deptmer.M.Ashley@uth.tmc.edu

S. E. Evans (✉)
Department of Pulmonary Medicine, University of Texas MD Anderson Cancer Center, Unit 1462, Houston, TX, USA
e-mail: seevans@mdanderson.org



A. O. Soubani (ed.), *Pulmonary and Critical Care Considerations of Hematopoietic Stem Cell Transplantation*, https://doi.org/10.1007/978-3-031-28797-8_7

radiographic findings, may not be present even in the setting of advanced bacterial infections.

In this chapter, we will explore the pathophysiologic mechanisms that contribute to bacterial pneumonia susceptibility, identify common causative pathogens and their temporal relationship to engraftment, recommend diagnostic strategies, discuss empiric approaches to treatment, and describe novel strategies to reduce the morbidity associated with bacterial pneumonias.

## Temporal Considerations in HSCT-Related Bacterial Pneumonia

The process of functional immune reconstitution following HSCT is determined by both intrinsic host factors and treatment-related factors, such as type of transplant (autologous vs. allogeneic), conditioning regimen (myeloablative vs. nonmyeloablative), source of transplant (peripheral blood, bone marrow, umbilical cord blood), and the presence of graft-versus-host disease (GVHD) [14, 18, 19]. Recognizing the typical patterns of leukocyte recovery, such as neutrophil counts recovering before lymphocyte recovery, can be helpful in anticipating likely bacterial pathogens causing respiratory infections. However, it is notable that leukocyte-mediated immunity may remain functionally impaired for months to years after transplant, even when counts have recovered to normal levels [20]. Such persistent qualitative defects may be specifically observed in bacterial pathogen detection and killing mechanisms of alveolar macrophages, neutrophils, and lung epithelial cells [14].

The peri-engraftment period (approximately day 0–30) is highlighted by both infectious and noninfectious pulmonary complications (NIPC) which can occur simultaneously. In the setting of severe neutropenia, persisting mucositis from the conditioning regimen frequently allows for bacterial translocation from the respiratory and alimentary tracts. Hence, these early pneumonias are commonly caused by Gram-negative bacterial organisms [21]. As an important corollary of bacterial translocation, recent studies indicate that the gut microbiota composition at the time of transplant may be predictive of pulmonary complications in the posttransplant setting [18].The innate and intrinsic immune defects associated with the peri-engraftment period are frequently paired with additional breaches to epithelial barrier integrity, such as indwelling vascular devices, nasogastric/PEG tubes, and endotracheal tubes, further facilitating bacterial infections [22]. Moreover, even as patients recover their neutrophil counts, many remain functionally neutropenic as common exposures such as corticosteroids, acidemia, and radiation therapy can impair neutrophil chemotaxis and respiratory burst [6].

In addition to systemic leukocytopenias, loss of alveolar macrophages results in impaired local pathogen surveillance in the lower respiratory tract in the peri-engraftment period, heightening the risk of bacterial pneumonias [23]. Importantly, epithelial mucociliary clearance of lower respiratory tract pathogens is also frequently impaired in the peri-engraftment period and may remain so even years after transplant [24]. The aggregate effect of these multiple forms of immune impairment results in relatively comparable bacterial pneumonia risks between allogeneic and autologous HSCT recipients in the peri-engraftment period, though the increased pneumonia risk generally persists longer for allogeneic HSCT recipients due to longer periods of functional leukocyte recovery and requirements for immunosuppressive therapies [25].

In the early post-engraftment period (roughly days 31–100), cellular and humoral immunity remain impaired, though neutrophil counts have often recovered. Following engraftment, NIPC such as idiopathic pneumonia syndrome (IPS) or posttransplant lymphoproliferative disease may present with radiographic abnormalities that mimic pneumonia. Alternatively, there may be evidence of delayed injury related to previous radiation or conditioning regimens. Among HSCT recipients that remain hospitalized in this period, the risk for nosocomial bacterial pneumonia is substantial [26]. Thus, it is important to recognize that NIPC and pulmonary infection may coexist, meriting consideration of bacterial pneumonias when evaluating patients with new respiratory symptoms, fever, or radiographic abnormalities.

Despite frequent quantitative recovery of leukocyte counts, the late post-engraftment period (>100 days) is notable for a persistent immunoglobulin deficiency, conferring increased risk for pneumonia caused by encapsulated bacterial organisms [27]. The risk is further heightened among allogeneic HSCT recipients with GVHD [4, 28]. Making the diagnosis of infectious pneumonias more challenging in this period, late posttransplant NIPC such as pulmonary veno-occlusive disease (PVOD), bronchiolitis obliterans syndrome (BOS), and pleuroparenchymal fibroelastosis (PPFE) may cause both radiographic abnormalities and worrisome respiratory symptoms that overlap with those of bacterial pneumonia [29].

## Imaging of Patients with Suspected Bacterial Pneumonia

Chest imaging is critical in the evaluation of HSCT recipients with new respiratory complaints and may be the only localizing finding when evaluating an unexplained episode of neutropenic fever. At least 60% of patients will develop pulmonary opacities in their posttransplant course [21, 30].

Although chest radiographs are often rapidly obtainable and, indeed, may reveal classical lobar consolidation in HSCT patients with bacterial pneumonias, the immune impairments of this population often render this modality insufficiently sensitive to reliably detect bacterial pneumonias [30, 31]. Compared to conventional chest radiography, computed tomography (CT) of the chest offers higher sensitivity and greater negative predictive value and allows for more precise procedural planning if pursuing bronchoscopy. Studies also suggest that CT can detect infiltrates up to 5 days earlier than chest radiography [32]. Thus, CT imaging is the preferred modality when evaluating for possible posttransplant bacterial pneumonia. Even with CT imaging, attenuated inflammatory responses may alter or delay the appearance of typical parenchymal infiltrates caused by bacterial pneumonia in HSCT patients [3, 21]. Further, the CT findings of bacterial pneumonia frequently overlap those of NIPC. Thus, there are no pathognomonic CT findings for posttransplant bacterial pneumonia [33]. Nonetheless, combining information derived from the clinical history with the observed CT patterns may provide insight into likely etiology.

As in other populations, airspace consolidation is the most characteristic CT pattern associated with bacterial pneumonia in HSCT patients, though these may not present as classical lobar consolidations [33]. Acute consolidation development is often associated with pneumonia caused by enteric Gram-negative organisms and common community-acquired Gram-positive pathogens. More subacute airspace consolidation development is often observed with infections caused by pathogens such as actinomycetes or mycobacteria, though rapid progression may occur with almost any bacterial respiratory pathogen in the peri-engraftment period.

Nodular lesions are another common CT manifestation of bacterial pneumonias in HSCT patients [33]. Although fungal pathogens are often considered first in the setting of well-defined nodules, *Pseudomonas* spp., *Stenotrophomonas* spp., *Klebsiella* spp., and *Nocardia* spp. are examples of pathogens that routinely present with nodules in this population [34, 35]. Further, while atypical bacteria and mycobacteria may be more likely to present with tree-in-bud patterns, they may alternately present with numerous nodules or even a miliary pattern [36].

Diffuse ground glass infiltrates observed during the pre-engraftment or early transplant phase could correspond with an almost unlimited number of possible bacterial, viral, or fungal infections. However, diffuse ground glass is not the pattern most often associated with bacterial pneumonias. In addition to considering alternate pathogens, this pattern should also prompt consideration of such entities as noninfectious causes of alveolar hemorrhage or peri-engraftment respiratory distress syndrome. Similarly, the presence of interstitial infiltrates does not exclude the diagnosis of bacterial pneumonia, but this pattern is more often observed in HSCT patients with viral infections or NIPC such as treatment toxicities, pulmonary edema, or PVOD.

## Laboratory Testing for Suspected Bacterial Pneumonia

Despite limitations of sensitivity, bronchoscopy with bronchoalveolar lavage (BAL) remains the gold standard for identification of bacterial respiratory pathogens in HSCT recipients [37]. Bronchoscopy allows visual inspection of the large airways and facilitates direct sampling of the lower respiratory tract for microbiologic and cytologic assessment. Although practices vary by center, relevant studies suggest that the greatest yield of pathogens from HSCT recipients occurs when BAL is obtained soon after onset of symptoms [38, 39]. As such, it is recommended that BAL be performed in a radiographically involved lung segment as soon as is practical in patients suspected of having an infectious pneumonia in the posttransplant period. Although prior delivery of antibiotics may reduce the BAL pathogen yield, it is not recommended to hold antibiotics in anticipation of a bronchoscopy unless the study can be completed immediately. The harm from delaying initiation of antibiotic therapy for hours or days likely outweighs the benefits of improved test performance [40–42]. Laboratory tests that potentially support the diagnosis of bacterial pneumonia, including those from BAL samples, are listed in Table 7.1.

**Table 7.1** Laboratory tests that support the diagnosis of bacterial pneumonia

| Sample source | Potential test strategy |
|---|---|
| Blood | Bacterial culture and sensitivity |
| Sputum | Gram stain |
| | Bacterial culture and sensitivity |
| | Ziehl-Neelsen acid-fast stain |
| | Modified Ziehl-Neelsen or Kinyoun acid-fast stain |
| Nasopharyngeal swab | PCR (multiplex) |
| | *Bordetella* culture |
| Bronchoalveolar lavage | Bacterial culture and sensitivity |
| | Mycobacterial culture |
| | *Legionella* culture |
| | Cell count and differential |
| | PCR (multiplex) |
| | Ziehl-Neelsen acid-fast stain |
| | Modified Ziehl-Neelsen or Kinyoun acid-fast stain |
| | *Legionella* immunofluorescence |
| Urine | Pneumococcal antigen |
| | *Legionella* antigen |

The role of transbronchial biopsies in HSCT recipients suspected of having bacterial pneumonia is not well established. While some have suggested that these biopsies may enhance the diagnostic yield of procedures performed in HSCT patients with fungal, viral, or mycobacterial infections, the incremental diagnostic benefit is even less clear in patients with bacterial infection [19]. Further, thrombocytopenia frequently precludes the safe completion of transbronchial biopsies in this population. The diagnostic yield of transbronchial cryobiopsies in the setting of bacterial pneumonia has not been reported, but this approach is similarly limited by thrombocytopenia.

Sputum cultures tend to be of low microbiologic yield in all populations. Moreover, although clinicians generally recognize that oropharyngeal contamination frequently results in detection of pneumonia-irrelevant microbes, the extreme susceptibility of peri-engraftment HSCT patients to opportunistic pathogens can make discernment of such irrelevant contaminants challenging. However, the detection of an established respiratory pathogen in sputum can aid in management of HSCT patients with bacterial pneumonia. For example, pathogens such as *Pseudomonas aeruginosa* or *Streptococcus pneumoniae* should never be dismissed as saliva contaminants and should generally prompt targeted antimicrobial therapy.

Multiplex nucleic acid amplification testing now offers the ability to detect a wide range of bacterial pathogens on nasopharyngeal swabs or washings. A recent guideline suggests the use of nucleic acid amplification testing on respiratory samples for viruses other than influenza in immunocompromised patients suspected of having community-acquired pneumonia [43]; however, there are no current recommendations regarding bacterial pneumonias, and there are very limited published data describing the utility of these tests in HSCT recipients. Few of these tests are currently FDA approved for use on BAL samples, but some institutions have adapted protocols for use in BAL samples.

Blood-based studies are of modest benefit in HSCT patients suspected of having bacterial pneumonia. Blood cultures are of generally low yield in most pneumonias but are routinely performed in HSCT patients suspected of having bacterial pneumonia and in those with febrile neutropenia of uncertain etiology. Detection of a respiratory pathogen on blood culture should always prompt initiation of appropriate antimicrobial therapy, as such patients are prone to rapid deterioration.

The role of procalcitonin levels in the evaluation of pneumonia remains controversial. It has been reported that elevated procalcitonin levels are predictive of increased mortality and longer hospital length of stay in the setting of bacterial pneumonia [44–46]. However, the value of a low level in excluding bacterial pneumonia is uncertain as is the impact of HSCT-related immune derangements on procalcitonin levels. Serum-based antigen detection (e.g., β-D-glucan, galactomannan) and PCR testing have been recommended for both diagnosis and surveillance of fungal pathogens in HSCT patients [47], but no blood-based molecular detection strategies are currently endorsed for bacterial pathogens in this population.

Additional biomarkers for bacterial infections have been previously investigated, including interleukin-6, C-reactive protein, and serum amyloid proteins. While some have been noted to be elevated in critically ill patients, none have demonstrated a convincing ability to discriminate bacterial pneumonia in HSCT (or other) populations from other conditions [48, 49]. Alternate scoring systems have been proposed as a means to predict the severity of pneumonia in HSCT patients based on standard clinical laboratory tests [50], and there have been recent attempts to use radiographic appearances to predict pneumonia outcomes in this population [51].

HSCT patients with bacterial pneumonia may present with parapneumonic effusions, though interestingly at a lower rate than the general population [52]. Although it is reported that the diagnostic yield of thoracentesis is often low in HSCT recipients [53], presumably due to the routine use of prophylactic antibiotics and the tendency of practitioners to promptly initiate broad spectrum antibiotics in these patients [54], sampling of unexplained pleural fluid collections remains important to excluding the presence of complicated parapneumonic effusions or empyema. This need must be balanced against the risk of bleeding associated with thrombocytopenia [53], but early detection of a pleural space infection may be lifesaving.

## Management of Bacterial Pneumonia in HSCT Patients

The foregoing diagnostic strategies derive their value from their ability to facilitate selection of effective antimicrobial therapies. Table 7.2 lists common respiratory bacterial pathogens to be considered in the initial antibiotic selection for HSCT recipients with suspected pneumonia. As

**Table 7.2** Common bacterial respiratory pathogens in HSCT patients

| |
|---|
| **Gram-negative bacteria** |
| *Acinetobacter baumannii* complex |
| *Alcaligenes/Achromobacter* spp. |
| *Burkholderia* spp. |
| *Citrobacter* spp. [a] |
| *Enterobacter cloacae* a |
| *Escherichia coli*[a,b] |
| *Klebsiella pneumonia* |
| *Moraxella catarrhalis*[b] |
| *Neisseria meningitides* |
| Nontypeable *Haemophilus influenzae*[b] |
| *Proteus* spp.[a] |
| *Pseudomonas* spp.[a,b] |
| *Stenotrophomonas maltophilia*[a] |
| *Serratia marcescens* |
| **Gram-positive bacteria** |
| *Actinomyces* spp. |
| *Enterococcus faecalis* |
| *Nocardia* spp. |
| *Rhodococcus equi* |
| *Streptococcus pneumoniae*[b] |
| *Streptococcus pyogenes*[b] |
| *Staphylococcus aureus*[a] |
| **Atypical bacteria** |
| *Chlamydophila pneumoniae*[b] |
| *Coxiella burnetii* |
| *Legionella* spp.[b] |
| *Mycoplasma pneumoniae*[b] |
| **Mycobacteria** |
| *Mycobacterium tuberculosis* |
| Nontuberculous mycobacteria |

[a]Increased risk for antimicrobial resistance
[b]Consider routinely in initial selection of antibiotics

shown, there is a broad range of potential bacterial pathogens to cover. At least as important in agent selection are the many contributing host factors. Therapeutic strategies must be directed by the patient's transplant-related immune status and his/her exposure history, both to pathogens and antimicrobials.

It is well established that delays in initiation of appropriate antimicrobial therapy increase risks of secondary complications and infection-associated deaths in immunocompromised patients. It is common practice to promptly initiate empiric or preemptive antibiotic therapy when bacterial pneumonia is suspected in HSCT patients [3, 55–57]. No formal consensus exists for the optimal time to first antibiotic dose in this unique population, although one study suggests that neutropenic fever outcomes are better when antibiotics are delivered within 104 min of presentation [58].

Initial antimicrobial therapy for febrile HSCT patients suspected of having pneumonia should include coverage of multidrug-resistant strains of *Staphylococcus aureus* and *Pseudomonas aeruginosa* [8, 17, 59–61]. Coverage for atypical organisms is also appropriate in HSCT patients admitted with suspected community-acquired pneumonia, with the selection of macrolide, fluoroquinolone, or doxycycline therapy largely dependent on the agent(s) initially chosen for coverage of drug-resistant pathogens and on the patient's prior prophylactic regimens [17, 62]. All antibiotic choices should consider available culture data, pneumonia severity, local antibiotic sensitivity profiles, prior antibiotic exposures, and patient immune status [17, 63].

Community-acquired pneumonia is defined by the development of new or worsening radiographic infiltrates in the setting of respiratory symptoms in a patient who has not been hospitalized or in a nursing home in the preceding 14 days [62]. Just as in all populations, HSCT recipients in the outpatient setting may acquire respiratory infections with typical community-acquired pneumonia pathogens. However, due to their frequent healthcare exposures, they also have opportunities to acquire bacterial strains that are typically associated with nosocomial pneumonias [15, 34, 64]. The designation of *healthcare-associated pneumonia* is no longer endorsed in major guidelines, due to the frequent clinical misapplication of this term promoting inappropriate antibiotic selection in other populations. However, the recognition that nonhospitalized HSCT patients are frequently at higher-than-average risk of infections caused by drug-resistant pathogens motivates the above recommendation for coverage of drug-resistant pathogens, particularly in HSCT patients with severe community-acquired pneumonia [34, 35].

Indeed, bacterial pathogens account for the greatest share of nosocomial pneumonias, most notably in the early post-engraftment period [26]. Empiric antibiotics for early hospital-acquired pneumonia (within 7 days of admission) should include coverage of *S. pneumoniae*, methicillin-resistant S. *aureus*, *Haemophilus influenzae*, and *Enterobacteriaceae* [65]. Recent evidence from HSCT centers reveals escalating incidence of extended spectrum beta lactamase (ESBL) producing and carbapenem-resistant organisms detected in the blood of HSCT patients with pneumonia [66, 67]. One study of multidrug-resistant *Acinetobacter baumannii* found the risk factors for infection with a carbapenem-resistant strain to include a recent ICU stay, recent central line placement, an abdominal drainage event, the number of previous antibiotics used, the presence of respiratory failure, and recent chemo- or radiotherapies [67, 68]. Initial regimens for patients with late hospital-acquired pneumonia or ventilator-associated pneumonia should ensure enhanced coverage for multidrug-resistant Gram-negative bacilli [56, 61, 65, 69]. Secondary antibiotic selections for patients with refractory hospital-acquired pneumonia or ventilator-associated pneumonia should be determined by institutional pathogen susceptibility profiles and on prior patient antimicrobial exposures [60, 61, 65, 70].

When possible, early de-escalation of broad empiric therapy is recommended as a universal element of antibiotic stewardship and may be considered in HSCT patients with bacterial pneumonia who demonstrate prompt clinical response and in whom granulocyte recovery has occurred, especially if a susceptible pathogen has been identified [71]. De-escalation should be undertaken with caution in patients with poor clinical response to antimicrobial therapy or those with persistent neutropenia [72]. Alternately, coverage can more confidently be rapidly narrowed if there is a significant improvement in the first 24 h, and PCR of the nares for methicillin-resistant S. *aureus* is negative, due to its high negative predictive value.

In addition to antimicrobial interventions for acute development of bacterial pneumonias, as described above, there are additional pathogens to consider when selecting therapy for more insidious onset bacterial respiratory infections. Mycobacterial infections are often observed in the late post-engraftment period, and therapy should generally be directed by laboratory-documented susceptibility testing whenever possible [36, 73, 74]. Expert guidance is recommended in the management of mycobacterial infections in this population due to the requirement for multiple antimicrobial agents over an extended period, the frequent occurrence of drug-drug interactions, and the need for ongoing follow-up [36].

Other tissue-destructive bacterial infections include those caused by *Nocardia* spp., *Rhodococcus* spp., and *Actinomyces* spp. that may present with a subacute or chronic onset. The most comprehensive data about these types of pathogens in HSCT patients are for *Nocardia* pneumonia. *Nocardia* tends to infect in the late post-engraftment period, with increased incidence in patients who underwent allogeneic HSCT with myeloablative conditioning, in those with ongoing steroid use, and in the absence of *Pneumocystis* prophylaxis at the time of diagnosis [75]. There is also evidence that *Nocardia* infections increase with previous parenchymal or airway diseases (cavitary lesion, bronchiolitis obliterans syndrome, COPD) and in patients with GVHD, often with concomitant infection with *S. aureus*, *Pseudomonas*, cytomegalovirus, or *Mycoplasma* spp. [75] The average time to diagnostic confirmation from cultures was 55.7 days, highlighting the difficulty in identifying this infection and how it is often mistaken for one of the coinfecting organisms listed. Therapy for patients in this category with slowly progressing disease is typically selected based on laboratory-derived susceptibilities, though these pathogens should also be considered when initial empiric therapy for acute pneumonia fails to result in clinical improvement.

## Host-Targeted Therapies

Despite the aggressive use of guideline-compliant broad-spectrum antibiotics, mortality rates remain unacceptably high in HSCT patients with bacterial pneumonia, particularly during the peri-engraftment and early post-engraftment periods. As many of these antibiotic failures arise from continuing posttransplant immune defects that prevent pathogen clearance, developing means to mitigate persisting immune defects remains an area of intensive investigation.

A major research focus has been correction of granulocytopenia. Preparations of granulocyte colony-stimulating factor (filgrastim, lenograstim, and pegfilgrastim) and granulocyte macrophage colony-stimulating factor (sargramostim and molgramostim) are available commercially. Both kinds of agents demonstrate efficacy in reducing the duration of neutropenia [76–79]. Although evidence supports using colony-stimulating factors to prevent some bacterial pneumonias [80, 81], they are not generally recommended in the treatment of established bacterial infections. Current guidelines recommend the administration of granulocyte colony-stimulating factor if the risk of developing febrile neutropenia is greater than 20% based on patient-specific risk factors [77, 82].

Infusion of donor granulocytes has also been proposed as an adjunct therapy in patients with febrile neutropenia [83]. Although this strategy holds promise, it remains investigational, and interpretation of the associated studies is challenging owing to heterogeneity of the populations and protocols [84]. However, some authors argue that severely ill neutropenic patients may benefit from granulocyte transfusion, particularly as a bridge until patients engaft [80, 83].

In addition to efforts to increase the absolute number of leukocytes in cytopenic patients, multiple groups have investigated the manipulation of existing leukocytes through the administration of recombinant cytokines. Exogenous interferon-gamma has demonstrated success in reducing some bacterial infections in patients with congenital neutropenia, and more recent studies suggest efficacy in patients with opportunistic infections after HSCT [85]. Potential mechanisms for this benefit include induction of surface molecules such as major histocompatibility complex class II, Fc receptor gamma and integrins, increased phagolysosomal superoxide production, and prolonged half-life of granulocytes. Administration of interleukin-12 has also been proposed as a strategy to protect against lung infections [86], potentially via interferon-gamma-dependent and tumor necrosis factor-dependent mechanisms.

Induction of innate antimicrobial responses directly from lung epithelial cells offers a novel alternate strategy to prevent, and possibly treat, pneumonias in HSCT patients. Lung epithelial cells are long-lived and relatively resistant to chemotherapy [87, 88]. Beyond their well-known barrier function, these cells also demonstrate a substantial capacity to detect pathogens, modulate local immune responses, and generate directly bactericidal responses through the production of antimicrobial peptides and reactive oxygen and nitrogen species [89, 90]. Advances in the understanding of the molecular mechanisms involved in recognition and signal transduction have allowed development of inhaled therapeutics that induce protective innate immune responses from the lung epithelium in animals. In animal models of pneumonia, this provides protection from lethal pathogens, even when there is concurrent neutropenia [88, 91, 92]. Preclinical animal studies of one such treatment, PUL-042, demonstrate protection against Gram-positive, Gram-negative, fungal, and viral pneumonias, and clinical trials are ongoing [88, 92, 93]. Augmentation of innate immune responses offers several hypothetical advantages in terms of rapidity of effect, breadth of pathogen specificity, and lack of known antimicrobial resistance [94], but efficacy has not been established in humans, and this approach is not presently approved in any population.

## Summary

HSCT patients are uniquely susceptible to bacterial pneumonias, due to defects of their recovering immune systems, breaches of barrier function due to prior and ongoing medical interventions, and exposure to a wide range of potentially drug-resistant pathogens. The diagnosis of bacterial pneumonia after HSCT is challenging due to both the frequent absence of characteristic clinical findings and the multiplicity of competing diagnoses. However, integration of traditional microbiologic techniques and targeted molecular diagnostics can facilitate prompt diagnosis. Consideration of the patient's unique immune status and exposure history can further aid in providing timely, evidence-based management strategies.

## References

1. Massaro KS, Macedo R, de Castro BS, et al. Risk factor for death in hematopoietic stem cell transplantation: are biomarkers useful to foresee the prognosis in this population of patients? Infection. 2014;42(6):1023–32.
2. Tomblyn M, Chiller T, Einsele H, et al. Guidelines for preventing infectious complications among hematopoietic cell transplantation recipients: a global perspective. Biol Blood Marrow Transplant. 2009;15(10):1143–238.
3. Wong JL, Evans SE. Bacterial pneumonia in patients with cancer: novel risk factors and management. Clin Chest Med. 2017;38(2):263–77.
4. Aguilar-Guisado M, Jimenez-Jambrina M, Espigado I, et al. Pneumonia in allogeneic stem cell transplantation recipients: a multicenter prospective study. Clin Transpl. 2011;25(6):E629–38.
5. Lossos IS, Breuer R, Or R, et al. Bacterial pneumonia in recipients of bone marrow transplantation. A five-year prospective study. Transplantation. 1995;60(7):672–8.
6. Safdar A, Armstrong D. Infectious morbidity in critically ill patients with cancer. Crit Care Clin. 2001;17(3):531–70, vii-viii.
7. Wong A, Marrie TJ, Garg S, Kellner JD, Tyrrell GJ, Group S. Increased risk of invasive pneumococcal

disease in haematological and solid-organ malignancies. Epidemiol Infect. 2010;138(12):1804–10.
8. Ashour HM, el-Sharif A. Microbial spectrum and antibiotic susceptibility profile of gram-positive aerobic bacteria isolated from cancer patients. J Clin Oncol. 2007;25(36):5763–9.
9. Joos L, Tamm M. Breakdown of pulmonary host defense in the immunocompromised host: cancer chemotherapy. Proc Am Thorac Soc. 2005;2(5):445–8.
10. Whimbey E, Goodrich J, Bodey GP. Pneumonia in cancer patients. Cancer Treat Res. 1995;79:185–210.
11. Kuderer NM, Dale DC, Crawford J, Cosler LE, Lyman GH. Mortality, morbidity, and cost associated with febrile neutropenia in adult cancer patients. Cancer. 2006;106(10):2258–66.
12. Chaoui D, Legrand O, Roche N, et al. Incidence and prognostic value of respiratory events in acute leukemia. Leukemia. 2004;18(4):670–5.
13. Lee CH, Huang CY, DeFor TE, Brunstein CG, Weisdorf DJ, Luo X. Semiparametric regression model for recurrent bacterial infections after hematopoietic stem cell transplantation. Stat Sin. 2019;29(3):1489–509.
14. Zinter MS, Hume JR. Effects of hematopoietic cell transplantation on the pulmonary immune response to infection. Front Pediatr. 2021;9:634566.
15. Dettenkofer M, Wenzler-Rottele S, Babikir R, et al. Surveillance of nosocomial sepsis and pneumonia in patients with a bone marrow or peripheral blood stem cell transplant: a multicenter project. Clin Infect Dis. 2005;40(7):926–31.
16. Steele RW. Managing infection in cancer patients and other immunocompromised children. Ochsner J. 2012;12(3):202–10.
17. Ramirez JA, Musher DM, Evans SE, et al. Treatment of community-acquired pneumonia in immunocompromised adults: a consensus statement regarding initial strategies. Chest. 2020;158(5):1896–911.
18. Harris B, Morjaria SM, Littmann ER, et al. Gut microbiota predict pulmonary infiltrates after allogeneic hematopoietic cell transplantation. Am J Respir Crit Care Med. 2016;194(4):450–63.
19. Harris B, Lowy FD, Stover DE, Arcasoy SM. Diagnostic bronchoscopy in solid-organ and hematopoietic stem cell transplantation. Ann Am Thorac Soc. 2013;10(1):39–49.
20. Gea-Banacloche J, Komanduri KV, Carpenter P, et al. National Institutes of Health hematopoietic cell transplantation late effects initiative: the immune dysregulation and pathobiology working group report. Biol Blood Marrow Transplant. 2017;23(6):870–81.
21. Harris B, Geyer AI. Diagnostic evaluation of pulmonary abnormalities in patients with hematologic malignancies and hematopoietic cell transplantation. Clin Chest Med. 2017;38(2):317–31.
22. Einsele H, Bertz H, Beyer J, et al. Infectious complications after allogeneic stem cell transplantation: epidemiology and interventional therapy strategies—guidelines of the Infectious Diseases Working Party (AGIHO) of the German Society of Hematology and Oncology (DGHO). Ann Hematol. 2003;82 Suppl 2(Suppl 2):S175–85.
23. Springmeyer SC, Silvestri RC, Sale GE, et al. The role of transbronchial biopsy for the diagnosis of diffuse pneumonias in immunocompromised marrow transplant recipients. Am Rev Respir Dis. 1982;126(5):763–5.
24. Cordonnier C, Gilain L, Ricolfi F, et al. Acquired ciliary abnormalities of nasal mucosa in marrow recipients. Bone Marrow Transplant. 1996;17(4):611–6.
25. Bjorklund A, Aschan J, Labopin M, et al. Risk factors for fatal infectious complications developing late after allogeneic stem cell transplantation. Bone Marrow Transplant. 2007;40(11):1055–62.
26. Gudiol C, Sabe N, Carratala J. Is hospital-acquired pneumonia different in transplant recipients? Clin Microbiol Infect. 2019;25(10):1186–94.
27. Marr KA. Delayed opportunistic infections in hematopoietic stem cell transplantation patients: a surmountable challenge. Hematology Am Soc Hematol Educ Program. 2012;2012:265–70.
28. Vento S, Cainelli F, Temesgen Z. Lung infections after cancer chemotherapy. Lancet Oncol. 2008;9(10):982–92.
29. Mo XD, Zhang XH, Xu LP, et al. Late-onset severe pneumonia after allogeneic hematopoietic stem cell transplantation: prognostic factors and treatments. Transpl Infect Dis. 2016;18(4):492–503.
30. Heussel CP, Kauczor HU, Heussel GE, et al. Pneumonia in febrile neutropenic patients and in bone marrow and blood stem-cell transplant recipients: use of high-resolution computed tomography. J Clin Oncol. 1999;17(3):796–805.
31. Cereser L, Zuiani C, Graziani G, et al. Impact of clinical data on chest radiography sensitivity in detecting pulmonary abnormalities in immunocompromised patients with suspected pneumonia. Radiol Med. 2010;115(2):205–14.
32. Chellapandian D, Lehrnbecher T, Phillips B, et al. Bronchoalveolar lavage and lung biopsy in patients with cancer and hematopoietic stem-cell transplantation recipients: a systematic review and meta-analysis. J Clin Oncol. 2015;33(5):501–9.
33. Escuissato DL, Gasparetto EL, Marchiori E, et al. Pulmonary infections after bone marrow transplantation: high-resolution CT findings in 111 patients. AJR Am J Roentgenol. 2005;185(3):608–15.
34. Yeshurun M, Gafter-Gvili A, Thaler M, Keller N, Nagler A, Shimoni A. Clinical characteristics of Stenotrophomonas maltophilia infection in hematopoietic stem cell transplantation recipients: a single center experience. Infection. 2010;38(3):211–5.
35. Srinivasan A, Wang C, Srivastava DK, et al. Timeline, epidemiology, and risk factors for bacterial, fungal, and viral infections in children and adolescents after allogeneic hematopoietic stem cell transplantation. Biol Blood Marrow Transplant. 2013;19(1):94–101.
36. Bergeron A, Mikulska M, De Greef J, et al. Mycobacterial infections in adults with haematological malignancies and haematopoietic stem cell

transplants: guidelines from the 8th European conference on infections in leukaemia. Lancet Infect Dis. 2022;22(12):e359–69.
37. Sampsonas F, Kontoyiannis DP, Dickey BF, Evans SE. Performance of a standardized bronchoalveolar lavage protocol in a comprehensive cancer center: a prospective 2-year study. Cancer. 2011;117(15):3424–33.
38. Yacoub AT, Thomas D, Yuan C, et al. Diagnostic value of bronchoalveolar lavage in leukemic and bone marrow transplant patients: the impact of antimicrobial therapy. Mediterr J Hematol Infect Dis. 2015;7(1):e2015002.
39. Shannon VR, Andersson BS, Lei X, Champlin RE, Kontoyiannis DP. Utility of early versus late fiberoptic bronchoscopy in the evaluation of new pulmonary infiltrates following hematopoietic stem cell transplantation. Bone Marrow Transplant. 2010;45(4):647–55.
40. Rosa RG, Goldani LZ. Cohort study of the impact of time to antibiotic administration on mortality in patients with febrile neutropenia. Antimicrob Agents Chemother. 2014;58(7):3799–803.
41. Mattison G, Bilney M, Haji-Michael P, Cooksley T. A nurse-led protocol improves the time to first dose intravenous antibiotics in septic patients post chemotherapy. Support Care Cancer. 2016;24(12):5001–5.
42. Kochanek M, Schalk E, von Bergwelt-Baildon M, et al. Management of sepsis in neutropenic cancer patients: 2018 guidelines from the infectious diseases working party (AGIHO) and intensive care working party (iCHOP) of the German Society of Hematology and Medical Oncology (DGHO). Ann Hematol. 2019;98(5):1051–69.
43. Evans SE, Jennerich AL, Azar MM, et al. Nucleic acid-based testing for noninfluenza viral pathogens in adults with suspected community-acquired pneumonia. An official American Thoracic Society clinical practice guideline. Am J Respir Crit Care Med. 2021;203(9):1070–87.
44. Chae H, Bevins N, Seymann GB, Fitzgerald RL. Diagnostic value of procalcitonin in transplant patients receiving immunosuppressant drugs: a retrospective electronic medical record-based analysis. Am J Clin Pathol. 2021;156(6):1083–91.
45. Bansal A, Jeyaraman P, Gupta SK, Dayal N, Naithani R. Clinical utility of procalcitonin in bacterial infections in patients undergoing hematopoietic stem cell transplantation. Am J Blood Res. 2020;10(6):339–44.
46. Shan M, Shen D, Song T, et al. The clinical value of procalcitonin in the neutropenic period after allogeneic hematopoietic stem cell transplantation. Front Immunol. 2022;13:843067.
47. Hage CA, Carmona EM, Epelbaum O, et al. Microbiological laboratory testing in the diagnosis of fungal infections in pulmonary and critical care practice. An official American Thoracic Society clinical practice guideline. Am J Respir Crit Care Med. 2019;200(5):535–50.
48. San Jose ME, Valdes L, Vizcaino LH, et al. Procalcitonin, C-reactive protein, and cell counts in the diagnosis of parapneumonic pleural effusions. J Invest Med. 2010;58(8):971–6.
49. von Lilienfeld-Toal M, Dietrich MP, Glasmacher A, et al. Markers of bacteremia in febrile neutropenic patients with hematological malignancies: procalcitonin and IL-6 are more reliable than C-reactive protein. Eur J Clin Microbiol Infect Dis. 2004;23(7):539–44.
50. Cao LQ, Zhou JR, Zhang XH, et al. A scoring system for predicting the prognosis of late-onset severe pneumonia after allogeneic hematopoietic stem cell transplantation. Transplant Cell Ther. 2021;27(10):870e871–7.
51. Sheshadri A, Godoy M, Erasmus JJ, et al. Progression of the radiologic severity index is associated with increased mortality and healthcare resource utilisation in acute leukaemia patients with pneumonia. BMJ Open Respir Res. 2019;6(1):e000471.
52. Modi D, Jang H, Kim S, et al. Incidence, etiology, and outcome of pleural effusions in allogeneic hematopoietic stem cell transplantation. Am J Hematol. 2016;91(9):E341–7.
53. Adam AK, Zamlut M, Soubani AO. The yield and safety of thoracentesis in hematopoietic stem cell transplantation recipients. Lung. 2007;185(5):257–62.
54. Yen KT, Lee AS, Krowka MJ, Burger CD. Pulmonary complications in bone marrow transplantation: a practical approach to diagnosis and treatment. Clin Chest Med. 2004;25(1):189–201.
55. Evans SE, Ost DE. Pneumonia in the neutropenic cancer patient. Curr Opin Pulm Med. 2015;21(3):260–71.
56. Carratala J, Roson B, Fernandez-Sevilla A, Alcaide F, Gudiol F. Bacteremic pneumonia in neutropenic patients with cancer: causes, empirical antibiotic therapy, and outcome. Arch Intern Med. 1998;158(8):868–72.
57. Brun-Buisson C, Lemaire F. Administration of antibiotics for pneumonia during respiratory failure: reaching the target. Am J Respir Crit Care Med. 2001;164(9):1554–5.
58. Lynn JJ, Chen KF, Weng YM, Chiu TF. Risk factors associated with complications in patients with chemotherapy-induced febrile neutropenia in emergency department. Hematol Oncol. 2013;31(4):189–96.
59. Vuotto F, Berthon C, Lemaitre N, et al. Risk factors, clinical features, and outcome of Pseudomonas aeruginosa bacteremia in patients with hematologic malignancies: a case-control study. Am J Infect Control. 2013;41(6):527–30.
60. Ghannam DE, Rodriguez GH, Raad II, Safdar A. Inhaled aminoglycosides in cancer patients with ventilator-associated gram-negative bacterial pneumonia: safety and feasibility in the era of escalating drug resistance. Eur J Clin Microbiol Infect Dis. 2009;28(3):253–9.
61. Wunderink RG, Niederman MS, Kollef MH, et al. Linezolid in methicillin-resistant Staphylococcus aureus nosocomial pneumonia: a randomized, controlled study. Clin Infect Dis. 2012;54(5):621–9.
62. Metlay JP, Waterer GW, Long AC, et al. Diagnosis and treatment of adults with community-acquired

pneumonia. An official clinical practice guideline of the American Thoracic Society and Infectious Diseases Society of America. Am J Respir Crit Care Med. 2019;200(7):e45–67.

63. Rabello LS, Silva JR, Azevedo LC, et al. Clinical outcomes and microbiological characteristics of severe pneumonia in cancer patients: a prospective cohort study. PloS One. 2015;10(3):e0120544.
64. Caselli D, Cesaro S, Ziino O, et al. Multidrug resistant Pseudomonas aeruginosa infection in children undergoing chemotherapy and hematopoietic stem cell transplantation. Haematologica. 2010;95(9):1612–5.
65. Kalil AC, Metersky ML, Klompas M, et al. Management of Adults with Hospital-acquired and ventilator-associated pneumonia: 2016 clinical practice guidelines by the Infectious Diseases Society of America and the American Thoracic Society. Clin Infect Dis. 2016;63(5):e61–e111.
66. Kim SH, Kwon JC, Choi SM, et al. Escherichia coli and Klebsiella pneumoniae bacteremia in patients with neutropenic fever: factors associated with extended-spectrum beta-lactamase production and its impact on outcome. Ann Hematol. 2013;92(4):533–41.
67. Kim SB, Min YH, Cheong JW, et al. Incidence and risk factors for carbapenem- and multidrug-resistant Acinetobacter baumannii bacteremia in hematopoietic stem cell transplantation recipients. Scand J Infect Dis. 2014;46(2):81–8.
68. Kim SY, Jung JY, Kang YA, et al. Risk factors for occurrence and 30-day mortality for carbapenem-resistant Acinetobacter baumannii bacteremia in an intensive care unit. J Korean Med Sci. 2012;27(8):939–47.
69. Bate J, Gibson F, Johnson E, et al. Neutropenic sepsis: prevention and management of neutropenic sepsis in cancer patients (NICE clinical guideline CG151). Arch Dis Child Educ Pract Ed. 2013;98(2):73–5.
70. Kiem S, Schentag JJ. Relationship of minimal inhibitory concentration and bactericidal activity to efficacy of antibiotics for treatment of ventilator-associated pneumonia. Semin Respir Crit Care Med. 2006;27(1):51–67.
71. Maschmeyer G, Carratala J, Buchheidt D, et al. Diagnosis and antimicrobial therapy of lung infiltrates in febrile neutropenic patients (allogeneic SCT excluded): updated guidelines of the infectious diseases working party (AGIHO) of the German Society of Hematology and Medical Oncology (DGHO). Ann Oncol. 2015;26(1):21–33.
72. Miedema KG, Tissing WJ, Abbink FC, et al. Risk-adapted approach for fever and neutropenia in paediatric cancer patients—a national multicentre study. Eur J Cancer. 2016;53:16–24.
73. Al-Anazi KA, Al-Jasser AM, Al-Anazi WK. Infections caused by non-tuberculous mycobacteria in recipients of hematopoietic stem cell transplantation. Front Oncol. 2014;4:311.
74. Al-Anazi KA, Al-Jasser AM, Alsaleh K. Infections caused by mycobacterium tuberculosis in recipients of hematopoietic stem cell transplantation. Front Oncol. 2014;4:231.
75. Shannon K, Pasikhova Y, Ibekweh Q, Ludlow S, Baluch A. Nocardiosis following hematopoietic stem cell transplantation. Transpl Infect Dis. 2016;18(2):169–75.
76. Dale DC. Colony-stimulating factors for the management of neutropenia in cancer patients. Drugs. 2002;62(Suppl 1):1–15.
77. Skoetz N, Bohlius J, Engert A, Monsef I, Blank O, Vehreschild JJ. Prophylactic antibiotics or G(M)-CSF for the prevention of infections and improvement of survival in cancer patients receiving myelotoxic chemotherapy. Cochrane Database Syst Rev. 2015;2015(12):CD007107.
78. Gale RP, Armitage JO. Use of molecularly-cloned haematopoietic growth factors in persons exposed to acute high-dose, high-dose rate whole-body ionizing radiations. Blood Rev. 2021;45:100690.
79. Weisdorf DJ, Verfaillie CM, Davies SM, et al. Hematopoietic growth factors for graft failure after bone marrow transplantation: a randomized trial of granulocyte-macrophage colony-stimulating factor (GM-CSF) versus sequential GM-CSF plus granulocyte-CSF. Blood. 1995;85(12):3452–6.
80. Estcourt LJ, Stanworth SJ, Hopewell S, Doree C, Trivella M, Massey E. Granulocyte transfusions for treating infections in people with neutropenia or neutrophil dysfunction. Cochrane Database Syst Rev. 2016;4(4):CD005339.
81. Damiani G, McCormick TS, Leal LO, Ghannoum MA. Recombinant human granulocyte macrophage-colony stimulating factor expressed in yeast (sargramostim): a potential ally to combat serious infections. Clin Immunol. 2020;210:108292.
82. Smith TJ, Bohlke K, Lyman GH, et al. Recommendations for the use of WBC growth factors: American Society of Clinical Oncology clinical practice guideline update. J Clin Oncol. 2015;33(28):3199–212.
83. Gea-Banacloche J. Granulocyte transfusions: a concise review for practitioners. Cytotherapy. 2017;19(11):1256–69.
84. Seidel MG, Peters C, Wacker A, et al. Randomized phase III study of granulocyte transfusions in neutropenic patients. Bone Marrow Transplant. 2008;42(10):679–84.
85. Safdar A, Rodriguez GH, Lichtiger B, et al. Recombinant interferon gamma1b immune enhancement in 20 patients with hematologic malignancies and systemic opportunistic infections treated with donor granulocyte transfusions. Cancer. 2006;106(12):2664–71.
86. Sun K, Salmon SL, Lotz SA, Metzger DW. Interleukin-12 promotes gamma interferon-dependent neutrophil recruitment in the lung and improves protection against respiratory Streptococcus pneumoniae infection. Infect Immun. 2007;75(3):1196–202.
87. Rawlins EL, Hogan BL. Ciliated epithelial cell lifespan in the mouse trachea and lung. Am J Physiol Lung Cell Mol Physiol. 2008;295(1):L231–4.

88. Leiva-Juarez MM, Ware HH, Kulkarni VV, Zweidler-McKay PA, Tuvim MJ, Evans SE. Inducible epithelial resistance protects mice against leukemia-associated pneumonia. Blood. 2016;128(7):982–92.
89. Bartlett JA, Fischer AJ, McCray PBJ. Innate immune functions of the airway epithelium. Contrib Microbiol. 2008;15:147–63.
90. Evans SE, Scott BL, Clement CG, et al. Stimulated innate resistance of lung epithelium protects mice broadly against bacteria and fungi. Am J Respir Cell Mol Biol. 2010;42(1):40–50.
91. Munoz N, Van Maele L, Marques JM, Rial A, Sirard JC, Chabalgoity JA. Mucosal administration of flagellin protects mice from Streptococcus pneumoniae lung infection. Infect Immun. 2010;78(10):4226–33.
92. Cleaver JO, You D, Michaud DR, et al. Lung epithelial cells are essential effectors of inducible resistance to pneumonia. Mucosal Immunol. 2014;7(1):78–88.
93. Duggan JM, You D, Cleaver JO, et al. Synergistic interactions of TLR2/6 and TLR9 induce a high level of resistance to lung infection in mice. J Immunol. 2011;186(10):5916–26.
94. Johnston SL, Goldblatt DL, Evans SE, Tuvim MJ, Dickey BF. Airway epithelial innate immunity. Front Physiol. 2021;12:749077.

# 8 Invasive Pulmonary Aspergillosis in Hematopoietic Stem Cell Transplantation

Geetha Sivasubramanian
and Pranatharthi H. Chandrasekar

## Introduction

Infections and graft-versus-host disease (GVHD) are major causes of morbidity and mortality in hematopoietic stem cell transplant (HSCT) recipients. Infections can happen during any of the treatment phases of HSCT: pre-engraftment, early post-engraftment, and late post-engraftment periods. Several factors such as host immune system, type of disease, time from transplant, etc. influence the microbiology of the infections. Invasive fungal infections account for a quarter of these infections including aspergillosis, candidiasis, mold infections such as those caused by zygomycetes, as well as cryptococcosis. This chapter will focus on invasive aspergillosis (IA) in HSCT recipients including risk factors, epidemiology, clinical features, diagnosis, and management.

## Mycology

*Aspergillus* species are ubiquitous in the environment. They are saprophytic fungi feeding on dead and decaying organic material. In the environment, they exist in mold forms with long hyphal stalks bearing the conidia or spores (Fig. 8.1). The size of these conidial spores (2–10 μm) and hydrophobicity aid in the aerosolization and inhalation by hosts [1]. They may be found in abundance in air conditioning units, composting, damp or flood damaged housing, and hospital building projects [2]. Invasive pulmonary aspergillosis (IPA) is most often caused by the species *Aspergillus fumigatus* [3]. Several factors seem to play a role in the virulence of *A. fumigatus* such as its structure, ability to grow and adaptation to stress conditions, and ability to evade the host immune system and cause damage to the host cells [4]. Other species known to cause invasive infections include *A. flavus*, *A. terreus*, *A.*

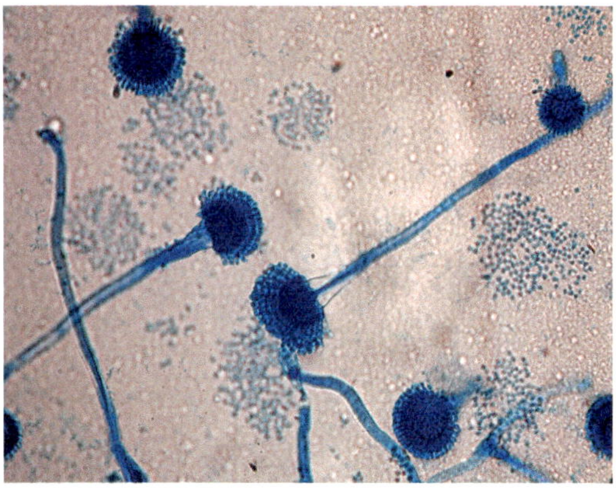

**Fig. 8.1** *Aspergillus fumigatus* conidia and hyphal stalk seen using Grocott's methenamine silver stain at 200× magnification

G. Sivasubramanian
Division of Infectious Diseases, University of California, San Francisco, Fresno, CA, USA

P. H. Chandrasekar (✉)
Division of Infectious Diseases, Wayne State University, Detroit, MI, USA
e-mail: pchandrasekar@med.wayne.edu



A. O. Soubani (ed.), *Pulmonary and Critical Care Considerations of Hematopoietic Stem Cell Transplantation*, https://doi.org/10.1007/978-3-031-28797-8_8

*niger*, and *A. nidulans* [5]. While *A. fumigatus* is most often recovered from lung samples, *A. flavus* and *A. niger* are often recovered from sinus passages [6]. *A. terreus* species tend to have higher minimal inhibitory concentration values to amphotericin B compared to other species and may be resistant to amphotericin therapy [7]. *Aspergillus nidulans* and *A. calidoustus* are resistant to multiple antifungal drugs including voriconazole and amphotericin B [8].

## Immunopathogenesis

Humans inhale about 200 *Aspergillus* conidial spores every day [9]. The primary route of infection is by inhalation of the spores into nasal, sinus, and lung passages. Once inhaled, the spores can germinate in the host tissues to hyphal forms which then invade the tissues and vasculature leading to destruction and damage. However, a sequential well-coordinated host immune response prevents this uncontrolled germination of *Aspergillus* conidia [10]. First the mucociliary clearance in proximal airways removes the inhaled conidia. Residual conidia are then encountered by columnar epithelial cells and pulmonary alveolar macrophages which can phagocytose and kill the conidia without eliciting a robust inflammatory response. Conidia that evade this and germinate into hyphae elicit a pro-inflammatory response attracting neutrophils which can ingest and kill the hyphae. Impairment in these host defenses such as neutropenia or corticosteroid-induced macrophage dysfunction plays a vital role in causing invasive infection along with *Aspergillus* species' capability to grow in the host environment. T cells are also important for host defense, and aberrations play an important role in allergic and chronic forms of infection.

## Epidemiology and Risk Factors

Traditional host factors for IPA include malignancies, hematopoietic and solid organ transplantation, and use of medications such as corticosteroids [11]. However, several nontraditional risk factors have emerged including COPD, HIV, postoperative states, intensive care unit stay, use of newer immunomodulatory therapies, and post-viral infections such as influenza and SARS-CoV-2 [12–19]. Exact contributory role of drugs such as ibrutinib is unclear. The incidence of IPA in HSCT recipients remains high and can be up to 23% with a high mortality approaching 20–75% despite effective antifungal prophylaxis and management strategies [20–23]. In patients who have undergone hematopoietic stem cell transplantation, several factors contribute to increased risk of IPA such as age, type of transplant, type of donor, timing since transplant, conditioning regimen, corticosteroids, duration of neutropenia, graft-versus-host disease (GVHD), cytomegalovirus (CMV) reactivation, antifungal prophylaxis, and hospital environment [20, 24–32] (Table 8.1). In recent decades, a significant num-

**Table 8.1** Risk factors for IPA[a] in HSCT[b] recipients

| Recipient related | Transplant related | Complications of transplant | Environmental exposure |
|---|---|---|---|
| Older age | Donor source (cord blood) | Lymphopenia | Construction sites |
| Underlying disease (multiple myeloma, aplastic anemia) | Type of donor (mismatched, haploidentical) | Neutropenia | Lack of HEPA[c] filter |
| Relapse of malignancy | Conditioning regimen | GVHD[d] | |
| Iron overload | Prolonged steroid use | Graft failure | |
| Comorbidities | Lack of antifungal prophylaxis | CMV[e] reactivation | |
| Genetic polymorphisms | Transplantation with T-cell depleted products | Respiratory virus infections | |

[a]Invasive pulmonary aspergillosis
[b]Hematopoietic stem cell transplantation
[c]High efficiency particulate air
[d]Graft-versus-host disease
[e]Cytomegalovirus

ber of IPA in HSCT recipients tend to occur in the late transplant periods (>100 days) [20, 25]. Many factors likely contributed to this shift including changes in transplantation procedures and supportive care variables such as antifungal prophylaxis and conditioning regimens. While neutropenia and acute GVHD play a significant role in early onset IPA, chronic GVHD, use of corticosteroids, CMV reactivation, and respiratory viral illnesses contribute to the development of late onset IPA [6].

## Clinical Features

Aspergillosis can present as a wide variety of clinical syndromes largely dependent on the host immune system (Table 8.2). The severity often correlates inversely with the extent of host immune impairment [33, 34]. IPA occurs in the lung following inhalation of conidia, germination to hyphae, and invasion of the pulmonary vasculature by hyphal forms. Symptoms of IPA include dry cough, dyspnea, pleuritic chest pain, fever despite broad spectrum antimicrobial agents, and hemoptysis. These symptoms may be very subtle in immunocompromised patients. Patients receiving steroids may not have a fever. Occasionally, untreated patients may progress to develop significant hypoxia and respiratory failure. Pleuritic chest pain, persistent fevers, and pulmonary infiltrate with hemoptysis in the setting of chemotherapy-induced neutropenia, particularly in patients with acute myelogenous leukemia, should significantly raise the suspicion for IPA. Physical examination may reveal signs related to pleural effusion or pneumothorax but may also be completely unrevealing. *Aspergillus* tracheobronchitis presentation is more common in lung transplant recipients and HIV patients [35].

*Aspergillus* tracheobronchitis is relatively uncommon in HSCT recipients and is seen more commonly in lung transplant recipients. It can present in one of three patterns, obstructive tracheobronchitis, ulcerative tracheobronchitis, or pseudomembranous tracheobronchitis. Whereas obstructive form causes thick mucosal plugs with *Aspergillus* hyphae, ulcerative form causes focal invasion of the mucosa/cartilage. Pseudomembranous form causes extensive inflammation and necrosis forming a pseudomembrane of debris. Common symptoms include cough, wheezing, and dyspnea with relatively normal chest imaging.

Aspergillosis of the paranasal sinuses can be invasive and present similar to rhino-cerebral mucormycosis. Initial presenting symptoms are facial pain, swelling, and nasal drainage. Necrosis may appear on the skin or in the palate as disease progresses appearing as black lesions (Fig. 8.2). As the disease progresses and involves deeper structures such as the orbit or cavernous sinuses, warning symptoms like proptosis, chemosis, vision changes, and cranial nerve deficits appear.

**Table 8.2** Aspergillosis clinical syndromes

| Clinical syndromes | Features | Host factors |
|---|---|---|
| Allergic aspergillosis | Asthma, allergic bronchopulmonary aspergillosis (ABPA), allergic sinusitis | Robust CD4 Th-2 response in the lungs, production of *Aspergillus* spp.—specific serum IgE; no risk of invasive disease |
| Aspergillus mycelial balls | Aspergillomas or fungal balls grow in areas of damaged lung tissue (Fig. 8.4) | Damaged lung tissue, bronchiectasis, cysts, preexisting cavities due to tuberculosis, etc., no allergy or invasion |
| Subacute aspergillosis or semi-invasive disease | Local disease but with progression of fibrosis and minimal fungal invasion; cavitary and fibrosing forms | Underlying lung disease, mild to moderate immunosuppression such as diabetes or corticosteroid use |
| Acute invasive aspergillosis | Invade sinus and pulmonary tissue causing severe disease; can disseminate to distant organs such as the skin, brain, spleen, and kidneys | Severe immunocompromised states such as transplant recipients, neutropenia, malignancy, or immunotherapy |

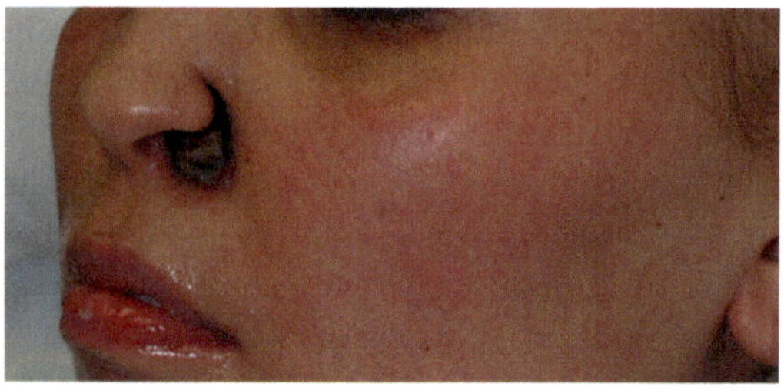

**Fig. 8.2** A 28-year-old allogeneic stem cell transplant recipient with sino-nasal aspergillosis

Angioinvasive disease can be disseminated by hematogenous spread to distant sites such as the central nervous system, skin, liver, spleen, and kidney and is usually associated with very high mortality.

CNS aspergillosis can occur either from hematogenous dissemination or local invasion from the sinuses. Patients may present with headache, seizures, or focal neurological deficits. Imaging findings may show ring enhancing lesions, strokes, or direct extension from sinuses (Fig. 8.3). CNS disease is associated with a very poor prognosis.

Cutaneous aspergillosis can be from dissemination or by direct inoculation. HSCT recipients often get skin involvement from dissemination or contiguous extension. The appearance of the lesion is usually a necrotic plaque or ulcer indistinguishable from other bacterial and fungal infections. Skin biopsy is necessary to make the diagnosis.

Laboratory features are often nonspecific such as elevation in lactate dehydrogenase and C-reactive protein. Radiological features may range from scattered pulmonary infiltrates to multiple diffuse nodular infiltrates (Figs. 8.4 and 8.5). Pleural effusions are common. Not chest radiography but a non-contrast enhanced computed tomography (CT) scan of the chest is the recommended mode of imaging in suspected IPA. During the early phase of the disease, usually during neutropenia, a halo of low attenuation (representing ischemia or hemorrhage) may surround a pulmonary nodular lesion (representing infarction). Later these turn into cavitary lesions with return of neutrophils, forming the air-crescent sign [36, 37] (Fig. 8.6). These classic findings along with others such as pleural-based wedge-shaped densities may not be commonly present. Occasionally, during the period of neutrophil recovery, imaging findings of IPA may progress (Fig. 8.7). The imaging

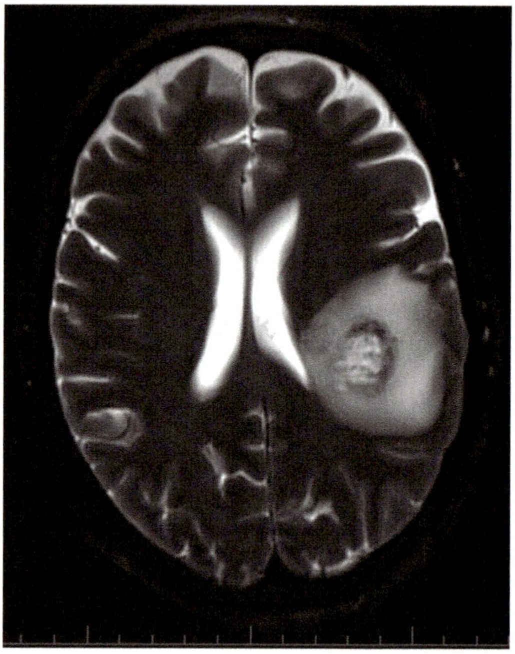

**Fig. 8.3** A 33-year-old allogeneic stem cell transplant recipient with invasive pulmonary aspergillosis, who later developed seizures and was found to have the intracranial lesion on MRI. Underwent resection; biopsy showed invasive aspergillosis

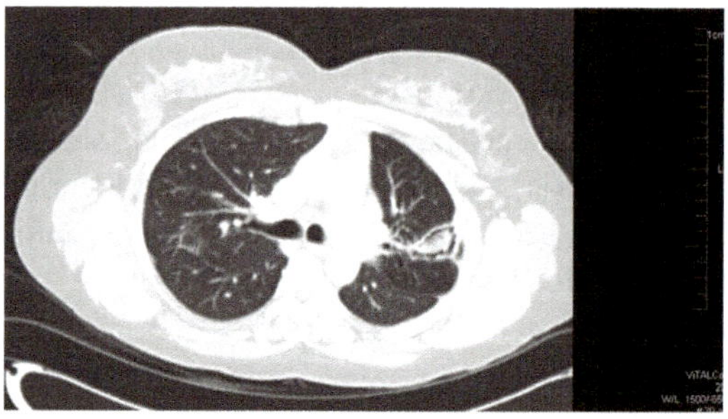

**Fig. 8.4** A 37-year-old woman with a long standing history of sarcoidosis developed intermittent hemoptysis. Chest CT scan revealed a left upper lobe soft tissue density within a cavity consistent with aspergilloma. Bronchoalveolar lavage revealed *Aspergillus* spp. (Courtesy: A. Soubani)

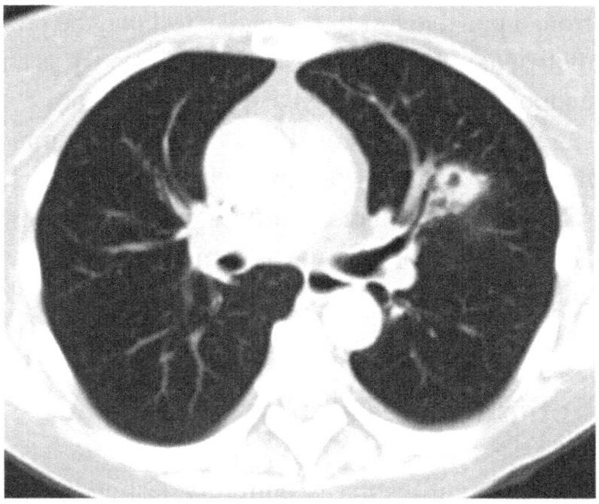

**Fig. 8.5** A 33-year-old allogeneic stem cell transplant recipient with invasive pulmonary aspergillosis: focal cavitary consolidation in left upper lobe (BAL fluid, galactomannan 2.2, culture—*Aspergillus fumigatus*)

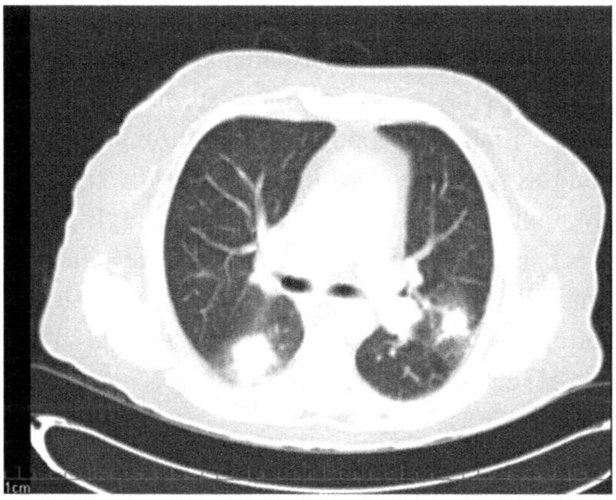


**Fig. 8.6** A 41-year-old allogeneic stem cell transplant recipient with invasive pulmonary aspergillosis during pre-engraftment neutropenia—large pulmonary nodules with surrounding ground glass infiltrates (halo sign)

findings should be interpreted with caution in this context prior to escalating antifungal therapy. The classic imaging findings of halo sign and air-crescent sign may also be seen in other angioinvasive fungal and bacterial infections. In patients with neutropenia lasting more than a week, with persistent fevers despite broad spectrum antibiotics and negative blood cultures, IPA should be suspected, warranting high resolution CT of the chest; contrast use is not required.

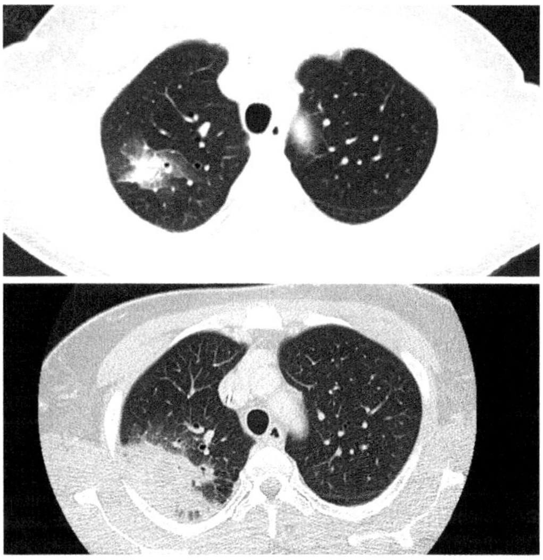

**Fig. 8.7** A 71-year-old-woman with acute myelogenous leukemia—post induction chemotherapy—top: acute invasive aspergillosis with large nodular infiltrate (neutrophil count 0, with fever and hemoptysis). Bottom: 12 days later, worsening infiltrate (neutrophil count 300/mm$^3$) but improved symptoms. Interpretation of CT needs to be based on neutrophil count

## Diagnosis

In appropriate hosts, clinical and radiological findings may raise suspicion for IPA. However, a proven diagnosis of IPA requires a tissue biopsy showing hyphal invasion along with positive cultures for *Aspergillus* species. A bronchoalveolar lavage (BAL) is recommended in patients with suspected invasive pulmonary aspergillosis [38]. A CT guided needle biopsy may be considered in peripheral lung lesions. Diagnosis may also be established if cultures are positive from a sterile site with a needle biopsy. Blood cultures are usually sterile. Obtaining a tissue biopsy may not always be possible in critically ill immunocompromised patients especially with coagulopathies. A probable diagnosis of IPA can be made by culturing *Aspergillus* species from respiratory samples such as BAL fluid in patients with compatible clinical and radiological features. Occasionally, in asymptomatic patients, presence of aspergillus in respiratory specimens may represent colonization. The difficulty in obtaining culture and tissue biopsy specimens has led to many non-culture methods to rapidly establish the diagnosis. Fungal cell wall components such as galactomannan (GM) and 1,3, beta-D-glucan (BDG) can be detected and are the most studied in invasive pulmonary aspergillosis [39]. Both serum and BAL specimens can be used to detect GM. Cross-reactivity with other fungi (*Penicillium*, *Fusarium*, *Histoplasma*) may lead to positive GM. During the early neutropenic phase, after chemotherapy, serial serum GM testing has good sensitivity and negative predictive value in detecting invasive aspergillosis [40]. However, the sensitivity is reduced during antifungal prophylaxis [41]. Also, the sensitivity of serum GM decreases in patients who are not neutropenic [42]. Presence of GM in circulation correlates with invasive growth of aspergillus through the pulmonary capillaries, and angioinvasion has been correlated with fungal burden and GM production [43]. Hence, the performance of GM may be variable in different patient populations. The burden is highest in the neutropenic setting and among infected stem cell recipients. In contrast, in solid organ recipients, as the burden may be low, the GM assay may perform relatively poorly. A declining serum GM value is a predictor of survival, whereas persistently elevated GM levels correlate with death. GM kinetics in the BAL fluid are poorly understood. Site of infection, sampling error, and nonstandardized BAL fluid collection are factors that may interfere with the test. In general, following serial GM value in the serum is recommended in patients with hematologic malignancies and stem cell recipients, with a raised GM at baseline to monitor disease progression, therapeutic response, and prediction of outcome.

While BDG is more sensitive, it is not specific for aspergillosis and may be detected in other fungal infections. BAL and serum *Aspergillus* lateral flow assay and polymerase chain reaction (PCR) assays are helpful as well. Availability of the PCR test in the USA is limited although it is commonly available in Europe. Data suggest that persistence of positive PCR results or a change from a positive test to a negative test may be predictive of outcome. Time to PCR negativity as an endpoint may be a promising clinical tool. In summary, diagnosis of IPA is based on a combination of clinical features, host risk factors, radiological features, culture, histopathology, and detection of the fungal components such as galactomannan.

## Antifungal Resistance

Routine antifungal susceptibility testing is not recommended when cultures grow *Aspergillus* species. Antifungal resistance could happen de novo or while on therapy. Azole resistance in *A. fumigatus* develops secondary to widespread antifungal use in agricultural industry, as well noted in Europe [10]. Antifungal susceptibility testing may be needed if patients do not respond to therapy or in case of some species known to have variable susceptibility to antifungal agents such as *A. terreus* (which is frequently resistant to amphotericin B) or in areas with high prevalence (>10%) of azole-resistant aspergillus. A tandem repeat in the gene promoter with a substitution of leucine for histidine at codon 98 ($TR_{34}$/L98H) causes pan-triazole resistance.

## Management

Early empiric antifungal therapy must be initiated in patients with strongly suspected IPA (e.g., persistently febrile neutropenic patient), while diagnostic evaluation is ongoing. Reducing the dose or completely withdrawing immunosuppression must be considered. Triazoles are preferred agents to treat invasive pulmonary aspergillosis, with voriconazole being the first-line preferred azole [38, 39, 44]. Posaconazole is used less commonly for primary therapy. Itraconazole is avoided as primary therapy for IPA. In patients receiving voriconazole, therapeutic drug monitoring (TDM) is recommended once steady state has been reached, to improve efficacy, minimize suboptimal drug exposure, and avoid toxicities attributable to azoles and drug interactions [38]. Isavuconazole is an approved alternative agent for primary treatment of IPA and appears to be better tolerated with fewer drug interactions [45]. Other options include liposomal amphotericin B or other lipid formulations. Conventional amphotericin B deoxycholate is best avoided. Combination antifungal therapy with voriconazole and an echinocandin may be considered in some patients such as those with prolonged neutropenia or cerebral aspergillosis. Primary monotherapy with an echinocandin is not recommended. Role for surgery is limited and may be considered in focal disease in a minimally immunosuppressed patient. Duration of treatment is a minimum of 6–12 weeks, but dependent on several factors such as the extent of immunosuppression, site of disease, and evidence of clinical/radiological improvement during follow-up. In addition to clinical and radiological parameters, serial serum GM testing can be considered especially if baseline level was elevated. Triazole-resistant aspergillus occurs in 5% of isolates in the USA and up to 20% of isolates in certain parts of Europe. Triazole-resistant IPA is associated with a higher mortality, and once identified, treatment should be switched to liposomal amphotericin B. Adverse events during triazole therapy may be seen and include hepatotoxicity, neurotoxicity such as hallucinations, QTc prolongation, cutaneous toxicities, photosensitivity, and drug interactions. Long term use of voriconazole may be associated with peripheral neuropathy, cognitive impairment, alopecia, and cutaneous malignancies. Drug level monitoring and dose adjustments may be necessary for certain drugs such as cyclosporine, sirolimus, and tacrolimus when given along with triazoles. Isavuconazole does not prolong the QTc interval and has a better safety profile among the triazoles.

Management must be individualized in patients with refractory or progressive disease. Factors to consider while evaluating patients who fail antifungal therapy include prior antifungal agents, host factors, pharmacokinetics, and possible antifungal resistance [46]. General principles in the management include switching to different antifungal, reducing immunosuppression, and possibly surgery for necrotic lesions.

After successful treatment, if further immunosuppression is needed as in cases of relapsing malignancy, secondary prophylaxis must be considered. Prior IPA is not a contraindication for subsequent chemotherapy or transplantation. The decision should be considered in individual patients weighing the risks of progressive aspergillosis versus progression of underlying malignancy.

## Prevention

Measures to reduce risk of at-risk hosts from acquiring aspergillus are recommended. These include pharmacologic and non-pharmacologic measures. Non-pharmacological measures include practices such as placing hospitalized allogeneic HSCT recipients in a protected environment to reduce mold exposure, admission to private rooms with no connection to construction sites, and not allowing plants or cut flowers to be brought into the patient's rooms [47].

Acceptable strategies for preventing IA in at-risk patients include primary prophylaxis with a mold-active azole along with serum biomarker (i.e., GM) monitoring. Primary prophylaxis should be considered in high-risk patients such as those anticipated to have profound and prolonged neutropenia or those with active graft-versus-host disease receiving immunosuppressive therapy [48]. Posaconazole and voriconazole are preferred agents for prophylaxis. Triazoles should be avoided with other agents known to reach potentially toxic levels with concurrent triazole administration (Table 8.3). Antifungal prophylaxis should be administered throughout the duration of immunosuppression in patients with chronic immunosuppression associated with GVHD. It is estimated that about 5–10% of patients receiving prophylaxis may develop probable or proven IPA. Measuring serum drug levels (posaconazole or voriconazole) at 2–5 days after starting prophylaxis is optimal.

**Table 8.3** Summary of invasive aspergillosis in stem cell transplant recipients

| |
|---|
| **A. When to Expect** |
| • Older age (usually >60 years); presence of GVHD[a]; steroid use |
| • Prolonged neutropenia (at transplant or graft failure) |
| • Haploidentical or mismatched recipients |
| **B. Symptoms/Signs** |
| • Persistent fever; pleuritic pain; hemoptysis (sign of angioinvasion) |
| • Nasal congestion, facial pain (sinus disease) |
| • Cacosmia (necrosis of nasal/sinus tissue) |
| • Orbital apex syndrome (ophthalmoplegia, vision loss) |
| • Neurologic deficits |
| **C. Radiology** |
| • Chest X-ray—unreliable; CT[b] findings may be nonspecific |
| • Typical CT nodules (pleural based), cavities |
| • Solitary or multiple CT lesions |
| • CT head—mass lesions/nodules |
| • Positron-emission tomography (PET-CT)[c]: may be useful in monitoring response to Rx |
| **D. Lab Tests** |
| • Serum galactomannan (GM)—if negative, infection not excluded |
| If positive, may be helpful to assess progress |
| • BAL galactomannan—useful (GM may be positive with other fungi, e.g., *Histoplasma, Fusarium*) |
| • Beta-D-glucan (BDG)—not specific for aspergillus |
| Watch for false positives (e.g., serum albumin, intravenous immune globulin, some antibiotics) |
| • PCR testing—may be helpful (concurrent galactomannan testing may be useful; may represent nonviable organisms); not widely available in the USA |
| **E. Management** |
| • **Prevention** |
| – Posaconazole (delayed release tablet)—not suspension or IV formulation |
| – Voriconazole—many adverse effects; isavuconazole—no data |
| – Useful in older age; prior transplant; neutropenia at transplant; haploidentical recipients; GVHD |
| – Avoid azole during preparative regimen (? alternative: micafungin) |
| • **Treatment** |
| – Voriconazole/isavuconazole/lipid amphotericin B |
| – Echinocandin—not for primary monotherapy |
| – Combination Rx (azole + echinocandin)—may be (1) in disseminated infection (2) with neutropenia (3) with concomitant steroid use |

[a]Graft-versus-host disease
[b]Computed tomography
[c]Positron emission tomography

## Future Directions

New risk factors for IA are emerging including ICU stays and respiratory viral illnesses. Novel diagnostic tests such as PCR and lateral flow assays with faster turnaround time are becoming available to aid in early diagnosis. As we battle invasive fungal infections in extended host populations, several new non-azole drugs such as ibrexafungerp, olorofim, rezafungin, and others with varying mechanisms of action are under intense scrutiny. Many have excellent anti-aspergillus activity and have superior pharmacokinetic or safety advantages over current azoles. These are welcome additions, particularly, at a time of rising azole resistance.

## References


1. Barnes PD, Marr KA. Aspergillosis: spectrum of disease, diagnosis, and treatment. Infect Dis Clin North Am. 2006;20:545–61.
2. Park JH, Ryu SH, Lee JY, Kim HJ, Kwak SH, Jung J, et al. Airborne fungal spores and invasive aspergillosis in hematologic units in a tertiary hospital during construction: a prospective cohort study. Antimicrob Resist Infect Control. 2019;8:88.
3. Kontoyiannis DP, Marr KA, Park BJ, Alexander BD, Anaissie EJ, Walsh TJ, et al. Prospective surveillance for invasive fungal infections in hematopoietic stem cell transplant recipients, 2001-2006: overview of the transplant-associated infection surveillance network (TRANSNET) database. Clin Infect Dis. 2010;50:1091–100.
4. Abad A, Fernández-Molina JV, Bikandi J, Ramírez A, Margareto J, Sendino J, et al. What makes aspergillus fumigatus a successful pathogen? Genes and molecules involved in invasive aspergillosis. Rev Iberoam Micol. 2010;27:155–82.
5. Balajee SA, Kano R, Baddley JW, Moser SA, Marr KA, Alexander BD, et al. Molecular identification of aspergillus species collected for the transplant-associated infection surveillance network 2009. J Clin Microbiol. 2009;7:3138–41.
6. Salman N, Budan B, Somer A. And solid organ transplantation invasive aspergillosis in hematopoietic stem cell and solid organ transplantation. Expert Rev Anti Infect Ther. 2011;9:307–15.
7. Steinbach WJ, Perfect JR, Schell WA, Walsh TJ, Benjamin DK. In vitro analyses, animal models, and 60 clinical cases of invasive Aspergillus terreus infection. Antimicrob Agents Chemother. 2004;48:3217–25.
8. Seroy J, Antiporta P, Grim SA, Proia LA, Singh K, Clark NM. Aspergillus calidoustus case series

and review of the literature. Transpl Infect Dis. 2017;19:e12755–62.
9. Dagenais TRT, Keller NP. Pathogenesis of aspergillus fumigatus in invasive aspergillosis. Clin Microbiol Rev. 2009;22:447–65.
10. Thompson GR 3rd, Young JH. Aspergillus infections. N Engl J Med. 2021;385:1496–509.
11. Baddley JW. Clinical risk factors for invasive aspergillosis. Med Mycol. 2011;49(Suppl) 1:S7–S12.
12. Dewi IM, Janssen NA, Rosati D, Bruno M, Netea MG, Brüggemann RJ, et al. Invasive pulmonary aspergillosis associated with viral pneumonitis. Curr Opin Microbiol. 2021;62:21–7.
13. Rouzé A, Lemaitre E, Martin-Loeches I, Povoa P, Diaz E, Nyga R, et al. Invasive pulmonary aspergillosis among intubated patients with SARS-CoV-2 or influenza pneumonia: a European multicenter comparative cohort study. Crit Care. 2022;26:11.
14. Tsiodras S, Samonis G, Boumpas DT, Kontoyiannis DP. Fungal infections complicating tumor necrosis factor alpha blockade therapy. Mayo Clin Proc. 2008;83:181–94.
15. Holding KJ, Dworkin MS, Wan PC, Hanson DL, Klevens RM, Jones JL, et al. Aspergillosis among people infected with human immunodeficiency virus: incidence and survival. Adult and adolescent spectrum of HIV disease project. Clin Infect Dis. 2000;31:1253–7.
16. Pasqualotto AC, Denning DW. Post-operative aspergillosis. Clin Microbiol. 2006;12:1060–76.
17. Denning DW. Aspergillosis in "nonimmunocompromised" critically ill patients. Am J Respir Crit Care Med. 2004;170:580–1.
18. Bulpa P, Dive A, Sibille Y. Invasive pulmonary aspergillosis in patients with chronic obstructive pulmonary disease. Eur Respir J. 2007;30:782–800.
19. Meersseman W, Lagrou K, Maertens J, Van Wijngaerden E. Invasive aspergillosis in the intensive care unit. Clin Infect Dis. 2007;45:205–16.
20. Robin C, Cordonnier C, Sitbon K, Raus N, Lortholary O. Mainly post-transplant factors are associated with invasive aspergillosis after allogeneic stem cell transplantation: a study from the Surveillance des Aspergilloses Invasives en France and Société Francophone de Greffe de Moelle et de Thérapie Cellulaire. Biol Blood Marrow Transplant. 2019;25:354–61.
21. Lortholary O, Gangneux J-P, Sitbon K, Lebeau B, de Monbrison F, Le Strat Y, et al. Epidemiological trends in invasive aspergillosis in France: the SAIF network (2005-2007). Clin Microbiol Infect. 2011;17:1882–9.
22. Neofytos D, Horn D, Anaissie E, Steinbach W, Olyaei A, Fishman J, et al. Epidemiology and outcome of invasive fungal infection in adult hematopoietic stem cell transplant recipients: analysis of multicenter prospective antifungal therapy (PATH) alliance registry. Clin Infect Dis. 2009;48:265–73.
23. Kuster S, Stampf S, Gerber B, Baettig V, Weisser M, Gerull S, et al. Incidence and outcome of invasive fungal diseases after allogeneic hematopoietic stem cell transplantation: a Swiss Transplant cohort study. Transpl Infect Dis. 2018;20:e12981.
24. Atalla A, Garnica M, Maiolino A, Risk MN. Risk factors for invasive mold diseases in allogeneic hematopoietic cell transplant recipients. Transpl Infect Dis. 2015;17:7–13.
25. Marr KA, Carter RA, Boeckh M, Martin P, Corey L. Invasive aspergillosis in allogeneic stem cell transplant recipients: changes in epidemiology and risk factors. Blood. 2002;100:4358–66.
26. Clark RA, Johnson FL, Klebanoff SJ, Thomas ED. Defective neutrophil chemotaxis in bone marrow transplant patients. J Clin Invest. 1976;58:22–31.
27. Storek J, Dawson MA, Storer B, Stevens-Ayers T, Maloney DG, Marr KA, et al. Immune reconstitution after allogeneic marrow transplantation compared with blood stem cell transplantation. Blood. 2001;97:3380–9.
28. Bensinger WI, Buckner CD, Anasetti C, Clift R, Storb R, Barnett T, et al. Allogeneic marrow transplantation for multiple myeloma: an analysis of risk factors on outcome. Blood. 1996;88:2787–93.
29. Baddley JW, Stroud TP, Salzman D, Pappas PG. Invasive mold infections in allogeneic bone marrow transplant recipients. Clin Infect Dis. 2001;32:1319–24.
30. Nichols WG, Corey L, Gooley T, Davis C, Boeckh M. High risk of death due to bacterial and fungal infection among cytomegalovirus (CMV)-seronegative recipients of stem cell transplants from seropositive donors: evidence for indirect effects of primary CMV infection. J Infect Dis. 2002;185:273–82.
31. Linder KA, McDonald PJ, Kauffman CA, Revankar SG, Chandrasekar PH, Miceli MH. Invasive aspergillosis in patients following umbilical cord blood transplant. Bone Marrow Transplant. 2019;54:308–11.
32. Narreddy S, Mellon-Reppen S, Abidi MH, Klein JL, Peres E, Heilbrun LK, et al. Non-bacterial infections in allogeneic non-myeloablative stem cell transplant recipients. Transpl Infect Dis. 2007;9:3–10.
33. Cadena J, Patterson TF. Aspergillosis. Infect Dis Clin North Am. 2021;35:415–34.
34. Sahu KK. Infectious disease in hematopoietic stem cell transplantation. Ther Adv Infect Dis. 2021;8:20499361211005600.
35. Barnes PD, Marr KA. Risks, diagnosis and outcomes of invasive fungal infections in haematopoietic stem cell transplant recipients. Br J Haematol. 2007;139:519–31.
36. Calandra T. Early diagnosis of invasive mould infections and disease. J Antimicrob Chemother. 2017;72(Suppl 1):i19–28.
37. Seyfarth H-J, Nenoff P, Winkler J, Krahl R, Klöppel R, Wirtz H, et al. Invasive pulmonary aspergillosis—CT findings in context with the clinical course. Rofo. 2002;174:1115–20.
38. Patterson TF, Thompson GR 3rd, Denning DW, Fishman JA, Hadley S, Herbrecht R, et al. Practice guidelines for the diagnosis and management

of Aspergillosis: 2016 update by the Infectious Diseases Society of America. Clin Infect Dis. 2016;63:e1–60.
39. Ullmann AJ, Aguado JM, Denning DW, Verweij PE, Arendrup MC, Bouza E, et al. Diagnosis and management of aspergillus diseases: executive summary of the 2017 ESCMID-ECMM-ERS guideline. Clin Microbiol Infect. 2018;24(Suppl 1):e1–e38.
40. Maertens JA, Klont R, Masson C, Theunissen K, Meersseman W, Lagrou K, et al. Optimization of the cutoff value for the aspergillus double-sandwich enzyme immunoassay. Clin Infect Dis. 2007;44:1329–36.
41. Duarte RF, Sánchez-Ortega I, Cuesta I, Arnan M, Patiño B, Fernández de Sevilla A, et al. Serum galactomannan-based early detection of invasive aspergillosis in hematology patients receiving effective antimold prophylaxis. Clin Infect Dis. 2014;59:1696–702.
42. Teering S, Verreth A, Peeters A, Van Regenmortel N, De Laet I, Schoonheydt K, et al. Prognostic value of serum galactomannan in mixed ICU patients: a retrospective observational study. Anaesthesiol Intensive Ther. 2014;46:145–54.
43. Thompson GR 3rd, Boulware DR, Bahr NC, Clancy CJ, Harrison TS, Kauffman CA, et al. Noninvasive testing and surrogate markers in invasive fungal diseases. Open Forum Infect Dis. 2022;9:ofac112.
44. Tissot F, Agrawal S, Pagano L, Petrikkos G, Groll AH, Skiada A, et al. ECIL-6 guidelines for the treatment of invasive transplant patients. Haematologica. 2017;102:433–44.
45. Maertens JA, Raad II, Marr KA, Patterson TF, Kontoyiannis DP, Cornely OA, et al. Isavuconazole versus voriconazole for primary treatment of invasive mould disease caused by aspergillus and other filamentous fungi (SECURE): a phase 3, randomised-controlled, non-inferiority trial. Lancet. 2016;387:760–9.
46. Nucci M, Perfect JR. When primary antifungal therapy fails. Clin Infect Dis. 2008;46:1426–33.
47. Méheust D, Le Cann P, Reboux G, Millon L, Gangneux J-P. Indoor fungal contamination: health risks and measurement methods in hospitals, homes and workplaces. Crit Rev Microbiol. 2014;40:248–60.
48. Cornely OA, Maertens J, Winston DJ, Perfect J, Ullmann AJ, Walsh TJ, et al. Posaconazole vs. fluconazole or itraconazole prophylaxis in patients with neutropenia. N Engl J Med. 2007;356:348–59.

# Other Respiratory Fungal Infections

9

Carol A. Kauffman and Marisa H. Miceli

## Introduction

Invasive pulmonary fungal infections are a major cause of morbidity and mortality among hematopoietic stem cell transplant (HSCT) recipients [1–4]. Infections caused by *Aspergillus* species are most common, but increasingly non-*Aspergillus* molds are reported as causing invasive pulmonary disease in this population [5, 6]. These molds primarily include organisms in the order *Mucorales*, *Fusarium* spp., *Scedosporium* spp., and *Lomentospora* spp. Not only serious pulmonary infections but also widespread dissemination is the hallmark of infections with these fungi in HSCT recipients. These molds share to differing extents increased virulence and/or antifungal resistance, making treatment difficult and outcomes dismal [6]. HSCT recipients also remain at increased risk of *Pneumocystis jirovecii* pneumonia in spite of widespread use of prophylaxis [1]. The diagnosis of this fungal infection is difficult to prove, and treatment can be problematic. In markedly immunosuppressed hosts, especially those who have graft-versus-host disease, persistent neutropenia, and high-dose corticosteroid treatment, many different environmental molds have been reported to cause invasive disease, but these are quite rare and will not be discussed in this chapter.

C. A. Kauffman (✉)
Division of Infectious Diseases, Department of Internal Medicine, LTC Charles S. Kettles Veterans Affairs Medical Center, University of Michigan Medical School, Ann Arbor, MI, USA
e-mail: ckauff@umich.edu

M. H. Miceli
Division of Infectious Diseases, Department of Internal Medicine, Transplant Infectious Diseases Program, University of Michigan, Ann Arbor, MI, USA
e-mail: mmiceli@med.umich.edu

## *Fusarium* Infections

### Pathogenesis

*Fusarium* species, found in the environment throughout the world, are primarily plant pathogens. Localized infections in humans can occur with minor trauma leading to inoculation through the skin or cornea. However, invasive pulmonary and disseminated infections occur almost entirely in highly immunocompromised persons [2, 7, 8]. Those at most risk for invasive fusariosis are patients who have a hematological malignancy or have received an allogeneic HSCT [2, 7]. Neutropenia, especially when prolonged and profound, is the greatest risk factor for disseminated infection, and corticosteroids also are a major risk factor for invasive fusariosis [7–10].

The primary mode of infection is inhalation of the conidia produced by the mold through the lungs or sinuses with subsequent tissue invasion; in markedly immunocompromised patients, widespread



A. O. Soubani (ed.), *Pulmonary and Critical Care Considerations of Hematopoietic Stem Cell Transplantation*, https://doi.org/10.1007/978-3-031-28797-8_9

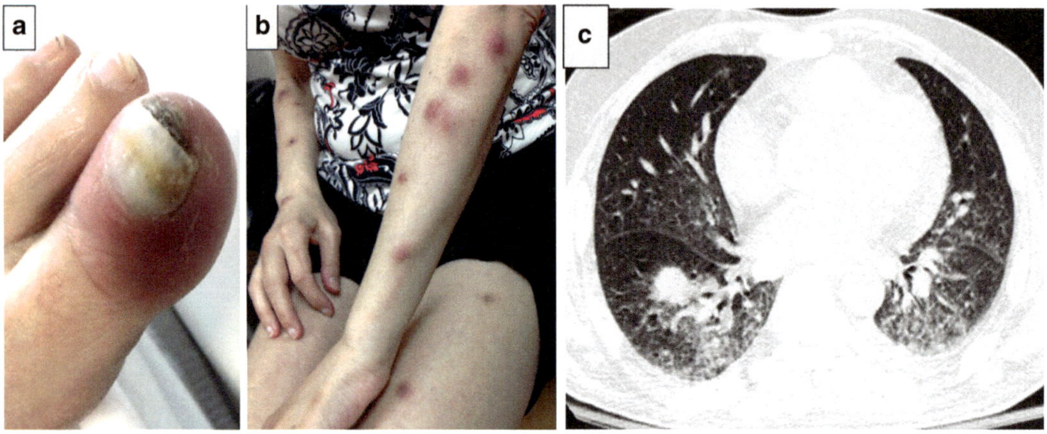


**Fig. 9.1** Clinical and radiological presentation of fusariosis. Onychomycosis of great toenail with adjacent skin and soft tissue involvement (**a**) and multiple subcutaneous painful nodules (**b**) in a neutropenic patient with disseminated fusariosis. Pulmonary nodules were present on CT of the thorax (**c**)

hematogenous dissemination often follows. Unique to patients with severe neutropenia is the ability of these organisms to disseminate widely from a simple paronychia or nail infection [10] (Fig. 9.1a). A hallmark of invasive fusariosis is angioinvasion, a property shared with *Aspergillus* species and the *Mucorales*. Angioinvasion culminates in hemorrhagic infarction and tissue necrosis [11].

## Clinical Aspects

The clinical presentation of pulmonary infection with *Fusarium* is similar to that noted with other molds. Fever, malaise, cough, and dyspnea occur and may be accompanied by pleuritic chest pain and hemoptysis.

Sinusitis due to *Fusarium* species presents in a similar fashion to that of infection with the *Mucorales* and *Aspergillus* species. Face pain is the cardinal symptom, accompanied by fever, swelling, and nasal discharge. Invasion of bone and necrosis of the palate and nasal turbinates can occur as the infection progresses.

Infection may remain localized to the lungs or sinuses, but *Fusarium* species often disseminate widely to other organs [12–14]. These non-pulmonary manifestations, especially skin lesions, can provide clues to the early diagnosis of fusariosis. The sudden appearance of painful skin pustules, nodules, or necrotic ecthyma-like lesions that may evolve to become hemorrhagic occurring in a neutropenic patient who has pulmonary infection points toward the diagnosis of fusariosis (Fig. 9.1b).

## Diagnosis

Thoracic computed tomography (CT) should be obtained when fever develops in an HSCT recipient who is neutropenic. The radiographic picture of invasive fusariosis is similar to that noted with other invasive mold infections. Typical findings are ground glass opacities, dense macronodules of varying sizes, and peribronchial consolidation (Fig. 9.1c) [11]. A halo sign is uncommon early in the infection, but can be seen later, as can cavitation of the nodules. Although there are subtle differences, the findings on CT scan are not specific enough to differentiate invasive fusariosis from invasive aspergillosis or other mold infections.

The diagnosis of proven invasive fusariosis in an immunocompromised host is established when the organism is isolated in culture from a sterile body site [15]. However, in most patients with clinical and radiological evidence typical for an invasive fungal infection, a positive culture is obtained from a non-sterile site, such as bronchoalveolar lavage (BAL) fluid or skin biopsy, and a diagnosis of probable invasive fusariosis is established [15].

*Fusarium* species, which grow readily in the laboratory on standard fungal media, have large banana-shaped (fusiform) macroconidia. These distinctive macroconidia allow clinical laboratories to easily identify the organism as belonging to the genus *Fusarium*. However, in most laboratories, further identification to the species level is generally not performed.

*Fusarium* is one of very few molds in which the organism can sporulate in vivo. Because of this, these molds are capable of growing in blood culture bottles. This is a valuable clue that is found in as many as 40%–50% of patients with invasive fusariosis and can help with an early differentiation of an invasive fungal pneumonia due to *Fusarium* species from that due to *Aspergillus* species [16].

Histopathological examination of biopsy material from skin lesions or other tissues shows non-pigmented hyphae that are septate and that branch at acute angles. Sometimes unusual hyphal forms are noted, but often the picture is indistinguishable from that of *Aspergillus* species. Culture is needed to define the specific mold that is causing disease.

False-positive results for *Aspergillus* galactomannan assays are seen frequently in patients with *Fusarium* infections [8, 17]. Invasive fusariosis should be a prime diagnostic consideration in patients who have a positive serum *Aspergillus* galactomannan test, but in whom *Aspergillus* has not been isolated. Beta-D-glucan, usually measured by the Fungitell assay, has also been detected in serum in patients with disseminated fusariosis but is nonspecific and cannot differentiate specific fungal infections [9].

There are no specific antibody or antigen detection tests available to aid in the diagnosis of invasive fusariosis. Several reference laboratories have reported on the use of polymerase chain reaction (PCR) methodology for the diagnosis of *Fusarium* infections, but this technique is not commercially available or standardized [18].

## Treatment

Invasive *Fusarium* infections are exceedingly difficult to treat because most species are resistant to many antifungal agents. The most active drugs appear to be amphotericin B, voriconazole, and posaconazole. Isavuconazole activity against *Fusarium* varies across species. Fluconazole and itraconazole are not active against most *Fusarium* species, and echinocandins have no activity against *Fusarium* species.

Recommended therapy is a lipid formulation of amphotericin B, voriconazole, or a combination of these two agents [19] (Table 9.1). Of the available mold-active azoles, the greatest experience is with

**Table 9.1** Treatment of non-*Aspergillus* fungal infections in HSCT recipients

| Fungal pathogen | Preferred treatment | Alternate/salvage treatment | Comments |
|---|---|---|---|
| *Fusarium* species | L-AmB: 5 mg/kg/day IV *plus* voriconazole: 6 mg/kg IV BID on day 1, then 4 mg/kg IV BID | *Step down:*<br>Voriconazole oral 200–300 mg PO BID<br>*Salvage:*<br>Posaconazole IV/PO 300 mg BID on day 1, then 300 mg QD | Drug-drug interactions are a major complication of azole therapy and should be carefully reviewed prior to starting these agents<br>Baseline EKG should be done before starting azole therapy<br>Oral voriconazole should be taken on an empty stomach<br>Serum trough concentrations of azoles should be obtained on day 5, as well as after any dose adjustment, to ensure adequate serum concentrations and to avoid toxicities<br>Goal serum trough concentration:<br>Posaconazole: 1.25–3 μg/mL<br>Voriconazole: 2–5.5 μg/mL<br>Isavuconazole: >1 μg/mL |
| *Scedosporium apiospermum* complex | Voriconazole: 6 mg/kg IV BID on day 1, then 4 mg/kg IV BID | *Step down*:<br>Voriconazole 200–300 mg PO BID<br>*Salvage:*<br>Posaconazole IV/PO 300 mg BID on day 1, then 300 mg QD | |
| *Lomentospora prolificans* | Voriconazole: 6 mg/kg IV BID on day 1, then 4 mg/kg IV BID *plus* terbinafine 500 mg PO QD | *Step down*:<br>Voriconazole 200–300 mg PO BID, *plus* terbinafine 500 mg PO QD | |
| *Mucorales* | L-AmB: 5 mg/kg/day IV<br>May have to increase dose to 10 mg/kg/day IV in severe cases | *Step down/salvage*:<br>Posaconazole 300 mg PO BID on day 1, then 300 mg QD, *or* isavuconazole IV/PO 200 mg TID for 2 days, then 200 mg QD | |

(continued)

**Table 9.1** (continued)

| Fungal pathogen | Preferred treatment | Alternate/salvage treatment | Comments |
|---|---|---|---|
| *Pneumocystis jirovecii* | TMP-SMX 15 mg/kg/day IV of TMP component given in three divided doses | *Second line agents:* Clindamycin 600 mg IV TID *plus* primaquine base 30 mg PO QD *or* pentamidine 4 mg/kg IV QD<br>*Step down:* TMP-SMX 15 mg/kg/day PO of TMP component in three divided doses | Add prednisone (or equivalent of methylprednisolone) when $PaO_2 < 70$ mmHg on room air, at dosage of 40 mg BID for 5 days, then 40 mg QD for 5 days, then 20 mg QD for 11 days |

*BID* twice daily, *IV* intravenous, *L-AmB* lipid formulation amphotericin B (Ambisome®/Albelcet®), *PO* oral, *QD* daily, *TID* three times daily, *TMP-SMX* trimethoprim-sulfamethoxazole

voriconazole [13, 19]. Posaconazole has been studied primarily as salvage or step-down therapy, and experience with isavuconazole has been minimal [19]. Combination therapy with a lipid formulation of amphotericin B and an azole, usually voriconazole, is often used as first-line therapy [8, 9, 12, 19, 20]. It is not clear that combination therapy is any more effective than monotherapy, but this approach is used frequently because susceptibility studies are not readily available and do not always reliably predict in vivo activity.

In patients who have *Fusarium* onychomycosis or paronychia, voriconazole should be given to prevent possible dissemination [10].

Survival rates are only 40–50% but overall are improved from earlier reports of only 10–20% survival [8, 9, 12, 14, 16]. However, among HSCT recipients, some series continue to show a mortality rate near 80% [5]. The best response rate is noted in the least immunosuppressed patients and in those with more localized disease. In general, patients who remain neutropenic throughout the course of therapy are unlikely to survive.

## *Scedosporium* and *Lomentospora* Infections

### Pathogenesis

The molds belonging to the genus *Scedosporium* occur in soil and water throughout the world. The major human pathogens belong to the *Scedosporium apiospermum* complex that is composed of at least five species [21–24]. *Scedosporium prolificans*, which differs in several fundamental aspects from other *Scedosporium* species, has been moved to a new genus and is now *Lomentospora prolificans*. *L. prolificans* is more geographically restricted than molds in the *S. apiospermum* complex; arid areas in Australia, southern Europe, and the southwestern USA account for the majority of cases of lomentosporiosis. The greatest concern is ascribed to this mold because of its resistance to most antifungal agents [20, 25].

Invasive pulmonary infections with *S. apiospermum* complex and *L. prolificans* occur in patients who have hematological malignancies and in HSCT recipients; neutropenia and T-cell suppression are important risk factors in these patients. Other at-risk groups include solid organ transplant recipients, burn victims, and near-drowning victims [22, 25]. *S. apiospermum* and less commonly *L. prolificans* are known to colonize the abnormal airways of patients with cystic fibrosis, form fungus balls, and uncommonly cause invasive disease, similar to that noted with *Aspergillus* species [26].

Infection follows inhalation of conidia into the alveoli and subsequent tissue invasion. Sinusitis also occurs but is less commonly seen than that caused by *Fusarium* or *Aspergillus*. Hematogenous spread to other organs, especially to the brain, is not uncommon following pulmonary invasion with these organisms.

### Clinical Aspects

Pulmonary infection caused by *S. apiospermum* complex or *L. prolificans* in immunocompromised patients has many similarities to infection with *Aspergillus* species [21]. Patients present with fever, cough, and shortness of breath; pleuritic chest pain and hemoptysis can occur.

Disseminated infection, often with brain abscesses, occurs commonly in HSCT recipients [25, 27]. Skin lesions occur, but are not painful, in contrast to disseminated infection with *Fusarium* species.

## Diagnosis

Thoracic CT scans should be done as soon as fever is manifested in an HSCT recipient. The findings of infection due *Scedosporium* or *Lomentospora* species are similar to those noted in other mold infections and include localized infiltrates and nodules with surrounding ground glass opacities (halo sign) and later cavitation (Fig. 9.2a) [22, 28, 29]. Progression to bilateral diffuse infiltrates can be quite rapid, especially with *Lomentospora* infection. Because of the risk of development of brain abscesses, MRI of the brain should be performed in patients with infections caused by these organisms (Fig. 9.2b).

The definitive diagnosis of scedosporiosis or lomentosporiosis is established by growing the organism from tissues or sterile body fluids. Growth of one of these molds from non-sterile body fluids, such as BAL fluid, in an immunocompromised patient whose CT scan shows typical radiographic evidence of an invasive fungal infection denotes probable scedosporiosis or lomentosporiosis [15]. Similar to *Fusarium* species, *L. prolificans* and, rarely, organisms of the *S. apiospermum* complex can sporulate in vivo, resulting in growth in blood cultures [30]. In markedly immunocompromised patients, such as HSCT recipients, fungemia with *Lomentospora* infection is common and can aid in diagnosis [29].

Histopathological examination of tissues infected with *Scedosporium* species demonstrates acutely branching septate hyphae that are seen best with methenamine-silver stain and that cannot be reliably differentiated from *Aspergillus* or *Fusarium* species. Many strains of *L. prolificans* are able to produce melanin and, because of this, appear as pigmented hyphae in tissues [30].

There are no specific antibody or antigen assays available to aid in the diagnosis of invasive infection with either *S. apiospermum* or *L. prolificans* infections. Serum beta-D-glucan has been reported to be positive in patients who have disseminated *Scedosporium* infection, but this assay is positive in many different fungal infections and not specific for *Scedosporium* [30]. PCR and in situ hybridization have been reported to be helpful for diagnosis, but these tests are not standardized nor are they commercially available [30].

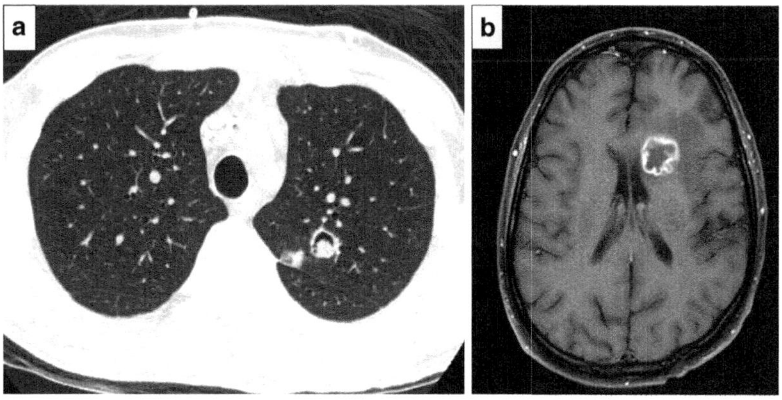


**Fig. 9.2** Radiological presentation of disseminated scedosporiosis. Several weeks after undergoing haploidentical HSCT, this patient developed disseminated infection due to *Scedosporium apiospermum*. CT thorax shows pulmonary nodules and patchy ground glass opacities (**a**), and a ring-enhancing left caudate/corpus callosum lesion was seen on the brain MRI (**b**)

## Treatment

*S. apiospermum* complex isolates are innately resistant to several antifungal agents; specifically, all species are resistant to amphotericin B, echinocandins, and fluconazole. However, these organisms are susceptible to mold-active azoles, and voriconazole has become the agent of choice for infections with *S. apiospermum* complex [19, 28, 29] (Table 9.1). Posaconazole has been used in fewer patients and appears to be effective; there is minimal experience with isavuconazole for scedosporiosis.

The mortality rates for scedosporiosis in HSCT recipients remain as high as 50–70% [19, 22]. Patients in other risk groups have lower mortality rates. Similar to fusariosis, patients who remain neutropenic have a very poor prognosis.

Treatment of lomentosporiosis remains problematic. Resistance to almost all antifungal agents is the hallmark of this organism [19, 21, 23, 31]. In vitro studies have shown synergistic activity when voriconazole is used in combination with terbinafine. Voriconazole at the doses noted for scedosporiosis plus terbinafine, 500 mg daily, has been reported to result in better outcomes than voriconazole alone [27, 32]. However, the outcome of infection with *L. prolificans*, regardless of the antifungal agents used, is dismal. Mortality rates greater than 80% are often seen and are especially high in HSCT recipients.

# Mucormycosis

## Pathogenesis

Invasive mucormycosis is a rare infection caused by molds of the order *Mucorales*. *Mucorales* are usually found in soil, decaying organic matter, and contaminated foods. Patients with uncontrolled diabetes and those who are immunosuppressed are at risk for this infection [33, 34]. Among immunocompromised patients, mucormycosis occurs most often in patients with hematologic malignancies, particularly those with prolonged neutropenia, and HSCT recipients, especially those who are receiving treatment for graft-versus-host disease [33, 35–37].

The primary mode of infection is inhalation of the spores that are produced by the mold through the lungs or sinuses. Direct skin inoculation secondary to trauma, or ingestion into the gastrointestinal tract, may also occur [37–40]. Spores germinate into hyphae, resulting in angioinvasion and subsequent hemorrhagic infarction and tissue necrosis. Angioinvasion also may lead to hematogenous dissemination and multiorgan involvement in HSCT recipients and other severely immunosuppressed patients [41].

## Clinical Aspects

Clinical presentation of mucormycosis depends on the organ involved and the immune status of the host. Rhino-orbital-cerebral infection, which is more common in patients with uncontrolled diabetes, is associated with fevers and localized symptoms that include headache, face pain, and nasal congestion. Progression of the infection with invasion of the orbit and palate and further extension to the brain result in loss of vision, cranial nerve palsies, and changes in mental status [37, 38].

Pulmonary infection is more common among patients with neutropenia that is related to a hematologic malignancy, HSCT recipients, and those who have received a solid organ transplant [33, 36]. Pulmonary mucormycosis presents with fever, chest pain, dyspnea, and hemoptysis. Contiguous spread of this aggressive infection can lead to involvement of surrounding structures, including the heart and mediastinum.

Cutaneous mucormycosis can be seen after trauma, including burns, and usually occurs in the immunocompetent host [39, 40]. Open wounds may show visible growth of the mold in severe cases. In patients with hematologic malignancies and HSCT recipients, skin lesions are secondary to hematogenous seeding and are a sign of disseminated disease [37, 41]. In this population, the skin lesions present as a necrotic eschar with surrounding painful erythema and induration. Gastrointestinal mucormycosis is rare and typically presents with gastrointestinal bleeding, gastric ulcerations, and/or bowel perforation.

## Diagnosis

Chest CT findings of pulmonary mucormycosis include multiple dense pulmonary infiltrates, nodules, and cavitary lesions; pleural effusions may develop [42, 43] (Fig. 9.3a). Although not always present, the "reverse halo" sign has been more commonly reported in pulmonary mucormycosis than in invasive pulmonary aspergillosis. This appears as a central ground glass opacification surrounded by a consolidative ring, reflective of central lung infarction surrounded by dense peripheral hemorrhage, that evolves into a cavitary lesion.

The definitive diagnosis of mucormycosis requires demonstration of characteristic wide, ribbonlike, nonseptate hyphae invading tissues on histopathology and growth of the mold from specimens of involved sites [44]. Unfortunately, culture of the *Mucorales* from tissues can be difficult, and the diagnosis often rests only on the characteristic histopathology (Fig. 9.3b). If the organism does grow in culture, species identification and antifungal susceptibilities are helpful in determining appropriate antifungal therapy.

Beta-D-glucan is not present in the cell wall of most *Mucorales*, and thus, this test is not helpful for the diagnosis of mucormycosis [44]. Serological tests for antigen or antibody are not available for the *Mucorales*.

PCR-based testing for the detection of *Mucorales* in tissue and in body fluids is an area of active investigation [45, 46]. Quantitative PCR assays for the detection of *Mucorales* DNA in serum, blood, and BAL have been tested in animal models and in patients with promising results [46]. However, similar to other fungal PCR assays, optimization of primers and DNA targets have not been standardized and are available only from research laboratories.

## Treatment

Mucormycosis is a life-threatening infection with ~50% mortality rate despite appropriate therapy. Early initiation of systemic antifungals has a direct impact on outcome. Therefore, when clinical suspicion for mucormycosis is high, appropriate antifungal therapy should be started immediately. Correcting the predisposing factors is pivotal in the management of patients with mucormycosis. However, eradication of the predisposing factor is often not possible in patients with hematological malignancies and in HSCT recipients.

A lipid formulation of amphotericin B is recommended for the initial treatment of mucormycosis [47] (Table 9.1). The usual dose for mucormycosis is 5 mg/kg/day, but doses as high as 10 mg/kg/day have been used in severe cases. However, at least one study found that higher daily doses did not improve outcome but did increase toxicity [48].

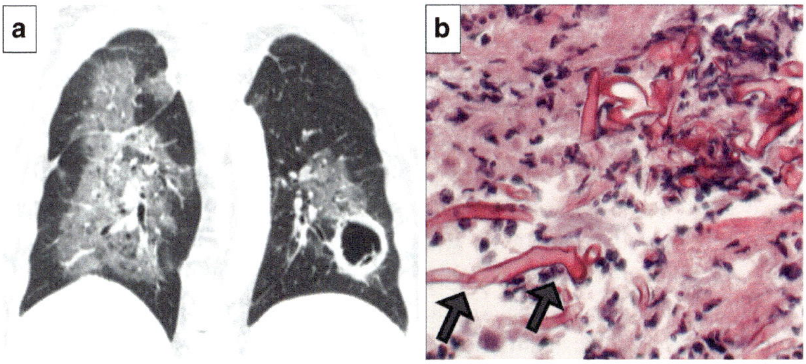


**Fig. 9.3** Radiological presentation of pulmonary mucormycosis. CT thorax shows bilateral patchy ground glass opacities and a large cavitary lesion in the left lower lobe in an allogeneic HSCT recipient (**a**). Histopathology of lung biopsy from a different patient with mucormycosis demonstrates ribbon-shaped nonseptate hyphae invading tissue (arrows) (**b**)

Of the currently available azoles, posaconazole and isavuconazole are active against most *Mucorales*; the organisms are innately resistant to voriconazole. Posaconazole is often used for step-down therapy once the infection is controlled with amphotericin B. Isavuconazole has been approved by the Food and Drug Administration for treatment of mucormycosis, based on results from an open-label clinical trial [49]. However, experience is limited for use as primary therapy, and it is preferable for use as step-down therapy.

Surgical debridement of necrotic tissue should be pursued urgently whenever possible. Surgical resection is very challenging in patients who have pulmonary mucormycosis, especially in those who have a hematological malignancy or have received a HSCT and have severe thrombocytopenia. Surgical debridement is a mainstay of therapy in most cases of rhino-orbital-cerebral and cutaneous mucormycosis [47, 50].

## *Pneumocystis* Infection

### Pathogenesis

*Pneumocystis jirovecii* has never been grown in vitro but has been classified taxonomically as a fungus based on ribosomal RNA and mRNA sequencing [51]. The environmental reservoir of *P. jirovecii* is unknown. It is thought that the organism is acquired by inhalation early in life with subsequent long-term persistence in the lungs in the cyst form [51, 52]. It is likely that most humans have been exposed to *P. jirovecii* and carry the organism in lung tissue with no symptoms.

Symptomatic infection occurs when *P. jirovecii* reactivates, assuming the trophozoite form in persons who have T-cell immune defects of various etiologies. Most affected are patients who have hematological malignancies, have received an allogeneic HSCT, or have been treated with high-dose corticosteroids or other immunosuppressive agents [53]. With the introduction of universal *P. jirovecii* prophylaxis after allogeneic HSCT, rates of *P. jirovecii* pneumonia have decreased from 5–16% to <5%, with most infections occurring within 5 months after HSCT [54].

Rates of *P. jirovecii* pneumonia among autologous HSCT recipients are much lower than among allogeneic HSCT recipients. Main risk factors for *P. jirovecii* pneumonia after autologous HSCT include underlying lymphoma, leukemia, or myeloma, especially if treatment includes purine analogs or high-dose corticosteroids [53, 54].

Aerosol transmission has been studied in animal models, and molecular typing of hospital outbreaks among solid organ transplant recipients have suggested that person-to-person transmission is possible, but such outbreaks are not common and have not been reported among HSCT recipients [51].

### Clinical Aspects

*Pneumocystis* pneumonia is a life-threatening infection among allogeneic HSCT recipients [53]. Clinical manifestations include fever, dry cough, and dyspnea. Severity of illness ranges from mild to severe. Infection can present as a subacute process but, in allogeneic HSCT recipients, can quickly progress to marked hypoxemia. Extrapulmonary *Pneumocystis* infection is extremely rare.

### Diagnosis

*P. jirovecii* pneumonia patterns seen on radiographs are indistinguishable from other interstitial lung processes. High-resolution CT of the chest usually shows early diffuse bilateral ground glass opacities, reticulation, and septal thickening that are often not seen on chest radiograph or standard chest CT scan [55]. Typically, infiltrates are most prominent in the peri-hilar region. Spontaneous pneumothorax has been described in HSCT recipients with *P. jirovecii* pneumonia. Unusual radiological presentations include pulmonary nodules, pleural effusion, and lobar consolidation [56].

The definitive diagnosis of *P. jirovecii* pneumonia is made by demonstrating the presence of *Pneumocystis* in the lung tissue, sputum, or BAL fluid. Lung tissue and BAL fluid are preferred over sputum because the yield of organisms is higher. The cysts can be visualized using a direct fluorescent antibody test or methenamine-silver stain. The sporozoites and trophozoites, which are the predominant form in active infection, can be observed using Giemsa, Wright's, or calcofluor stains. However, direct visualization of *Pneumocystis* in HSCT patients is challenging because of the low burden of organisms that is usually present in sputum or BAL fluid in these patients [56, 57].

Many medical centers now use PCR assays on respiratory specimens for the diagnosis of *P. jirovecii* infection. BAL fluid gives the best yield, and thus, bronchoscopy as soon as *Pneumocystis* infection is suspected is crucial. However, PCR techniques are not standardized and vary from laboratory to laboratory. PCR is highly specific but gives many false-positive results [56, 57].

A positive serum beta-D-glucan result supports the diagnosis of *Pneumocystis* pneumonia in patients at risk who have a compatible clinical and radiological presentation. Serum levels tend to be very high with *Pneumocystis* infection [58, 59]. However, a negative test result does not rule out the diagnosis of *P. jirovecii* pneumonia in patients at risk. Use of the beta-D-glucan assay on BAL fluid has not proven helpful in the diagnosis of *P. jirovecii* pneumonia [60].

Invasive diagnostic procedures, such as lung biopsy, are rarely pursued in the HSCT population because of thrombocytopenia. When obtained, histopathological examination of biopsy material from infected lung tissue shows airspaces filled with a foamy eosinophilic exudate. The intra-alveolar exudate consists of aggregates of trophozoites surrounded by surface glycoprotein and proteinaceous debris from the lungs and inflammatory cells.

## Treatment

Treatment options for *P. jirovecii* pneumonia are summarized in Table 9.1. Trimethoprim-sulfamethoxazole (TMP-SMX), either oral or IV, is considered to be first-line treatment for *P. jirovecii* infection. However, the use of TMP-SMX in HSCT recipients is limited by the risk of bone marrow toxicity and potential graft loss. Alternative treatment in HSCT recipients with mild *P. jirovecii* pneumonia is atovaquone and in those with moderate to severe disease is clindamycin and primaquine. Recommended duration of therapy is 2–3 weeks for mild infection and 3 weeks for moderate to severe disease.

The use of adjuvant corticosteroids in the setting of severe hypoxemia with *P. jirovecii* pneumonia is routinely used to dampen the inflammatory response, which has been documented to worsen hypoxemia as antimicrobial therapy is initiated [51]. In patients receiving corticosteroids for other reasons, including graft-versus-host disease, the dose can be increased during acute infection and then tapered to the baseline dose.

*Pneumocystis* pneumonia is considered a preventable complication after HSCT. Thus, strategies to prevent disease (primary prophylaxis) or to prevent reinfection or reactivation after recent infection (secondary prophylaxis) are recommended in this patient population [54]. Primary *P. jirovecii* prophylaxis in HSCT recipients should be administered from engraftment until at least 6 months after HSCT and should be continued for longer than 6 months in patients who continue to receive immunosuppressive drugs. Recurrence of *P. jirovecii* pneumonia in HSCT recipients is rare. Nonetheless, secondary prophylaxis for *P. jirovecii* should be continued lifelong or until immunosuppression is resolved.

The preferred regimen for *P. jirovecii* prophylaxis is TMP-SMX, but TMP-SMX can delay engraftment and thus is not usually administered before engraftment occurs. Many transplant programs use alternative regimens, including oral dapsone, aerosolized or intravenous pentamidine, or oral atovaquone.

## References

1. Rahi MS, Jindal V, Pednekar P, et al. Fungal infections in hematopoietic stem-cell transplant patients: a review of epidemiology, diagnosis, and management. Ther Adv Infect Dis. 2021;8:1–26.
2. Young AY, Juarez MMK, Evans SE. Fungal pneumonia in patients with hematologic malignancy and hematopoietic stem cell transplant. Clin Chest Med. 2017;38(3):479–91.
3. Omrani AS, Almaghrabi RS. Complications of hematopoietic stem cell transplantation: fungal infections. Hematol Oncol Stem Cell Ther. 2017;10:239–44.
4. Miceli MH, Churay T, Braun T, et al. Risk factors and outcomes of invasive fungal infections in allogeneic hematopoietic cell transplant recipients. Mycopathologia. 2017;182:495–504.
5. Riches ML, Trifilio S, Chen M, et al. Risk factors and impact of non-*aspergillus* mold infections following allogeneic HCT: a CIBMTR infection and immune reconstitution analysis. Bone Marrow Transplant. 2016;51:177–82.
6. Larcher R, Platon L, Amalric M, et al. Emerging invasive fungal infections in critically ill patients: incidence, outcomes, and prognostic factors, a case-control study. J Fungi. 2021;7:330. https://doi.org/10.3390/jof7050330.
7. Garnica M, Oliveira de Cunha M, Portugal R, et al. Risk factors for invasive fusariosis in patients with acute myeloid leukemia and in hematopoietic cell transplant recipients. Clin Infect Dis. 2015;60(6):875–80.
8. Horn DL, Freifeld AG, Schuster MG, et al. Treatment and outcomes of invasive fusariosis: review of 65 cases from the PATH Alliance registry. Mycoses. 2014;57:652–8.
9. Fernandez-Cruz A, Semiglia MA, Guinea J, et al. A retrospective cohort of invasive fusariosis in the era of antimould prophylaxis. Med Mycol. 2020;58:300–8.
10. Varon AG, Nouer SA, Barreiros G, et al. Antimold prophylaxis may reduce the risk of invasive fusariosis in hematologic patients with superficial skin lesions with positive culture for *Fusarium*. Antimicrob Agents Chemother. 2016;60(12):7290–4.
11. Sassi C, Stanzani M, Lewis RE, et al. Radiologic findings of *Fusarium* pneumonia in neutropenic patients. Mycoses. 2017;60(2):73–8.
12. Nucci M, Marr KA, Vehreschild MJGT, et al. Improvement in the outcome of invasive fusariosis in the last decade. Clin Microbiol Infect. 2014;20:580–5.
13. Lortholary O, Obenga G, Biswas P, et al. International retrospective analysis of 73 cases of invasive fusariosis treated with voriconazole. Antimicrob Agents Chemother. 2010;54:4446–50.
14. Stempel JM, Hammond SP, Sutton DA, et al. Invasive fusariosis in the voriconazole era: single-center 13-year experience. Open Forum Infect Dis. 2015;2(3):ofv099. https://doi.org/10.1093/ofid/ofv099.
15. Donnelly PJ, Chen S, Kauffman CA, et al. Revision and update of the consensus definitions of invasive fungal disease from the European Organization for Research and Treatment of Cancer and the Mycoses Study Group Education and Research Consortium. Clin Infect Dis. 2020;71:1367–76.
16. Nucci F, Nouer SA, Capone D, et al. Invasive mould disease in haematologic patients: comparison between fusariosis and aspergillosis. Clin Microbiol Infect. 2018;24:1105.e1–4.
17. Nucci M, Carlesse F, Cappellano P, et al. Earlier diagnosis of invasive fusariosis with *Aspergillus* serum galactomannan testing. PloS One. 2014;9:e87784.
18. Springer J, Walther G, Rickerts V, et al. Detection of *Fusarium* species in clinical specimens by probe-based real-time PCR. J Fungi. 2019;5:105. https://doi.org/10.3390/jof5040105.
19. Hoenigl M, Salmanton-Garcia J, Walsh TJ, et al. Global guideline for the diagnosis and management of rare mould infections: an initiative of the European Confederation of Medical Mycology in cooperation with the International Society for Human and Animal Mycology and the American Society for Microbiology. Lancet Infect Dis. 2021;21:e246. https://doi.org/10.1016/S1473-3099(20)30784-2.
20. McCarthy MW, Katragkou A, Iosifidis E, et al. Recent advances in the treatment of scedosporiosis and fusariosis. J Fungi. 2018;4:73. https://doi.org/10.3390/jof4020073.
21. Cobo F, Lara-Oya A, Rodriguez-Granger J, et al. Infections caused by *Scedosporium/Lomentospora* species: clinical and microbiological findings in 21 cases. Med Mycol. 2018;56:917–25.
22. Jacobs SE, Wengenack NL, Walsh TJ. Non-*aspergillus* hyaline molds: emerging causes of sinopulmonary fungal infections and other invasive mycoses. Semin Respir Crit Care Med. 2020;41:115–30.
23. Ramirez-Garcia A, Pellon A, Rementeria A, et al. *Scedosporium* and *Lomentospora*: updated overview of underrated opportunists. Med Mycol. 2018;56(suppl 1):102–25.
24. Rammaert B, Putade M, Cornely OA, et al. Perspectives on *Sedosporium* species and *Lomentospora prolificans* in lung transplantation: results of an international practice survey from ESCMID fungal infection study group and study group for infections in immunocompromised hosts and European Confederation of Medical Mycology. Transpl Infect Dis. 2019;21(5):e13141.
25. Bronniman D, Garcia-Hermoso D, Dromer F, et al. Scedosporiosis/lomentosporiosis observational study: clinical significance of *Scedosporium* species identification. Med Mycol. 2021;59:486–97.
26. Schwarz C, Brandt C, Antweiler E, et al. Prospective multicenter German study on pulmonary colonization with *Scedosporium/Lomentspora* species in cystic fibrosis: epidemiology and new associations. PloS One. 2017;12:e0171485.
27. Penteado FD, Litvinov N, Sztajnbok J, et al. *Lomentospora prolificans* fungemia in hematopoietic stem cell transplant patients: first report in South

America and literature review. Transpl Infect Dis. 2018;20(4):e12908.
28. Seidel D, Meissner A, Lackner M, et al. Prognostic factors in 264 adults with invasive *Scedosporium* spp. and *Lomentospora prolificans* invasive infections reported in the literature and FungiScope. Crit Rev Microbiol. 2019;45(1):1–21.
29. Seidel D, Hassler A, Salmanton-Garcia J, et al. Invasive *Scedosporium* spp. and *Lomentospora prolificans* infections in pediatric patients: analysis of 55 patients from FungiScope and the literature. Int J Infect Dis. 2019;92:114–22.
30. Chen SC-A, Halliday CL, Hoenigl M, et al. *Scedosporium* and *Lomentospora* infections: contemporary microbiological tools for the diagnosis of invasive disease. J Fungi. 2021;7:23. https://doi.org/10.3390/jof701002.
31. Jenks JD, Seidel D, Cornely OA, et al. Clinical characteristics and outcomes of invasive *Lomentospora prolificans* infections: analysis of patients in the FungiScope® registry. Mycoses. 2020;63:437–42.
32. Jenks JD, Seidel D, Cornely OA, et al. Voriconazole plus terbinafine combination antifungal therapy for invasive *Lomentospora prolificans* infections: analysis of 41 patients from the FungiScope® registry 2008-2019. Clin Microbiol Infect. 2020;26:781–4.
33. Park BJ, Pappas PG, Wannemuehler KA, et al. Invasive non-*aspergillus* mold infections in transplant recipients, United States, 2001-2006. Emerg Infect Dis. 2011;17(10):1855–64.
34. Azie N, Neofytos D, Pfaller M, et al. The PATH (prospective antifungal therapy) Alliance registry and invasive fungal infections: update 2012. Diagn Microbiol Infect Dis. 2012;73(4):293–300.
35. Jeong W, Keighley C, Wolfe R, et al. The epidemiology and clinical manifestations of mucormycosis: a systematic review and meta-analysis of case reports. Clin Microbiol Infect. 2019;25(1):26–34.
36. Kontoyiannis DP, Marr KA, Park BJ, et al. Prospective surveillance for invasive fungal infections in hematopoietic stem cell transplant recipients, 2001-2006: overview of the transplant-associated infection surveillance network (TRANSNET) database. Clin Infect Dis. 2010;50(8):1091–100.
37. Petrikkos G, Skiada A, Lortholary O, et al. Epidemiology and clinical manifestations of mucormycosis. Clin Infect Dis. 2012;54(Suppl 1):S23–34.
38. Reid G, Lynch JP 3rd, Fishbein MC, et al. Mucormycosis. Semin Respir Crit Care Med. 2020;41(1):99–114.
39. Neblett Fanfair R, Benedict K, Bos J, et al. Necrotizing cutaneous mucormycosis after a tornado in Joplin, Missouri, in 2011. N Engl J Med. 2012;367(23):2214–25.
40. Warkentien T, Rodriguez C, Lloyd B, et al. Invasive mold infections following combat-related injuries. Clin Infect Dis. 2012;55(11):1441–9.
41. Petrikkos G, Tsioutis C. Recent advances in the pathogenesis of mucormycoses. Clin Ther. 2018;40(6):894–902.
42. Jung J, Kim MY, Lee HJ, et al. Comparison of computed tomographic findings in pulmonary mucormycosis and invasive pulmonary aspergillosis. Clin Microbiol Infect. 2015;21(7):684.e11–8.
43. Hammer MM, Madan R, Hatabu H. Pulmonary mucormycosis: radiologic features at presentation and over time. Am J Roentgenol. 2018;210(4):742–7.
44. Walsh TJ, Gamaletsou MN, McGinnis MR, et al. Early clinical and laboratory diagnosis of invasive pulmonary, extrapulmonary, and disseminated mucormycosis (zygomycosis). Clin Infect Dis. 2012;54(Suppl 1):S55–60.
45. Hammond SP, Bialek R, Milner DA, et al. Molecular methods to improve diagnosis and identification of mucormycosis. J Clin Microbiol. 2011;49(6):2151–3.
46. Dadwal SS, Kontoyiannis DP. Recent advances in the molecular diagnosis of mucormycosis. Expert Rev Mol Diagn. 2018;18(10):845–54.
47. Cornely OA, Alastruey-Izquierdo A, Arenz D, et al. Global guideline for the diagnosis and management of mucormycosis: an initiative of the European Confederation of Medical Mycology in cooperation with the mycoses study group education and research consortium. Lancet Infect Dis. 2019;19(12):e405–21.
48. Lanternier F, Poiree S, Elie C, et al. Prospective pilot study of high-dose (10 mg/kg/day) liposomal amphotericin B (L-AMB) for the initial treatment of mucormycosis. J Antimicrob Chemother. 2015;70(11):3116–23.
49. Marty FM, Ostrosky-Zeichner L, Cornely OA, et al. Isavuconazole treatment for mucormycosis: a single-arm open-label trial and case control analysis. Lancet Infect Dis. 2016;16(7):828–37.
50. Vironneau P, Kania R, Morizot G, et al. Local control of rhino-orbito-cerebral mucormycosis dramatically impacts survival. Clin Microbiol Infect. 2014;20(5):336–9.
51. Fishman J. Pneumocystis jiroveci. Semin Respir Crit Care Med. 2020;41:141–57.
52. Köhler JR, Hube B, Puccia R, et al. Fungi that infect humans. Microbiol Spectr. 2017;5(3). https://doi.org/10.1128/microbiolspec.FUNK-0014-2016.
53. Cordonnier C, Cesaro S, Maschmeyer G, et al. *Pneumocystis jirovecii* pneumonia: still a concern in patients with haematological malignancies and stem cell transplant recipients. J Antimicrob Chemother. 2016;71(9):2379–85.
54. Tomblyn M, Chiller T, Einsele H, et al. Guidelines for preventing infectious complications among hematopoietic cell transplantation recipients: a global perspective. Biol Blood Marrow Transplant. 2009;15(10):1143–238.
55. Kanne JP, Yandow DR, Meyer CA. *Pneumocystis jirovecii* pneumonia: high resolution computed tomography findings in patients with and without HIV infection. Am J Roentgenol. 2012;198(6):W555–61.
56. Lagrou K, Chen S, Masur H, et al. *Pneumocystis jirovecii* disease: basis for the revised EORTC/MSGERC invasive fungal disease definitions in indi-

viduals without human immunodeficiency virus. Clin Infect Dis. 2021;72(Suppl 2):S114–20.
57. Alanio A, Hauser PM, Lagrou K, et al. ECIL guidelines for the diagnosis of *Pneumocystis jirovecii* pneumonia in patients with haematological malignancies and stem cell transplant recipients. J Antimicrob Chemother. 2016;71:2386–96.
58. Finkelman MA. Specificity influences in Beta (1->3)-D-glucan-supported diagnosis of invasive fungal disease. J Fungi. 2021;7:14. https://doi.org/10.3390/jof7010014.
59. Bateman M, Oladele R, Kolls JK. Diagnosing *pneumocystis jirovecii* pneumonia: a review of current methods and novel approaches. Med Mycol. 2020;58(8):1015–28.
60. Zhou S, Linder KA, Kauffman CA, et al. Diagnostic performance of bronchoalveolar lavage (1,3)-β-D-glucan assay for *pneumocystis jirovecii* pneumonia. J Fungi. 2020;6(4):200. https://doi.org/10.3390/jof6040200.

# 10 Cytomegalovirus Diseases in Hematopoietic Cell Transplant Recipients

Alexander Franklin, Amy Spallone, and Roy F. Chemaly

## Introduction: General Principles

Since the early days of hematopoietic cell transplantation (HCT), cytomegalovirus (CMV), a highly seroprevalent human herpesvirus, has remained one of the most notable posttransplant infectious complications encountered in this highly vulnerable patient population. Transplant care providers are frequently faced with challenging clinical scenarios regarding the management and treatment of CMV, especially in the critical care setting. CMV can adversely affect outcomes through both direct and indirect mechanisms. Reactivation of CMV can lead to invasive single or multi-organ diseases, such as pneumonia, gastrointestinal (GI) disease, central nervous system (CNS) disease, and retinitis, among others, either early (≤3 months) or later (>3 months) post-HCT [1]. Furthermore, a patient's CMV serostatus and development of viremia have been associated with increased posttransplant non-relapse mortality and overall mortality [2, 3]. In addition, CMV has been closely associated with increased incidence of graft-versus-host disease (GVHD) and graft failure [4, 5], as well as secondary invasive fungal and bacterial infections attributed to modulation of the host immune response and serious toxicities (mainly myelosuppression) of some of the commercially available anti-CMV agents [6–10]. Despite recent advances in the prevention of CMV reactivation, such as the US Food and Drug Administration (FDA) approval of letermovir for primary prophylaxis, our understanding of CMV is still evolving, and a need for enhanced diagnostics, immune-monitoring tools, and effective and well-tolerated anti-CMV therapies, especially for patients with critical illnesses, remains unmet [11].

## Pathophysiology of CMV

As a member of the herpes virus subfamily *Betaherpesvirinae*, which is ubiquitous in humans, CMV can efficiently infect several cell types, including endothelial cells, epithelial cells, smooth muscle cells, fibroblasts, leukocytes, and dendritic cells [8, 12]. The coevolution of CMV and the immune system is highlighted in the virus's ability to adapt to and evade elimination during the height of the immunocompetent host's

A. Franklin
Department of Infectious Diseases, Infection Control and Employee Health, Unit 1460, The University of Texas MD Anderson Cancer Center, Houston, TX, USA

Section of Infectious Diseases, Baylor College of Medicine, Houston, TX, USA

A. Spallone · R. F. Chemaly (✉)
Department of Infectious Diseases, Infection Control and Employee Health, Unit 1460, The University of Texas MD Anderson Cancer Center, Houston, TX, USA
e-mail: rfchemaly@mdanderson.org


A. O. Soubani (ed.), *Pulmonary and Critical Care Considerations of Hematopoietic Stem Cell Transplantation*, https://doi.org/10.1007/978-3-031-28797-8_10

cellular response to the infection, which merely results in lifelong viral latency in predominantly myeloid cells [13]. Following HCT, CMV can reactivate during T-cell deficiency or dysfunction episodes, resulting in loss of CMV immune containment. Although not completely understood, the attendant suppression of CMV on the host immune system in HCT recipients can be attributed to its effect on leukocyte antigen expression, cytokine production, and adhesion molecules. These cellular immune alterations may partly explain the increased incidence of invasive fungal and bacterial infections and GVHD following CMV reactivation in HCT recipients [7, 8].

## Risk Factors for CMV Reactivation and Disease

Without anti-CMV prophylaxis, about 60–70% of CMV-seropositive HCT recipients will experience CMV infection following transplantation [14]. These patients are at particular risk for poor outcomes because of enhanced immunosuppression, limited treatment options, frequent drug toxicities, and the development of viral resistance, which all lead to increased morbidity and mortality rates [7, 15]. A robust body of literature has described the risk factors for developing CMV infection (also referred to as CMV viremia), clinically significant CMV infection (CS-CMVi) (that requires treatment), and CMV end-organ involvement (also referred to as CMV disease). The primary risk factors can be stratified into transplant-related factors, host-related factors, and laboratory markers, including novel tools used to assess CMV risk.

### Transplant-Related Factors

In allogeneic HCT recipients, the main and most consistent risk factor for CMV infection is the pretransplant serostatus of the donor (D) and the recipient (R) (Fig. 10.1). At the highest risk are those with CMV-negative donor cells transplanted into a CMV-positive recipient (D−/R+). These patients will receive a CMV-naïve immune system grafted into a recipient with a latent CMV reservoir. In addition, these patients are at increased risk for repeat CMV reactivation and CMV disease [16]. In the modern transplant era, CMV reactivation rates in this group are about 36% [17]. Compared with CMV R− patients, CMV R+ patients have increased risk, regardless of donor status [17–19]. However, studies have shown that CMV D+/R− transplant recipients may be at lower risk for CMV infection, with rates estimated at around 13% [17, 20], and these patients have much lower rates of CMV disease [21]. CMV D−/R− transplants carry a low overall risk of CMV infection (3%) [17]; however, they are still at risk for primary infection and require leukoreduced blood or blood products from CMV seronegative donors for transfusions [22, 23].

Allogeneic transplantation carries a higher risk than autologous transplantation, to the extent that routine serum CMV monitoring is not recommended following autologous transplantation [24]. Other risk factors for CMV infection include myeloablative chemotherapy, conditioning regimens containing fludarabine or antithymocyte globulin, umbilical cord blood transplants, haploidentical and matched unrelated donor transplants, total body irradiation, T cell-depleted stem cells or use of anti-T-cell antibodies (e.g., alemtuzumab), GVHD, high-dose steroids, posttransplant cyclophosphamide, low CD4 count, and undetectable CMV-specific T-cell immunity [7, 25–32]. Elevated tacrolimus troughs have also been associated with increased risk, whereas the use of sirolimus appears to be protective against CMV, possibly in a dose-dependent manner [33].

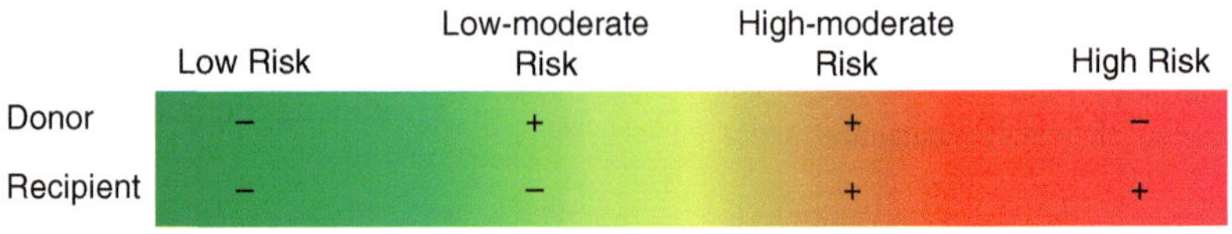


**Fig. 10.1** CMV risk of HCT recipients based on donor and recipient CMV serostatus

## Host-Related Risk Factors

In some studies, underlying malignancy has been associated with an increased risk of CMV infections after transplantation. Specifically, although not consistently associated with initial CMV infection, patients receiving transplants for lymphoma or myeloma may be at high risk for recurrent CMV infections [29]. Older age has been studied extensively as a potential risk factor but remains controversial. CMV-positive serostatus increases with older age, but when controlling for serostatus and transplant type, the effect of age may be minimal [19, 28].

## Laboratory Studies and Novel Tools

Lymphopenia, CMV-specific T-cell responses, and low natural killer cell counts have been identified as potential markers for CMV risk [34–39]. More recently, interest in investigating more refined markers of CMV risk has increased and includes the development of interferon-γ release assays such as enzyme-linked immunospot assays (ELISPOT and T-Track) and enzyme-linked immunoassays (QuantiFERON-CMV) [36–39]. These assays have demonstrated utility in predicting CMV risk status but have not yet gained widespread use.

Investigators have also studied risk factors for CMV disease. However, CMV disease is much less common than CMV infection in the modern transplant era (generally estimated to be ~7%) [17, 26]. Nevertheless, a high viral load, slow resolution of viremia, and a refractory CMV infection may increase the risk of progression to CMV disease [40–43]. Additionally, few studies have identified persistent leukopenia, CMV serostatus, and acute GVHD as risk factors for progression from viremia to disease or de novo CMV disease [26, 40, 44, 45].

## Prevention

The choice of CMV preventive strategy is dictated by the underlying risk factors, such as transplant type and serostatus of the allogeneic HCT donor and recipient (Fig. 10.1). As stated previously, CMV D−/R− transplants are at risk from primary exposure; as such, using leukoreduced blood products or blood products from CMV-negative donors is a sufficient precaution [22]. On the other hand, CMV D+/R− allogeneic HCT recipients are at intermediate risk. Therefore, serial monitoring with early preemptive therapy (PET) of viremia to halt progression to CMV disease is sometimes employed as a prevention strategy for this group.

For adult allogeneic HCT recipients with CMV-positive serostatus, the FDA approval of the DNA terminase inhibitor complex letermovir was a major advancement in CMV prevention. Over the past few decades, PET with (val) ganciclovir or foscarnet has been the primary strategy for preventing CMV disease. While PET reduced the incidence of CMV disease, recent studies demonstrated the negative impact of any level of CMV viremia on nonrelapse mortality or overall survival, which could be only partially explained by the serious side effects of the anti-CMV drugs, such as exposure-dependent myelosuppression and nephrotoxicity [6, 19, 43, 46–48]. On the other hand, letermovir has a safer profile, lacks the cytotoxic effects associated with (val)ganciclovir and foscarnet, and was shown to consistently reduce the rates of viremia and CS-CMVi in CMV-seropositive allogeneic HCT recipients [11, 49–51], especially in the high-risk D−/R+ group [52, 53]. In an analysis of phase III trial data, when compared with a placebo, letermovir was also associated with shorter hospital stays and fewer rehospitalizations in CMV-seropositive HCT recipients, leading to lower overall healthcare costs [54].

Further analysis showed that letermovir use for CMV prophylaxis was a more cost-effective option than no prophylaxis. The base-case analysis demonstrated an incremental cost-effectiveness ratio of $25,046 per quality-adjusted life-year gained [55]. While studies have demonstrated the positive impact of letermovir through transplant day +100, recent real-world studies suggested that longer durations of letermovir prophylaxis should be considered to prevent viral reactivation in certain high-risk patients, such as those with delayed T-cell reconstitution [56, 57]. A randomized clinical trial investigating the safety and efficacy of letermovir beyond day +100 post allogeneic HCT is ongoing (NCT03930615). Finally, letermovir chemoprophylaxis shifted the paradigm from CMV PET to primary prophylaxis in the appropriate allogeneic HCT population.

## CMV Infection or Reactivation: Diagnosis and Treatment

CMV infection is defined by the isolation of CMV in culture or detection of viral proteins or nucleic acids in the blood without end-organ involvement [58]. Multiple diagnostic methods identify CMV infection, such as viral antigen assays, to detect CMV phosphoprotein 65 in neutrophils and polymerase chain reaction (PCR) assays to detect CMV DNA in blood [7]. CMV phosphoprotein 65 is a semiquantitative correlate of viral replication that often rises during the first week of therapy for CMV infection and should be interpreted with caution during this period. Overall, it is inexpensive to perform, but a lack of standardization in interpreting its results and a need for an adequate neutrophil count greater than 1000 cells/mL for sensitivity make it less practical in the early periods after transplantation [7]. Molecular methods such as quantitative CMV DNA detection using PCR have largely replaced antigen assays owing to their high sensitivity and quantitative measurements in monitoring viral replication and response to therapy [59].

While treatment of CMV viremia can prevent the development of CMV disease and other complications associated with viremia, the optimal CMV viral load cutoffs that warrant treatment have yet to be established. Therefore, most experts advocate adopting a strategy similar to the one used in the phase III trial of letermovir, in which a patient's risk factors determine the CMV viral load cutoffs above which therapy is recommended [14, 49]. Figure 10.2 depicts the University of Texas MD Anderson Cancer Center's CMV treatment recommendations according to patient characteristics, risk factors, and CMV viral load cutoffs. In the high-risk group, therapy is recommended for a CMV viral load greater than 150 IU/mL according to PCR or three consecutive PCRs positive at any level below 150 IU/mL. For moderate-risk HCT recipients, treatment is recommended for a CMV viral load of at least 500 IU/μL or two consecutive positive values with at least a twofold increase in PCR values from the previous level and greater than 1000 IU/μL. Finally, treatment is recommended for low-risk recipients following two consecutive positive values with at least a fivefold increase in PCR values.

The main agents used to treat CMV infections are (val)ganciclovir, foscarnet, and cidofovir. Unfortunately, these agents can have significant adverse effects, frequently limiting their use. Ganciclovir and valganciclovir are associated with

| | Low Risk | Moderate Risk | High Risk |
|---|---|---|---|
| Patient Characteristics | MRD<br>GVHD (steroid dose <1mg/kg/day)<br>Autologous<br>>Day +100 post-Allo HCT | MUD<br>Mismatched<br>GVHD >1mg/kg/day) | Cord blood<br>Haploidentical<br>Mismatched + post-cy<br>T-cell depleted<br>Alemtuzumab |
| CMV PCR Treatment Value | >1000 IU/mL-or-<br>>5-fold increase from previous value | >500 IU/mL-or-<br>>2-fold increase from previous value | >150 IU/mL-or-<br>3 consecutive values |

Abbreviation. MRD, match-related donor; GVHD, graft-versus-host-disease; HCT, hematopoietic cell transplant; Allo, allogeneic; MUD, matched-unrelated donor; IU, international units; Post-cy, post-transplant cyclophosphamide.

**Fig. 10.2** Indications for treatment of CMV infection by HCT patient risk group and CMV PCR value adapted from the University of Texas MD Anderson Cancer Center's Guidelines of Care (GC11.6 CMV Treatment and Management, updated 4/7/2020). *MRD* match-related donor, *allo* allogeneic HCT, *MUD* matched-unrelated donor, *Post-cy* post-transplant cyclophosphamide

**Table 10.1** CMV infection treatment, duration, and secondary prophylaxis recommendations by HCT recipient risk group

Low Risk → Moderate Risk → High Risk

| | | | |
|---|---|---|---|
| Induction | Ganciclovir, valganciclovir, or foscarnet for 7-14 days **-and-** | | |
| | CMV PCR ≤ 150 IU/mL | | CMV PCR negative |
| Maintenance and/or Secondary prophylaxis | Ganciclovir, valganciclovir, or foscarnet, followed by valacyclovir prophylaxis | Ganciclovir, valganciclovir, or foscarnet, followed by valacyclovir prophylaxis -or- Consider letermovir secondary prophylaxis* immediately following induction therapy and continue through HCT day +100 | |
| Total duration of induction + maintenance | ≥3 weeks | ≥3 weeks | |

*CMV PCR value must be undetectable or have ≥2 consecutive PCR values ≤150 IU/mL prior to starting secondary prophylaxis
Abbreviation. CMV, cytomegalovirus; HCT, hematopoietic cell transplant; IU, international units.

cytopenias, foscarnet with nephrotoxicity and electrolyte abnormalities, and cidofovir with all of these adverse effects [60–63]. Head to head trials of (val)ganciclovir versus foscarnet demonstrated similar efficacy, with prevention of CMV disease or death within 180 days post-HCT and low overall rates of serious nephrotoxicity with foscarnet when used with close monitoring [64, 65]. An individualized approach is recommended when selecting initial therapy, considering whether the patient is in the pre-engraftment or peri-engraftment period, the risk of graft failure, and the probability of serious nephrotoxicity and renal failure. A multidisciplinary approach for critically ill patients with CMV infections should include critical care and transplant providers, nephrologists, and infectious diseases specialists. Table 10.1 outlines the University of Texas MD Anderson Cancer Center's recommendations for the duration of therapy based on risk stratification and CMV viral loads according to PCR values [66].

## CMV Disease: Presentation, Diagnosis, and Therapy

### CMV Pneumonia

CMV pneumonia or pneumonitis is one of the most serious and potentially fatal manifestations of CMV disease, with mortality rates approaching 30–50% [67–70]. Most CMV pneumonia cases are generally diagnosed in the early post-transplant period (i.e., within the first 100 days post-HCT). However, recent studies showed an increase in late presentation (i.e., after day +100 post-HCT) [67, 69]. Lymphocytopenia, male sex, and severe acute GVHD have all been associated with fatal CMV pneumonia [71]. In addition, patients with CMV pneumonia may present with rapid progression of fever, hypoxia, shortness of breath, and cough [72]. Radiographic findings include bilateral interstitial infiltrates on chest X-ray, although plain films may not show any findings early in the disease course [25, 67]. Common chest computed tomography findings include ground-glass opacities, small centrilobular nodules, and airspace opacities, more often with central and peripheral distributions than in either distribution alone [73]. However, other viral infections, such as influenza, RSV, SARS-CoV-2, adenovirus, and parainfluenza, may appear similarly on chest radiographs [74, 75].

The diagnosis of proven CMV pneumonia requires clinical symptoms and signs, such as radiographic evidence of pulmonary viral infection, along with detection of CMV in lung parenchyma by virus isolation, rapid culture, histopathology and immunohistochemistry, or DNA hybridization techniques [58]. Lung biopsy with a histopathologic examination revealing CMV within cells or atypical intranuclear inclusions, supported by immunohistochemical staining or in situ hybridization for CMV, is the gold standard for diagnosis [76]. However, this is rarely feasible for critically ill HCT recipients due to concerns regarding respiratory failure and thrombocytopenia-associated complications such as bleeding. In addition, it should be recognized that qualitative detection of CMV DNA in lung specimens using nucleic acid testing assays lacks specificity as viral shedding in the lower respiratory tract does occur, even in the absence of CMV pneumonia, and may represent asymptomatic infection [58, 77]. Also, the correlation between CMV viral load in blood specimens and diagnosis of CMV pneumonia is not optimal in many instances [78, 79]. Multiple studies have demonstrated good sensitivity and specificity of quantitative PCR using bronchoalveolar lavage; however, the ideal cutoff values varied significantly in previous studies [70, 79–82].

Studies in the 1980s showed better survival in patients with CMV pneumonia treated with pooled intravenous immunoglobulin (IVIG) or CMV-specific immunoglobulins and ganciclovir compared to either therapy alone. However, these studies were of limited quality, with small sample sizes, and historical controls were used for comparison groups. More recent studies failed to demonstrate a significant impact on mortality with the addition of IVIG to anti-CMV agents [67, 69]. In the absence of high-quality evidence, the addition of IVIG to anti-CMV agents in severely ill patients with CMV pneumonia is still utilized (Table 10.2).

## CMV Gastrointestinal Disease

CMV GI disease may occur early or late after HCT, with a median onset around day +90 with a wide range (17–1099 days post-HCT) [83, 84]. Allogeneic HCT recipients with CMV GI disease may present with a variety of symptoms related to the area of GI involvement, including diarrhea (59%) that can be profuse and either watery or bloody, nausea (51%), and vomiting (33%) [85]. Other symptoms include odynophagia, dysphagia, persistent substernal chest pain, fever, and abdominal pain. Although CMV can involve any part of the GI tract, one study showed that upper GI involvement is more common in HCT transplant recipients (upper GI CMV, 14/18 [78%]) [83]. Upon endoscopic evaluation, CMV GI manifestations may appear as erosive and/or ulcerative conditions and can occur anywhere along the GI tract from the mouth to the rectum [85]. Common sites of CMV GI disease in HCT and cancer patients include the stomach, esophagus, colon/rectum, liver, and duodenum [71, 86]. In one study, 11% of HCT recipients had multiple GI sites of CMV disease, and 39% had disseminated disease involving other organs [83].

In allogeneic HCT recipients, CMV GI disease can be difficult to distinguish from GI GVHD relying solely on symptomatology. Additionally, GI GVHD and GI CMV disease can be present in these patients, complicating the diagnosis and treatment of both diseases [83]. Diagnosing and distinguishing GI CMV from GI GVHD requires an endoscopic evaluation and tissue biopsy confirming both entities [76]. Proven CMV GI disease requires GI symptoms in addition to macroscopic mucosal lesions plus CMV in histopathology, virus isolation, rapid culture, immunohistochemistry, or DNA hybridization techniques [58]. CMV detection in blood or tissue biopsy specimens using PCR or the presence of antigenemia is not sufficient for diagnosing CMV GI disease. However, quantitative tissue PCR has been investigated as a potential diagnostic tool, and preliminary studies report a high sensitivity and specificity [58, 78, 84, 87, 88].

In HCT recipients with CMV GI disease, the treatment of choice includes induction phase therapy with (val)ganciclovir or foscarnet for a minimum of 2 weeks with improvement in symptoms (and resolution of positive serum CMV PCR if this was present at diagnosis), followed by secondary prophylaxis therapy with (val)ganciclovir or foscarnet until at least day +90 after HCT or for a minimum of 8 weeks, whichever is longer (Table 10.2). In patients with significant GI involvement resulting in diarrhea or vomiting, caution should be taken when switching to an oral antiviral agent. Poor GI

**Table 10.2** Recommendations for CMV disease treatment in HCT recipients by end-organ involvement adapted from the University of Texas MD Anderson Cancer Center's Guidelines of Care[a]

| | 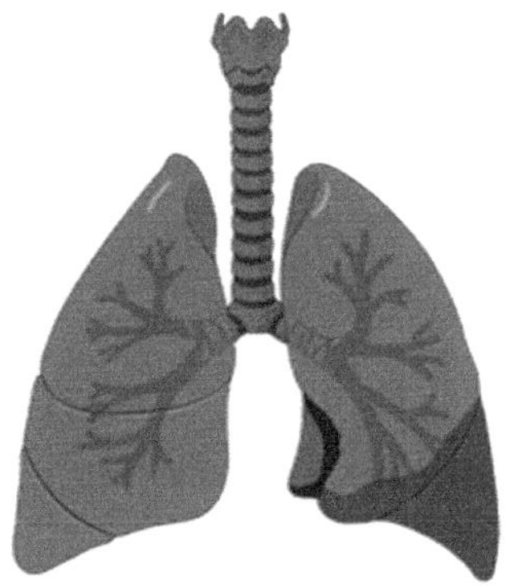 Pneumonia | 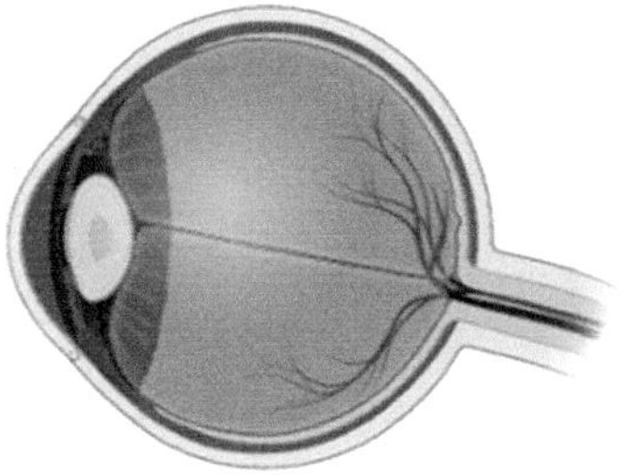 Retinitis | 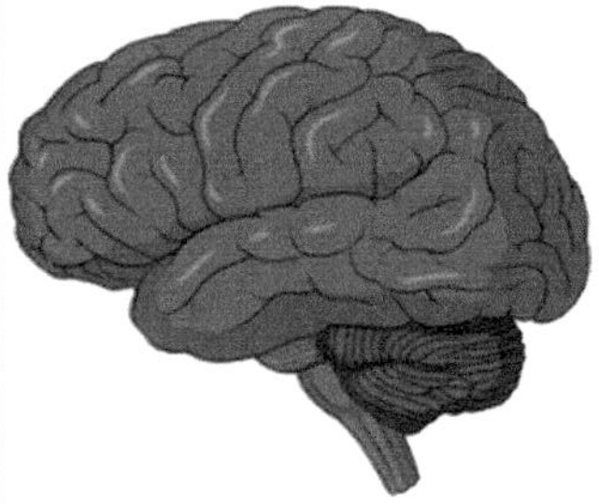 CNS/encephalitis | 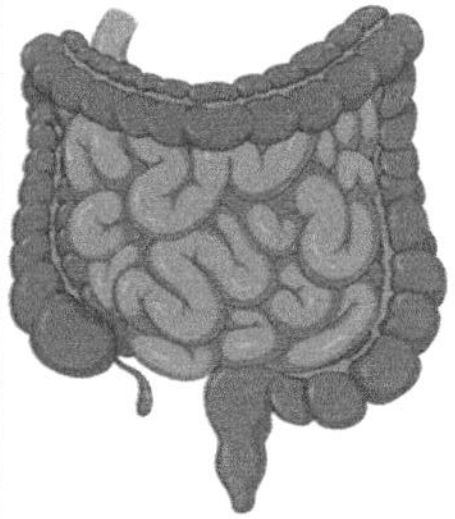 Any CMV disease[b] |
|---|---|---|---|---|
| Induction | Ganciclovir or foscarnet for $\geq$2 weeks<br>**-and-**<br>Patient has improvement in symptoms<br>**-and-**<br>CMV PCR is negative | | | |
| Special treatment considerations | 0.5 mg/kg IVIG (adjusted body weight) every other day for 7–14 days may be considered for CMV pneumonia | Ganciclovir intravitreal implant in addition to systemic induction and secondary prophylaxis is an option if deemed appropriate by ophthalmology | Include CMV resistance testing of CMV PCR-positive CSF specimens, and consider combination therapy while awaiting results | Consider a longer duration of secondary prophylaxis until risk factors subside |
| Maintenance | Ganciclovir, valganciclovir, or foscarnet until day+90 post-HCT<br>**-or-**<br>For $\geq$8 weeks, whichever duration is longer and recommended by ID specialist | | | |

(continued)

**Table 10.2** (continued)

| | |
|---|---|
| Novel or adjunctive therapies | Maribavir for resistant and refractory CMV disease |
| | CMV-specific CTLs |
| | Leflunomide[c,d] in addition to other antiviral agents |
| | Cidofovir as monotherapy[e] (weekly dosing for 2–3 weeks of induction followed by every-other-week secondary prophylaxis dosing with probenecid and hydration with each dose) |
| | Letermovir[f] in addition to other antiviral agents **if** no improvement after ≥4 weeks of appropriate treatment with first- or second-line agents **or** serious toxicity precludes use of other standard therapies **or** documented multidrug resistance **or** patient ineligible for CMV CTLs or available treatment protocols |

*ID* infectious diseases, *CTLs* cytotoxic T lymphocytes
[a]GC11.6 CMV treatment and management, updated 4/7/2020
[b]Including but not limited to CMV pneumonia, retinitis, GI disease, and CMV CNS disease
[c]Adverse effects may include anemia, thrombocytopenia, diarrhea, nausea, hepatotoxicity, and neuropathy
[d]Not recommended for patients with preexisting liver disease or with alanine aminotransferase levels more than two times the upper limit of normal. Contraindicated for patients with severe hepatic impairment
[e]Use limited by nephrotoxicity and cross-resistance conferred by UL54 mutation against valganciclovir
[f]Does not prevent viral DNA synthesis, and CMV DNA PCR and phosphoprotein 65 antigen are not useful markers of acute treatment response. If no decrease in CMV PCR after 21 days of treatment, consider changing therapy

absorption can lead to virologic failure and the development of CMV resistance [89]. The use of IVIG remains controversial, as no mortality benefit has been observed compared to anti-CMV medications alone, and it is not recommended for CMV GI disease [66, 90].

## CMV Retinitis

Most commonly a clinical complication of human immunodeficiency virus (HIV), CMV retinitis has been infrequently reported in HCT recipients (1–3%) [43, 91, 92]. Traditionally, retinitis has been reported as a late manifestation of CMV infection, with most cases occurring after day +100 posttransplant and at a median occurrence at 8 to 9 months [91, 93]. However, more recent studies suggest that an active approach to surveillance, such as with ophthalmological screening based on positive CMV infection, before developing symptoms among patients with viremia may lead to earlier diagnosis and better outcomes [41, 94]. Symptoms typically include unilateral or bilateral visual complaints such as diminished visual acuity, floaters, and photophobia [93, 94]. In addition, reported risk factors include lymphopenia and CMV seropositivity [94].

CMV retinitis is diagnosed primarily via fundoscopic examination by an experienced ophthalmologist and confirmed using CMV PCR analysis of aqueous or vitreous humor specimens. Typical fundoscopic findings include yellow-white retinal exudates and/or hemorrhage. Other findings include branch vessel occlusion, vessel sheathing, anterior uveitis, and retinal edema. In severe cases, retinal necrosis and/or detachment can occur [93–95]. Investigators have studied the utility of CMV PCR from aqueous humor specimens in patients with advanced HIV and found it to have good sensitivity [96]. Although retinitis is associated with CMV reactivation and high peak CMV blood levels [41], not all patients present with CMV viremia at diagnosis [97–100].

Ganciclovir and foscarnet are the most widely used systemic therapies for CMV retinitis in HCT recipients [99]. In addition to systemic antiviral therapy, intravitreal ganciclovir injections and ganciclovir implants should be considered in the treatment of CMV retinitis (Table 10.2). Intravitreal ganciclovir injection results in high retinal tissue concentrations [101], but few case series on its use in HCT recipients have been published [97, 98, 102, 103]. Intravitreal foscarnet has also demonstrated efficacy in clearing CMV retinitis in HCT recipients and may be used in patients with peripheral cytopenias or those who have not previously responded to systemic treatment with (val)ganciclovir [99]. Systemic cidofovir, which is approved for CMV retinitis in HIV, is used as an alternative CMV therapy in HCT recipients with CMV disease (Table 10.2). However, intravitreal cidofovir injections have a narrow therapeutic index and are not commonly used due to their toxicity profile and poor tolerance [101].

## CMV Central Nervous System Disease/Encephalitis

CMV disease of the central nervous system (CNS) is associated with high mortality rates, even in the modern transplant era, with poor neurologic recovery in survivors [104–106]. Onset is usually late, with most cases occurring beyond day +100 after HCT [104, 107, 108]. Overall, the incidence of CMV CNS disease in HCT recipients has not been established, but in a large multicenter study of HCT recipients with viral encephalitis, CMV encephalitis was rare (6%) [109]. Reported risk factors in HCT recipients include delayed engraftment, haploidentical HCT, T-cell depleting agents, and GVHD [58]. In this population, CMV CNS disease typically manifests as encephalitis or ventriculoencephalitis with rapid progression of symptoms, such as encephalopathy and cognitive dysfunction, which ranges from mild confusion to extreme lethargy and coma [100, 104, 107, 110]. In a review of published CMV CNS cases in HCT recipients, approximately half of the patients presented with concomitant CMV disease in other organs (e.g., retinitis, pneumonitis, colitis) [104].

Regarding diagnosis, mild to moderate cerebrospinal fluid (CSF) pleocytosis with a lymphocytic predominance is common, although this may not be consistent in patients with severe leukopenia. Hypoglycorrhachia and mild to moderate elevation of protein levels in the CSF may be present [104, 105]. Magnetic resonance imaging (MRI) findings include subependymal and periventricular inflammation, but these are not pathognomonic [104, 105]. Furthermore, MRI findings suggesting ventriculitis with fluid-attenuated inversion recovery demonstrating abnormal periventricular hypersensitivity have also been described [111]. Quantitative CMV by PCR in the CSF from an atraumatic lumbar puncture, either as a stand-alone test or as part of a multi-array panel, has excellent sensitivity and should be performed to aid in diagnosis and to monitor treatment response [105]. The definition of proven CMV CNS disease includes evidence of tissue involvement via histopathology, immunohistochemical staining, culture, or tissue CMV PCR; however, brain tissue is rarely obtained [58]. Compatible signs and symptoms in the setting of a positive CMV by PCR from the CSF are sufficient to establish a clinical diagnosis in the absence of an alternate etiology.

Compartmentalized resistance has been described in the setting of CMV encephalitis, such that resistant virus may be isolated from CSF in the absence of resistant virus in the serum [105, 110, 112]. Therefore, testing for CMV resistance from a CSF specimen is recommended (Table 10.2). The optimal therapy for CMV CNS disease in HCT recipients is not well established. However, ganciclovir and foscarnet could be used in combination, as foscarnet may have variable CSF penetration, and ganciclovir's CSF penetration is not well studied [105].

### Other CMV Disease Manifestations

Other infrequently reported CMV disease manifestations include hepatitis, nephritis, cystitis, and myocarditis/pericarditis [58]. Because they are rare, few reports describe their clinical presentation and incidence in HCT recipients. Diagnosing proven CMV disease in any of these organ systems includes compatible signs and symptoms and detection of CMV via virus isolation, rapid culture, immunohistochemistry, or in situ hybridization in infected tissue, together with identification of histologic features of CMV infection [58]. Because of the rarity of these CMV end-organ diseases, more common etiologies should be considered and ruled out when making treatment decisions [58].

## Resistant and Refractory CMV Infection and Disease

### Definitions

Definitions of resistant/refractory (R/R) CMV infections were developed by the Resistant Definitions Working Group of the Cytomegalovirus Drug Development Forum to assist in clinical trial designs and standardize the results of epidemiologic studies [113]. After the first week of induction antiviral therapy, an increase in viral load up to twice the initial level is not unusual [30]. This contrasts with refractory CMV infection, defined as viremia that increases by at least 1 log after 2 weeks of appropriately routed and correctly dosed antiviral therapy [113]. Therefore, an increase in CMV level during the first 2 weeks of therapy of up to 1 log can be considered probable refractory infection and may warrant investigation. Refractory CMV disease can occur with or without refractory viremia, defined as worsening signs and symptoms after 2 weeks of appropriate therapy or development of organ involvement after 2 weeks of treatment of viremia.

A lack of improvement in signs and symptoms of end-organ involvement without worsening can be considered probable refractory CMV disease. Of note is that not all refractory CMV infections result from virologic resistance. Many risk factors for CMV viremia can also contribute to delays in response to antiviral therapy [89, 114]. These include delayed and poor engraftment, intensive conditioning regimens, and immunosuppression for the treatment or prevention of GVHD. Therefore,

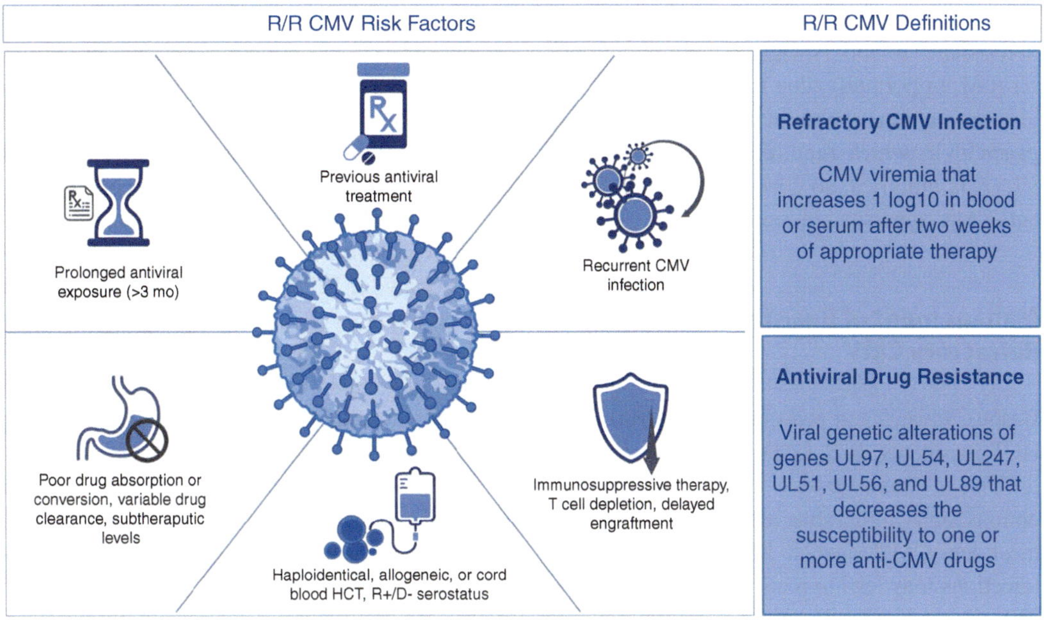


**Fig. 10.3** Definitions of and risk factors for resistant and refractory CMV infections [114]

testing for mutations conferring resistance to the available antiviral agents is recommended if a patient meets the criteria for proven or probable refractory CMV infection or disease [89].

CMV resistance is defined by identifying genetic mutations in specific areas of the CMV genome that decrease susceptibility to one or more antiviral drugs [89, 113, 114]. Resistance was traditionally assessed using phenotypic assays; however, these have been replaced by genotypic assays, including PCR and next-generation sequencing, which provide more timely results [89]. Resistance most commonly occurs following extended antiviral treatment, poor medication adherence, underdosing, or poor absorption leading to inadequate drug levels (Fig. 10.3). Rates of CMV resistance in the HCT population range from 1.7% to 14.5%, while rates of refractory CMV infections are as high as 29% to 39% in HCT recipients [30, 114–119].

## Mechanisms of CMV Resistance

Ganciclovir, valganciclovir, foscarnet, and cidofovir act through various cellular pathways by inhibiting the viral DNA polymerase UL54; (val) ganciclovir, however, must be phosphorylated by the CMV UL97 protein kinase (pUL97) before its activity at UL54. Therefore, specific mutations on the UL54 subunits can confer resistance to one or more of these drugs, while specific mutations on UL97 confer resistance to (val)ganciclovir (Fig. 10.3) [114]. Letermovir acts on the CMV UL56/89/51 terminase complex, and resistance to letermovir is most often mediated by mutations on UL56 [89], although mutations on UL51 and UL89 have been described but less frequently [114].

Maribavir is an inhibitor of pUL97-mediated phosphorylation of nuclear lamin A/C, which is responsible for CMV DNA synthesis, gene expression, and viral encapsulation. Resistance to maribavir is mediated by mutations to pUL97, similar to (val)ganciclovir. However, the amino acid substitutions described for maribavir resistance are mostly different from those that confer resistance to (val)ganciclovir, although some substitutions, such as M460V/I, result in CMV mutant resistance to (val)ganciclovir and hypersensitivity to maribavir (half-maximal inhibitory concentration, 4.8 nM) [114, 120]. Others, such as C480F, F342Y, P521L, and V466G, can result in resistance to both (val)ganciclovir and maribavir [66]. Importantly, due to maribavir's mechanism of action, the antiviral activity of (val) ganciclovir, which requires phosphorylation by UL97, is inhibited, so coadministration of these anti-CMV agents is not recommended.

## Management of Resistant/Refractory CMV

Despite advances in prevention and treatment in HCT recipients, R/R CMV infections are often difficult to manage due to limited treatment options and intolerable side effect profiles of most anti-CMV agents. Moreover, R/R CMV infections may lead to recurrent infections [121]. Therefore, changes in initial therapy should be guided by resistance testing if refractory CMV infection is suspected. If no resistance is detected, ensuring appropriate dosing, the optimal route of administration to mitigate the risk of poor absorption, and compliance should all be considered.

Changing therapy empirically while awaiting resistance testing is appropriate. An empiric change or additional anti-CMV agents may be necessary for patients at high risk for severe complications of CMV disease or those who already have refractory disease with severe manifestations. Foscarnet is usually the drug of choice for patients initially treated with ganciclovir. High-dose ganciclovir (7.5–10.0 mg/kg twice daily) has been studied in solid organ transplant (SOT) recipients and advanced HIV populations with some success. However, high-dose ganciclovir is less well studied in the HCT population, for whom the risk of significant cytopenias may limit this approach. High-dose ganciclovir administration may be considered for HCT recipients with known mutations conferring low-level resistance to ganciclovir, such as the UL97 mutations C592G and A591V [122]. Similarly, treatment with cidofovir has had some success in the SOT population, but the experience with cidofovir in HCT recipients is limited [114].

In late 2021, the FDA approved maribavir for the treatment of posttransplant CMV infection and disease that is refractory or resistant to treatment with (val)ganciclovir, foscarnet, or cidofovir. Their decision stemmed from data from phase II and III trials demonstrating its safety and efficacy in adult and pediatric patients with R/R CMV infection and/or disease. Specifically, in the phase II randomized, dose-ranging trial, maribavir was assessed for efficacy as an alternative therapy for R/R CMV infections in HCT and SOT recipients [123]. Sixty-seven percent of patients met the primary endpoint of confirmed undetectable CMV DNA within 6 weeks of treatment at a dose of 400 mg twice daily, which was as effective as the higher doses. In addition, maribavir was well tolerated, with no renal or cytotoxic effects. However, dysgeusia (65%), nausea (34%), and vomiting (29%) were common in the higher dose arms [123, 124]. In the phase III open-label, randomized, multicenter, active-controlled trial comparing maribavir to investigator-assigned therapy, the primary endpoint of superior viral clearance at week 8 after starting the study drug on the maribavir arm was achieved (55.7% vs. 23.9%, $p < 0.0001$) [125]. The FDA approved maribavir for children (aged $\geq$ 12 years and weighing $\geq$35 kg) and adults with posttransplant R/R CMV infections or disease on November 23, 2021 [126]. Maribavir is an important new treatment option that may soon become the first line of therapy for R/R CMV infection in HCT and SOT recipients based on its favorable results in clinical trials.

## Other Agents and Novel Therapies

The use of donor-derived CMV-specific cytotoxic T lymphocytes (CTLs) dates to the early 2000s. Multiple case series demonstrated success with this approach, but confirmation trials are lacking thus far [127–130]. Initial challenges to this approach included delays in obtaining cells due to time spent culturing or processing them. However, more recent efforts have focused on developing "off-the-shelf" CTLs from partially human leukocyte antigen-matched donors to reduce the delays in initiating therapy [131–133]. A phase II trial designed to determine the efficacy of donor CMV-specific CTLs in HCT recipients is ongoing (NCT02210078) [130].

Leflunomide, a drug initially used for rheumatoid arthritis, has shown some promise for CMV management in HCT recipients. Investigators demonstrated its activity in vitro due to its effects on virion assembly rather than DNA synthesis [100, 114]. For CMV infection/disease, we recommend leflunomide as adjunctive therapy with another CMV antiviral agent. Adult dosing consists of an initial loading dose of 100 mg daily for 5 days, followed by 40 mg daily thereafter. Dosing should then be adjusted based on serum levels of its active metabolite teriflunomide [134]. Recent case reports described its use for R/R CMV infections combined with conventional therapy [134, 135]. Adverse effects of leflunomide include anemia, thrombocytopenia, hepatotoxicity, and neuropathy, which may limit its use in critically ill HCT recipients. In addition, pulmonary hypertension has occurred in patients after long-term use, and it is not recommended for patients with elevated liver enzymes or severe hepatic impairment (Table 10.2) [135].

Agents derived from artesunate, an antimalarial drug, have shown in vitro and in vivo activity against CMV via an unknown mechanism of action [136]. Case reports describing its use for R/R CMV in HCT patients have shown mixed results [136–139].

In several small case series, authors have reported on the use of letermovir for R/R CMV combined with other therapies, mostly in SOT recipients. The doses used in these series were often higher than those used for prophylaxis, ranging from 280 to 960 mg daily, with little toxicity reported [140–142].

## Conclusion

CMV is one of the most pathogenic viruses in humans and frequently occurs in critically ill HCT recipients, with devastating outcomes. The prevention and treatment of CMV infection/disease after HCT have changed greatly over the past decade with the approval of letermovir for primary CMV prophylaxis in adult CMV-seropositive HCT recipients and maribavir for HCT and SOT recipients with R/R CMV infection/disease. However, despite these major advancements, breakthrough CMV reactivation and the development of R/R CMV infections continue to lead to devastating outcomes in HCT recipients.

## References


1. Boeckh M, Ljungman P. How we treat cytomegalovirus in hematopoietic cell transplant recipients. Blood. 2009;113(23):5711–9.
2. Schmidt-Hieber M, Tridello G, Ljungman P, Mikulska M, Knelange N, Blaise D, et al. The prognostic impact of the cytomegalovirus serostatus in patients with chronic hematological malignancies after allogeneic hematopoietic stem cell transplantation: a report from the infectious diseases working party of EBMT. Ann Hematol. 2019;98(7):1755–63. https://doi.org/10.1007/s00277-019-03669-z.
3. Gimenez E, Torres I, Albert E, Pinana JL, Hernandez-Boluda JC, Solano C, et al. Cytomegalovirus (CMV) infection and risk of mortality in allogeneic hematopoietic stem cell transplantation (Allo-HSCT): a systematic review, meta-analysis, and meta-regression analysis. Am J Transplant. 2019;19(9):2479–94. https://doi.org/10.1111/ajt.15515.
4. Cantoni N, Hirsch HH, Khanna N, Gerull S, Buser A, Bucher C, et al. Evidence for a bidirectional relationship between cytomegalovirus replication and acute graft-versus-host disease. Biol Blood Marrow Transplant. 2010;16(9):1309–14. https://doi.org/10.1016/j.bbmt.2010.03.020.
5. Ghobadi A, Milton DR, Gowda L, Rondon G, Chemaly RF, Hamdi A, et al. HLA-DP mismatch and CMV reactivation increase risk of aGVHD independently in recipients of allogeneic stem cell transplant. Curr Res Transl Med. 2019;67(2):51–5. https://doi.org/10.1016/j.retram.2019.01.001.
6. Teira P, Battiwalla M, Ramanathan M, Barrett AJ, Ahn KW, Chen M, et al. Early cytomegalovirus reactivation remains associated with increased transplant-related mortality in the current era: a CIBMTR analysis. Blood. 2016;127(20):2427–38. https://doi.org/10.1182/blood-2015-11-679639.
7. Ariza-Heredia EJ, Nesher L, Chemaly RF. Cytomegalovirus diseases after hematopoietic stem cell transplantation: a mini-review. Cancer Lett. 2014;342(1):1–8. https://doi.org/10.1016/j.canlet.2013.09.004.
8. Nichols WG, Corey L, Gooley T, Davis C, Boeckh M. High risk of death due to bacterial and fungal infection among cytomegalovirus (CMV)—seronegative recipients of stem cell transplants from seropositive donors: evidence for indirect effects of primary

CMV infection. J Infect Dis. 2002;185(3):273–82. https://doi.org/10.1086/338624.
9. Marchesi F, Pimpinelli F, Di Domenico EG, Renzi D, Gallo MT, Regazzo G, et al. Association between CMV and invasive fungal infections after autologous stem cell transplant in lymphoproliferative malignancies: opportunistic partnership or cause-effect relationship? Int J Mol Sci. 2019;20(6):19. https://doi.org/10.3390/ijms20061373.
10. Lavallée C, Labbé AC, Talbot JD, Alonso CD, Marr KA, Cohen S, et al. Risk factors for the development of Clostridium difficile infection in adult allogeneic hematopoietic stem cell transplant recipients: a single-center study in Québec, Canada. Transpl Infect Dis. 2017;19(1). https://doi.org/10.1111/tid.12648.
11. Sassine J, Khawaja F, Shigle TL, Handy V, Foolad F, Aitken SL, et al. Refractory and resistant cytomegalovirus after hematopoietic cell transplant in the Letermovir primary prophylaxis era. Clin Infect Dis. 2021;73(8):1346–54. https://doi.org/10.1093/cid/ciab298.
12. Minton K. How CMV bypasses immune memory. Nat Rev Immunol. 2010;10(5):288–9.
13. La Rosa C, Diamond DJ. The immune response to human CMV. Futur Virol. 2012;7(3):279–93.
14. Einsele H, Ljungman P, Boeckh M. How I treat CMV reactivation after allogeneic hematopoietic stem cell transplantation. Blood. 2020;135(19):1619–29. https://doi.org/10.1182/blood.2019000956.
15. Avery RK, Arav-Boger R, Marr KA, Kraus E, Shoham S, Lees L, et al. Outcomes in transplant recipients treated with foscarnet for ganciclovir-resistant or refractory cytomegalovirus infection. Transplantation. 2016;100(10):e74.
16. Beck JC, Wagner JE, DeFor TE, Brunstein CG, Schleiss MR, Young J-A, et al. Impact of cytomegalovirus (CMV) reactivation after umbilical cord blood transplantation. Biol Blood Marrow Transplant. 2010;16(2):215–22.
17. Styczynski J. Who is the patient at risk of CMV recurrence: a review of the current scientific evidence with a focus on hematopoietic cell transplantation. Infect Dis Ther. 2018;7(1):1–16. https://doi.org/10.1007/s40121-017-0180-z.
18. Reusser P, Fisher LD, Buckner CD, Thomas ED, Meyers JD. Cytomegalovirus infection after autologous bone marrow transplantation: occurrence of cytomegalovirus disease and effect on engraftment. Blood. 1990;75(9):1888–94. https://doi.org/10.1182/blood.V75.9.1888.1888.
19. Lam S, Boan P, Polistena P, Cannell P, Cooney J, Wright M, et al. High dose valaciclovir to prevent cytomegalovirus infection in allogeneic haematopoietic stem cell transplant recipients. Transpl Infect Dis. 2021;23:e13633. https://doi.org/10.1111/tid.13633.
20. Ljungman P, Brand R, Hoek J, de la Camara R, Cordonnier C, Einsele H, et al. Donor cytomegalovirus status influences the outcome of allogeneic stem cell transplant: a study by the European group for blood and marrow transplantation. Clin Infect Dis. 2014;59(4):473–81.
21. Boeckh M, Nichols WG. The impact of cytomegalovirus serostatus of donor and recipient before hematopoietic stem cell transplantation in the era of antiviral prophylaxis and preemptive therapy. Blood. 2004;103(6):2003–8.
22. Ziemann M, Thiele T. Transfusion-transmitted CMV infection–current knowledge and future perspectives. Transfus Med. 2017;27(4):238–48.
23. Ljungman P. The role of cytomegalovirus serostatus on outcome of hematopoietic stem cell transplantation. Curr Opin Hematol. 2014;21(6):466–9.
24. Bilgrami S, Aslanzadeh J, Feingold JM, Bona RD, Clive J, Dorsky D, et al. Cytomegalovirus viremia, viruria and disease after autologous peripheral blood stem cell transplantation: no need for surveillance. Bone Marrow Transplant. 1999;24(1):69–73.
25. Pande A, Dubberke ER. Cytomegalovirus infections of the stem cell transplant recipient and hematologic malignancy patient. Infect Dis Clin North Am. 2019;33(2):485–500. https://doi.org/10.1016/j.idc.2019.02.008.
26. Lindsay J, Othman J, Kerridge I, Fay K, Stevenson W, Arthur C, et al. Cytomegalovirus (CMV) management in allogeneic hematopoietic cell transplantation: pre-transplant predictors of survival, reactivation, and spontaneous clearance. Transpl Infect Dis. 2021;23(3):e13548. https://doi.org/10.1111/tid.13548.
27. Beauvais D, Drumez E, Blaise D, Peffault de Latour R, Forcade E, Ceballos P, et al. Scoring system for clinically significant CMV infection in seropositive recipients following allogenic hematopoietic cell transplant: an SFGM-TC study. Bone Marrow Transplant. 2021;56(6):1305–15. https://doi.org/10.1038/s41409-020-01178-6.
28. Lin CH, Su YJ, Hsu CY, Wang PN, Teng CJ. Haploidentical allogeneic hematopoietic stem cell transplantation increases the risk of cytomegalovirus infection in adult patients with acute leukemia. Transpl Infect Dis. 2019;21(4):e13096. https://doi.org/10.1111/tid.13096.
29. Cohen L, Yeshurun M, Shpilberg O, Ram R. Risk factors and prognostic scale for cytomegalovirus (CMV) infection in CMV-seropositive patients after allogeneic hematopoietic cell transplantation. Transpl Infect Dis. 2015;17(4):510–7.
30. Nichols WG, Corey L, Gooley T, Drew WL, Miner R, Huang M-L, et al. Rising pp65 antigenemia during preemptive anticytomegalovirus therapy after allogeneic hematopoietic stem cell transplantation: risk factors, correlation with DNA load, and outcomes. Blood. 2001;97(4):867–74.
31. Goldsmith SR, Abid MB, Auletta JJ, Bashey A, Beitinjaneh A, Castillo P, et al. Posttransplant cyclophosphamide is associated with increased cytomegalovirus infection: a CIBMTR analysis. Blood.

2021;137(23):3291–305. https://doi.org/10.1182/blood.2020009362.
32. Chemaly RF, El Haddad L, Winston DJ, Rowley SD, Mulane KM, Chandrasekar P, et al. Cytomegalovirus (CMV) cell-mediated immunity and CMV infection after allogeneic hematopoietic cell transplantation: the REACT study. Clin Infect Dis. 2020;71(9):2365–74. https://doi.org/10.1093/cid/ciz1210.
33. Pinana JL, Perez-Pitarch A, Guglieri-Lopez B, Gimenez E, Hernandez-Boluda JC, Terol MJ, et al. Sirolimus exposure and the occurrence of cytomegalovirus DNAemia after allogeneic hematopoietic stem cell transplantation. Am J Transplant. 2018;18(12):2885–94. https://doi.org/10.1111/ajt.14754.
34. Cao K, Marin D, Sekine T, Rondon G, Zhao W, Smith NT, et al. Donor NKG2C copy number: an independent predictor for CMV reactivation after double cord blood transplantation. Front Immunol. 2018;9:2444. https://doi.org/10.3389/fimmu.2018.02444.
35. Meesing A, Razonable RR. Absolute lymphocyte count thresholds: a simple, readily available tool to predict the risk of cytomegalovirus infection after transplantation. Open forum. Open Forum Infect Dis. 2018;5(10):ofy230. https://doi.org/10.1093/ofid/ofy230.
36. Nesher L, Shah DP, Ariza-Heredia EJ, Azzi JM, Siddiqui HK, Ghantoji SS, et al. Utility of the enzyme-linked immunospot interferon-γ- release assay to predict the risk of cytomegalovirus infection in hematopoietic cell transplant recipients. J Infect Dis. 2016;213(11):1701–7. https://doi.org/10.1093/infdis/jiw064.
37. El Haddad L, Ariza-Heredia E, Shah DP, Jiang Y, Blanchard T, Ghantoji SS, et al. The ability of a cytomegalovirus ELISPOT assay to predict outcome of low-level CMV reactivation in hematopoietic cell transplant recipients. J Infect Dis. 2019;219(6):898–907. https://doi.org/10.1093/infdis/jiy592.
38. Krawczyk A, Ackermann J, Goitowski B, Trenschel R, Ditschkowski M, Timm J, et al. Assessing the risk of CMV reactivation and reconstitution of antiviral immune response post bone marrow transplantation by the QuantiFERON-CMV-assay and real time PCR. J Clin Virol. 2018;99–100:61–6. https://doi.org/10.1016/j.jcv.2018.01.002.
39. Wagner-Drouet E, Teschner D, Wolschke C, Janson D, Schäfer-Eckart K, Gärtner J, et al. Standardized monitoring of cytomegalovirus-specific immunity can improve risk stratification of recurrent cytomegalovirus reactivation after hematopoietic stem cell transplantation. Haematologica. 2021;106(2):363–74. https://doi.org/10.3324/haematol.2019.229252.
40. Jang JE, Hyun SY, Kim YD, Yoon SH, Hwang DY, Kim SJ, et al. Risk factors for progression from cytomegalovirus viremia to cytomegalovirus disease after allogeneic hematopoietic stem cell transplantation. Biol Blood Marrow Transplant. 2012;18(6):881–6. https://doi.org/10.1016/j.bbmt.2011.10.037.
41. Jeon S, Lee WK, Lee Y, Lee DG, Lee JW. Risk factors for cytomegalovirus retinitis in patients with cytomegalovirus viremia after hematopoietic stem cell transplantation. Ophthalmology. 2012;119(9):1892–8.
42. Liu J, Kong J, Chang YJ, Chen H, Chen YH, Han W, et al. Patients with refractory cytomegalovirus (CMV) infection following allogeneic haematopoietic stem cell transplantation are at high risk for CMV disease and non-relapse mortality. Clin Microbiol Infect. 2015;21(12):1121–e9.
43. Green ML, Leisenring W, Xie H, Mast TC, Cui Y, Sandmaier BM, et al. Cytomegalovirus viral load and mortality after haemopoietic stem cell transplantation in the era of pre-emptive therapy: a retrospective cohort study. Lancet Haematol. 2016;3(3):e119–e27. https://doi.org/10.1016/S2352-3026(15)00289-6.
44. Ljungman P, Perez-Bercoff L, Jonsson J, Avetisyan G, Sparrelid E, Aschan J, et al. Risk factors for the development of cytomegalovirus disease after allogeneic stem cell transplantation. Haematologica. 2006;91(1):78–83.
45. Meng XY, Fu HX, Zhu XL, Wang JZ, Liu X, Yan CH, et al. Comparison of different cytomegalovirus diseases following haploidentical hematopoietic stem cell transplantation. Ann Hematol. 2020;99(11):2659–70. https://doi.org/10.1007/s00277-020-04201-4.
46. Wilhelm K, Chemaly R, Saliba R, Gulbis A, Saunders I, Cool R, et al. The impact of pre-transplant valganciclovir on early cytomegalovirus reactivation after allogeneic hematopoietic stem cell transplantation. J Oncol Pharm Pract. 2014;20(4):257–62. https://doi.org/10.1177/1078155213501360.
47. Hill JA, Pergam SA, Cox E, Xie H, Leisenring WM, Boeckh M, et al. A modified intensive strategy to prevent cytomegalovirus disease in seropositive umbilical cord blood transplantation recipients. Biol Blood Marrow Transplant. 2018;24(10):2094–100. https://doi.org/10.1016/j.bbmt.2018.05.008.
48. Chen K, Cheng MP, Hammond SP, Einsele H, Marty FM. Antiviral prophylaxis for cytomegalovirus infection in allogeneic hematopoietic cell transplantation. Blood Adv. 2018;2(16):2159–75. https://doi.org/10.1182/bloodadvances.2018016493.
49. Marty FM, Ljungman P, Chemaly RF, Maertens J, Dadwal SS, Duarte RF, et al. Letermovir prophylaxis for cytomegalovirus in hematopoietic-cell transplantation. N Engl J Med. 2017;377(25):2433–44. https://doi.org/10.1056/NEJMoa1706640.
50. Anderson A, Raja M, Vazquez N, Morris M, Komanduri K, Camargo J. Clinical "Real-world" experience with letermovir for prevention of cytomegalovirus infection in allogeneic hematopoietic cell transplant recipients. Clin Transpl. 2020;34(7):e13866. https://doi.org/10.1111/ctr.13866.
51. Chemaly RF, Ullmann AJ, Stoelben S, Richard MP, Bornhaüser M, Groth C, et al. Letermovir for cytomegalovirus prophylaxis in hematopoietic-cell

transplantation. N Engl J Med. 2014;370(19):1781–9. https://doi.org/10.1056/NEJMoa1309533.
52. Johnsrud JJ, Nguyen IT, Domingo W, Narasimhan B, Efron B, Brown JW. Letermovir prophylaxis decreases burden of cytomegalovirus (CMV) in patients at high risk for CMV disease following hematopoietic cell transplant. Biol Blood Marrow Transplant. 2020;26(10):1963–70. https://doi.org/10.1016/j.bbmt.2020.07.002.
53. Sharma P, Gakhar N, MacDonald J, Abidi MZ, Benamu E, Bajrovic V, et al. Letermovir prophylaxis through day 100 post transplant is safe and effective compared with alternative CMV prophylaxis strategies following adult cord blood and haploidentical cord blood transplantation. Bone Marrow Transplant. 2020;55(4):780–6. https://doi.org/10.1038/s41409-019-0730-y.
54. Golan Y, Tang Y, Mt-Isa S, Wan H, Teal V, Badshah C, et al. Impact of Letermovir use for cytomegalovirus prophylaxis on re-hospitalization following allogeneic hematopoietic stem cell transplantation: an analysis of a phase III randomized clinical trial. PharmacoEcon Open. 2021;5(3):469–73. https://doi.org/10.1007/s41669-021-00264-9.
55. Alsumali A, Chemaly RF, Graham J, Jiang Y, Merchant S, Miles L, et al. Cost-effectiveness analysis of cytomegalovirus prophylaxis in allogeneic hematopoietic cell transplant recipients from a US payer perspective. J Med Virol. 2021;93(6):3786–94. https://doi.org/10.1002/jmv.26462.
56. Sperotto A, Candoni A, Gottardi M, Facchin G, Stella R, De Marchi R, et al. Cytomegalovirus prophylaxis versus pre-emptive strategy: different CD4+ and CD8+ T cell reconstitution after allogeneic hematopoietic stem cell transplantation. Transplant Cell Therapy. 2021;27(6):518e1–4.
57. Bansal R, Gordillo CA, Abramova R, Assal A, Mapara MY, Pereira MR, et al. Extended letermovir administration, beyond day 100, is effective for CMV prophylaxis in patients with graft versus host disease. Transpl Infect Dis. 2021;23(2):e13487. https://doi.org/10.1111/tid.13487.
58. Ljungman P, Boeckh M, Hirsch HH, Josephson F, Lundgren J, Nichols G, et al. Definitions of cytomegalovirus infection and disease in transplant patients for use in clinical trials. Clin Infect Dis. 2017;64(1):87–91. https://doi.org/10.1093/cid/ciw668.
59. Engelmann I, Alidjinou EK, Lazrek M, Pouillaude J-M, Ogiez J, Rose F, et al. Comparison of two commercial quantitative PCR assays for EBV DNA detection and their correlation with the first WHO international standard for EBV. J Med Microbiol. 2018;67(4):529–36.
60. Curran M, Noble S. Valganciclovir. Drugs. 2001;61(8):1145–50.
61. Matsumoto K, Shigemi A, Ikawa K, Kanazawa N, Fujisaki Y, Morikawa N, et al. Risk factors for ganciclovir-induced thrombocytopenia and leukopenia. Biol Pharm Bull. 2015;38(2):235. https://doi.org/10.1248/bpb.b14-00588.
62. Deray G, Martinez F, Katlama C, Levaltier B, Beaufils H, Danis M, et al. Foscarnet nephrotoxicity: mechanism, incidence and prevention. Am J Nephrol. 1989;9(4):316. https://doi.org/10.1159/000167987.
63. Ljungman P, Deliliers GL, Platzbecker U, Matthes-Martin S, Bacigalupo A, Einsele H, et al. Cidofovir for cytomegalovirus infection and disease in allogeneic stem cell transplant recipients. Blood. 2001;97(2):388. https://doi.org/10.1182/blood.V97.2.388.
64. Moretti S, Zikos P, Van Lint MT, Tedone E, Occhini D, Gualandi F, et al. Foscarnet vs ganciclovir for cytomegalovirus (CMV) antigenemia after allogeneic hemopoietic stem cell transplantation (HSCT): a randomised study. Bone Marrow Transplant. 1998;22(2):175–80.
65. Reusser P, Einsele H, Lee J, Volin L, Rovira M, Engelhard D, et al. Randomized multicenter trial of foscarnet versus ganciclovir for preemptive therapy of cytomegalovirus infection after allogeneic stem cell transplantation. Blood. 2002;99(4):1159–64.
66. Yong MK, Shigle TL, Kim Y-J, Carpenter PA, Chemaly RF, Papanicolaou GA. American Society for Transplantation and Cellular Therapy Series:# 4-cytomegalovirus treatment and management of resistant or refractory infections after hematopoietic cell transplantation. Transplant Cell Therapy. 2021;27(12):957–67.
67. Travi G, Pergam SA. Cytomegalovirus pneumonia in hematopoietic stem cell recipients. J Intensive Care Med. 2013;29(4):200–12. https://doi.org/10.1177/0885066613476454.
68. Boeckh M, Nichols WG, Papanicolaou G, Rubin R, Wingard JR, Zaia J. Cytomegalovirus in hematopoietic stem cell transplant recipients: current status, known challenges, and future strategies. Biol Blood Marrow Transplant. 2003;9(9):543–58. https://doi.org/10.1016/S1083-8791(03)00287-8.
69. Erard V, Guthrie KA, Seo S, Smith J, Huang M, Chien J, et al. Reduced mortality of cytomegalovirus pneumonia after hematopoietic cell transplantation due to antiviral therapy and changes in transplantation practices. Clin Infect Dis. 2015;61(1):31–9. https://doi.org/10.1093/cid/civ215.
70. Boeckh M, Stevens-Ayers T, Travi G, Huang M-L, Cheng G-S, Xie H, et al. Cytomegalovirus (CMV) DNA quantitation in bronchoalveolar lavage fluid from hematopoietic stem cell transplant recipients with CMV pneumonia. J Infect Dis. 2017;215(10):1514–22. https://doi.org/10.1093/infdis/jix048.
71. Torres H, Aguilera E, Safdar A, Rohatgi N, Raad I, Sepulveda C, et al. Fatal cytomegalovirus pneumonia in patients with haematological malignancies: an autopsy-based case–control study. Clin Microbiol Infect. 2008;14(12):1160–6.

72. Vigil KJ, Adachi JA, Chemaly RF. Analytic review: viral pneumonias in immunocompromised adult hosts. J Intensive Care Med. 2010;25(6):307–26.
73. Gasparetto EL, Ono SE, Escuissato D, Marchiori E, Roldan L, Marques HL, et al. Cytomegalovirus pneumonia after bone marrow transplantation: high resolution CT findings. Br J Radiol. 2004;77(921):724. https://doi.org/10.1259/bjr/70800575.
74. Franquet T, Rodriguez S, Martino R, Giménez A, Salinas T, Hidalgo A. Thin-section CT findings in hematopoietic stem cell transplantation recipients with respiratory virus pneumonia. Am J Roentgenol. 2006;187(4):1085. https://doi.org/10.2214/AJR.05.0439.
75. Bao C, Liu X, Zhang H, Li Y, Liu J. Coronavirus disease 2019 (COVID-19) CT findings: a systematic review and meta-analysis. J Am Coll Radiol. 2020;17(6):701. https://doi.org/10.1016/j.jacr.2020.03.006.
76. Ljungman P, Griffiths P, Paya C. Definitions of cytomegalovirus infection and disease in transplant recipients. Clin Infect Dis. 2002;34(8):1094–7.
77. Schmidt GM, Horak DA, Niland JC, Duncan SR, Forman SJ, Zaia JA, et al. A randomized, controlled trial of prophylactic ganciclovir for cytomegalovirus pulmonary infection in recipients of allogeneic bone marrow transplants. N Engl J Med. 1991;324(15):1005–11.
78. Ruell J, Barnes C, Mutton K, Foulkes B, Chang J, Cavet J, et al. Active CMV disease does not always correlate with viral load detection. Bone Marrow Transplant. 2007;40(1):55–61. https://doi.org/10.1038/sj.bmt.1705671.
79. Westall GP, Michaelides A, Williams TJ, Snell GI, Kotsimbos TC. Human cytomegalovirus load in plasma and bronchoalveolar lavage fluid: a longitudinal study of lung transplant recipients. J Infect Dis. 2004;190(6):1076–83. https://doi.org/10.1086/422327.
80. Beam E, Germer JJ, Lahr B, Yao JDC, Limper AH, Binnicker MJ, et al. Cytomegalovirus (CMV) DNA quantification in bronchoalveolar lavage fluid of immunocompromised patients with CMV pneumonia. Clin Transpl. 2018;32(1). https://doi.org/10.1111/ctr.13149.
81. Tan SK, Burgener EB, Waggoner JJ, Gajurel K, Gonzalez S, Chen SF, et al. Molecular and culture-based bronchoalveolar lavage fluid testing for the diagnosis of cytomegalovirus pneumonitis. Open Forum Infect Dis. 2016;3(1):ofv212. https://doi.org/10.1093/ofid/ofv212.
82. Chemaly RF, Yen-Lieberman B, Castilla EA, Reilly A, Arrigain S, Farver C, et al. Correlation between viral loads of cytomegalovirus in blood and bronchoalveolar lavage specimens from lung transplant recipients determined by histology and immunohistochemistry. J Clin Microbiol. 2004;42(5):2168–72.
83. Torres HA, Kontoyiannis DP, Bodey GP, Adachi JA, Luna MA, Tarrand JJ, et al. Gastrointestinal cytomegalovirus disease in patients with cancer: a two decade experience in a tertiary care cancer center. Eur J Cancer. 2005;41(15):2268–79.
84. Suarez-Lledo M, Marcos MA, Cuatrecasas M, Bombi JA, Fernandez-Aviles F, Magnano L, et al. Quantitative PCR is faster, more objective, and more reliable than immunohistochemistry for the diagnosis of cytomegalovirus gastrointestinal disease in allogeneic stem cell transplantation. Biol Blood Marrow Transplant. 2019;25(11):2281–6. https://doi.org/10.1016/j.bbmt.2019.07.016.
85. Fisher CE, Alexander J, Bhattacharya R, Rakita RM, Kirby KA, Boeckh M, et al. Sensitivity of blood and tissue diagnostics for gastrointestinal cytomegalovirus disease in solid organ transplant recipients. Transpl Infect Dis. 2016;18(3):372–80.
86. Ko JH, Peck KR, Lee WJ, Huh K, Yoo JR, Kim K, et al. Risk factors for cytomegalovirus gastrointestinal diseases in adult patients with cancer. Eur J Clin Microbiol Infect Dis. 2014;33(10):1847–53. https://doi.org/10.1007/s10096-014-2107-x.
87. Mavropoulou E, Ternes K, Mechie N-C, Bremer SCB, Kunsch S, Ellenrieder V, et al. Cytomegalovirus colitis in inflammatory bowel disease and after haematopoietic stem cell transplantation: diagnostic accuracy, predictors, risk factors and disease outcome. BMJ Open Gastroenterol. 2019;6(1):e000258. https://doi.org/10.1136/bmjgast-2018-000258.
88. Obeid KM, Cober E, Abounader D, Gerds AT, Mossad SB. Cytomegalovirus infection in the era of preemptive strategy in allogeneic hematopoietic cell transplant recipients: progression from viremia to disease remains rare but unpredictable. Infect Dis Clin Pract. 2019;27(1):32–5. https://doi.org/10.1097/IPC.0000000000000523.
89. El Chaer F, Shah DP, Chemaly RF. How I treat resistant cytomegalovirus infection in hematopoietic cell transplantation recipients. Blood. 2016;128(23):2624–36. https://doi.org/10.1182/blood-2016-06-688432.
90. Ljungman P, Cordonnier C, Einsele H, Bender-Götze C, Bosi A, Dekker A, et al. Use of intravenous immune globulin in addition to antiviral therapy in the treatment of CMV gastrointestinal disease in allogeneic bone marrow transplant patients: a report from the European Group for Blood and Marrow Transplantation (EBMT). Bone Marrow Transplant. 1998;21(5):473–6.
91. Crippa F, Corey L, Chuang EL, Sale G, Boeckh M. Virological, clinical, and ophthalmologic features of cytomegalovirus retinitis after hematopoietic stem cell transplantation. Clin Infect Dis. 2001;32(2):214–9. https://doi.org/10.1086/318447.
92. Song WK, Min YH, Kim YR, Lee SC. Cytomegalovirus retinitis after hematopoietic stem cell transplantation with alemtuzumab. Ophthalmology. 2008;115(10):1766–70.
93. Eid AJ, Bakri SJ, Kijpittayarit S, Razonable RR. Clinical features and outcomes of cytomegalovirus retinitis after transplantation.

Transpl Infect Dis. 2008;10(1):13–8. https://doi.org/10.1111/j.1399-3062.2007.00241.x.
94. Mori T, Kikuchi T, Koh M, Koda Y, Yamazaki R, Sakurai M, et al. Cytomegalovirus retinitis after allogeneic hematopoietic stem cell transplantation under cytomegalovirus antigenemia-guided active screening. Bone Marrow Transplant. 2021;56(6):1266–71. https://doi.org/10.1038/s41409-020-01176-8.
95. Murray HW, Knox DL, Green WR, Susel RM. Cytomegalovirus retinitis in adults. A manifestation of disseminated viral infection. Am J Med. 1977;63(4):574. https://doi.org/10.1016/0002-9343(77)90203-0.
96. Mao F, Sun H, Li D, Wang S, Lu D. Polymerase chain reaction analysis of aqueous humor specimens in the diagnosis of cytomegalovirus retinitis in AIDS patients. Eur J Ophthalmol. 2020;30(4):738–42.
97. Jeon S, Lee WK. Cytomegalovirus retinitis in a human immunodeficiency virus-negative cohort: long-term management and complications. Ocul Immunol Inflamm. 2015;23(5):392–9. https://doi.org/10.3109/09273948.2014.985385.
98. Zhang Y, Ruan X, Yang W, Li L, Xian Z, Feng Q, et al. High ocular CMV copies and mismatched receipts may predict poor visual prognosis in CMV retinitis patients following allogeneic haematopoietic stem cell transplantation. BMC Ophthalmol. 2017;17(1):224. https://doi.org/10.1186/s12886-017-0622-0.
99. Vassallo F, Nuzzi R, Cattani I, Dellacasa C, Giaccone L, De Rosa FG, et al. CMV retinitis in a stem cell transplant recipient treated with foscarnet intravitreal injection and CMV specific immunoglobulins. Ther Adv Hematol. 2020;11:2040620720975651. https://doi.org/10.1177/2040620720975651.
100. Camargo JF. Cytomegalovirus in hematopoietic stem cell transplant recipients: prevention, diagnosis, and treatment. In: Emerging transplant infections: clinical challenges and implications; 2020. p. 1–44.
101. Stewart MW. Optimal management of cytomegalovirus retinitis in patients with AIDS. Clin Ophthalmol. 2010;4:285.
102. Miao H, Tao Y, Jiang Y-r, Li X-x. Multiple intravitreal injections of ganciclovir for cytomegalovirus retinitis after stem-cell transplantation. Graefes Arch Clin Exp Ophthalmol. 2013;251(7):1829–33.
103. Zöllner SK, Herbrüggen H, Kolve H, Mihailovic N, Schubert F, Reicherts C, et al. Cytomegalovirus retinitis in children and adolescents with acute leukemia following allogeneic hematopoietic stem cell transplantation. Transpl Infect Dis. 2019;21(5):e13089.
104. Reddy SM, Winston DJ, Territo MC, Schiller GJ. CMV central nervous system disease in stem-cell transplant recipients: an increasing complication of drug-resistant CMV infection and protracted immunodeficiency. Bone Marrow Transplant. 2010;45(6):979–84.
105. Baghban A, Malinis M. Ganciclovir and foscarnet dual-therapy for cytomegalovirus encephalitis: a case report and review of the literature. J Neurol Sci. 2018;388:28–36. https://doi.org/10.1016/j.jns.2018.02.029.
106. Zhang XH, Zhang JM, Han W, Chen H, Chen YH, Wang FR, et al. Viral encephalitis after haploidentical hematopoietic stem cell transplantation: causative viral spectrum, characteristics, and risk factors. Eur J Haematol. 2017;98(5):450–8.
107. Wolf DG, Lurain NS, Zuckerman T, Hoffman R, Satinger J, Honigman A, et al. Emergence of late cytomegalovirus central nervous system disease in hematopoietic stem cell transplant recipients. Blood. 2003;101(2):463–5.
108. Sarva H, Graber J, Remanan R, Rosenblum M, Omuro A. CMV encephalitis in BMT recipients. Bone Marrow Transplant. 2012;47(2):318–20.
109. Schmidt-Hieber M, Schwender J, Heinz WJ, Zabelina T, Kühl JS, Mousset S, et al. Viral encephalitis after allogeneic stem cell transplantation: a rare complication with distinct characteristics of different causative agents. Haematologica. 2011;96(1):142–9. https://doi.org/10.3324/haematol.2010.029876.
110. Jeong T-D, Sung H, Choi S-H, Lee S-O, Yoon H-K, Kim M-N, et al. Cytomegalovirus ventriculoencephalitis with compartmentalization of antiviral-resistant cytomegalovirus in a T cell–depleted haploidentical peripheral blood stem cell transplant recipient. Diagn Microbiol Infect Dis. 2012;74(3):307–10.
111. Lee S, Kim S-H, Choi S-M, Lee D-G, Kim S-Y, Lee J-W, et al. Cytomegalovirus ventriculoencephalitis after unrelated double cord blood stem cell transplantation with an alemtuzumab-containing preparative regimen for Philadelphia-positive acute lymphoblastic leukemia. J Korean Med Sci. 2010;25(4):630–3.
112. Piret J, Schibler M, Pham VD, Hantz S, Giannotti F, Masouridi-Levrat S, et al. Compartmentalization of a multidrug-resistant cytomegalovirus UL54 mutant in a stem cell transplant recipient with encephalitis. J Infect Dis. 2019;220(8):1302–6.
113. Chemaly RF, Chou S, Einsele H, Griffiths P, Avery R, Razonable RR, et al. Definitions of resistant and refractory cytomegalovirus infection and disease in transplant recipients for use in clinical trials. Clin Infect Dis. 2019;68(8):1420–6. https://doi.org/10.1093/cid/ciy696.
114. Khawaja F, Batista MV, El Haddad L, Chemaly RF. Resistant or refractory cytomegalovirus infections after hematopoietic cell transplantation: diagnosis and management. Curr Opin Infect Dis. 2019;32:565. https://doi.org/10.1097/QCO.0000000000000607.
115. Shmueli E, Or R, Shapira MY, Resnick IB, Caplan O, Bdolah-Abram T, et al. High rate of cytomegalovirus drug resistance among patients receiving preemptive antiviral treatment after haploidentical stem cell transplantation. J Infect Dis. 2014;209(4):557–61.
116. Hantz S, Garnier-Geoffroy F, Mazeron M-C, Garrigue I, Merville P, Mengelle C, et al. Drug-resistant cytomegalovirus in transplant recipients: a French cohort study. J Antimicrob Chemother. 2010;65(12):2628–40.

117. Allice T, Busca A, Locatelli F, Falda M, Pittaluga F, Ghisetti V. Valganciclovir as pre-emptive therapy for cytomegalovirus infection post-allogenic stem cell transplantation: implications for the emergence of drug-resistant cytomegalovirus. J Antimicrob Chemother. 2009;63(3):600–8.
118. Almyroudis N, Jakubowski A, Jaffe D, Sepkowitz K, Pamer E, O'Reilly R, et al. Predictors for persistent cytomegalovirus reactivation after T-cell-depleted allogeneic hematopoietic stem cell transplantation. Transpl Infect Dis. 2007;9(4):286–94.
119. Nakamura R, Battiwalla M, Solomon S, Follmann D, Chakrabarti S, Cortez K, et al. Persisting posttransplantation cytomegalovirus antigenemia correlates with poor lymphocyte proliferation to cytomegalovirus antigen and predicts for increased late relapse and treatment failure. Biol Blood Marrow Transplant. 2004;10(1):49–57.
120. Shannon-Lowe CD, Emery VC. The effects of maribavir on the autophosphorylation of ganciclovir resistant mutants of the cytomegalovirus UL97 protein. Herpesviridae. 2010;1(1):4. https://doi.org/10.1186/2042-4280-1-4.
121. Guiu A, López-Aladid R, Cardeñoso L, Mosquera MM, de la Cámara R, Marcos MA. Study of cytomegalovirus resistance in allogeneic hematopoietic cell transplant recipients. Med Clin. 2020;154(11):433–9. https://doi.org/10.1016/j.medcli.2019.07.027.
122. Chou S, Ercolani RJ, Vanarsdall AL. Differentiated levels of ganciclovir resistance conferred by mutations at codons 591 to 603 of the cytomegalovirus UL97 kinase gene. J Clin Microbiol. 2017;55(7):2098–104. https://doi.org/10.1128/JCM.00391-17.
123. Papanicolaou GA, Silveira FP, Langston AA, Pereira MR, Avery RK, Uknis M, et al. Maribavir for refractory or resistant cytomegalovirus infections in hematopoietic-cell or solid-organ transplant recipients: a randomized, dose-ranging, double-blind, phase 2 study. Clin Infect Dis. 2019;68(8):1255–64. https://doi.org/10.1093/cid/ciy706.
124. Maertens J, Cordonnier C, Jaksch P, Poiré X, Uknis M, Wu J, et al. Maribavir for preemptive treatment of cytomegalovirus reactivation. N Engl J Med. 2019;381(12):1136–47. https://doi.org/10.1056/NEJMoa1714656.
125. Avery RK, Alain S, Alexander BD, Blumberg EA, Chemaly RF, Cordonnier C, et al. Maribavir for refractory cytomegalovirus infections with or without resistance post-transplant: results from a phase 3 randomized clinical trial. Clin Infect Dis. 2022;75:690. https://doi.org/10.1093/cid/ciab988.
126. Kang C. Maribavir: first approval. Drugs. 2022;82:335–40.
127. Bao L, Cowan MJ, Dunham K, Horn B, McGuirk J, Gilman A, et al. Adoptive immunotherapy with CMV-specific cytotoxic T lymphocytes for stem cell transplant patients with refractory CMV infections. J Immunother. 2012;35(3):293. https://doi.org/10.1097/CJI.0b013e31824300a2.
128. Peggs KS, Verfuerth S, Pizzey A, Khan N, Guiver M, Moss PA, et al. Adoptive cellular therapy for early cytomegalovirus infection after allogeneic stem-cell transplantation with virus-specific T-cell lines. Lancet. 2003;362(9393):1375. https://doi.org/10.1016/S0140-6736(03)14634-X.
129. Ke P, Bao X, Zhou J, Li X, Zhuang J, He X, et al. Donor CMV-specific cytotoxic T lymphocytes successfully treated drug-resistant cytomegalovirus encephalitis after allogeneic hematopoietic stem cell transplantation. Hematology. 2020;25(1):43–7.
130. Neill L, Peggs K. Cell therapy for cytomegalovirus infection. Expert Opin Biol Ther. 2021;21(5):649–59. https://doi.org/10.1080/14712598.2021.1857720.
131. O'Reilly RJ, Prockop S, Hasan AN, Koehne G, Doubrovina E. Virus-specific T-cell banks for 'off the shelf' adoptive therapy of refractory infections. Bone Marrow Transplant. 2016;51(9):1163–72. https://doi.org/10.1038/bmt.2016.17.
132. Tzannou I, Papadopoulou A, Naik S, Leung K, Martinez CA, Ramos CA, et al. Off-the-shelf virus-specific T cells to treat BK virus, human herpesvirus 6, cytomegalovirus, Epstein-Barr virus, and adenovirus infections after allogeneic hematopoietic stem-cell transplantation. J Clin Oncol. 2017;35(31):3547–57. https://doi.org/10.1200/JCO.2017.73.0655.
133. Tzannou I, Watanabe A, Naik S, Daum R, Kuvalekar M, Leung KS, et al. "mini" bank of only 8 donors supplies CMV-directed T cells to diverse recipients. Blood Adv. 2019;3(17):2571–80. https://doi.org/10.1182/bloodadvances.2019000371.
134. Wang E, Jan AS, Doan VP, Ferguson JB, Yeh JC. Leflunomide therapy for refractory cytomegalovirus infections in hematopoietic stem cell transplant recipients. J Oncol Pharm Pract. 2019;25(7):1731–7. https://doi.org/10.1177/1078155218796188.
135. El Chaer F, Mori N, Shah D, Oliver N, Wang E, Jan A, et al. Adjuvant and salvage therapy with leflunomide for recalcitrant cytomegalovirus infections in hematopoietic cell transplantation recipients: a case series. Antiviral Res. 2016;135:91–6. https://doi.org/10.1016/j.antiviral.2016.08.027.
136. Wolf DG, Shimoni A, Resnick IB, Stamminger T, Neumann AU, Chou S, et al. Human cytomegalovirus kinetics following institution of artesunate after hematopoietic stem cell transplantation. Antiviral Res. 2011;90(3):183. https://doi.org/10.1016/j.antiviral.2011.03.184.
137. Lau PKH, Woods ML, Ratanjee SK, John GT. Artesunate is ineffective in controlling valganciclovir-resistant cytomegalovirus infection. Clin Infect Dis. 2011;52:279.
138. Germi R, Mariette C, Alain S, Lupo J, Thiebaut A, Brion JP, et al. Success and failure of artesunate treatment in five transplant recipients with disease caused by drug-resistant cytomegalovirus. Antiviral Res. 2014;101(1):57. https://doi.org/10.1016/j.antiviral.2013.10.014.

139. Gantt S, Huang ML, Magaret A, Bunts L, Selke S, Wald A, et al. An artesunate-containing antimalarial treatment regimen did not suppress cytomegalovirus viremia. J Clin Virol. 2013;58(1):276. https://doi.org/10.1016/j.jcv.2013.06.008.
140. Phoompoung P, Ferreira VH, Tikkanen J, Husain S, Viswabandya A, Kumar D, et al. Letermovir as salvage therapy for cytomegalovirus infection in transplant recipients. Transplantation. 2020;104:404–9. https://doi.org/10.1097/TP.0000000000002785.
141. Kaul DR, Stoelben S, Cober E, Ojo T, Sandusky E, Lischka P, et al. First report of successful treatment of multidrug-resistant cytomegalovirus disease with the novel anti-CMV compound AIC246. Am J Transplant. 2011;11(5):1079. https://doi.org/10.1111/j.1600-6143.2011.03530.x.
142. Turner N, Strand A, Grewal DS, Cox G, Arif S, Baker AW, et al. Use of letermovir as salvage therapy for drug-resistant cytomegalovirus retinitis. Antimicrob Agents Chemother. 2019;63(3):e02337. https://doi.org/10.1128/AAC.02337-18.

# 11 Respiratory Viral Infections

Zeinab El Boghdadly, Chikara Ogimi, and Michael Boeckh

## Introduction

Respiratory viral infections (RVIs) are well-established causes of serious morbidity and mortality among hematopoietic cell transplantation (HCT) recipients [1–4]. Given their impaired humoral and cell-mediated immunity, they are at risk for rapid progression of upper respiratory tract infection (URTI) to lower respiratory tract infection (LRTI) [5–8]. Furthermore, RVIs can result in late noninfectious pulmonary complications, including airflow decline and bronchiolitis obliterans syndrome [9–11]. Recent data using multiplex molecular detection platforms show that RVIs are common in allogeneic HCT recipients (Fig. 11.1). In this chapter, we focus on contemporary data published on RVIs in HCT recipients in the last ~5 years, addressing updated management strategies in the field and highlighting unmet needs. As data primarily come from adults, some information may not be applicable to children. We cover both RNA and DNA respiratory viruses, including influenza virus, adenovirus, respiratory syncytial virus (RSV), human metapneumovirus (HMPV), parainfluenza viruses (PIV), human rhinoviruses (HRV), and human coronaviruses (HCoV) other than SARS-CoV-2.

Z. El Boghdadly (✉)
Division of Infectious Diseases, The Ohio State University Wexner Medical Center, Columbus, OH, USA
e-mail: Zeinab.elboghdadly@osumc.edu

C. Ogimi
Division of Infectious Diseases, Department of Medical Subspecialties, National Center for Child Health and Development, Tokyo, Japan

Vaccine and Infectious Disease Division, Fred Hutchinson Cancer Center, Seattle, WA, USA

M. Boeckh
Vaccine and Infectious Disease Division, Fred Hutchinson Cancer Center, Seattle, WA, USA

Clinical Research Division, Fred Hutchinson Cancer Center, Seattle, WA, USA

Division of Allergy and Infectious Disease, Department of Medicine, University of Washington, Seattle, WA, USA



A. O. Soubani (ed.), *Pulmonary and Critical Care Considerations of Hematopoietic Stem Cell Transplantation*, https://doi.org/10.1007/978-3-031-28797-8_11

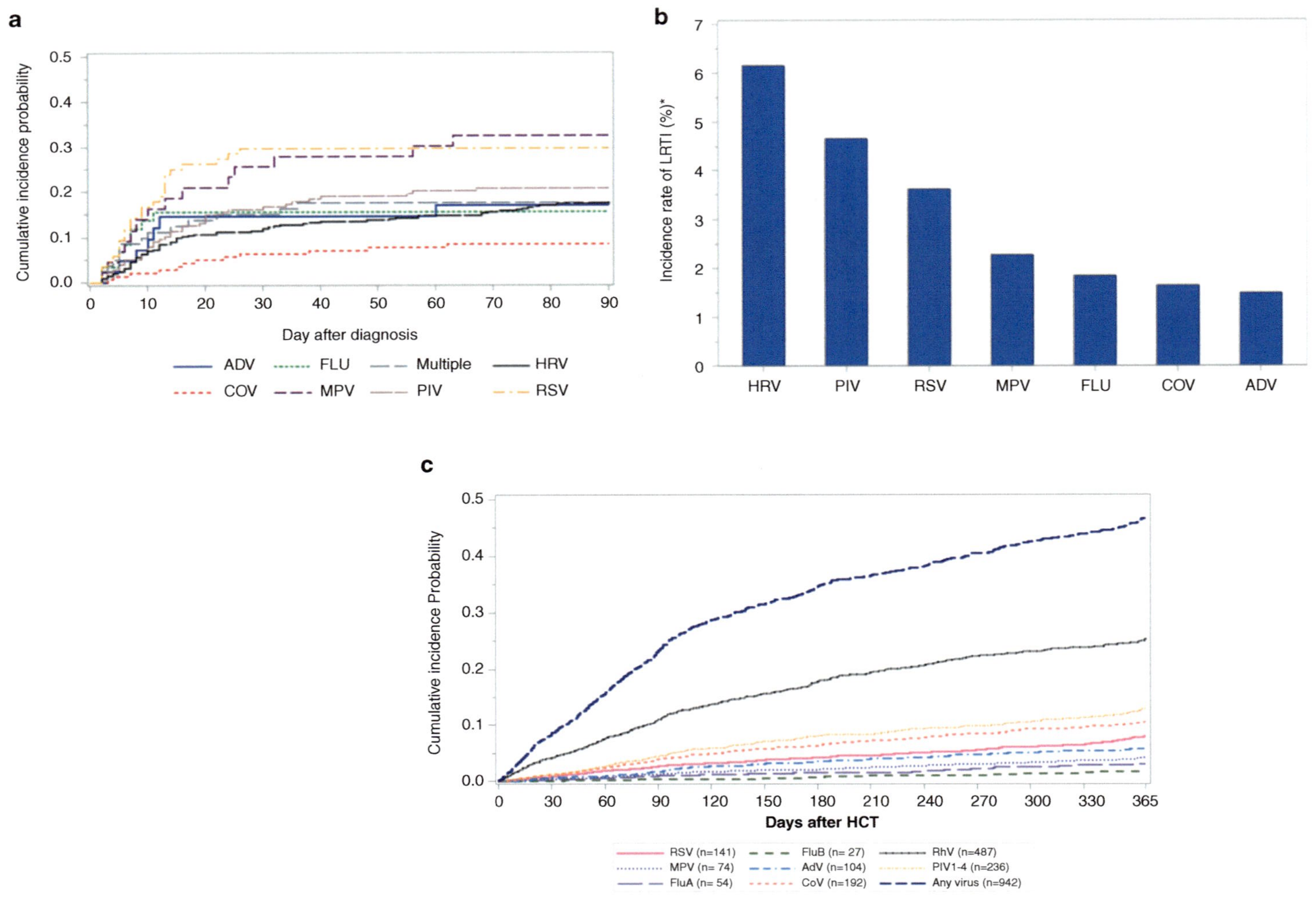


**Fig. 11.1** Epidemiology of respiratory virus infections at Fred Hutchinson Cancer Center. Cumulative incidence of progression to LRTI within 90 days among patients presenting with first viral URTI (**a**), incidence rate of LRTI after first infection by each virus among 2552 allogeneic hematopoietic cell transplantation recipients (**b**), time to first viral infection by 1 year after allogeneic hematopoietic cell transplantation (**c**). Panel (**a**) and (**b**) were reproduced from Ogimi, C. *et al. Bone Marrow Transplant* 57, 649–657 (2022); Panel (**c**): data generated from the same cohort

## Diagnostic Considerations

Over the past two decades, molecular assays for the diagnosis of RVIs have improved dramatically, leading to more accessible testing, shorter turnaround time, standardization, and higher sensitivity and/or specificity compared to viral cultures and immunofluorescence assays [12]. Nucleic acid-based detection assays have become the gold standard [13, 14], and multiplex polymerase chain reaction (PCR) assays have further added the advantage of simultaneous detection of multiple respiratory viral and bacterial pathogens [13]. However, to date, many licensed PCR assays do not provide validated quantitative results [13, 15]. Discordant results of PCR between upper and lower respiratory tract samples have been described, with discrepancies occurring in both directions; thus, it is encouraged to perform bronchoalveolar lavage (BAL) when LRTI is highly suspected, especially with a negative result from the nasopharyngeal sample [16]. Routine chest computed tomography is not required in patients without lower respiratory tract symptoms; however, it can capture subtle pulmonary changes undetected on a chest X-ray: patchy ground glass opacities, centrilobular nodules, peribronchial thickening, and airspace consolidation. Viral pneumonia can radiographically mimic other noninfectious pulmonary complications such as pulmonary edema, sirolimus-induced pneumonitis, interstitial pneumonitis, and diffuse alveolar hemorrhage [17, 18], further supporting the use of BAL to definitely establish a diagnosis.

## Specific Viral Infections

### Influenza Viruses

Influenza virus is an RNA virus that belongs to the family *Orthomyxovidae,* which is further classified based on hemagglutinin and neuraminidase. Influenza A and influenza B are the types that are relevant to human infections. Influenza A viruses are subject to antigenic drifts and antigenic shifts, which results in pandemics. Patients with hematologic malignancies and HCT recipients with influenza are at risk for severe outcomes, including progression to LRTI up to 46% and in-hospital mortality of 19.55% [95% CI, 10.59–29.97%] as noted in a recent meta-analysis [19]. The incidence of influenza LRTI and progression to LRTI after allogeneic HCT is shown in Fig. 11.1. In a 5-year multicenter prospective study of seasonal influenza in HCT (autologous and allogeneic) and solid organ transplant recipients, 26.5% of HCT recipients developed LRTI, and 10.8% required intensive care unit (ICU) admission [20]. Viral loads were significantly higher among unvaccinated patients, those admitted to the ICU, and those with LRTI. Using Ct values as a surrogate for viral load, higher progression rates among adult allogeneic HCT recipients with higher viral loads were also noted in another recent study [7]. Influenza vaccination remains a powerful tool for primary prevention in this population. The vaccine series usually starts around 6 months post-HCT; however, it can be given as early as 3 months during community outbreaks [21, 22]. Live attenuated influenza vaccine should not be given to HCT households or recipients within the first 2 years or to those on treatment for active graft versus host disease (GvHD) [23]. Despite suboptimal vaccine response, overall benefits are still tangible in terms of reducing total numbers of RVIs (51 vs 36 %, $p = 0.036$), LRTI (16 vs 2%, $P = 0.01$) and lowering progression rates to LRTI (30 vs 7%, $P < 0.01$) compared to unvaccinated HCT recipients [24]. Multiple vaccine strategies [25] have been adopted to augment immunogenicity, including high-dose trivalent vaccines [26], two-dose vaccine schedules [27, 28], and the use of adjuvants [29]. Although the high-dose inactivated vaccine resulted in higher titers for the H3N2 strain compared to the standard dose, the trial was not powered adequately to compare immunogenicity [26]. National societies recommend annual influenza vaccination with either an inactivated or recombinant vaccine [30] with no favoring of one vaccine type over the other [31, 32]. Multiple studies emphasized the importance of early antiviral treatment (within 48 h of the symptom onset) to improve clinical outcomes [20]; however, given the high risk for worse outcomes [33], a later initiation may still be beneficial [34]. The typical course is 5 days of standard dose oseltamivir. Longer oseltamivir duration (10 days) and high-dose oseltamivir (150 mg BID) have been used in critically ill patients, but no solid evidence exists to suggest the superiority of higher doses [2, 35–37]. Another agent is inhaled zanamivir (active against influenza A and B), which is active against oseltamivir-resistant strains [1]. An intravenous formulation is approved in Europe, is being explored in clinical trials for children, and is available for compassionate use through the United States Food and Drug Administration [38]. Baloxavir is a novel single-dose drug for influenza, approved in 2018 for both post-exposure prophylaxis and treatment [39]. Some reports showed superior effectiveness against influenza B compared to oseltamivir [40], but the emergence of baloxavir-related resistance poses a clinical and epidemiological challenge, as demonstrated in multiple trials [40, 41]. More recently, the FLAGSTONE study showed rapid virologic clearance but no clinical benefit of baloxavir and neuraminidase inhibitors in combination compared with neuraminidase inhibitors alone in patients with severe influenza [42]. Some experts argue combination therapy may be beneficial in immunocompromised hosts [41, 43–45], but there are to date no randomized clinical trials demonstrating the superiority of this approach.

Peramivir is a single-dose intravenous antiviral agent that is approved in the United States for influenza infection. Studies did not show the superiority of oseltamivir [46, 47], and it also lacks activity against oseltamivir-resistant strains (H275Y mutation) [48]. Serious neuropsychiatric adverse events have been described.

The role of polyclonal intravenous immunoglobulin (IVIG) remains unclear in HCT recipients with influenza. In one European clinical trial, no additional benefit of adjunct IVIG to oseltamivir was found [49, 50]. We illustrate the management of influenza and other RVIs in Fig. 11.2.

## Adenoviruses

Adenovirus is a DNA virus and a member of the *Adenoviridae* family that circulates throughout the year. It is further classified into seven species (A-G) with variable disease severity [43]. Infection in HCT recipients can either be primarily acquired following exogenous exposure or reactivation of latent infection. Infections can range from asymptomatic DNAemia to serious pneumonia that can progress to acute respiratory failure requiring mechanical ventilation. In contrast to other RVIs, infection is not limited to the respiratory tract and can disseminate, causing enterocolitis, esophagitis, hemorrhagic cystitis, interstitial nephritis/renal failure, hepatitis/liver failure, and encephalitis and carrying a very high mortality rate [51].

Infection is more commonly seen in pediatric HCT recipients compared to adults [52]. In the AdVance multinational study, the incidence of any adenovirus infection was about 32% and 6% among pediatric and adult centers, respectively [53]. The majority of adenovirus infections in that study occurred in the first 100 days post-HCT, and use of T cell depletion, young age, and donor types other than matched related were all associated with the development of high-grade viremia >1000 copies/mL [53]. Despite the high mortality of this infection, there are no specific approved antiviral drugs against adenovirus [51, 52]. Cidofovir has been the only antiviral used for adenovirus treatment [51, 54]. It causes significant nephrotoxicity, leading to acute renal failure. There is no consensus on a specific adenovirus viral load cutoff to initiate cidofovir. A threshold of >1000 copies/ml is the most frequently used and was also endorsed in the position statement by the European Society of Blood and Marrow Transplantation [52]. Duration of antiviral therapy is dependent on the resolution of DNAemia, end organ disease recovery, and immune reconstitution. Based on our anecdotal experience, HCT recipients with asymptomatic low-level DNAemia or mild URTI do not necessarily require antiviral therapy. Pursuing supportive measures such as reducing the level of

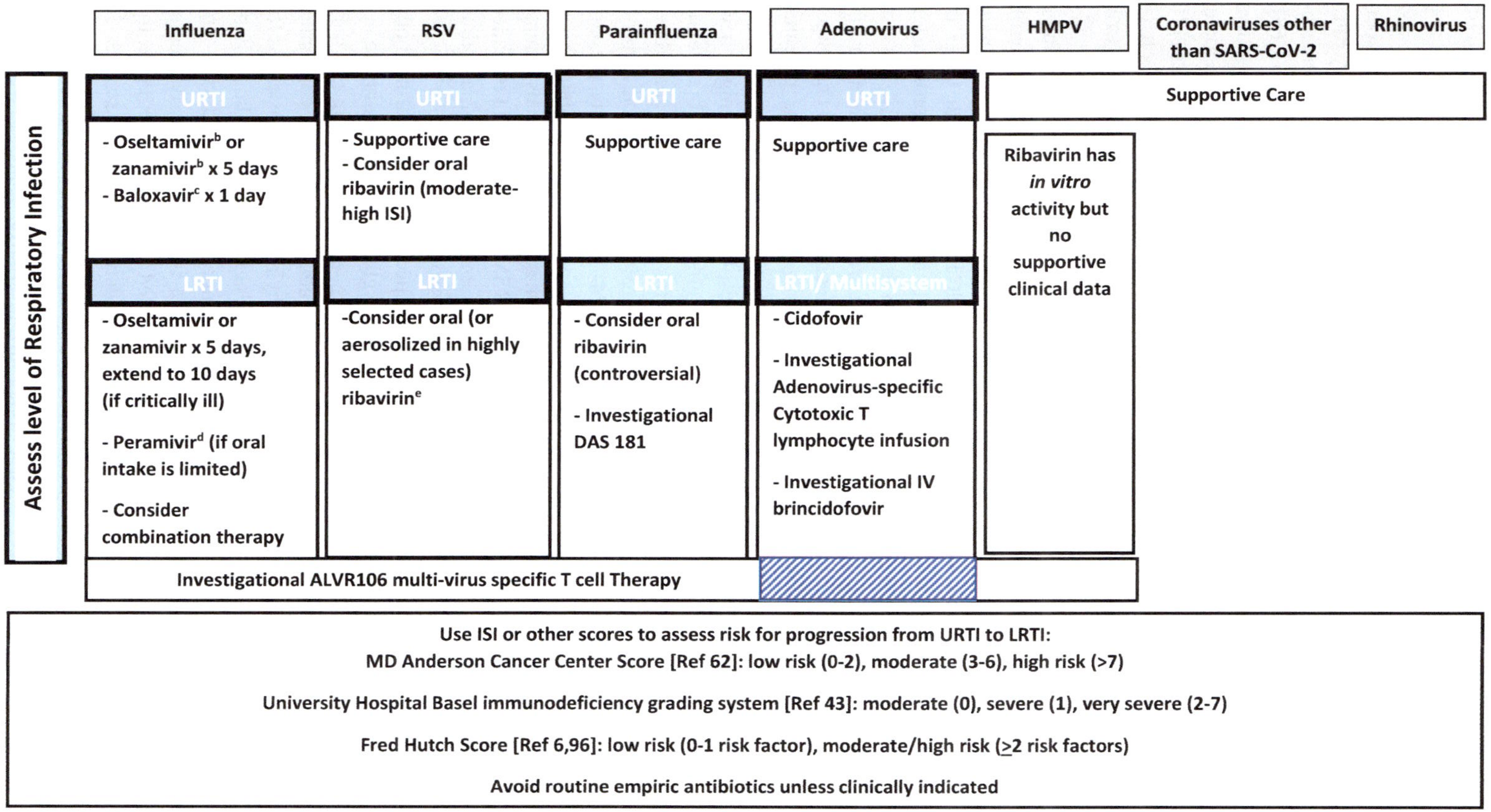


[a] HMPV, human metapneumovirus; ISI, immunodeficiency scoring index; IV, intravenous; LRTI, lower respiratory tract infection; SARS, severe acute respiratory syndrome; RSV, respiratory syncytial virus; URTI, upper respiratory tract infection

[b] Neuraminidase inhibitor against strains A and B

[c] Interferes with endonuclease activity (cap snatching) and causes reduction in viral shedding, active against some oseltamivir-resistant strains

[d] Neuroaminidase inhibitor against Influenza A and B

[e] There are limited data on dosing oral ribavirin especially for young children

**Fig. 11.2** Summary of management of respiratory viral infections[a]

immunosuppression (if feasible) with vigilant monitoring for progression to moderate-to-severe disease is recommended. Some studies have shown in vitro activity of ribavirin against adenovirus species C [55, 56], but clinical data are lacking, and ribavirin is not routinely recommended as antiviral therapy [52]. Brincidofovir (CMX001), an oral lipid conjugate prodrug of cidofovir [57, 58], is no longer available for compassionate use in the US, although it was approved for human smallpox disease in 2021. An intravenous formulation is presently being studied (ClinicalTrials.gov NCT04706923).

## Respiratory Syncytial Virus (RSV)

RSV belongs to the *Pneumoviridae* RNA virus family, further classified into types A and B. Infection occurs throughout the year, with a higher incidence in the winter [43]. The incidence of RSV infection also varies by transplant type, time since transplant, and age, and some reports demonstrate that up to 17% of HCT recipients suffered from RSV infection [59]. HCT recipients with RSV URTI are at high risk for rapid progression to LRTI with rates ranging from 33% to 61% [60] (Fig. 11.1).

Researchers have developed scoring systems to assess the degree of immunosuppression in adult HCT recipients with RSV infection and stratify risk for progression to LRTI. The University Hospital Basel Immunodeficiency grading system [61] and the MD Anderson Cancer Center immunodeficiency scoring index (ISI) [62] are commonly used scoring systems, and a simplified approach to determining the number of risk factors at the time of URTI has been recently proposed [6]. Some of the clinical and laboratory criteria are overlapping in these scoring systems. These include but are not limited to myeloablative conditioning regimen, timing after allogeneic HCT, presence of GvHD, use of systemic corticosteroids, prior lymphodepletion, and degree of neutropenia $<0.5 \times 10^9$/l, lymphopenia ($<0.2$ vs $0.1 \times 10^9$/l) [43, 61, 62]. These scoring systems were initially created to assess the outcome of RSV but, due to the overlapping risk factors, were later applied to other viruses, including HMPV, influenza, PIV, HRV, and seasonal HCoVs [6, 63–66]. Additional risk factors such as monocytopenia, hypoalbuminemia, multiple transplants, and hyperglycemia were recently found to be associated with progression to LRTI [6]. Mortality rates are higher among patients with higher ISI, reaching more than 50% in some studies [3, 62, 67, 68]. To date, the primary RSV treatment is supportive care, including bronchodilators (if appropriate, predominantly in adults) and antipyretics [2]. Several studies from large transplant centers have shown a potential mortality benefit of ribavirin (aerosolized or oral) in HCT recipients with LRTI compared to no antivirals [69–71]. However, large randomized controlled trials are lacking. Ribavirin is currently endorsed by some experts for the treatment of RSV in HCT recipients with LRTI or those with URTI with a higher risk of progression (e.g., moderate-high risk ISI) [4, 60, 72].

Aerosolized ribavirin is neither widely available nor routinely recommended due to challenges associated with drug administration, potential adverse events, and its extraordinarily high cost [73]. Although aerosolized ribavirin might have stronger protective effects compared to systemic ribavirin [70], several retrospective studies have shown comparable results with oral and aerosolized formulations [74–76]. Most recently, presatovir (GS-5806), an oral fusion inhibitor, was evaluated in two phase 2 clinical trials among HCT recipients for RSV URTI and LRTI but failed to meet the primary endpoints [77, 78], and drug development was discontinued.

Palivizumab, a specific monoclonal antibody against the RSV F glycoprotein, was originally approved for the prevention of RSV in newborn infants born ≤29 weeks or those with congenital heart disease. Prophylaxis may be considered for children younger than 24 months who will be profoundly immunocompromised during the RSV season [79]. It is neither routinely recommended nor approved in adults with RSV, as the efficacy is inconclusive in multiple studies, in addition to its high cost [70, 80–83]. Data on polyclonal IVIG are limited given the lack of large randomized control trials. Few reports showed potential benefit [69, 84], but retrospective studies and systematic analyses have shown no improved outcomes compared to placebo [70, 85]. Similarly to other RVIs, the use of empiric antibiotics should be avoided unless bacterial co-infection is suspected or confirmed. Exposure to antibiotics, especially with anaerobic activity, was associated with progression to LRTI in allogeneic HCT patients with PIV, RSV, HMPV, and HRV after adjusting for other confounders [86, 87]. Although direct causation is difficult to prove, antibiotics have a known impact on microbiome diversity and subsequent poor transplant outcomes [88].

## Human Metapneumovirus (HMPV)

HMPV belongs to the *Pneumovirinae* subfamily within the *Paramyxoviridae* family and was first identified in 2001. It circulates more in the late winter and early spring seasons [89]. It can cause both URTI and LRTI, with a progression rate similar to that of RSV (Fig. 11.1). In a recent systematic review, HMPV incidence was about 7% among HCT recipients, which was similar to nontransplant patients with hematologic malignancies; 34% of cases progressed to LRTI with a mortality rate up to 27% [90]. Lymphopenia and high-dose steroids (≥1 mg/kg) increased the risk of progression to LRTI [91]; however, viral load in nasopharyngeal samples at the time of diagnosis of URTI was not predictive of progression to LRTI [7]. There is no proven antiviral therapy against HMPV, and current guidelines only recommend supportive care. Although some centers have anecdotally used ribavirin and polyclonal IVIG in high-risk patients, their role remains controversial [2, 4, 92, 93].

## Parainfluenza Virus (PIV)

PIV is a member of the *Paramyxoviridae* family (serotypes 1-4) with PIV serotype 3 being the most common. PIV serotype 3 circulates throughout the year compared to PIV serotypes 1 and 2, which occur mainly in the fall and winter [94, 95]. PIV infection primarily causes URTI and it shares similar risk factors for progression to LRTI with other RVIs [96–99]. The risk for progression to LRTI ranges between 20 and 39% among HCT recipients, with an associated pooled mortality rates up of 30% [94]. PIV LRTI can predispose to long-term pulmonary dysfunction [100]. Management is primarily focused on supportive care given the lack of any efficaciously approved antivirals or vaccines. Off-label use of ribavirin has been observed given its *in vitro* activity against PIV [1, 2, 4, 101]; however, there is no evidence to support its routine use, as noted in a recent meta-analysis showing a lack of any benefits of aerosolized or intravenous forms on mitigating risk of progression or mortality [94]. DAS181 is an investigational inhaled sialidase fusion protein inhibitor that blocks the virus entry into respiratory epithelial cells. Reports of compassionate use showed improved lung function and viral load reduction [102–104]. It is presently studied in a phase 3 randomized, placebo-controlled, multicenter clinical trial (STOP PIV) based on the results of a phase 2 trial [105] (clinicaltrials.gov NCT03808922).

## Human Rhinovirus

HRV is a member of the *Picornaviridae* family, part of the *Enterovirus* genus. HRV is divided into 3 species (A-C) with numerous serotypes >100, which makes the development of a targeted vaccine challenging. HRV circulates throughout the year; however, more cases occur in spring and autumn, and it is the most common cause of common cold [106]. It accounts for the majority of the RVIs in HCT recipients, with a cumulative incidence of ~20% within the first year post-HCT (Fig. 11.1) [107]. HRV is known for prolonged shedding among HCT recipients compared to other viruses with a median of 3 weeks but can last beyond 3 months in some patients [107, 108]. One study found a possible correlation between initial high viral load and increased risk for prolonged viral shedding [109]. Majority of HRV infections are limited to URTI but severe cases of LRTI requiring ICU care have been reported with mortality rates similar to those associated with

RSV, PIV, or influenza virus, even in the absence of other co-infections [110, 111]. Figure 11.1 shows a relatively low progression rate of HRV to LRTI; however, given the highest incidence of the infection, the number of LRTI cases was the highest post-HCT. HRV also shares similar risk factors for progression to LRTI compared to other RVIs. In a large retrospective study, allogeneic HCT, prior HRV URTI events, lymphocyte count < $100 \times 10^6$ cells/l, positive recipient CMV serostatus, statin use, and steroid use ≥2 mg/kg/day were identified as risk factors for progression to LRTI [66]. There are currently no effective antiviral therapies [2, 4]; however, several drug and immunotherapy development programs are ongoing [2, 112–114].

## Human Coronaviruses Other Than SARS-CoV-2 (HCoVs)

Seasonal HCoVs belong to the *Coronaviridae* family, with either the *Alphacoronavirus* (229E and NL63) or *Betacoronavirus* (OC43 and HKU1) genera, and are considered the second most common cause of common colds following HRV [43, 115]. Their progression to LRTI is infrequent compared to other RVIs, as depicted in Fig. 11.1. *Gammacoronavirus* and *Deltacoronavirus* genera mainly infect animals and are well recognized as zoonotic diseases. Severe acute respiratory syndrome (SARS), Middle East respiratory syndrome (MERS), and the ongoing SARS-CoV-2 pandemic are described in other chapters. In addition to the common risk factors associated with progression to viral LRTI, hypoalbuminemia, and steroid-induced hyperglycemia were found to increase the risk, while no correlation with an initial high viral load was noted [115]. A recent study showed that the presence of HCoVs in BAL samples in HCT recipients was significantly associated with high rates of respiratory support (oxygen use and mechanical ventilation) and mortality, similar to well-established virulent respiratory viruses including RSV, influenza virus, and PIV [116]. Prolonged viral shedding has also been described among HCT recipients with HCoV [107, 117, 118]. In one study, prolonged viral shedding occurred in 59% of patients with a median duration of 4 weeks (range 0–30 weeks) [119], but no specific serotype was significantly associated with prolonged viral shedding [117, 119] and no evolution of the viral genome occurred [117]. In a recent international study among allogeneic HCT with HCoVs, the 3-month overall mortality was 7% in the entire cohort and 16% in those with LRTI [118]. Risk factors associated with higher mortality were an absolute lymphocyte count <$0.1 \times 10^9$/ml, corticosteroid use, and ICU admission [118]. Treatment consists of supportive care as vaccines, monoclonal antibodies, or direct-acting antivirals are not available.

## Special Considerations for HCT Recipients with Respiratory Viruses

### Pretransplant Respiratory Viral Infections

Given the negative impact of respiratory viral infections on HCT outcomes [120], optimizing the proper timing of transplant following recent exposure or a confirmed RVI in HCT candidates is paramount. In HCT candidates with confirmed RVIs due to RSV, HMPV, PIV, influenza, and adenoviruses, deferral of HCT or cellular therapy should be considered as advised by the consensus recommendations [4, 72, 92]; however, these recommendations are primarily based on small case series and anecdotal experience. For the past few years, there has been uncertainty on whether pretransplant HRV and HCoV infections also require deferral of HCT [120]. However, a recent large retrospective study exploring the consequences of pretransplant RVIs according to the location of the infection and the strength of the conditioning regimen provided stronger evidence [121]. In that study, HCT candidates with HRV or HCoVs URTI did not have worse post-HCT outcomes than those without pre-HCT RVIs, in contrast to prior observations in another study [120]. However, myeloablative conditioning and pre-HCT LRTI with any virus were independent risk factors for increased mortality [121].

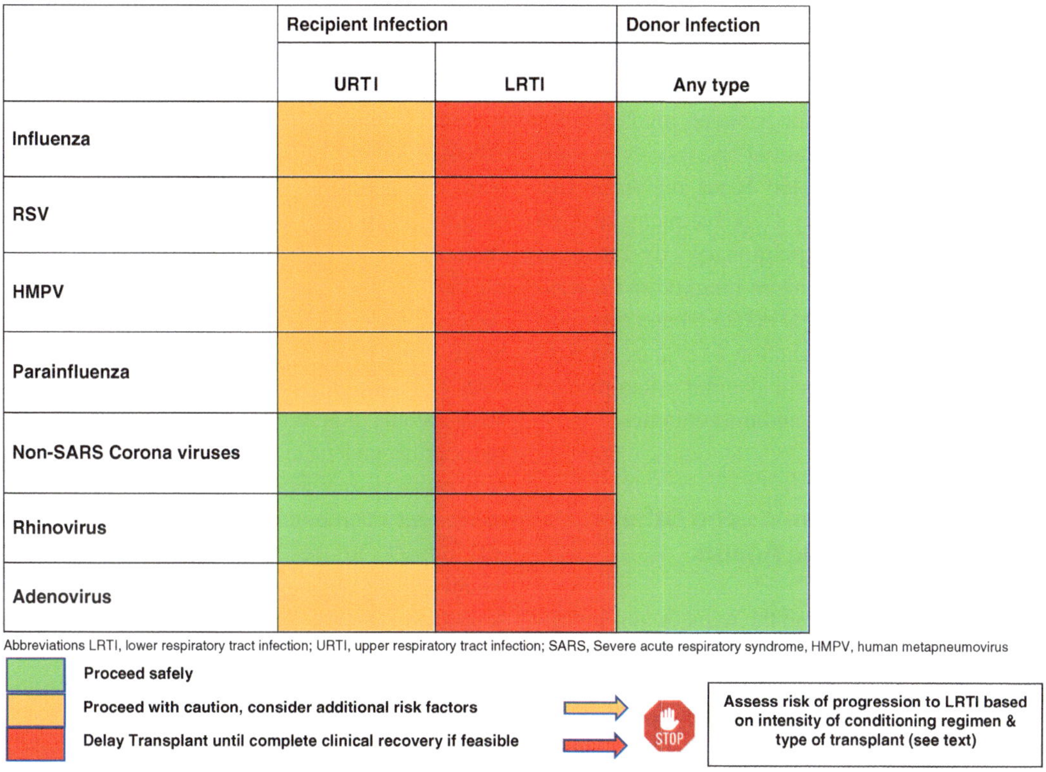


**Fig. 11.3** Pretransplant respiratory viral infections in allogeneic hematopoietic stem cell transplant candidates (expert opinion)

In HCT candidates who have persistently positive PCR results following clinical recovery from RVIs, confirmation of a "test of cure" is often neither practical nor a prerequisite to proceeding with HCT. However, the practice has been variable among cancer centers, and some may require a negative pre-HCT PCR, especially in those with persistent respiratory symptoms, given the risk of poor HCT outcomes [121]. Consensus guidelines do not routinely recommend universal nasopharyngeal PCR screening for respiratory viruses in asymptomatic HCT candidates [4]. For high-risk HCT candidates who are exposed to the influenza virus, antiviral prophylaxis with once-daily oseltamivir, once-daily inhaled zanamivir or one-time baloxavir can be considered [31, 122]. In Fig. 11.3, we summarize our expert opinion on how to tackle some common scenarios related to pre-HCT RVIs among allogeneic HCT candidates. Key decision variables are the type of virus, the location of the infection, and the strength of the conditioning regimen. Proper timing for HCT is dependent on the urgency of transplantation, recovery from respiratory illness, and overall clinical performance.

## Clinical Sequelae of Respiratory Viral Illness

The negative implications of RVIs in HCT recipients extend beyond the initial acute phase, as they can increase the future risk for superimposed infections including bacteria (*Staphylococcus*, *Streptococcus*, *Haemophilus*, *Pseudomonas*) and mold (*Aspergillus* species) [123–125]. There are emerging data that link RVIs to alloimmune post-HCT pulmonary syndromes [126], such as idiopathic pneumonia syndrome, late airflow decline, bronchiolitis obliterans syndrome, and cryptogenic organizing pneumonia [9, 11, 127]. One study showed that prior RVI with RSV, PIV, or influenza is associated with at least a 10% decline in post-RVI forced expiratory volume in the first second (FEV1) from pre-infection baseline values, which was an independent predictor for 2-year nonrelapse mortality [9].

Future research should focus on innovative tools that better identify HCT recipients at high risk for post-RVI pulmonary dysfunction. Examples include relying on longitudinal assessment of home-based viral detection and quantitation [128] and lung function [129], as well as measuring serum, bronchoalveolar inflammatory markers, lung viromes, and microbiomes.

## Adjunct Corticosteroids and Other Immunosuppressive Agents

We generally recommend the reduction of immunosuppression as clinically feasible to facilitate clinical recovery and mitigate the risk of progression to LRTI and prolonged shedding. Impact of steroids on progression to LRTI varies by pathogen and has been, especially at high doses, an independent risk factor for overall mortality for most RVIs, but the correlation is less clear for influenza [2, 94, 111].

Use of corticosteroids is not generally recommended, although theoretically it may abate a virus-induced hyper-inflammatory response. Corticosteroids are widely used for the management of GvHD, and their impact on respiratory virus outcomes has been examined in many studies. Moderate doses of steroids (up to 1 mg/kg) may not increase the risk of progression to LRTI, but it remains unclear if they are beneficial (summarized in [2]). Administration of dexamethasone has become the standard practice in severe cases of SARS-CoV-2 requiring supplemental oxygen [130]. Although its utility in other RVIs has not been fully explored, some studies have reported benefits in patients with influenza, as described in one review [2], but the impact has been deemed inconclusive by others [131, 132].

## Summary and Future Directions

RVIs among HCT candidates and recipients still represent a therapeutic dilemma given the limited efficaciousness of antiviral and monoclonal antibody options. Recently identified risk factors for progression, such as hyperglycemia, hypoalbuminemia, CMV infection (in some cases), and use of antibiotics, require validation and could be incorporated in revised progression scoring indices. Some of these factors are also potentially modifiable. Future grading scores should also focus on virus-specific humoral and cell-mediated immunity. Further understanding of the interplay between respiratory viruses, viral load in different compartments, gut microbiome, pulmonary microbiome, and impact on the immune-inflammatory axis would provide insight into determinants of RVI severity and apply sensitive predictive models to identify high-risk patients. Given the potentially important role of T-cell immunity in controlling RVIs, the use of adoptive T-cell therapy is increasingly investigated in early-phase clinical trials. Promising results in patients with adenovirus have been reported [133–135], and the utility and safety of parainfluenza-specific T-cells are also being investigated [136]. ALVR106 is an off-the-shelf, multi-virus-specific therapy that targets RSV, influenza, PIV, and HMPV and is being explored in a Phase 1/2, randomized double-blind trial (ClinicalTrials.gov NCT04933968). The successful development of long-lasting monoclonal antibodies against SARS-CoV-2 and recently also against RSV emphasizes the potential need for developing monoclonal antibodies against multiple respiratory viruses, providing unprecedented prophylactic and therapeutic options in this vulnerable population [137, 138]. Also, new antiviral drugs are needed for respiratory viruses, and existing drugs for SARS-CoV-2 should be examined for their efficacy against seasonal HCoVs. In Fig. 11.4, we illustrate our holistic approach on how to address current knowledge gaps with proposed exploratory research venues that focus on diagnostic, preventive, therapeutic, immunologic, and microbiologic

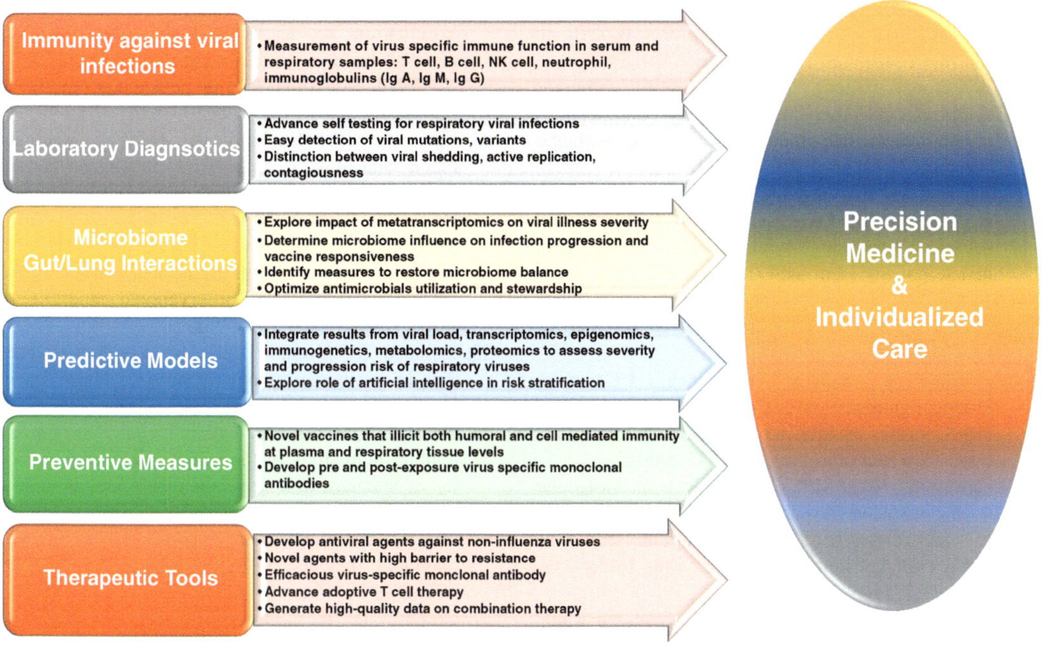


**Fig. 11.4** Gaps of knowledge and unmet clinical needs in respiratory viral infections in HCT recipients

pathways. In the absence of effective antiviral drugs and vaccines for the majority of RVIs, strict infection control measures remain essential tools to mitigate the morbidity of RVIs. Lastly, more pediatric-specific data are warranted, as the majority of the data come from adult patients, and the application of the management guidance to children may need caution.

## References

1. Chemaly RF, Shah DP, Boeckh MJ. Management of respiratory viral infections in hematopoietic cell transplant recipients and patients with hematologic malignancies. Clin Infect Dis. 2014;59:S344–51.
2. Waghmare A, Englund JA, Boeckh M. How I treat respiratory viral infections in the setting of intensive chemotherapy or hematopoietic cell transplantation. Blood. 2016;127:2682–92.
3. Vakil E, Sheshadri A, Faiz SA, et al. Risk factors for mortality after respiratory syncytial virus lower respiratory tract infection in adults with hematologic malignancies. Transpl Infect Dis. 2018;20:e12994.
4. Hirsch HH, Martino R, Ward KN, Boeckh M, Einsele H, Ljungman P. Fourth European Conference on Infections in Leukaemia (ECIL-4): guidelines for diagnosis and treatment of human respiratory syncytial virus, parainfluenza virus, metapneumovirus, rhinovirus, and coronavirus. Clin Infect Dis. 2013;56:258–66.
5. Boeckh M, Campbell A, Xie H, et al. Progression, shedding patterns, and clinical disease associated with respiratory virus infections after allogeneic hematopoietic cell transplantation (HCT). Blood. 2013;122:3278.
6. Ogimi C, Xie H, Waghmare A, et al. Novel factors to predict respiratory viral disease progression in allogeneic hematopoietic cell transplant recipients. Bone Marrow Transplant. 2022;57:649–57.
7. Ogimi C, Xie H, Waghmare A, et al. Correlation of initial upper respiratory tract viral burden with progression to lower tract disease in adult allogeneic hematopoietic cell transplant recipients. J Clin Virol. 2022;150–151:105152.
8. Kim Y-J, Guthrie KA, Waghmare A, et al. Respiratory syncytial virus in hematopoietic cell transplant recipients: factors determining progression to lower respiratory tract disease. J Infect Dis. 2014;209:1195–204.
9. Sheshadri A, Chemaly RF, Alousi AM, et al. Pulmonary impairment after respiratory viral infec-

tions is associated with high mortality in allogeneic hematopoietic cell transplant recipients. Biol Blood Marrow Transplant. 2019;25:800–9.
10. Bergeron A, Cheng G-S. Bronchiolitis obliterans syndrome and other late pulmonary complications after allogeneic hematopoietic stem cell transplantation. Clin Chest Med. 2017;38:607–21.
11. Versluys AB, Rossen JWA, van Ewijk B, Schuurman R, Bierings MB, Boelens JJ. Strong association between respiratory viral infection early after hematopoietic stem cell transplantation and the development of life-threatening acute and chronic alloimmune lung syndromes. Biol Blood Marrow Transplant. 2010;16:782–91.
12. Charlton CL, Babady E, Ginocchio CC, et al. Practical guidance for clinical microbiology laboratories: viruses causing acute respiratory tract infections. Clin Microbiol Rev. 2019;32:e00042.
13. Hanson KE, Azar MM, Banerjee R, et al. Molecular testing for acute respiratory tract infections: clinical and diagnostic recommendations from the IDSA's Diagnostics Committee. Clin Infect Dis. 2020;71:2744–51.
14. Vos LM, Bruning AHL, Reitsma JB, et al. Rapid molecular tests for influenza, respiratory syncytial virus, and other respiratory viruses: a systematic review of diagnostic accuracy and clinical impact studies. Clin Infect Dis. 2019;69:1243–53.
15. Bouzid D, Vila J, Hansen G, et al. Systematic review on the association between respiratory virus realtime PCR cycle threshold values and clinical presentation or outcomes. J Antimicrob Chemother. 2021;76:iii33–49.
16. Boonyaratanakornkit J, Vivek M, Xie H, et al. Predictive value of respiratory viral detection in the upper respiratory tract for infection of the lower respiratory tract with hematopoietic stem cell transplantation. J Infect Dis. 2020;221:379–88.
17. Peña E, Souza CA, Escuissato DL, et al. Noninfectious pulmonary complications after hematopoietic stem cell transplantation: practical approach to imaging diagnosis. RadioGraphics. 2014;34:663–83.
18. Ahya VN. Noninfectious acute lung injury syndromes early after hematopoietic stem cell transplantation. Clin Chest Med. 2017;38:595–606.
19. Atalla E, Kalligeros M, Mylona EK, et al. Impact of influenza infection among adult and pediatric populations with hematologic malignancy and hematopoietic stem cell transplant: a systematic review and meta-analysis. Clin Ther. 2021;43:e66–85.
20. Kumar D, Ferreira VH, Blumberg E, et al. A 5-year prospective multicenter evaluation of influenza infection in transplant recipients. Clin Infect Dis. 2018;67:1322–9.
21. Rubin LG, Levin MJ, Ljungman P, et al. 2013 IDSA clinical practice guideline for vaccination of the immunocompromised host. Clin Infect Dis. 2014;58:e44–e100.
22. Cordonnier C, Einarsdottir S, Cesaro S, et al. Vaccination of haemopoietic stem cell transplant recipients: guidelines of the 2017 European Conference on Infections in Leukaemia (ECIL 7). Lancet Infect Dis. 2019;19:e200–12.
23. Carpenter PA, Englund JA. How I vaccinate blood and marrow transplant recipients. Blood. 2016;127(23):2824–32.
24. Piñana JL, Pérez A, Montoro J, et al. Clinical effectiveness of influenza vaccination after allogeneic hematopoietic stem cell transplantation: a cross-sectional, prospective, observational study. Clin Infect Dis. 2019;68:1894–903.
25. Bosaeed M, Kumar D. Seasonal influenza vaccine in immunocompromised persons. Hum Vaccin Immunother. 2018;14:1311–22.
26. Halasa NB, Savani BN, Asokan I, et al. Randomized double-blind study of the safety and immunogenicity of standard-dose trivalent inactivated influenza vaccine versus high-dose trivalent inactivated influenza vaccine in adult hematopoietic stem cell transplantation patients. Biol Blood Marrow Transplant. 2016;22:528–35.
27. Cordero E, Roca-Oporto C, Bulnes-Ramos A, et al. Two doses of inactivated influenza vaccine improve immune response in solid organ transplant recipients: results of TRANSGRIPE 1-2, a randomized controlled clinical trial. Clin Infect Dis. 2017;64:829–38.
28. Karras NA, Weeres M, Sessions W, et al. A randomized trial of one versus two doses of influenza vaccine after allogeneic transplantation. Biol Blood Marrow Transplant. 2013;19:109–16.
29. Natori Y, Humar A, Lipton J, et al. A pilot randomized trial of adjuvanted influenza vaccine in adult allogeneic hematopoietic stem cell transplant recipients. Bone Marrow Transplant. 2017;52:1016–21.
30. Dunkle LM, Izikson R, Patriarca P, et al. Efficacy of recombinant influenza vaccine in adults 50 years of age or older. N Engl J Med. 2017;376:2427–36.
31. Uyeki TM, Bernstein HH, Bradley JS, et al. Clinical practice guidelines by the Infectious Diseases Society of America: 2018 update on diagnosis, treatment, chemoprophylaxis, and institutional outbreak management of seasonal influenza. Clin Infect Dis. 2019;68:895–902.
32. Grohskopf LA, Blanton LH, Ferdinands JM, et al. Prevention and control of seasonal influenza with vaccines: recommendations of the advisory committee on immunization practices - United States, 2022-23 influenza season. MMWR Recomm Rep. 2022;71:1–28.
33. Louie JK, Yang S, Acosta M, et al. Treatment with neuraminidase inhibitors for critically ill patients with influenza A (H1N1)pdm09. Clin Infect Dis. 2012;55:1198–204.
34. Choi S-M, Boudreault AA, Xie H, Englund JA, Corey L, Boeckh M. Differences in clinical outcomes after 2009 influenza A/H1N1 and seasonal

influenza among hematopoietic cell transplant recipients. Blood. 2011;117:5050–6.
35. Casper C, Englund J, Boeckh M. How I treat influenza in patients with hematologic malignancies. Blood. 2010;115:1331–42.
36. Lee N, Hui DSC, Zuo Z, et al. A prospective intervention study on higher-dose oseltamivir treatment in adults hospitalized with influenza a and B infections. Clin Infect Dis. 2013;57:1511–9.
37. South East Asia Infectious Disease Clinical Research Network. Effect of double dose oseltamivir on clinical and virological outcomes in children and adults admitted to hospital with severe influenza: double blind randomised controlled trial. BMJ. 2013;346:f3039.
38. Weller S, Jones LS, Lou Y, Peppercorn A, Ng-Cashin J. Pharmacokinetics of zanamivir following intravenous administration to subjects with and without renal impairment. Antimicrob Agents Chemother. 2013;57:2967–71.
39. Hayden FG, Sugaya N, Hirotsu N, et al. Baloxavir marboxil for uncomplicated influenza in adults and adolescents. N Engl J Med. 2018;379:913–23.
40. Ison MG, Portsmouth S, Yoshida Y, et al. Early treatment with baloxavir marboxil in high-risk adolescent and adult outpatients with uncomplicated influenza (CAPSTONE-2): a randomised, placebo-controlled, phase 3 trial. Lancet Infect Dis. 2020;20:1204–14.
41. Ison MG, Hayden FG, Hay AJ, et al. Influenza polymerase inhibitor resistance: assessment of the current state of the art - a report of the isirv Antiviral Group. Antivir Res. 2021;194:105158.
42. Kumar D, Ison MG, Mira J-P, et al. Combining baloxavir marboxil with standard-of-care neuraminidase inhibitor in patients hospitalised with severe influenza (FLAGSTONE): a randomised, parallel-group, double-blind, placebo-controlled, superiority trial. Lancet Infect Dis. 2022;22(5):718–30.
43. Ison MG, Hirsch HH. Community-acquired respiratory viruses in transplant patients: diversity, impact, unmet clinical needs. Clin Microbiol Rev. 2019;32:e00042. https://doi.org/10.1128/CMR.00042-19.
44. Angelidakis G, Khawaja F, Mulanovich VE, Dailey-Garnes N, Ariza-Heredia E, Chemaly RF. Combination of baloxavir and oseltamivir for treatment of severe influenza infection in hematopoietic cell transplant recipients: a novel treatment strategy for a high-risk population. Microbes Infect. 2022;24:104895.
45. Ison MG. Respiratory viral infections in the immunocompromised. Curr Opin Pulm Med. 2022;28:205–10.
46. de Jong MD, Ison MG, Monto AS, et al. Evaluation of intravenous peramivir for treatment of influenza in hospitalized patients. Clin Infect Dis. 2014;59:e172–85.
47. Zhao Y, Huang G, He W, et al. Efficacy and safety of single-dose antiviral drugs for influenza treatment: a systematic review and network meta-analysis. J Med Virol. 2022;94:3270–302.
48. Higgins RR, Beniprashad M, Chong-King E, et al. Recovery of influenza B virus with the H273Y point mutation in the neuraminidase active site from a human patient. J Clin Microbiol. 2012;50:2500–2.
49. Davey RT, Fernández-Cruz E, Markowitz N, et al. Anti-influenza hyperimmune intravenous immunoglobulin for adults with influenza A or B infection (FLU-IVIG): a double-blind, randomised, placebo-controlled trial. Lancet Respir Med. 2019;7:951–63.
50. Onodera H, Urayama T, Hirota K, et al. Neutralizing activities against seasonal influenza viruses in human intravenous immunoglobulin. Biologics. 2017;11:23–30.
51. Lindemans CA, Leen AM, Boelens JJ. How I treat adenovirus in hematopoietic stem cell transplant recipients. Blood. 2010;116(25):5476–85. Available https://ashpublications.org/blood/article/116/25/5476/28618/How-I-treat-adenovirus-in-hematopoietic-stem-cell. Accessed 13 May 2022.
52. Hiwarkar P, Kosulin K, Cesaro S, et al. Management of adenovirus infection in patients after haematopoietic stem cell transplantation: state-of-the-art and real-life current approach: a position statement on behalf of the Infectious Diseases Working Party of the European Society of Blood and Marrow Transplantation. Rev Med Virol. 2018;28:e1980.
53. Sedláček P, Petterson T, Robin M, et al. Incidence of adenovirus infection in hematopoietic stem cell transplantation recipients: findings from the advance study. Biol Blood Marrow Transplant. 2019;25:810–8.
54. Matthes-Martin S, Feuchtinger T, Shaw PJ, et al. European guidelines for diagnosis and treatment of adenovirus infection in leukemia and stem cell transplantation: summary of ECIL-4 (2011). Transpl Infect Dis. 2012;14:555–63.
55. Lion T. Adenovirus infections in immunocompetent and immunocompromised patients. Clin Microbiol Rev. 2014;27:441–62.
56. Morfin F, Dupuis-Girod S, Frobert E, et al. Differential susceptibility of adenovirus clinical isolates to cidofovir and ribavirin is not related to species alone. Antivir Ther. 2009;14:55–61.
57. Grimley MS, Chemaly RF, Englund JA, et al. Brincidofovir for asymptomatic adenovirus viremia in pediatric and adult allogeneic hematopoietic cell transplant recipients: a randomized placebo-controlled phase II trial. Biol Blood Marrow Transplant. 2017;23:512–21.
58. Ehlert K, Schulte JH, Kühl J-S, Lang P, Eggert A, Voigt S. Efficacy of brincidofovir in pediatric stem cell transplant recipients with adenovirus infections. J Pediatric Infect Dis Soc. 2021;2021:72.
59. Shah JN, Chemaly RF. Management of RSV infections in adult recipients of hematopoietic stem cell transplantation. Blood. 2011;117:2755–63.
60. Khawaja F, Chemaly RF. Respiratory syncytial virus in hematopoietic cell transplant recipi-

ents and patients with hematologic malignancies. Haematologica. 2019;104:1322–31.
61. Khanna N, Widmer AF, Decker M, et al. Respiratory syncytial virus infection in patients with hematological diseases: single-center study and review of the literature. Clin Infect Dis. 2008;46:402–12.
62. Shah DP, Ghantoji SS, Ariza-Heredia EJ, et al. Immunodeficiency scoring index to predict poor outcomes in hematopoietic cell transplant recipients with RSV infections. Blood. 2014;123:3263–8.
63. Kmeid J, Vanichanan J, Shah DP, et al. Outcomes of influenza infections in hematopoietic cell transplant recipients: application of an immunodeficiency scoring index. Biol Blood Marrow Transplant. 2016;22:542–8.
64. Piñana JL, Hernández-Boluda JC, Calabuig M, et al. A risk-adapted approach to treating respiratory syncytial virus and human parainfluenza virus in allogeneic stem cell transplantation recipients with oral ribavirin therapy: a pilot study. Transpl Infect Dis. 2017;19:4.
65. Khawaja F, Chemaly RF. Predicting risk of progression to lower respiratory tract infection in allogeneic hematopoietic cell transplant recipients with respiratory viral infections: where are we now? Bone Marrow Transplant. 2022;57:701–2.
66. Waghmare A, Xie H, Kuypers J, et al. Human rhinovirus infections in hematopoietic cell transplant recipients: risk score for progression to lower respiratory tract infection. Biol Blood Marrow Transplant. 2019;25:1011–21.
67. Wang L, Allen J, Diong C, et al. Respiratory virus infection after allogeneic hematopoietic stem cell transplant in a tropical center: predictive value of the immunodeficiency scoring index. Transpl Infect Dis. 2017;19:e12693.
68. Damlaj M, Bartoo G, Cartin-Ceba R, et al. Corticosteroid use as adjunct therapy for respiratory syncytial virus infection in adult allogeneic stem cell transplant recipients. Transpl Infect Dis. 2016;18:216–26.
69. Shah DP, Ghantoji SS, Shah JN, et al. Impact of aerosolized ribavirin on mortality in 280 allogeneic haematopoietic stem cell transplant recipients with respiratory syncytial virus infections. J Antimicrob Chemother. 2013;68:1872–80.
70. Waghmare A, Campbell AP, Xie H, et al. Respiratory syncytial virus lower respiratory disease in hematopoietic cell transplant recipients: viral RNA detection in blood, antiviral treatment, and clinical outcomes. Clin Infect Dis. 2013;57:1731–41.
71. Boeckh M, Englund J, Li Y, et al. Randomized controlled multicenter trial of aerosolized ribavirin for respiratory syncytial virus upper respiratory tract infection in hematopoietic cell transplant recipients. Clin Infect Dis. 2007;44:245–9.
72. Tomblyn M, Chiller T, Einsele H, et al. Guidelines for preventing infectious complications among hematopoietic cell transplant recipients: a global perspective. Bone Marrow Transpl. 2009;44:453–5.
73. Chemaly RF, Aitken SL, Wolfe CR, Jain R, Boeckh MJ. Aerosolized ribavirin: the most expensive drug for pneumonia. Transpl Infect Dis. 2016;18:634–6.
74. Foolad F, Aitken SL, Shigle TL, et al. Oral versus aerosolized ribavirin for the treatment of respiratory syncytial virus infections in hematopoietic cell transplant recipients. Clin Infect Dis. 2019;68:1641–9.
75. Gorcea CM, Tholouli E, Turner A, et al. Effective use of oral ribavirin for respiratory syncytial viral infections in allogeneic haematopoietic stem cell transplant recipients. J Hosp Infect. 2017;95:214–7.
76. Park S-Y, Baek S, Lee S-O, et al. Efficacy of oral ribavirin in hematologic disease patients with paramyxovirus infection: analytic strategy using propensity scores. Antimicrob Agents Chemother. 2013;57:983–9.
77. Chemaly RF, Dadwal SS, Bergeron A, et al. A phase 2, randomized, double-blind, placebo-controlled trial of presatovir for the treatment of respiratory syncytial virus upper respiratory tract infection in hematopoietic-cell transplant recipients. Clin Infect Dis. 2020;71:2777–86.
78. Marty FM, Chemaly RF, Mullane KM, et al. A phase 2b, randomized, double-blind, placebo-controlled multicenter study evaluating antiviral effects, pharmacokinetics, safety, and tolerability of presatovir in hematopoietic cell transplant recipients with respiratory syncytial virus infection of the lower respiratory tract. Clin Infect Dis. 2020;71:2787–95.
79. Kimberlin DW, Barnett ED, Lynfield R, Sawyer MH, Committee on Infectious Diseases. Respiratory syncytial virus. In: Red book: 2021–2024 report of the committee on infectious diseases. Itasca: American Academy of Pediatrics; 2021.
80. Boeckh M, Berrey MM, Bowden RA, Crawford SW, Balsley J, Corey L. Phase 1 evaluation of the respiratory syncytial virus-specific monoclonal antibody palivizumab in recipients of hematopoietic stem cell transplants. J Infect Dis. 2001;184:350–4.
81. Ye X, Iwuchukwu OP, Avadhanula V, et al. Comparison of palivizumab-like antibody binding to different conformations of the RSV F protein in RSV-infected adult hematopoietic cell transplant recipients. J Infect Dis. 2018;217:1247–56.
82. Permpalung N, Mahoney MV, McCoy C, et al. Clinical characteristics and treatment outcomes among respiratory syncytial virus (RSV)-infected hematologic malignancy and hematopoietic stem cell transplant recipients receiving palivizumab. Leuk Lymphoma. 2019;60:85–91.
83. Seo S, Campbell AP, Xie H, et al. Outcome of respiratory syncytial virus lower respiratory tract disease in hematopoietic cell transplant recipients receiving aerosolized ribavirin: significance of stem cell source and oxygen requirement. Biol Blood Marrow Transplant. 2013;19:589–96.
84. Balassa K, Salisbury R, Watson E, et al. Treatment stratification of respiratory syncytial virus infection in allogeneic stem cell transplantation. J Infect. 2019;78:461–7.

85. Sanders SL, Agwan S, Hassan M, van Driel ML, Del Mar CB. Immunoglobulin treatment for hospitalised infants and young children with respiratory syncytial virus infection. Cochrane Database Syst Rev. 2019;8:CD009417.
86. Ogimi C, Krantz EM, Golob JL, et al. Antibiotic exposure prior to respiratory viral infection is associated with progression to lower respiratory tract disease in allogeneic hematopoietic cell transplant recipients. Biol Blood Marrow Transplant. 2018;24:2293–301.
87. Ogimi C, Krantz EM, Golob JL, et al. Exposure to antibiotics with anaerobic activity before respiratory viral infection is associated with respiratory disease progression after hematopoietic cell transplant. Bone Marrow Transplant. 2022;57(12):1765–73.
88. Haak BW, Littmann ER, Chaubard J-L, et al. Impact of gut colonization with butyrate-producing microbiota on respiratory viral infection following allo-HCT. Blood. 2018;131:2978–86.
89. Haas LEM, Thijsen SFT, van Elden L, Heemstra KA. Human metapneumovirus in adults. Viruses. 2013;5:87–110.
90. Shah DP, Shah PK, Azzi JM, El Chaer F, Chemaly RF. Human metapneumovirus infections in hematopoietic cell transplant recipients and hematologic malignancy patients: a systematic review. Cancer Lett. 2016;379:100–6.
91. Seo S, Gooley TA, Kuypers JM, et al. Human metapneumovirus infections following hematopoietic cell transplantation: factors associated with disease progression. Clin Infect Dis. 2016;63:178–85.
92. Dignan FL, Clark A, Aitken C, et al. BCSH/BSBMT/UK clinical virology network guideline: diagnosis and management of common respiratory viral infections in patients undergoing treatment for haematological malignancies or stem cell transplantation. Br J Haematol. 2016;173:380–93.
93. Renaud C, Xie H, Seo S, et al. Mortality rates of human metapneumovirus and respiratory syncytial virus lower respiratory tract infections in hematopoietic cell transplantation recipients. Biol Blood Marrow Transplant. 2013;19:1220–6.
94. Shah DP, Shah PK, Azzi JM, Chemaly RF. Parainfluenza virus infections in hematopoietic cell transplant recipients and hematologic malignancy patients: a systematic review. Cancer Lett. 2016;370:358–64.
95. Chemaly RF, Hanmod SS, Rathod DB, et al. The characteristics and outcomes of parainfluenza virus infections in 200 patients with leukemia or recipients of hematopoietic stem cell transplantation. Blood. 2012;119:2738–45.
96. Seo S, Xie H, Leisenring WM, et al. Biol Blood Marrow Transplant. 2019;25:163–71.
97. Nichols WG, Corey L, Gooley T, Davis C, Boeckh M. Parainfluenza virus infections after hematopoietic stem cell transplantation: risk factors, response to antiviral therapy, and effect on transplant outcome. Blood. 2001;98:573–8.
98. Seo S, Xie H, Campbell AP, et al. Parainfluenza virus lower respiratory tract disease after hematopoietic cell transplant: viral detection in the lung predicts outcome. Clin Infect Dis. 2014;58:1357–68.
99. Ustun C, Slabý J, Shanley RM, et al. Human parainfluenza virus infection after hematopoietic stem cell transplantation: risk factors, management, mortality, and changes over time. Biol Blood Marrow Transplant. 2012;18:1580–8.
100. Erard V, Chien JW, Kim HW, et al. Airflow decline after myeloablative allogeneic hematopoietic cell transplantation: the role of community respiratory viruses. J Infect Dis. 2006;193:1619–25.
101. Moscona A, Porotto M, Palmer S, et al. A recombinant sialidase fusion protein effectively inhibits human parainfluenza viral infection in vitro and in vivo. J Infect Dis. 2010;202:234–41.
102. Dhakal B, D'Souza A, Pasquini M, et al. DAS181 treatment of severe parainfluenza virus 3 pneumonia in allogeneic hematopoietic stem cell transplant recipients requiring mechanical ventilation. Case Rep Med. 2016;2016:8503275.
103. Waghmare A, Wagner T, Andrews R, et al. Successful treatment of parainfluenza virus respiratory tract infection with DAS181 in 4 immunocompromised children. J Pediatric Infect Dis Soc. 2015;4:114–8.
104. Salvatore M, Satlin MJ, Jacobs SE, et al. DAS181 for treatment of parainfluenza virus infections in hematopoietic stem cell transplant recipients at a single center. Biol Blood Marrow Transplant. 2016;22:965–70.
105. Chemaly RF, Marty FM, Wolfe CR, et al. DAS181 treatment of severe lower respiratory tract parainfluenza virus infection in immunocompromised patients: a phase 2 randomized, placebo-controlled study. Clin Infect Dis. 2021;73:e773–81.
106. Heikkinen T, Järvinen A. The common cold. Lancet. 2003;361:51–9.
107. Milano F, Campbell AP, Guthrie KA, et al. Human rhinovirus and coronavirus detection among allogeneic hematopoietic stem cell transplantation recipients. Blood. 2010;115:2088–94.
108. Zlateva KT, de Vries JJC, Coenjaerts FEJ, et al. Prolonged shedding of rhinovirus and re-infection in adults with respiratory tract illness. Eur Respir J. 2014;44:169–77.
109. Ogimi C, Xie H, Leisenring WM, et al. Initial high viral load is associated with prolonged shedding of human rhinovirus in allogeneic hematopoietic cell transplant recipients. Biol Blood Marrow Transplant. 2018;24:2160–3.
110. Sim SA, Leung VKY, Ritchie D, Slavin MA, Sullivan SG, Teh BW. Viral respiratory tract infections in allogeneic hematopoietic stem cell transplantation recipients in the era of molecular testing. Biol Blood Marrow Transplant. 2018;24:1490–6.
111. Seo S, Waghmare A, Scott EM, et al. Human rhinovirus detection in the lower respiratory tract of hematopoietic cell transplant recipients: association with mortality. Haematologica. 2017;102:1120–30.

112. Sun L, Meijer A, Froeyen M, et al. Antiviral activity of broad-spectrum and enterovirus-specific inhibitors against clinical isolates of enterovirus D68. Antimicrob Agents Chemother. 2015;59:7782–5.
113. Lanko K, Sun L, Froeyen M, et al. Comparative analysis of the molecular mechanism of resistance to vapendavir across a panel of picornavirus species. Antivir Res. 2021;195:105177.
114. Coultas JA, Cafferkey J, Mallia P, Johnston SL. Experimental antiviral therapeutic studies for human rhinovirus infections. J Exp Pharmacol. 2021;13:645–59.
115. Ogimi C, Xie H, Waghmare A, et al. Risk factors for seasonal human coronavirus lower respiratory tract infection after hematopoietic cell transplantation. Blood Adv. 2021;5:1903–14.
116. Ogimi C, Waghmare AA, Kuypers JM, et al. Clinical significance of human coronavirus in bronchoalveolar lavage samples from hematopoietic cell transplant recipients and patients with hematologic malignancies. Clin Infect Dis. 2017;64:1532–9.
117. Ogimi C, Greninger AL, Waghmare AA, et al. Prolonged shedding of human coronavirus in hematopoietic cell transplant recipients: risk factors and viral genome evolution. J Infect Dis. 2017;216:203–9.
118. Piñana JL, Xhaard A, Tridello G, et al. Seasonal human coronavirus respiratory tract infection in recipients of allogeneic hematopoietic stem cell transplantation. J Infect Dis. 2021;223:1564–75.
119. Eichenberger EM, Soave R, Zappetti D, et al. Incidence, significance, and persistence of human coronavirus infection in hematopoietic stem cell transplant recipients. Bone Marrow Transplant. 2019;54:1058–66.
120. Campbell AP, Guthrie KA, Englund JA, et al. Clinical outcomes associated with respiratory virus detection before allogeneic hematopoietic stem cell transplant. Clin Infect Dis. 2015;61:192–202.
121. Kim Y, Waghmare A, Xie H, et al. Respiratory viruses in hematopoietic cell transplant candidates: impact of preexisting lower tract disease on outcomes. Blood Adv. 2022;6(18):5307–16.
122. Welliver R, Monto AS, Carewicz O, et al. Effectiveness of oseltamivir in preventing influenza in household contacts: a randomized controlled trial. JAMA. 2001;285:748–54.
123. Magira EE, Chemaly RF, Jiang Y, Tarrand J, Kontoyiannis DP. Outcomes in invasive pulmonary aspergillosis infections complicated by respiratory viral infections in patients with hematologic malignancies: a case-control study. open forum. Infect Dis. 2019;6:ofz247.
124. Sharma A, Mishra T, Kumar N, Soubani AO. Influenza-associated aspergillosis: nationwide trends, predictors and outcomes from 2005 to 2014. Chest. 2020;158:1857–66.
125. Brunel A-S, Wójtowicz A, Lamoth F, et al. Pentraxin-3 polymorphisms and invasive mold infections in acute leukemia patients receiving intensive chemotherapy. Haematologica. 2018;103:e527–30.
126. Zinter MS, Lindemans CA, Versluys BA, et al. The pulmonary metatranscriptome prior to pediatric HCT identifies post-HCT lung injury. Blood. 2021;137:1679–89.
127. Versluys B, Bierings M, Murk JL, et al. Infection with a respiratory virus before hematopoietic cell transplantation is associated with alloimmune-mediated lung syndromes. J Allergy Clin Immunol. 2018;141:697–703.e8.
128. Waghmare A, Krantz EM, Baral S, et al. Reliability of self-sampling for accurate assessment of respiratory virus viral and immunologic kinetics. J Infect Dis. 2020;2020:451.
129. Turner J, He Q, Baker K, et al. Home spirometry telemonitoring for early detection of bronchiolitis obliterans syndrome in patients with chronic graft-versus-host disease. Transplant Cell Ther. 2021;27(616):e1–616.e6.
130. The RECOVERY Collaborative Group. Dexamethasone in hospitalized patients with Covid-19. N Engl J Med. 2021;384:693–704.
131. Boudreault AA, Xie H, Leisenring W, Englund J, Corey L, Boeckh M. Impact of corticosteroid treatment and antiviral therapy on clinical outcomes in hematopoietic cell transplant patients infected with influenza virus. Biol Blood Marrow Transplant. 2011;17:979–86.
132. Lansbury L, Rodrigo C, Leonardi-Bee J, Nguyen-Van-Tam J, Lim WS. Corticosteroids as adjunctive therapy in the treatment of influenza. Cochrane Database Syst Rev. 2019;2:CD010406.
133. Tzannou I, Papadopoulou A, Naik S, et al. Off-the-shelf virus-specific T cells to treat BK virus, human herpesvirus 6, cytomegalovirus, Epstein-Barr virus, and adenovirus infections after allogeneic hematopoietic stem-cell transplantation. J Clin Oncol. 2017;35:3547–57.
134. Baugh KA, Tzannou I, Leen AM. Infusion of cytotoxic T lymphocytes for the treatment of viral infections in hematopoetic stem cell transplant patients. Curr Opin Infect Dis. 2018;31:292–300.
135. Rubinstein JD, Zhu X, Leemhuis T, et al. Virus-specific T cells for adenovirus infection after stem cell transplantation are highly effective and class II HLA restricted. Blood Adv. 2021;5:3309–21.
136. McLaughlin LP, Lang H, Williams E, et al. Human parainfluenza virus-3 can be targeted by rapidly ex vivo expanded T lymphocytes. Cytotherapy. 2016;18:1515–24.
137. Boonyaratanakornkit J, Boeckh M, Waghmare A. Monoclonal antibodies for prophylaxis and treatment of respiratory viral infections. Curr Opin Infect Dis. 2022;35:280–7.
138. Muller WJ, Madhi SA, Seoane Nuñez B, et al. MELODY Study Group. Nirsevimab for Prevention of RSV in Term and Late-Preterm Infants. N Engl J Med. 2023. https://doi.org/10.1056/NEJMc2214773. Epub ahead of print. PMID: 37018470

# 12 COVID-19 and Hematopoietic Stem Cell Transplantation

Chiara Oltolini, Raffaella Greco, and Maria Teresa Lupo Stanghellini

*Raffaella Greco and Maria Teresa Lupo Stanghellini contributed equally with all other contributors.*

## Incidence and Pathophysiology

Severe acute respiratory syndrome coronavirus-2 (SARS-CoV-2) has spread rapidly since December 2019, and the World Health Organization (WHO) declared Coronavirus disease 2019 (COVID-19) a global pandemic causing a public health crisis. At the time of this report, 404,910,528 cases were reported worldwide with 5,783,776 deaths [1]. Infected individuals develop several symptoms, mainly affecting the respiratory system. The disease course can range from mild to life-threatening, in the latter case because of an inflammatory reaction and a microvascular pulmonary thrombosis leading to a progressive endothelial thrombo-inflammatory syndrome that takes place after alveolar viral damage and, potentially involving other vital organs, can lead to multiple organ failure and death [2].

## Clinical Presentation and Risk Factors

In the general population, risk factors for severe COVID-19 are older age, male sex, and comorbidities such as cardiovascular disease, obesity, or cancer. Moreover, the individual predisposition may play a role, with at least 10% of critical COVID-19 pneumonia cases being proven to be secondary to autosomal inborn errors of type I interferon immunity, autoantibodies against these cytokines, and X-linked recessive toll-like receptor-7 deficiency [3, 4]. COVID-19 severity is classified according to the World Health Organization (WHO) scale, a measure of patient clinical progression through the health-care system (Table 12.1) [5].

Hematopoietic stem cell transplant (HSCT) or chimeric antigen receptor T-cell (CAR-T) therapy recipients have a higher risk of mortality with COVID-19 owing to profound immune dysregulation. Mathew et al. revealed the existence of three immune types displaying different patterns of lymphocyte responses in hospitalized patients

Raffaella Greco: On behalf of the European Society for Blood and Marrow Transplantation (EBMT) Autoimmune Diseases Working Party (ADWP).

C. Oltolini
Clinic of Infectious Diseases, Division of Immunology, Transplantation and Infectious Diseases, IRCCS San Raffaele Scientific Institute, Milano, Italy

R. Greco (✉) · M. T. L. Stanghellini
Hematology and Bone Marrow Transplantation Unit, IRCCS San Raffaele Scientific Institute, Milano, Italy
e-mail: greco.raffaella@hsr.it


A. O. Soubani (ed.), *Pulmonary and Critical Care Considerations of Hematopoietic Stem Cell Transplantation*, https://doi.org/10.1007/978-3-031-28797-8_12

with COVID-19. These three patterns may each represent a different suboptimal response, ranging from a robust active CD4+ or CD8+ T-cell activity to a lack of activated B and T-cell reactivity, reflecting different clinical patterns and disease severity [6]. Most immunocompromised patients likely represent the immune type without a valid immune activation, suggesting that a timely treatment directed towards viral clearance could be beneficial. In these years of the pandemic, great efforts have been made to collect data on the impact of COVID-19 on hematological patients and transplant recipients, both autologous stem cell transplant (ASCT) and allogeneic HSCT (allo-HSCT). Table 12.2 summarizes the most relevant studies.

**Table 12.1** Classification of COVID-19 severity according to the WHO scale, a measure of patient clinical progression through the health-care system (adapted from the 'WHO Working Group on the Clinical Characterization and Management of COVID-19 infection') [5]

| Patient state | Descriptor | Score |
|---|---|---|
| Uninfected | Uninfected; no viral RNA detected | 0 |
| Ambulatory: mild disease | Asymptomatic; viral RNA detected<br>Symptomatic; independent<br>Symptomatic; assistance needed | 1<br>2<br>3 |
| Hospitalized: moderate disease | Hospitalized; no oxygen therapy<br>Hospitalized; oxygen by mask or nasal prongs | 4<br>5 |
| Hospitalized: severe disease | Hospitalized; oxygen by NIV or high flow<br>Intubation and mechanical ventilation, $PaO_2/FiO_2 \geq 150$ or $SpO_2/FiO_2 \geq 200$<br>Mechanical ventilation $PaO_2/FiO_2 < 150$ ($SpO_2/FiO_2 < 200$) or vasopressors<br>Mechanical ventilation $PaO_2/FiO_2 < 150$ and vasopressors, dialysis, or ECMO | 6<br>7<br>8<br>9 |
| Dead | Death | 10 |

*COVID-19* Coronavirus disease 2019, *ECMO* extracorporeal membrane oxygenation, *NIV* noninvasive ventilation, *$PaO_2/FiO_2$ ratio* ratio of arterial oxygen partial pressure ($PaO_2$ in mmHg) to fractional inspired oxygen ($FiO_2$ expressed as a fraction), *$SpO_2/FiO_2$* oxygen saturation to fraction of inspired oxygen ratio, *WHO* World Health Organization

The ITA-HEMA-COV group performed a multicenter study on behalf of all Italian societies dealing with hematology, reporting the outcome of 536 adults with hematological malignancy and symptomatic COVID-19 during the first wave of the pandemic. Overall, 84% of patients required hospitalization, and 37% died, a worse outcome than both the general Italian population with COVID-19 (standardized mortality ratio of 2.04 in the whole study cohort and of 3.72 in individuals <70 years) and the adults with hematological malignancies without COVID-19 (standardized mortality ratio of 41.3). In multivariable analysis, older age [hazard ratio (HR) 1.03], progressive disease status (2.10), diagnosis of acute myeloid leukemia (AML) (3.49), indolent non-Hodgkin lymphoma (NHL) (2.19), aggressive NHL (2.56), or multiple myeloma (MM) (2.48), and severe COVID-19 (4.08) were associated with worse survival. Among 536 patients, 15% were transplant recipients (51 ASCT, 31 allo-HSCT), with a mortality rate in allo-HSCT of 35% [7].

The first large-scale study on transplant recipients was conducted by the Center for International Blood and Marrow Transplant Research, analyzing 318 patients (184 allo-HSCT, 134 ASCT) diagnosed with symptomatic COVID-19. The median time from transplant to COVID-19 was 17 months for allo-HSCT and 23 months for ASCT, and the median follow-up of survivors was 21 days for allo-HSCT and 25 days for ASCT. Overall, disease severity was mild in 49% of patients, while it was severe in 14%. At 30 days, after COVID-19 diagnosis, overall survival was 68% for allo-HSCT and 67% for ASCT. In allo-HSCT recipients, higher mortality was observed in older patients (HR 2.53), male sex (3.53), and those who developed COVID-19 within 12 months of transplant (2.67) [8]. Soon after, the European Society for Blood and Marrow Transplantation (EBMT) published data on 382 transplant recipients (236 allo-HSCT, 146 ASCT) diagnosed with COVID-19. Overall, 91% experienced symptomatic disease, the median age was 54 years for allo-HSCT and 61 years for ASCT, and the median time from transplant to COVID-19 was 16 months for allo-

**Table 12.2** Clinical observational studies of Coronavirus disease 2019 in allogeneic hematopoietic stem cell transplant and chimeric antigen receptor T-cell therapy recipients

| Reference | Location/year Study population | COVID-19 severity | COVID-19 treatment | Outcome (mortality) | Risk factors for mortality in multivariable analysis |
|---|---|---|---|---|---|
| Passamonti et al. (2020) [7] | Multicenter retrospective, Italy<br>First wave (Feb-20, May-20)<br>536 hematological patients with symptomatic COVID-19<br>51 ASCT, 31 allo-HSCT (16 recent transplant[a]) | 85 patients in out-patient setting:<br>• 84 mild disease<br>• 1 severe disease<br>451 patients hospitalized:<br>• 184 mild disease<br>• 193 severe disease<br>• 74 critical disease (50 immediate ICU admission) | 188 antivirals [114 LPV/r, 62 DRV, 8 RDV, 5 oseltamivir (single or in combination)]<br>295 hydroxy-chloroquine<br>40 tocilizumab | Overall 37% (198/536)<br>In allo-HSCT 35% (11/31) | Older age (HR 1.03)<br>Progressive disease status (HR 2.1)<br>Diagnosis of:<br>• AML (HR 3.49)<br>• indolent NHL (HR 2.19)<br>• aggressive NHL (HR 2.56)<br>• plasma cell neoplasms (HR 2.48)<br>Severe-critical COVID (HR 4.08) |
| Sharma et al. (2021) [8] | Multicenter, CIBMTR (mainly USA)<br>First wave (Mar-20, Aug-20)<br>318 transplant recipients with symptomatic COVID-19<br>134 ASCT, 184 allo-HSCT | Mild disease (no oxygen supply): 155 transplant recipients<br>Moderate disease (oxygen supply): 49 allo-HSCT (27%), 27 ASCT (20%)<br>Severe disease (mechanical ventilation): 28 allo-HSCT (15%), 17 ASCT (13%)[b] | 44 antivirals (38 RDV, 6 oseltamivir)<br>40 hydroxy-chloroquine<br>7 tocilizumab<br>19 convalescent plasma | In allo-HSCT 22% [40/184 (37 COVID-related mortality, 3 disease-related)]<br>In ASCT 19% [26/134 (19 COVID-related mortality, 4 disease-related)] | In allo-HSCT:<br>• Age ≥50 years (HR 2.53)<br>• Male sex (HR 3.53)<br>• COVID <12 months of transplant (HR 2.67)<br>In ASCT:<br>• Disease [lymphoma > myeloma (HR 2.41)] |
| Ljungman et al. (2021) [9] | Multicenter prospective, EBMT-GETH<br>First wave (Mar-20, Jul-20)<br>146 ASCT (132 symptomatic COVID-19), 236 allo-HSCT (216 symptomatic COVID-19) | Asymptomatic disease: 8.9% of patients<br>Hospitalization: 74.4% of patients<br>• Oxygen supply: 76 allo-HSCT (32%), 56 ASCT (38%)<br>• No details about a severe, critical disease | 61 antivirals (44 LPV/r, 14 RDV, 3 favipiravir)<br>81 hydroxy-chloroquine<br>48 corticosteroids, 40 tocilizumab, 15 anakinra, 2 siltuximab<br>5 convalescent plasma | In allo-HSCT: 66 deaths<br>In ASCT: 41 deaths<br>Overall COVID-related: 25%<br>Survival at 6 weeks:<br>• In allo-HSCT 78%<br>• In ASCT 72% | Older age (HR 1.21)<br>Better PS (HR 0.83)<br>Need for ICU (HR 3.17)<br>Moderate-high ISI score (HR 1.84) |

(continued)

**Table 12.2** (continued)

| Reference | Location/year Study population | COVID-19 severity | COVID-19 treatment | Outcome (mortality) | Risk factors for mortality in multivariable analysis |
|---|---|---|---|---|---|
| Daudt et al. (2022) [10] | Multicenter cross-sectional, Brazil<br>First wave (Mar-20, Sep-20)<br>25 ASCT, 61 allo-HSCT<br>62 adults, 24 children | Asymptomatic disease: 10 patients (12%)<br>Hospitalization: 61 patients (71%)<br>ICU admission: 12 patients (14%) | 21 antivirals (19 oseltamivir, 2 GCV)<br>12 hydroxy-chloroquine<br>24 corticosteroids, 1 tocilizumab<br>2 convalescent plasma | Overall 30% (26/86):<br>• COVID-related 18/26<br>• superinfection-related 5/26<br>COVID-related:<br>• Overall 21%<br>• In allo-HSCT 15%<br>• In ASCT 36% | *Multivariate Correspondence Analysis model*:<br>• COVID-19 severity (asymptomatic/mild versus severe/critical)<br>• Acute renal injury (urea ≤50 versus >50 mg/dl)<br>• ECOG PS (0-2 versus >2) |
| Pagano et al. (2021) [11] | Multicenter observational, EHA<br>First-second waves (Mar-20, Dec-20)<br>3801 hematological patients with COVID-19<br>292 ASCT, 265 allo-HSCT, 24 CAR-T (74 ASCT, 173 allo-HSCT, 21 CAR-T performed within 3 months) | Asymptomatic disease: 675 patients (18%)<br>Mild disease: 658 patients (17%)<br>Severe disease: 1736 patients (46%)<br>Critical disease[c]: 689 patients (18%)<br>Hospitalization: 2778 patients (73%)<br>• ICU admission (689/2778) | Not reported | Overall 31% (1185/3801)<br>• COVID-related 58%<br>• Hematological disease-related 15%<br>• Both 13%<br>In ASCT 27% (20/74) deaths in allo-HSCT 25% (43/173)<br>In CAR-T 48% (10/21)<br>Lower mortality in second wave [41% vs 25% ($p < 0.0001$)] | Older age (HR 1.03)<br>Active underlying disease (HR 1.86)<br>Acute myeloid leukemia (HR 2.05)<br>Severe COVID-19 (HR 1.68)<br>Critical COVID-19 (HR 4.23)<br>Chronic cardiac disease (HR 1.41)<br>Liver disease (HR 1.39)<br>Chronic kidney disease (HR 1.40)<br>Lymphocytes >0.5 × $10^9/mm^3$ (HR 0.60) |
| Mushtaq et al. (2021) [12] | Single-center prospective, USA<br>First-second waves (Mar-20, May-21)<br>23 ASCT, 32 allo-HSCT, 3 CAR-T (3 ASCT, 8 allo-HSCT, 2 CAR-T within 100-day) | Mild disease: 29 patients<br>Moderate-severe disease: 20 patients<br>Critical disease: 9 patients<br>ICU admission: 11 patients (19%) | 24 antivirals (24 RDV)<br>13 dexamethasone, 2 tocilizumab<br>20 convalescent plasma, 11 mAb | In allo-HSCT 28% (9/32)<br>In ASCT 0% (0/23)<br>In CAR-T 0% (0/3) | *Univariate logistic regression analysis for predictors of COVID severity*:<br>• allo-HSCT (OR 3.6)<br>• grade II-IV a-GVHD (OR 4.6)<br>• concurrent IST (OR 5.9) |

(continued)

**Table 12.2** (continued)

| Reference | Location/year Study population | COVID-19 severity | COVID-19 treatment | Outcome (mortality) | Risk factors for mortality in multivariable analysis |
|---|---|---|---|---|---|
| Spanjaart et al. (2021) [13] | Multicenter observational, EHA-EBMT First-second waves (Mar-20-May-21) 56 CAR-T | Hospitalization: 45/56 patients (80%) Oxygen supply: 24/56 patients (43%) ICU admission: 22/56 patients (39%) | 21 antivirals (20 RDV, 1 LPV/r) 1 hydroxy-chloroquine 12 corticosteroids, 8 tocilizumab, 2 baricitinib 17 convalescent plasma | Overall 45% (25/56) COVID-related 41% (23/56) | Older age (10-year-effect, HR 1.39) Not being in complete remission at COVID diagnosis (HR 2.40) Metabolic comorbidities (HR 2.75) Better PS (10-point effect, HR 0.71) |

*COVID-19* coronavirus disease 2019, *ASCT* autologous stem cell transplant, *allo-HSCT* allogeneic hematopoietic stem cell transplant, *ICU* intensive care unit, *HR* hazard ratio, *NHL* non-Hodgkin lymphoma, *LPV/r* lopinavir/ritonavir, *DRV* darunavir, *RDV* remdesivir, *GCV* ganciclovir, *CIBMTR* Center for International Blood and Marrow Transplant Research, *USA* United States of America, *EBMT* European Society for Blood and Marrow Transplantation, *GETH* Spanish Group of Hematopoietic Stem Cell Transplantation, *ISI* immunodeficiency scoring index, *EHA* European Hematology Association, *a-GVHD* acute graft-versus host disease, *IST* immunosuppressive therapy, *ECOG PS* Eastern Cooperative Oncology Group Performance status, *mAb* monoclonal antibodies

[a] Recent transplant: performed within 6 and 3 months for allo-HSCT and ASCT, respectively

[b] No information about COVID-19 severity in 42 patients

[c] COVID-19 classification according to WHO scale

HSCT and 25 months for ASCT. Moreover, 83% developed lower respiratory tract disease (LRTD), and 22% were admitted to an intensive care unit (ICU). Survival at 6 weeks after COVID-19 diagnosis was 78% and 72% in allo-HSCT and ASCT recipients, respectively. In multivariable analysis, older age (HR 1.21), need for ICU (3.17), and moderate/high immunodeficiency index (1.84) increased the risk of death; other factors such as the underlying diagnosis, time from transplant, graft-versus-host disease (GVHD), or ongoing immunosuppressive therapy (IST) did not seem to influence survival [9]. A national survey from Brazil reported data on 86 transplant recipients (61 allo-HSCT, 25 ASCT; 62 adults, 24 children). The COVID-related mortality rate was 36% in ASCT and 15% in allo-HSCT. Transplant recipients with COVID-19 displayed a high mortality rate if they were adults and had critical disease at admission [10]. One additional single-center prospective study analyzed the outcome of 58 adults (32 allo-HSCT, 23 ASCT, 3 CAR-T therapy) who were diagnosed with COVID-19 during both the first and second waves of the pandemic. The median time from treatment to SARS-CoV-2 infection was 18 months, and 22% of patients acquired SARS-CoV-2 within 100 days posttreatment. Active GVHD and current IST were noted in 31% and 36% of patients, respectively; co-infections were observed in 19%. Overall, 28% of patients developed severe COVID, and 19% experienced ICU admission. In univariate analysis, significant predictors of COVID-19 severity included allo-HSCT (OR 3.6), history of grade II-IV acute GVHD (OR 4.6), and concurrent IST (OR 5.9). After a median follow-up of 6 months, the overall mortality rate was 16% (28% in allo-HSCT). Among allo-HSCT recipients, 16% developed pulmonary chronic GVHD, necessitating additional IST. The median duration of viral shedding was 7.7 weeks, and two patients had persistent infection for >5 months post-CAR-T therapy [12].

Deriving data from the second pandemic wave, the European Hematology Association

(EHA) performed the largest survey on 3801 patients affected by hematological cancer diagnosed with COVID-19 [NHL $n$ = 1084, MM $n$ = 684, chronic lymphoid leukemia (CLL) $n$ = 474, AML $n$ = 497, and myelodysplastic syndromes (MDS) $n$=279]. Considering the last treatment strategy before COVID-19, 173, 74, and 21 patients underwent allo-HSCT, ASCT, and CAR-T therapy, respectively. Overall, 64% of patients developed severe COVID-19, requiring hospitalization in 73% of cases and ICU admission in 18%. Death occurred in 31% of patients (COVID-19 as the primary cause of death in 58% of cases). The highest mortality was observed in AML (40%) and MDS (42%); interestingly, the mortality rate significantly decreased between the first (Mar–May 2020) and second wave (Oct–Dec 2020) [41% vs 25% ($p < 0.0001$)], and it was higher in CAR-T recipients than in allo-HSCT recipients [47% (10/21) vs 25% (43/173)]. In multivariable analysis, age, active malignancy, chronic cardiac disease, liver or renal impairment, smoking history, and ICU stay correlated with mortality [11].

Finally, EBMT and EHA joined forces to provide data about COVID-19 in CAR-T recipients, reporting 56 cases. CAR-T therapy was given mainly for NHL (82%); most patients were in complete remission after CAR-T (62%). The median time from CAR-T infusion to COVID-19 was 7 months. Overall, 32% of patients had metabolic comorbidities, 80% were hospitalized for COVID-19, 43% needed oxygen supply, and 39% required an ICU stay. The mortality rate was 45%, with most deaths COVID-related (23/25). In multivariable analysis, older age (HR = 1.39), not being in complete remission at COVID-19 diagnosis (2.40), and metabolic comorbidities (2.75) were associated with higher mortality; conversely, sex, time from CAR-T to COVID-19, and occurrence of neurotoxicity or cytokine release syndrome after CAR-T did not have a relevant effect on mortality [13].

## Management and Therapeutic Treatments for COVID-19

In the setting of hospitalized patients requiring supplemental oxygen (WHO score 5), the first drug exhibiting a survival benefit was dexamethasone, as shown in the controlled open-label Recovery trial [mortality within 28 days: 23% dexamethasone vs 26% standard of care (SOC); rate ratio 0.82] [14]. Also, a 5-day course of the antiviral remdesivir is recommended unless high-flow oxygen is needed, even if the results from the studies were conflicting. The most consistent trial on remdesivir was ACTT-1, a large, randomized placebo-controlled study showing that remdesivir improved time to recovery and lowered mortality within 29 days [HR for death 0.30 (0.14–0.64)] [15]; a post hoc analysis demonstrated that the clinical benefit of remdesivir was most evident in those with symptoms for ≤10 days. Two open-label controlled trials (Solidarity, Discovery) reported no difference in the rate of in-hospital deaths, percentage of those who progressed to mechanical ventilation (MV), or length of hospital stay between patients who received remdesivir and those who received SOC [16, 17].

Regarding anticoagulants, three open-label randomized trials compared the use of therapeutic to prophylactic or intermediate doses of heparin in hospitalized patients who did not require ICU-level care (entry criteria: requirement of supplemental oxygen, elevated D-dimer levels, not being at risk of major bleeding events) [18–20]. The largest trial showed an increase in the number of organ support-free days in the therapeutic heparin arm, but no difference in mortality or length of hospitalization [18]. So, in this setting (WHO score of 5), a therapeutic dose of heparin for COVID-19 could be considered and should be further evaluated.

In the setting of hospitalized patients who require rapidly increasing oxygen supplementation (WHO score 6–7), a second immunomodulatory drug [IL-6 inhibitors (tocilizumab, sarilumab) or Janus kinase (JAK) inhibitors (baricitinib)] should be considered in addition to dexamethasone, weighing the risk of opportunistic infections. The analyses of different trials have not clearly defined which patients in this heterogeneous group are most likely to benefit from using corticosteroids with another immune modulator. The Recovery trial showed that in patients on low-flow oxygen and with evidence of systemic inflammation (C-reactive protein ≥75 mg/L), those who received tocilizumab plus dexamethasone had a lower incidence of 28-day mortality than those who received SOC including dexamethasone [21]. Data on JAK inhibitors are conflicting; the Cov-Barrier trial did not find a significant benefit for baricitinib in patients on low-flow oxygen (WHO score 5), whereas in the ACTT-2 placebo-controlled trial, among patients receiving high-flow oxygen (WHO score 6), baricitinib plus remdesivir was superior to remdesivir alone (corticosteroids were not yet SOC) in reducing recovery time [22, 23]. In patients on invasive MV or extracorporeal membrane oxygenation (WHO score 7–9), treatment with baricitinib compared with placebo (with SOC including corticosteroids) significantly reduced 28-day and 60-day mortality [24]. Regarding anticoagulants in this setting (WHO score 6–7), therapeutic doses of anticoagulants are not recommended unless venous thromboembolism is confirmed.

Nonhospitalized patients with COVID-19 at risk of progression to severe disease (WHO score 2–3) should receive antivirals (ritonavir-boosted nirmatrelvir, remdesivir, molnupiravir) and/or monoclonal antibodies against SARS-2-CoV [mAb (primarily sotrovimab)], the choice of which must take into account various aspects [clinical efficacy, activity against SARS-2-CoV variants of concern (VOC), availability, feasibility of administering parenteral drugs (mAb, remdesivir), drug-drug interactions (ritonavir-boosted nirmatrelvir)]. The preferred option is oral antiviral ritonavir-boosted nirmatrelvir, which was studied in the randomized placebo-controlled EPIC-HR trial enrolling 2246 unvaccinated adults with symptomatic COVID-19 within 5 days after symptoms' onset. In the modified intention-to-treat population that included patients treated within 3 days of symptom onset who did not receive mAb, the Kaplan-Meier estimated event rates for COVID-19-related hospitalization or any-cause death through day 28 were 0.7% with ritonavir-boosted nirmatrelvir vs 6.5% with placebo [25]. The second option is intravenous sotrovimab, which retains activity against the last-emerging Omicron (B.1.1.529) VOC, whose data derived from the COMET-ICE trial, which included adults with mild to moderate COVID-19 within 5 days of symptoms' onset. Endpoint events (hospitalization or death from any cause by day 29) occurred in 3 of 291 participants (1%) in the sotrovimab arm and in 21 of 292 participants (7%) in the placebo arm ($p$ = 0.002), resulting in an 85% relative reduction in risk of hospitalization or death [26]. The third option is remdesivir, which has been studied in the PINETREE trial in patients with mild to moderate COVID-19: a 3-day course of remdesivir within 7 days of symptoms' onset resulted in an 87% relative reduction in risk of hospitalization or death compared to placebo [27]. Finally, molnupinavir is recommended only if these three options are unavailable because of its lower efficacy (reducted rate of hospitalization or death by 30% compared to placebo [28]) and potential risk for genotoxicity. All these three antivirals are expected to be active against Omicron (B.1.1.529) VOC. Importantly, there are currently no clinical trial data that (1) directly compare the clinical efficacy of these four therapies, (2) explore the use of combinations of antivirals and/or anti-SARS-CoV-2 mAb, and (3) focus on the impact of these therapies in immunocompromised patients because in registration trials, enrolled patients had mainly metabolic or cardiovascular diseases (0-5% of the trials' population was affected by cancer or immunocompromised).

The abovementioned studies on transplant recipients do not assess the impact of all these therapeutic interventions because they are based on the data from the first wave of the pandemic. In the setting of immunosuppressed transplant recipients, the ideal approach is to try to avoid the progression from upper to lower respiratory tract infection with an early therapy directed towards viral clearance (antivirals, neutralizing mAb); only data that will emerge from the second wave onwards will tell us how these interventions will have been able to modify the course of COVID-19 in immunocompromised patients. The validity of this approach has partially emerged from the study of *Spanjaart*, where a positive effect of convalescent plasma on overall survival was observed in univariate analysis when only looking at patients who were hospitalized (HR 0.37, $p = 0.03$); unfortunately, the number of patients was too small to observe any effect of treatments on the outcome [13].

Finally, in ASCT, allo-HSCT, and CAR-T recipients, current and future therapeutic perspectives regard the role of (1) post-exposure prophylaxis with ritonavir-boosted nirmatrelvir (EPIC-PEP randomized placebo-controlled trial ongoing, NCT05047601) and (2) pre-exposure prophylaxis with the mAb combination tixagevimab-cilgavimab that is recommended for high-risk patients with absence of IgG antibodies against SARS-2-CoV spike protein [29].

## EBMT Recommendations

The new coronavirus SARS-CoV-2 caused unprecedented stress on the health-care system, including programs performing HSCT and CAR-T. Since 2020, EBMT has provided clear recommendations for the management of transplant recipients, their donors, and patients undergoing CAR-T therapy [30], addressing various aspects of clinical management and providing specific suggestions to guide the delivery of HSCT through different stages of the pandemic. The evolution of the global pandemic has been rapid with great impact on many hospital services and health-care workers (HCWs) [31]. The learning curve has extended into longer-term modifications in clinical practice, with 'restoration and recovery' or 'reset' periods, including SARS-CoV-2 minimization pathways, and the possibility of further 'resurges' and peaks. Consequently, HSCT programs have been ready to rapidly adapt to change, following the course of the pandemic and adopting a prioritization process to deliver HSCT according to clinical urgency, strictly depending on [32]:

1. *Virus-related factors*: local prevalence of the virus in the community, the reproduction rate (R-rate), national and regional alert status. Key epidemiological parameters are the R-rate, which defines the average number of secondary cases generated by one primary case, thus reflecting the infectious potential of the disease, and the growth rate of the epidemic [33]. In case of "resurges" and peaks or local outbreaks, HSCT for some indications (i.e., nonmalignant disorders) was postponed; patients and families have been counseled about the possibility of short notice cancellation of their planned HSCT.
2. *Hospital-related factors*: availability of infection prevention and control (IPC) and personal protective equipment (PPE) for staff, testing and tracing of staff and patients, ability to create COVID-secure facilities with clear pathways to separate patients from those that may have COVID, adequate supportive services for the HSCT program, including ICU beds; suitable isolation facilities, including single rooms with en-suite facilities and for patients that tested positive for SARS-CoV-2, rooms with negative pressure or neutral pressure if this is not possible; back-log of patients with hematological malignancies, who will take priority. In many countries, HSCT follows established pathways for adult elective care, but patients may also need to access services urgently (i.e., post-discharge complications, non-admitted emergency care, outpatient procedures and diagnostics). Where possible and clinically appropriate, separate care pathways for urgent and planned care have been arranged with the aim of eliminating the risk of nosocomial infection. All patients have been screened at the hospital entrance with a questionnaire and temperature

checks. Access to appropriate expertise was maintained, and pathways have been compliant with JACIE measures. Most hospitals have developed physically separate zones and cohorted staffing to reduce movement between COVID-protected and non-protected areas.

3. *Patient-related factors*: individual risk/benefit assessment and ability to give fully informed consent; ability to self-isolate, PPE compliance, home infrastructure to allow self-isolation and agreement to comply with the need to self-isolate; financial factors pertinent to the need to work from home for the first few months following HSCT; ability to attend clinical appointments without using public transportation.

Before starting the transplant procedure, the availability of adequately trained staff, ICU beds, ventilators, as well as the stem cell product have been ensured. All patients have been tested for SARS-CoV-2. A negative test result was required before the start of conditioning, regardless of whether upper respiratory symptoms were present. Patients planned to be admitted for transplant or to undergo CAR-T therapy have been recommended to minimize the risk by going into home isolation 14 days before the start of transplant conditioning [30].

In cases where potential recipients test positive for SARS-CoV-2, transplant has been delayed as advised in EBMT guidelines, having an additional negative swab before start of conditioning, full recovery of lung function, considering the gravity of SARS-CoV-2 infection and underlying hematological disease.

During the high-risk phases of the pandemic, access to a stem cell donor was restricted either due to the donor becoming infected, logistical reasons at the harvest centers in the middle of a strained health-care system, or travel restrictions across international borders. Indeed, it was strongly recommended to secure stem cell product access by freezing the product before the start of conditioning and, when not possible, to have an alternative donor as a backup. Peripheral blood has been preferentially used, unless in cases with strong indications for bone marrow, since it is more complicated to cryopreserve. Each center is still addressing the issue of the graft on an individual basis.

Patients have been advised to strictly adhere to prevention practices such as hand hygiene and social distancing after HSCT [34], at least until a full immune reconstitution. Vaccination is covered in a separate part of this chapter, but vaccinated patients have been informed to continue following guidelines to decrease the risk of contracting SARS-CoV-2, especially early after transplantation and with ongoing immunosuppression and/or active GVHD.

In this context, nurses have played a key role in explaining all precautions and providing written information for patients and caregivers. Patients have received guidance on how to minimize the risk of infection and advice for household members; a dedicated caregiver with low risk of COVID-19 exposure was strongly recommended for the first few months after HSCT. Visitors have not been admitted to transplant wards during peaks of the pandemic, and methods for communication between recipients, family members, and HCWs, such as video-calls, have been supported. Outpatient visits have been facilitated at home via telehealth if deemed appropriate and feasible. Since the COVID-19 situation varies substantially between and within countries, centers have been mandated to follow guidelines, policies, and procedures decided by national authorities as well as local and institutional policies.

A specific 'COVID-19 Task Force' with transversal participation across different EBMT groups and committees was created to support patients and the transplant community throughout the pandemic. Information has been constantly updated on the EBMT website (https://www.ebmt.org/covid-19-and-bmt) and through disease-specific publications (i.e., acute leukemias and autoimmune diseases) [32, 35], promptly adapting them to available updates on COVID-19 epidemiology and clinical outcome. EBMT started early in the pandemic to collect data regarding the impact of COVID-19 on HSCT recipients and on CAR-T treated patients.

Currently, more than 1350 patients have been registered. The 6-week mortality in the first wave [9] was approximately 25%. Preliminary data from the second wave supports an improvement in outcome, showing a mortality rate a bit below 20%.

The recent EBMT activity survey [36] described this pandemic challenge within the transplant community, who continued to provide patients access to treatment. In allo-HSCT, the use of haploidentical donors and cord blood units increased, together with the use of non-myeloablative conditioning. Reductions have been more pronounced in nonmalignant disorders for allo-HSCT and in autoimmune diseases for autologous procedures since nonurgent transplants have been deferred for nonmalignant disorders, mainly in 2020. Moreover, in 29% of EBMT centers, CAR-T therapy [37] was delayed for at least one patient due to the pandemic.

## ASH: ASTCT Recommendations

Similarly to EBMT, the American Society for Transplantation and Cellular Therapy (ASTCT), in a joint effort with the American Society of Hematology (ASH), has provided support to clinicians and patients during the pandemic.

Recommendations are periodically updated according to the evolution of the pandemic, therapeutic options, and strategy of prevention [38]. Based on COVID-19 transplant and immunotherapy, centers have modulated their activity: some centers never decreased their activity, while others curtailed clinical activity while preparing for or responding to a COVID-19 surge. At the last survey follow-up, many centers were back to normal patient numbers. As a general consideration, in the case of ongoing or increasing levels of COVID-19 activity, deferring of nonurgent patients is still an option.

Similarly, patients who are positive for SARS-CoV-2 and are candidates for cellular therapies should have the procedure delayed until the viral test is negative. Immunocompromised patients typically shed the virus for longer than 4 weeks, advocating for careful monitoring of patients after COVID-19. Of note, for patients with a persistently low level PCR positivity, transplant practices are evolving and vary by centers; not enough evidence is available to make any recommendations.

Rigorous preventable measures for the safety of patients undergoing cellular therapies are warranted: testing of patients, limitations of visitors, and screening of medical staff that are measures still crucial to preventing infections and nosocomial cross infection.

Cryopreservation of cells collected is an option; prospective studies evaluating the impact on major outcomes are ongoing and will better clarify the real cost-effectiveness. So far, there is geographic variability.

An important consideration was designated for patients with GVHD: no adjustment of GVHD treatment due to COVID-19 risk or actual infection is recommended. The current therapeutic guideline recommendation for the use of dexamethasone as the standard of care for hypoxemia in COVID-19 pneumonia or the anti-inflammatory treatment of specific COVID-19 manifestations, makes it unlikely that the reduction of immunosuppressive treatment in patients with GVHD will be necessary.

## Vaccination

Starting from the general consideration that vaccination is the cornerstone for the prevention of infectious diseases, the advent of a vaccine specific for SARS-CoV-2 was one of the major achievements during the pandemic. The prevention of SARS-CoV-2 infection is based on strict infection control measures coupled with vaccinations that have shown high efficacy in reducing community transmission, hospitalization, and deaths due to severe COVID-19 disease in the general population.

Multiple vaccines have advanced to the clinic [39]. For immunocompromised patients and patients with hematological malignancies, mRNA-based vectors have been the most commonly used.

Several vaccine candidates were tested in phase II/III trials for the general population, but so far data on safety and efficacy in immunocompromised patients remain scarce [40]. Definitive information on different immunocompromised patient populations is not yet available.

As a general consideration, to generate optimal protective immunity post vaccine, it is crucial to have a preserved antigen presentation system, functional B- and T-cell activation, and plasma B-cell antibody generation. A fully protective immune response to vaccines is linked to a functional adaptive immune system. Both HSCT and CAR-T treatments are well known to highly compromise the functionality of the adaptive and innate immune systems.

A prospective study among immunocompromised vulnerable patients [41–43] confirmed that adverse events were generally mild, proving the safety in immunocompromised patients [41, 42] and that the rate of seroconversion was substantially lower than in healthy controls [41]. Among immunocompromised patients, those with hematological malignancies showed the worst performance for what concerns the humoral response despite a competitive T cell response [43]. Repeated mRNA vaccination against SARS-CoV-2 elicits a robust polyfunctional T cell response in allo-HSCT recipients [44], proving to be safe and effective in HSCT recipients, especially in those who are immunosuppression-free [45]. Of note, SARS-CoV-2 mRNA vaccines induce meaningful cellular immunity in patients with isolated B-cell deficiency due to anti-CD19 CAR-T therapy [46, 47]. A dissertation on the features of each vaccine approved for immunocompromised patients is beyond the scope of the present chapter.

Recently the 9th European Conference on Infections in Leukemia (ECIL 9) [48] paved the way with recommendations for the management of vaccination in patients with hematological malignancies or hematopoietic cell transplantation. Similarly, the principal scientific societies involved in the field of transplantation and cellular therapies have constantly supported the scientific community through recommendations and guidelines: both EBMT [49] and the ASTCT—NMPD (National Marrow Donor Program)—ASH with the CDC (Center for Disease Control and Prevention) [50] have implemented specific recommendations on vaccine in immunocompromised patients after HSCT and cellular therapy. Both the European and American recommendations strongly support vaccination for vulnerable HSCT-CAR-T patients, along with their caregivers, families, and household contacts—in line with local regulatory approval for specific age groups. Patients should receive a full vaccination program (Table 12.3) with the most immediately available, locally approved vaccine, except in specific conditions where the expected response rate is very low. Whatever the actual measured vaccine response, patients should be informed of the ongoing risk of SARS-CoV-2/COVID-19 despite vaccination and adhere to the hygiene and social distancing recommendations of their community or country.

**Table 12.3** Recommended COVID-19 vaccination schedule for HSCT and CAR-T patients (adapted from "Use of COVID-19 vaccines in the United States"—Centers for Disease Control and Prevention) [51]

| Primary vaccination | Age group | No. of primary vaccine doses | No. of booster doses | Interval between the first and second dose | Interval between 2nd and 3rd dose | Interval between 3rd and 4th dose |
|---|---|---|---|---|---|---|
| Pfizer-BioNTech | 5–11 years | 3 | NA | 3 weeks | ≥4 weeks | NA |
| Pfizer-BioNTech | ≥12 years | 3 | 1 | 3 weeks | ≥4 weeks | ≥3 months |
| Moderna | ≥18 years | 3 | 1 | 4 weeks | ≥4 weeks | ≥3 months |
| Janssen | ≥18 years | 1 Janssen, followed by 1 mRNA | 1 | 4 weeks | >2 months | NA |

*COVID-19* coronavirus disease 2019, *HSCT* hematopoietic stem cell transplant, *CAR-T* chimeric antigen receptor T-cell

According to the ECIL9 recommendation, HSCT recipients should receive the COVID-19 vaccine, preferably initiating at least 6 months after HSCT if transmission of SARS-CoV-2 in the community is low. Moreover, m-RNA vaccines are preferred over the adenovirus vector-based vaccine for primary and booster vaccination. Of note, both the EBMT and the ASTCT-NMDP-ASH recommendations outlined that the current mRNA SARS-CoV-2 vaccines could be offered as early as 3 months post-transplantation to HCST and CAR T cell recipients to prevent infection and severe disease, though efficacy may not be optimal as suggested in situations of influenza community outbreaks.

Risk factors associated with poor efficacy (viz., insufficient humoral response) of SARS-CoV-2 vaccination are immunosuppressive drugs [52–56], active GVHD [55–57], low lymphocyte counts [52, 54, 57], older age (>65 years) [53], and early time after HSCT (<12 months) [53, 54, 57]. An important consideration is that a deficiency of SARS-CoV-2-specific T-cell immunity can also translate into insufficient humoral responses [58].

Based on data from other vaccines, it is likely that immunity obtained from either pre-transplant SARS-CoV-2 infection or vaccination will be wiped out by the transplant procedure. However, no data currently exists regarding this issue. However, it seems logical from a risk/benefit assessment that such patients should have a full-dose new vaccine schedule (a primary series of 3 doses plus the 4th booster dose; the m-RNA vaccine is recommended) after transplantation. HSCT patients with previous SARS-CoV-2/COVID-19 should be vaccinated with the full program.

In the case of COVID-19 infection prior to the second dose, the CDC recommends delaying the second dose of the m-RNA COVID-19 vaccine series until the symptoms have resolved and isolation precautions are discontinued. There is no indication so far of vaccine-associated enhanced disease (VAED) or other serious adverse events.

In the case of therapy with SARS-CoV-2 monoclonal antibodies or convalescent plasma in HCT and CAR T-cell recipients, despite the limited published report, based on the CDC recommendations, COVID-19 vaccination should not be deferred after receipt of convalescent plasma or monoclonal antibodies directed at SARS CoV-2 for post-exposure prophylaxis or treatment. Conversely, due to the restrictions from the regulatory agency for Evusheld (tixagevimab/cilgavimab), administration of Evusheld should be delayed for two weeks after vaccine administration.

Patients who are exposed to or develop SARS-CoV-2 infection after receiving the COVID-19 vaccine are eligible for monoclonal antibodies that retain neutralizing activity against the circulating variant(s) for post-exposure prophylaxis or treatment with COVID-19. All the scientific societies confirm that COVID-19 vaccines should not be used for treatment. Of note, routine post-transplant vaccines can be given concomitantly with COVID-19 vaccines, and no limitation is related to immunoglobulin intravenous administration.

Data on efficacy are constantly increasing; of note—as underlined by the ECIL9 recommendation—the response rate to two doses of mRNA vaccine varied between 69 and 85% among HSCT patients and 0–36% among CAR-T patients, pointing out as risk factors for poor response early after cellular therapy: lower lymphocyte count, B-cell aplasia, active GVHD, and ongoing (or recently discontinued) immunosuppression.

ECIL9 confirmed that the vaccine safety events were similar in non-transplanted hematology patients and in healthy individuals, both in frequency and type, and were mostly local (pain, redness, swelling) and rarely systemic (fatigue, headache, fever). Of interest, most reported studies show similar rates of side effects among HSCT patients as in healthy controls. However, as outlined by both the ECIL9 recommendation—EBMT recommendation and ASTCT/ASH recommendation, there is a risk for worsening/eliciting GVHD in allo-HSCT recipients. This risk needs to be considered when deciding about the timing of vaccination.

There is no specific recommendation for vaccinating stem cell donors for any other purpose than protecting the donor. However, previous vaccination of the donor might reduce the risk of jeopardizing the donation. Moreover, the recent emergence of new variants may require vaccine modifications and strategies to improve efficacy in these vulnerable patients.

## Conclusions and Future Directions

Summarizing available data, the overall mortality rate in allo-HSCT and ASCT recipients with COVID-19 is around 25–30%, lower than in non-transplanted hematological patients. The following aspects may explain in part the lower mortality in the transplant setting: patients undergoing allo-HSCT are by definition younger and healthier than overall onco-hematological patients, and generally, transplantation is performed with an underlying controlled disease [11]. Conversely, patients undergoing CAR-T infusion displayed worse clinical outcome that needs further investigation [11, 13]. However, even if adults with hematological malignancies and after transplantation have a substantial mortality rate for COVID-19, formal comparisons to the general population are lacking. Such a comparison deserves to be investigated because, for example, in the setting of solid-organ transplant recipients, the building evidence suggests that they are not at increased risk of mortality from COVID-19 when compared with age- and comorbidity-matched controls [59].

Moreover, it should be considered that by displaying protracted SARS-2-CoV shedding and prolonged symptoms' duration, transplant recipients are also at risk for promoting the generation of highly mutated viruses that could render treatments ineffective, as for one of the latest VOC, Omicron 2 (B.1.1.529.2), that is resistant to sotrovimab and for which the newest mAb bebtelovimab is upcoming [60, 61].

Finally, given the essential roles of IgM and IgA in the control and elimination of SARS-CoV-2 infection, mucosal immunity could be exploited for therapeutic and prophylactic purposes; so IgM, IgA, and bispecific antibodies anti-SARS-2-CoV are currently under investigation, as well as the possibility to exploit adoptive SARS-2-CoV-specific T-cell therapy in immunocompromised hosts at risk of severe COVID-19 [62, 63].

**Acknowledgements** RG contributes this article on behalf of the Autoimmune Diseases Working Party (ADWP) of the European Society for Blood and Marrow Transplantation (EBMT). We acknowledge the ADWP for the support of working party activities and all EBMT member centers and their clinicians, data managers, and patients for their valuable contributions to the EBMT registry.

## References

1. Ministero della Salute (IT). Available http://www.salute.gov.it/portale/home.html. Accessed Feb 11, 2022.
2. Ciceri F, Beretta L, Scandroglio AM, Colombo S, Landoni G, Ruggeri A, et al. Microvascular COVID-19 lung vessels obstructive thromboinflammatory syndrome (MicroCLOTS): an atypical acute respiratory distress syndrome working hypothesis. Crit Care Resusc. 2020;22(2):95–7.
3. Bastard P, Rosen LB, Zhang Q, Michailidis E, Hoffmann HH, Zhang Y, et al. Autoantibodies against type I IFNs in patients with life-threatening COVID-19. Science. 2020;370:6515. https://doi.org/10.1126/science.abd4585.
4. Asano T, Boisson B, Onodi F, Matuozzo D, Moncada-Velez M, Maglorius Renkilaraj MRL, et al. X-linked recessive TLR7 deficiency in ~1% of men under 60 years old with life-threatening COVID-19. Sci Immunol. 2021;6:62. https://doi.org/10.1126/sciimmunol.abl4348.
5. WHO Working Group on the Clinical Characterisation and Management of COVID-19 Infection. A minimal common outcome measure set for COVID-19 clinical research. Lancet Infect Dis. 2020;20(8):e192–7. https://doi.org/10.1016/S1473-3099(20)30483-7.
6. Mathew D, Giles JR, Baxter AE, Oldridge DA, Greenplate AR, Wu JE, et al. Deep immune profiling of COVID-19 patients reveals distinct immunotypes with therapeutic implications. Science. 2020;369:6508. https://doi.org/10.1126/science.abc8511.
7. Passamonti F, Cattaneo C, Arcaini L, Bruna R, Cavo M, Merli F, et al. Clinical characteristics and risk factors associated with COVID-19 severity in patients with haematological malignancies in Italy: a retrospective, multicentre, cohort study. Lancet Haematol. 2020;7(10):e737–45. https://doi.org/10.1016/S2352-3026(20)30251-9.
8. Sharma A, Bhatt NS, St Martin A, Abid MB, Bloomquist J, Chemaly RF, et al. Clinical char-

acteristics and outcomes of COVID-19 in haematopoietic stem-cell transplantation recipients: an observational cohort study. Lancet Haematol. 2021;8(3):e185–93. https://doi.org/10.1016/S2352-3026(20)30429-4.

9. Ljungman P, de la Camara R, Mikulska M, Tridello G, Aguado B, Zahrani MA, et al. COVID-19 and stem cell transplantation; results from an EBMT and GETH multicenter prospective survey. Leukemia. 2021;35(10):2885–94. https://doi.org/10.1038/s41375-021-01302-5.
10. Daudt LE, Corso MCM, Kerbauy MN, de Assis L, Rechenmacher C, Colturato I, et al. COVID-19 in HSCT recipients: a collaborative study of the Brazilian Society of Marrow Transplantation (SBTMO). Bone Marrow Transplant. 2022;57(3):453–9. https://doi.org/10.1038/s41409-021-01561-x.
11. Pagano L, Salmanton-Garcia J, Marchesi F, Busca A, Corradini P, Hoenigl M, et al. COVID-19 infection in adult patients with hematological malignancies: a European Hematology Association Survey (EPICOVIDEHA). J Hematol Oncol. 2021;14(1):168. https://doi.org/10.1186/s13045-021-01177-0.
12. Mushtaq MU, Shahzad M, Chaudhary SG, Luder M, Ahmed N, Abdelhakim H, et al. Impact of SARS-CoV-2 in hematopoietic stem cell transplantation and chimeric antigen receptor T cell therapy recipients. Transpl Cell Ther. 2021;27(9):796. https://doi.org/10.1016/j.jtct.2021.07.005.
13. Spanjaart AM, Ljungman P, de La Camara R, Tridello G, Ortiz-Maldonado V, Urbano-Ispizua A, et al. Poor outcome of patients with COVID-19 after CAR T-cell therapy for B-cell malignancies: results of a multicenter study on behalf of the European Society for Blood and Marrow Transplantation (EBMT) Infectious Diseases Working Party and the European Hematology Association (EHA) Lymphoma Group. Leukemia. 2021;35(12):3585–8. https://doi.org/10.1038/s41375-021-01466-0.
14. Group RC, Horby P, Lim WS, Emberson JR, Mafham M, Bell JL, et al. Dexamethasone in hospitalized patients with Covid-19. N Engl J Med. 2021;384(8):693–704. https://doi.org/10.1056/NEJMoa2021436.
15. Beigel JH, Tomashek KM, Dodd LE, Mehta AK, Zingman BS, Kalil AC, et al. Remdesivir for the treatment of Covid-19 - final report. N Engl J Med. 2020;383(19):1813–26. https://doi.org/10.1056/NEJMoa2007764.
16. Pan H, Peto R, Henao-Restrepo AM, Preziosi MP, Sathiyamoorthy V, et al. Repurposed antiviral drugs for Covid-19 - interim WHO solidarity trial results. N Engl J Med. 2021;384(6):497–511. https://doi.org/10.1056/NEJMoa2023184.
17. Ader F, Bouscambert-Duchamp M, Hites M, Peiffer-Smadja N, Poissy J, Belhadi D, et al. Remdesivir plus standard of care versus standard of care alone for the treatment of patients admitted to hospital with COVID-19 (DisCoVeRy): a phase 3, randomised, controlled, open-label trial. Lancet Infect Dis. 2022;22(2):209–21. https://doi.org/10.1016/S1473-3099(21)00485-0.
18. Lawler PR, Goligher EC, Berger JS, Investigators A, Investigators AC-C, Investigators R-C. Therapeutic anticoagulation with heparin in noncritically ill patients with Covid-19. N Engl J Med. 2021;385(9):790–802. https://doi.org/10.1056/NEJMoa2105911.
19. Sholzberg M, Tang GH, Rahhal H, AlHamzah M, Kreuziger LB, Ainle FN, et al. Effectiveness of therapeutic heparin versus prophylactic heparin on death, mechanical ventilation, or intensive care unit admission in moderately ill patients with covid-19 admitted to hospital: RAPID randomised clinical trial. BMJ. 2021;375:n2400. https://doi.org/10.1136/bmj.n2400.
20. Spyropoulos AC, Goldin M, Giannis D, Diab W, Wang J, Khanijo S, et al. Efficacy and safety of therapeutic-dose heparin vs standard prophylactic or intermediate-dose heparins for thromboprophylaxis in high-risk hospitalized patients with COVID-19: the HEP-COVID randomized clinical trial. JAMA Intern Med. 2021;181(12):1612–20. https://doi.org/10.1001/jamainternmed.2021.6203.
21. Group RC. Tocilizumab in patients admitted to hospital with COVID-19 (RECOVERY): a randomised, controlled, open-label, platform trial. Lancet. 2021;397(10285):1637–45. https://doi.org/10.1016/S0140-6736(21)00676-0.
22. Marconi VC, Ramanan AV, de Bono S, Kartman CE, Krishnan V, Liao R, et al. Efficacy and safety of baricitinib for the treatment of hospitalised adults with COVID-19 (COV-BARRIER): a randomised, double-blind, parallel-group, placebo-controlled phase 3 trial. Lancet Respir Med. 2021;9(12):1407–18. https://doi.org/10.1016/S2213-2600(21)00331-3.
23. Kalil AC, Patterson TF, Mehta AK, Tomashek KM, Wolfe CR, Ghazaryan V, et al. Baricitinib plus remdesivir for hospitalized adults with Covid-19. N Engl J Med. 2021;384(9):795–807. https://doi.org/10.1056/NEJMoa2031994.
24. Ely EW, Ramanan AV, Kartman CE, de Bono S, Liao R, Piruzeli MLB, et al. Efficacy and safety of baricitinib plus standard of care for the treatment of critically ill hospitalised adults with COVID-19 on invasive mechanical ventilation or extracorporeal membrane oxygenation: an exploratory, randomised, placebo-controlled trial. Lancet Respir Med. 2022;10(4):327–36. https://doi.org/10.1016/S2213-2600(22)00006-6.
25. Hammond J, Leister-Tebbe H, Gardner A, Abreu P, Bao W, Wisemandle W, et al. Oral nirmatrelvir for high-risk, nonhospitalized adults with Covid-19. N Engl J Med. 2022;386(15):1397–408. https://doi.org/10.1056/NEJMoa2118542.
26. Gupta A, Gonzalez-Rojas Y, Juarez E, Crespo Casal M, Moya J, Falci DR, et al. Early treatment for Covid-19 with SARS-CoV-2 neutralizing antibody sotrovimab. N Engl J Med. 2021;385(21):1941–50. https://doi.org/10.1056/NEJMoa2107934.
27. Gottlieb RL, Vaca CE, Paredes R, Mera J, Webb BJ, Perez G, et al. Early remdesivir to prevent progression to severe Covid-19 in outpatients. N Engl J

Med. 2022;386(4):305–15. https://doi.org/10.1056/NEJMoa2116846.
28. Food and Drug Administration. Fact sheet for healthcare providers: emergency use authorization for molnupiravir. 2021. Available https://www.fda.gov/media/155054/download.
29. Author. Tixagevimab and Cilgavimab (Evusheld) for pre-exposure prophylaxis of COVID-19. JAMA. 2022;327(4):384–5. https://doi.org/10.1001/jama.2021.24931.
30. Ljungman P, Mikulska M, de la Camara R, Basak GW, Chabannon C, Corbacioglu S, et al. The challenge of COVID-19 and hematopoietic cell transplantation; EBMT recommendations for management of hematopoietic cell transplant recipients, their donors, and patients undergoing CAR T-cell therapy. Bone Marrow Transplant. 2020;55(11):2071–6. https://doi.org/10.1038/s41409-020-0919-0.
31. Ueda M, Martins R, Hendrie PC, McDonnell T, Crews JR, Wong TL, et al. Managing cancer care during the COVID-19 pandemic: agility and collaboration toward a common goal. J Natl Compr Cancer Netw. 2020;2020:1–4. https://doi.org/10.6004/jnccn.2020.7560.
32. Greco R, Alexander T, Burman J, Del Papa N, de Vries-Bouwstra J, Farge D, et al. Hematopoietic stem cell transplantation for autoimmune diseases in the time of COVID-19: EBMT guidelines and recommendations. Bone Marrow Transplant. 2021;56(7):1493–508. https://doi.org/10.1038/s41409-021-01326-6.
33. https://royalsociety.org/-/media/policy/projects/set-c/set-covid-19-R-estimates.pdf.
34. Zhang R, Li Y, Zhang AL, Wang Y, Molina MJ. Identifying airborne transmission as the dominant route for the spread of COVID-19. Proc Natl Acad Sci U S A. 2020;117(26):14857–63. https://doi.org/10.1073/pnas.2009637117.
35. Brissot E, Labopin M, Baron F, Bazarbachi A, Bug G, Ciceri F, et al. Management of patients with acute leukemia during the COVID-19 outbreak: practical guidelines from the acute leukemia working party of the European Society for Blood and Marrow Transplantation. Bone Marrow Transplant. 2021;56(3):532–5. https://doi.org/10.1038/s41409-020-0970-x.
36. Passweg JR, Baldomero H, Chabannon C, Corbacioglu S, de la Camara R, Dolstra H, et al. Impact of the SARS-CoV-2 pandemic on hematopoietic cell transplantation and cellular therapies in Europe 2020: a report from the EBMT activity survey. Bone Marrow Transplant. 2022;57(5):742–52. https://doi.org/10.1038/s41409-022-01604-x.
37. Ghorashian S, Malard F, Yuksel MK, Mauff K, Hoogenboom JD, Urbano-Ispizua A, et al. Defining the impact of SARS-COV-2 on delivery of CAR T-cell therapy in Europe: a retrospective survey from the CTIWP of the EBMT. Bone Marrow Transplant. 2022;57(2):299–301. https://doi.org/10.1038/s41409-021-01483-8.
38. COVID-19 and hematopoietic cell transplantation: frequently asked question. https://www.hematology.org/covid-19/covid-19-and-hct-version-2.0. Accessed 1 April 2022.
39. Rotshild V, Hirsh-Raccah B, Miskin I, Muszkat M, Matok I. Comparing the clinical efficacy of COVID-19 vaccines: a systematic review and network meta-analysis. Sci Rep. 2021;11(1):22777. https://doi.org/10.1038/s41598-021-02321-z.
40. General principles of COVID-19 vaccines for immunocompromised patients. www.hematology.org/covid-19-version-6.1. Accessed 14 April 2022.
41. Bergman P, Blennow O, Hansson L, Mielke S, Nowak P, Chen P, et al. Safety and efficacy of the mRNA BNT162b2 vaccine against SARS-CoV-2 in five groups of immunocompromised patients and healthy controls in a prospective open-label clinical trial. EBioMedicine. 2021;74:103705. https://doi.org/10.1016/j.ebiom.2021.103705.
42. Lupo-Stanghellini MT, Di Cosimo S, Costantini M, Monti S, Mantegazza R, Mantovani A, et al. mRNA-COVID19 vaccination can be considered safe and tolerable for frail patients. Front Oncol. 2022;12:855723. https://doi.org/10.3389/fonc.2022.855723.
43. Corradini P, Agrati C, Apolone G, Mantovani A, Giannarelli D, Marasco V, et al. Humoral and T-cell immune response after three doses of mRNA SARS-CoV-2 vaccines in fragile patients: the Italian VAX4FRAIL study. Clin Infect Dis. 2022;76(3):e426–38. https://doi.org/10.1101/2022.01.12.22269133.
44. Harrington P, Doores KJ, Saha C, Saunders J, Child F, Dillon R, et al. Repeated vaccination against SARS-CoV-2 elicits robust polyfunctional T cell response in allogeneic stem cell transplantation recipients. Cancer Cell. 2021;39(11):1448–9. https://doi.org/10.1016/j.ccell.2021.10.002.
45. Shem-Tov N, Yerushalmi R, Danylesko I, Litachevsky V, Levy I, Olmer L, et al. Immunogenicity and safety of the BNT162b2 mRNA COVID-19 vaccine in haematopoietic stem cell transplantation recipients. Br J Haematol. 2022;196(4):884–91. https://doi.org/10.1111/bjh.17918.
46. Jarisch A, Wiercinska E, Huenecke S, Bremm M, Cappel C, Hauler J, et al. Immune responses to SARS-CoV-2 vaccination in young patients with anti-CD19 CAR-T-induced B-cell aplasia. Transpl Cell Ther. 2022;28(7):366.e1–7. https://doi.org/10.1016/j.jtct.2022.04.017.
47. Ram R, Freund T, Halperin T, Ben-Ami R, Amit O, Bar-On Y, et al. Immunogenicity of a third dose of the BNT162b2 mRNA Covid-19 vaccine in patients with impaired B cell reconstitution after cellular therapy-a single center prospective cohort study. Transpl Cell Ther. 2022;28(5):278. https://doi.org/10.1016/j.jtct.2022.02.012.
48. Cesaro S, Ljungman P, Mikulska M, Hirsch HH, von Lilienfeld-Toal M, Cordonnier C, et al. Recommendations for the management of COVID-19 in patients with haematological malignancies or haematopoietic cell transplantation, from

the 2021 European Conference on Infections in Leukaemia (ECIL 9). Leukemia. 2022;36(6):1467–80. https://doi.org/10.1038/s41375-022-01578-1.
49. COVID-19 vaccines. Version 8, January 2, 2022. https://www.ebmt.org/covid-19-and-bmt.
50. ASH-ASTCT COVID-19 vaccination for HCT and CAR-T cell recipients - version 5.0. https://www.hematology.org/covid-19/ash-astct-covid-19-vaccination-for-hct-and-car-t-cell-recipients. Accessed 22 March 2022.
51. https://www.cdc.gov/vaccines/covid-19/clinical--considerations/interim-considerations-us.html. Accessed 21 April 2022.
52. Leclerc M, Redjoul R, Le Bouter A, Beckerich F, Robin C, Parinet V, et al. Determinants of SARS-CoV-2 waning immunity in allogeneic hematopoietic stem cell transplant recipients. J Hematol Oncol. 2022;15(1):27. https://doi.org/10.1186/s13045-022-01250-2.
53. Huang A, Cicin-Sain C, Pasin C, Epp S, Audige A, Muller NJ, et al. Antibody response to SARS-CoV-2 vaccination in patients following allogeneic hematopoietic cell transplantation. Transpl Cell Ther. 2022;28(4):214. https://doi.org/10.1016/j.jtct.2022.01.019.
54. Maillard A, Redjoul R, Klemencie M, Labussiere Wallet H, Le Bourgeois A, D'Aveni M, et al. Antibody response after 2 and 3 doses of SARS-CoV-2 mRNA vaccine in allogeneic hematopoietic cell transplant recipients. Blood. 2022;139(1):134–7. https://doi.org/10.1182/blood.2021014232.
55. Yeshurun M, Pasvolsky O, Shargian L, Yahav D, Ben-Zvi H, Rubinstein M, et al. Humoral serological response to the BNT162b2 vaccine after allogeneic haematopoietic cell transplantation. Clin Microbiol Infect. 2022;28(2):303. https://doi.org/10.1016/j.cmi.2021.10.007.
56. Canti L, Humblet-Baron S, Desombere I, Neumann J, Pannus P, Heyndrickx L, et al. Predictors of neutralizing antibody response to BNT162b2 vaccination in allogeneic hematopoietic stem cell transplant recipients. J Hematol Oncol. 2021;14(1):174. https://doi.org/10.1186/s13045-021-01190-3.
57. Pinana JL, Lopez-Corral L, Martino R, Montoro J, Vazquez L, Perez A, et al. SARS-CoV-2-reactive antibody detection after SARS-CoV-2 vaccination in hematopoietic stem cell transplant recipients: prospective survey from the Spanish Hematopoietic Stem Cell Transplantation and Cell Therapy Group. Am J Hematol. 2022;97(1):30–42. https://doi.org/10.1002/ajh.26385.
58. Einarsdottir S, Martner A, Waldenstrom J, Nicklasson M, Ringlander J, Arabpour M, et al. Deficiency of SARS-CoV-2 T-cell responses after vaccination in long-term allo-HSCT survivors translates into abated humoral immunity. Blood Adv. 2022;6(9):2723–30. https://doi.org/10.1182/bloodadvances.2021006937.
59. Goldman JD, Robinson PC, Uldrick TS, Ljungman P. COVID-19 in immunocompromised populations: implications for prognosis and repurposing of immunotherapies. J Immunother Cancer. 2021;9(6):e002630. https://doi.org/10.1136/jitc-2021-002630.
60. Lafarge A, Mabrouki A, Yvin E, Bredin S, Binois Y, Clere-Jehl R, et al. Coronavirus disease 2019 in immunocompromised patients: a comprehensive review of coronavirus disease 2019 in hematopoietic stem cell recipients. Curr Opin Crit Care. 2022;28(1):83–9. https://doi.org/10.1097/MCC.0000000000000907.
61. Iketani S, Liu L, Guo Y, Liu L, Chan JF, Huang Y, et al. Antibody evasion properties of SARS-CoV-2 Omicron sublineages. Nature. 2022;604(7906):553–6. https://doi.org/10.1038/s41586-022-04594-4.
62. Zhang J, Zhang H, Sun L. Therapeutic antibodies for COVID-19: is a new age of IgM, IgA and bispecific antibodies coming? MAbs. 2022;14(1):2031483. https://doi.org/10.1080/19420862.2022.2031483.
63. Bonifacius A, Tischer-Zimmermann A, Santamorena MM, Mausberg P, Schenk J, Koch S, et al. Rapid manufacturing of highly cytotoxic clinical-grade SARS-CoV-2-specific T cell products covering SARS-CoV-2 and its variants for adoptive T cell therapy. Front Bioeng Biotechnol. 2022;10:867042. https://doi.org/10.3389/fbioe.2022.867042.

# Sepsis and Septic Shock: Special Considerations in the Hematopoietic Stem Cell Transplantation Patient

13

Sammar R. Alsunaid and Ayman O. Soubani

## Abbreviations

| | |
|---|---|
| ARDS | Acute respirator distress syndrome |
| GVHD | Graft versus host disease |
| HFNC | High flow nasal cannula |
| HSCT | Hematopoietic stem cell transplantation |
| MAP | Mean arterial pressure |
| MEWS | Modified early warning score |
| NEWS | National early warning score |
| NIV | Noninvasive ventilation |
| PLR | Passive leg raise |
| PEEP | Positive end expiratory pressure |
| POCUS | Point of care ultrasonography |
| qSOFA | Quick sequential organ failure score |
| SSC | Surviving sepsis campaign |
| SIRS | Systemic inflammatory response syndrome |
| SOFA | Sequential organ failure score |

S. R. Alsunaid (✉)
Department of Cardiothoracic and Vascular Surgery, Montefiore Medical Center, The University Hospital of the Albert Einstein College of Medicine, Bronx, NY, USA
e-mail: salsunaid@montefiore.org

A. O. Soubani
Division of Pulmonary, Critical Care Medicine and Sleep Medicine, Wayne State University School of Medicine, Detroit, MI, USA
e-mail: asoubani@med.wayne.edu

## Introduction

Major advances in the care of hematopoietic stem cell transplantation (HSCT) patients through improved transplant procedures and the use of reduced intensity conditioning regimens have led to improved outcomes [1]. Despite this, mortality following HSCT remains high, especially in patients with allogeneic (allo-HSCT), reaching as high as 51.7% based on a systematic review by Saillard et al. [2]. The review also showed a reduction in mortality when looking at data from 2004 onwards. Infectious complications are a major factor leading to morbidity and mortality in this patient population. Given the immunological compromises associated with HSCT, including neutropenia, neutrophils and lymphocytes dysfunction, the break in mucosal barriers associated with mucositis, and graft versus host disease (GVHD), infections are commonly associated with sepsis that could quickly progress to septic shock. Improved prophylactic measures against infections, earlier diagnosis, and more effective antimicrobial therapies have improved the outcomes associated with infections as well as sepsis [2]. The advances in the management of different infections following HSCT are detailed in other chapters. This chapter will focus on the approach to the management of sepsis and septic shock, providing specifics related to HSCT recipients whenever applicable.



A. O. Soubani (ed.), *Pulmonary and Critical Care Considerations of Hematopoietic Stem Cell Transplantation*, https://doi.org/10.1007/978-3-031-28797-8_13

## Definition and Screening for Sepsis

Early recognition and prompt initiation of therapeutic measures, including appropriate antibiotics, hemodynamic support, and source control, are key to improved outcomes of sepsis [3]. In order to do so, standardized and current definitions are needed, as sepsis and septic shock definitions have evolved since their first introduction in 1991 [4]. In 2016, the Sepsis-3 committee defined sepsis as a life-threatening condition caused by a dysregulated host response to infection, resulting in organ dysfunction. Septic shock, on the other hand, is characterized by circulatory, cellular, and metabolic abnormalities in septic patients, presenting as fluid-refractory hypotension requiring vasopressor therapy with associated tissue hypoperfusion (manifested in different ways, including lactate >2 mmol/L) [5]. These definitions were used in the most recent updated 2021 surviving sepsis campaign (SSC) guidelines [6].

HSCT patients are at increased risk of developing sepsis and septic shock compared to non-transplant patients. The risk is highest for allo-HSCT recipients. These are at an even greater risk for complications if the diagnosis was missed or delayed [7]. Their immune system may respond to or handle infection differently secondary to prior cancer therapies, neutropenia, or immunosuppressive therapies [8]. Furthermore, other common post-transplant complications such as engraftment syndrome, anemia, transfusion reactions, idiopathic pneumonia syndrome, acute kidney injury, and drug side effects can present in a similar fashion to sepsis [9].

The immunocompromised state associated with HSCT poses an increased risk for critical illness in these patients. When the clinical signs and symptoms point towards organ dysfunction related to sepsis, it is important for the treating team to be able to recognize and initiate treatments quickly. Severe neutropenia (absolute neutrophil count <500/μL) and neutropenia lasting longer than 7 days are known to increase sepsis risk in addition to prolonged hospital stay, prior surgery, advanced disease, delay in ICU admission, presence of long-term catheters, and pre-treatment with antibiotics or chemotherapy, all of which are associated with increased infection, sepsis, and septic shock [8, 10]. Studies have also linked the occurrence of sepsis and its progression to septic shock with the presence of hypophosphatemia (<0.8 mmol/L), hypoproteinemia (<62 g/L) [11], febrile neutropenia, tachypnea, elevated procalcitonin (PCT ≥1.5 ng/ml), lactate level (>3 mmol/L), low bicarbonate (<17 mmol/L), low antithrombin (<70%), or factor VIIa (<0.8 ng/mL) [8].

It is strongly recommended by the SSC that sepsis screening programs for acutely ill or high-risk patients be part of standard operating procedures to improve morbidity and reduce mortality [12].

Multiple tools for screening are available, including the systemic inflammatory response syndrome (SIRS) criteria [4], the quick sequential organ failure score (qSOFA) [5], the sequential organ failure score (SOFA) [13], the national early warning score (NEWS) [14], and the modified early warning score (MEWS) [15], all with variable sensitivity and specificity that help in early identification and timely intervention (Table 13.1). Because of these variations, the 2021 SSC guidelines strongly recommend with moderate quality evidence, against using qSOFA compared to SIRS, NEWS, or MEWS as a single screening tool [12]. This can be further understood by reviewing a recent retrospective analysis by Lind et al. [9] that looked at the predictive values of qSOFA (cutoff ≥2), SIRS (cutoff ≥2), and NEWS (cutoff ≥7) with respect to short-term mortality in allo-HSCT patients during the first 100 days specifically, measured at 10-day and 28-days post infection in both inpatient and outpatient settings. They observed a 10.7% mortality, which was similar to previously published rates in US transplant centers [16]. The study showed that NEWS had a balanced performance but suboptimal sensitivity, with its sensitivity and specificity being 78.3% and 70.2%, respectively. SIRS maintained the highest sensitivity at 91.3% but with a poor specificity of 35.0%, while qSOFA was the opposite, with the highest specificity of 90.5% but the least sensitive at 47.8%. In the HCT patients specifically, these scores performed worse, with low positive predictive values and likelihood ratios. These limitations indicate the need for new, population-specific criteria in this population [9]. This prevented SSC from recommending one screening tool over the other, but rather, a comprehensible assessment for each patient should be utilized. In summary, screening for sepsis in allo-HSCT patients may be more challenging compared to the general population. The current available screening tools are helpful, but none appears to be more superior.

**Table 13.1** Surviving sepsis campaign major recommendations for the management of sepsis and septic shock

| Recommendation | Strength | Quality of evidence |
|---|---|---|
| Hospital to adopt programs to screen acutely ill and high-risk patients for sepsis | Strong | Moderate |
| Recommendation against using qSOFA compared with SIRS, NEWS, or MEWS as a single-screening tool for sepsis or septic shock | Strong | Moderate |
| When suspecting sepsis, suggest measuring serum blood lactate | Weak | Low |
| When hypoperfusion is present, suggest that at least 30 mL/kg of IV crystalloid fluid should be given within the first 3 h of resuscitation | Weak | Low |
| Suggest using dynamic measures to guide fluid resuscitation, over physical examination, or static parameters alone | Weak | Very low |
| Suggest guiding resuscitation to decrease serum lactate in patients with elevated lactate levels over not using serum lactate | Weak | Low |
| When on vasopressors, recommend an initial target mean arterial pressure (MAP) of 65 mm Hg over higher MAP targets | Strong | Moderate |
| When unconfirmed infection, recommend continuously reevaluating and searching for alternative diagnoses and discontinuing empiric antimicrobials if an alternative cause of illness is demonstrated or strongly suspected | Best practice | |
| Recommend administering antimicrobials immediately, ideally within 1 hour of recognition | Strong | Weak |
| Suggest against using procalcitonin plus clinical evaluation to decide when to start antimicrobials, as compared to clinical evaluation alone. | Weak | Very low |
| Recommend prompt removal of intravascular access devices that are a possible source of sepsis or septic shock after other vascular access has been established | Best practice | |
| Recommend using crystalloids as first-line fluid for resuscitation. | Strong | Moderate |
| Suggest using balanced crystalloids instead of normal saline for resuscitation | Weak | Very low |
| Suggest using albumin in patients who received large volumes of crystalloids | Weak | Moderate |
| Recommend against using starches for resuscitation | Strong | High |
| Recommend using norepinephrine as the first-line agent over other vasopressors | Strong | Low to high against other vasopressors |
| When on norepinephrine with inadequate mean arterial pressure levels, suggest adding vasopressin instead of escalating the dose of norepinephrine | Weak | Moderate |
| When inadequate mean arterial pressure levels persist despite norepinephrine and vasopressin, suggest adding epinephrine | Weak | Low |
| When cardiac dysfunction is associated with persistent hypoperfusion despite adequate volume status and arterial blood pressure, suggest either adding dobutamine to norepinephrine or using epinephrine alone | Weak | Low |
| Suggest invasive monitoring of arterial blood pressure over noninvasive monitoring, as soon as practical and if resources are available | Weak | Very low |
| Suggest starting vasopressors peripherally to restore mean arterial pressure rather than delaying initiation until central venous access is secured | Weak | Very low |
| Insufficient evidence to make a recommendation on the use of restrictive versus liberal fluid strategies in the first 24 h of resuscitation in patients who still have signs of hypoperfusion and volume depletion after the initial resuscitation | No recommendation | |
| For sepsis-induced hypoxemic respiratory failure, we suggest the use of high-flow nasal oxygen over noninvasive ventilation | Weak | Low |
| With ongoing requirement for vasopressor therapy, we suggest using IV corticosteroids | Weak | Moderate |
| Recommend using a restrictive transfusion strategy over a liberal transfusion strategy | Strong | Moderate |
| Recommend initiating insulin therapy at a glucose level of ≥180 mg/dL | Strong | Moderate |
| Suggest against using IV vitamin C | Weak | Low |

In most cancer centers, sepsis screening is part of the daily rounds as the presentation can be atypical. General screening parameters include fever or hypothermia, new or increased tachycardia, dyspnea and/or tachypnea, and altered mentation [8, 17]. Once sepsis is diagnosed, further evaluation and treatment steps should be started immediately, these often include measurement of lactate level, blood cultures, administration of broad-spectrum antibiotics, rapid fluid administration, and possibly vasopressors to maintain blood pressure, source control, and additional supportive therapies [8]. These measures are detailed below and summarized in Table 13.2.

**Table 13.2** Variables of some of the validated sepsis and septic shock screening tools

| | | | | | | | | | |
|---|---|---|---|---|---|---|---|---|---|
| | Temperature (°C) | | Heart rate (beats/min) | Respiratory rate (breaths/min) | WBC count (cells/mm³) | | | | |
| SIRS (≥2) | <36 or > 38 | | >90 | >20 | <4000 or >12,000 or a 10% increase in immature (band) forms | | | | |
| qSOFA (≥2) | Respiratory rate ≥22 breaths/min | | Altered mental status | | Systolic blood pressure (SBP) ≤100 mmHg | | | | |
| SOFA (each scored 0–4 re-calculate every 24 h) | $PaO_2$/ $FiO_2$ | $SpO_2$/ $FiO_2$ | MAP | Bilirubin (mg/dL) | Creatinine (mg/dL) | Platelets (×10³/mm³) | GCS score | | |
| | >400 | >302 | ≥70 mmHg | <1.2 | <1.2 | ≥150 | 15 | | |
| | <400 | <302 | <70 mmHg | 1.2–1.9 | 1.2–1.9 | <150 | 13–14 | | |
| | <300 | <221 | Dopamine ≤ 5 or any dobutamine | 2.0–5.9 | 2.0–3.4 | <100 | 10–12 | | |
| | <200 | <142 | Dopamine >5 Norepi/Epi ≤ 0.1 Phenylephrine ≤ 0.8 | 6.0–11.9 | 3.5–4.9 | <50 | 6–9 | | |
| | <100 | <67 | Dopamine >15 Norepi/Epi >0.1 Phenylephrine > 0.8 | >12 | >5.0 | <20 | <6 | | |
| NEWS<br>Low 1–4<br>Medium 5–6<br>High >6 | Respiratory rate (breaths/min) | | Oxygen saturation | SBP (mmHg) | Pulse rate (beats/min) | LOC or new confusion | Temperature (°C) | | |
| | 12–20 (0) | | ≥96% (0) | 111–219 (0) | 51–90 (0) | Alert (0) | 36.1–38.0 (0) | | |
| | 9–11 (1) | | 94–95% (1) | 101–110 (1) | 41–50 0r 91–110 (1) | | 35.1–36.0 or 38.1–39.0 (1) | | |
| | 21–24 (2) | | 92–93% (2) | 91–100 (2) | 111–130 (2) | | ≥39.1 (2) | | |
| | ≤8 or ≥25 (3) | | ≤91% (3) | ≤90 or ≥200 (3) | ≤40 or ≥131 (3) | CVPU (3) | ≤35.0 (3) | | |
| MEWS (≥5) | Respiratory rate (breaths/min) | | Saturation | Heat rate (beats/min) | SBP (mmHg) | Temperature (°C) | Consciousness | UOP | Nurse worried |
| | 9–14 (0) | | <90% (3) | 51–100 (0) | 101–200 (0) | 36.5–37.5 (0) | Alert (0) | <75 ml in 4 h (1–3) | 1 point |
| | 15–20 (1) | | | 40–50 or 101–110 (1) | 81–100 (1) | 35.1–36.5 or >37.5 (1) | Voice (1) | | |
| | <9 or 21–30 (2) | | | <40 or 111–130 (2) | 70–80 (2) | <35.1 (2) | Pain (2) | | |
| | >30 (3) | | | >130 (3) | <70 (3) | | Unresponsive (3) | | |

*SIRS* systemic inflammatory response syndrome, *qSOFA* quick sequential organ failure score, *SOFA* sequential organ failure score, *NEWS* National early warning score, *MEWS* modified early warning score, *WBC* white blood cells, *MAP* mean arterial pressure, *GCS* Glasco coma score, *LOC* level of consciousness, *CVPU* confusion, voice, pain, unresponsive, *UOP* urine output

## Initial Resuscitation and Fluid Management

Once sepsis or septic shock are suspected, timely resuscitation is important. When there is evidence of hypoperfusion, it is suggested by SSC to give 30 ml/kg of intravenous balanced crystalloid fluid over normal saline within the first 3 hours [12]. While the strength of the recommendation was downgraded to weak based on the lack of prospective intervention studies comparing outcomes at different fluid volumes, there is evidence from a retrospective analysis of higher in-hospital mortality for patients presenting to emergency departments with sepsis and septic shock who did not receive 30 ml/kg within 3 hours that supports its use [18]. There is no evidence that using a colloid such as albumin improves the outcome of patients with sepsis or septic shock. Albumin's use is suggested by SSC only in patients requiring large volumes of crystalloids, while starches are contraindicated [12, 19]. Following initial resuscitation, patients should be evaluated for additional volume needs; this becomes more challenging as the risk of volume overload increases. Dynamic guides, including the passive leg raise (PLR) test, fluid bolus, stroke volume, stroke volume variation, pulse pressure variation, and point-of-care ultrasonography, are recommended over static measures such as central venous pressure, where only extreme values can be helpful [12, 20]. Capillary refill time and serial lactate levels are additional resources that can guide fluid recusation, with the objective being to identify volume responders from nonresponders where early start of vasopressor may be needed [12, 20]. The goal of volume resuscitation is to maintain adequate cardiac output and tissue perfusion, which should take into consideration the severity of illness and cardiac function, especially since many HSCT patients may have baseline cardiac dysfunction from comorbidities or prior cancer therapies [2, 20].

Hypervolemia increases intravascular pressure, promoting edema; increase in pulmonary artery pressure, which can contribute to right ventricular failure; increase in central venous pressure, which may impair organ perfusion, and increase in intra-abdominal pressure, which may impair renal function [20]. It should be noted that the presence of edema does not exclude the need for fluids [21]. Circling back to the prediction of fluid responsiveness, the dynamic measures can be used in two main categories: methods that mimic a fluid challenge (fluid bolus or mini bolus, PLR) and methods that measure variations in cardiac preload by mechanical ventilation (pulse pressure and stroke volume variation) [20]. To conclude, fluid management should be individualized according to the patient's condition and hemodynamics. This should include appropriate amounts of fluids during the resuscitation and maintenance phases, followed by fluid removal after stabilization once organ recovery starts [3, 20, 22].

## Vasopressors

In fluid nonresponders or when adequate organ perfusion is not achieved despite appropriate resuscitative measures, the use of vasoactive medications is needed. These should be started promptly to restore and maintain mean arterial pressure (MAP) >65 mmHg. In the absence of central access, these medications should be started peripherally and not delayed till access is secured [3, 12]. Norepinephrine is the preferred first-line vasopressor in sepsis and septic shock, as it has demonstrated survival benefit and reduced risk of arrhythmia [23]. While two systematic reviews [23, 24] found no difference in clinical outcomes and mortality with norepinephrine vs epinephrine, vasopressin, terlipressin, or phenylephrine, the stronger evidence from multicenter randomized controlled trials favors norepinephrine, making it the first-line recommendation from SSC guidelines [12]. When norepinephrine treatment fails to achieve the targeted MAP, it is recommended to add a second pressor over an escalating norepinephrine dose. Both vasopressin and epinephrine are recommended as second-line agents by the SSC guidelines. Septic shock involves a relative vasopressin deficiency; adding vasopressin has been shown to have a sparing effect on norepinephrine, resulting in lower doses being needed [3]. Epinephrine is a strong alpha- and beta-adrenergic agonist, which increases MAP by increasing cardiac output and vasomotor tone. Its use is limited by the significant risk of tachycardia, arrhythmia, and lactic acidosis [25]. When cardiac dysfunction is present in septic shock patients and hypoperfusion persists despite adequate volume status and arterial blood pressure, the addition of dobutamine to norepinephrine or the use of epinephrine alone is recommended. With the use of vasopressors, invasive monitoring of arterial blood pressure is recommended [12].

## Antimicrobial Treatment and Source Control

After initial stabilization and while awaiting infectious work up results to reveal potential sources, it is important to decide on the appropriate empiric antimicrobial therapy. It is recommended by the SSC guidelines to administer antimicrobials immediately, ideally within one hour of sepsis recognition after obtaining appropriate samples for culture [12]. The initial choice should be broad spectrum, covering all likely pathogens, considering the site of infection, previous antibiotic use, local pathogen susceptibility patterns, risk factors for resistant organisms, and the immunocompromised state [3]. Rising antibiotic resistance rates may impact the efficiency of empiric treatment; a recent cross-sectional study, including 14 US cancer centers, the "BISHOP" study [26], prospectively identified blood stream infections in high-risk febrile neutropenia patients, including HSCT patients, found that cefepime and piperacillin-tazobactam were the most commonly prescribed and that they remain effective as empirical treatment, maintaining high pathogen susceptibility and excellent outcomes. Adding methicillin-resistant *Staphylococcus aureus* (MRSA) coverage is recommended, as is the use of two antimicrobial gram-negative coverage agents versus a single agent when there is a high risk of multidrug-resistant organisms [12]. It is also important to consider antifungal coverage in allo-HSCT patients in septic shock, as they are at an increased risk for fungal infections given their immunocompromised state and likely recent antibiotic exposure [3]. Antiviral or anti-*Pneumocystis jirovecii* pneumonia (PJP) treatment should be considered in the appropriate situations [27]. Timely consultation with infectious disease specialists with expertise in HSCT patients is recommended.

Another key aspect of sepsis and septic shock management is the identification and elimination of the likely source of infection as soon as logistically and medically possible; this includes the prompt removal of indwelling catheters and intravascular access devices after other access has been established, the drainage of purulent collections, and the debridement of necrotic tissue when applicable [12, 28]. In the past, a more conservative approach to catheter removal was suggested in cytopenic patients for fear of complications from new catheter insertion. This is no longer the case with the availability, feasibility, and improved clinician skill with the use of bedside ultrasound [29]. Tunneled catheters should also be removed if they are suspected sources of infection, and a temporary non-tunneled catheter should be placed in the meantime. This is especially true for infections with non-fermenting gram-negative bacilli, candida species, and *Staphylococcus aureus* infections. Only in rare cases where there is no alternative, the use of systemic antibiotics and an antibiotic lock can be considered to salvage the catheter [28, 29].

A multidisciplinary team approach is needed to choose the least invasive procedures that guarantee maximal source control while avoiding additional damage or creating long-term disability. Keeping in mind that sometimes temporizing strategies are needed to overcome certain limitations, for example, patient factors; severity of illness, hemodynamic instability, respiratory, and metabolic status, abnormal labs; coagulation profile, location; extent of infection; and collateral damage associated with source control interventions [28].

Ongoing assessments for de-escalation of antimicrobial therapies are recommended over a fixed duration of therapy without de-escalation; shorter courses are preferred over longer courses, especially when cultures are negative and no identifiable infection is identified [12]. A retrospective analysis in HSCT patients with febrile neutropenia and a negative infectious workup done by Rearigh et al. [30]. where early empiric antibiotics were de-escalated to prophylactic therapy 24 hours prior to neutrophilic recovery when patients were afebrile 48 hours later found that mortality rates, new infections, and clinical decompensation requiring ICU transfer within 30-days were similar to standard of care, leading to less broad-spectrum antibiotic exposure.

## Mechanical Ventilation

HSCT patients in septic shock often develop respiratory failure, including acute respiratory distress syndrome (ARDS), and require mechanical ventilation. It is recommended to apply lung protective strategies with low tidal volume (6 ml/kg of ideal body weight), addition of PEEP with limitation of plateau pressure (<30 $cmH_2O$). Other strategies for the management of severe ARDS include prone positioning for >12 h/day [12].

## Additional Therapies

Additional supportive measures for HSCT patients with septic shock include the use of intravenous stress-dose corticosteroids (hydrocortisone <300 mg daily) [12]. An updated meta-analysis found that systemic corticosteroids accelerated the resolution of shock and increased vasopressor-free days [31]. These desirable benefits outweigh the undesirable effects such as neuromuscular weakness, and as such, the SSC guidelines continue to suggest their use when adequate volume resuscitation and vasopressors are unable to restore hemodynamic stability [12].

Hyperglycemia (>180 mg/dL), hypoglycemia (<70 mg/dL), and frequent glycemic variability are associated with increased mortality in the critically ill [32]. It is recommended that insulin therapy be initiated when blood sugar levels are >180 mg/dL and that it be titrated to a target range of 140–180 mg/dL [12].

The use of IV vitamin C, which is known to have anti-inflammatory properties, in septic shock was recommended after a single-center study in 2017 reported a mortality benefit and shorter vasopressor duration when used in combination with corticosteroids and thiamine [33]. The SSC group analyzed systematic reviews and meta-analyses from multiple RCTs published since, which showed that the overall size of any desirable effect was small and recommended against its use in septic shock based on the current data [12]. No data is available for HSCT patients specifically.

Sodium bicarbonate is not routinely recommended to improve hemodynamics or reduce vasopressor requirements unless there is severe metabolic acidemia (pH ≤7.2) and acute kidney injury [12].

Early administration of enteral nutrition in sepsis and septic shock patients has physiologic benefits in maintaining gut integrity and preventing intestinal permeability, dampening the inflammatory response, and modulating metabolic responses that may reduce insulin resistance [34]. It is recommended that in septic shock patients who can be fed eternally, nutrition be started within 72 h [12].

Finally, in assessing short-term mortality of critically ill allo-HSCT patients admitted to the ICU, Saillard et al. [2] identified the following prognostic factors as being associated with increased mortality: mechanical ventilation, vasopressor need, renal replacement therapy, ICU admission for respiratory failure, acute kidney injury, and acute graft-versus-host disease. In contrast, single organ failure, neurological failure, and reduced conditioning regimens were associated with increased ICU survival [2].

## Conclusion

HSCT patients are at an increased risk of infection leading to sepsis or septic shock. Early identification and prompt management of sepsis and septic shock are essential in all patients and particularly in HSCT recipients given their compromised immune system. Figure 13.1 sum-

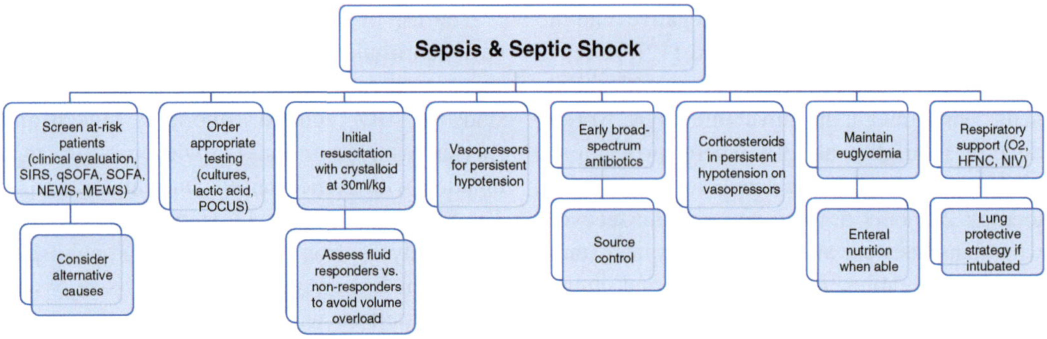


**Fig. 13.1** Initial management of sepsis and septic shock in HSCT patients

marizes the main components suggested by SSC for the initial management of sepsis and septic shock. We believe that the components of this bundle apply to the HSCT patient with sepsis or septic shock. Strong collaboration between the transplant specialist, intensivist, and other specialists is critical in improving the outcome of these patients.

## References

1. Gooley TA, et al. Reduced mortality after allogeneic hematopoietic-cell transplantation. N Engl J Med. 2010;363:2091–101.
2. Saillard C, et al. Critically ill allogeneic HSCT patients in the intensive care unit: a systematic review and meta-analysis of prognostic factors of mortality. Bone Marrow Transplant. 2018;53:1233–41.
3. Dugar S, Choudhary C, Duggal A. Sepsis and septic shock: guideline-based management. CCJM. 2020;87:53–64.
4. Bone RC, et al. Definitions for sepsis and organ failure and guidelines for the use of innovative therapies in sepsis. The ACCP/SCCM Consensus Conference Committee American College of Chest Physicians/Society of Critical Care Medicine. Chest. 1992;101:1644–55.
5. Singer M, et al. The third international consensus definitions for sepsis and septic shock (sepsis-3). JAMA. 2016;315:801–10.
6. Evans L, et al. Executive summary: surviving sepsis campaign: international guidelines for the management of sepsis and septic shock 2021. Crit Care Med. 2021;49:1974–82.
7. Dadwal SS, et al. A dynamic machine-learning based prediction model for sepsis in patients undergoing hematopoietic stem cell transplantation. Biol Blood Marrow Transplant. 2018;24:S373–4.
8. Kochanek M, et al. Management of sepsis in neutropenic cancer patients: 2018 guidelines from the Infectious Diseases Working Party (AGIHO) and Intensive Care Working Party (iCHOP) of the German Society of Hematology and Medical Oncology (DGHO). Ann Hematol. 2019;98:1051–69.
9. Lind ML, et al. Predictive value of 3 clinical criteria for sepsis (quick sequential organ failure assessment, systemic inflammatory response syndrome, and national early warning score) with respect to short-term mortality in allogeneic hematopoietic cell transplant recipients with suspected infections. Clin Infect Dis. 2021;72(7):1220–9.
10. Tolsma V, et al. Sepsis severe or septic shock: outcome according to immune status and immunodeficiency profile. Chest. 2014;146:1205–13.
11. Jeddi R, et al. Factors associated with severe sepsis: prospective study of 94 neutropenic febrile episodes. Hematology. 2010;15:28–32.
12. Evans L, et al. Surviving sepsis campaign: international guidelines for management of sepsis and septic shock 2021. Crit Care Med. 2021;49:e1063.
13. Vincent JL, et al. The SOFA (sepsis-related organ failure assessment) score to describe organ dysfunction/failure. On behalf of the Working Group on Sepsis-Related Problems of the European Society of Intensive Care Medicine. Intensive Care Med. 1996;22:707–10.
14. Jones M. NEWSDIG: The National Early Warning Score Development and Implementation Group. Clin Med. 2012;12:501–3.
15. Subbe CP, Kruger M, Rutherford P, Gemmel L. Validation of a modified early warning score in medical admissions. QJM. 2001;94:521–6.
16. Majhail NS, et al. Transplant center characteristics and survival after allogeneic hematopoietic cell transplantation in adults. Bone Marrow Transplant. 2020;55:906–17.
17. Oczkowski S, et al. Surviving sepsis campaign guidelines 2021: highlights for the practicing clinician. Pol Arch Intern Med. 2022;132:16290.
18. Kuttab HI, et al. Evaluation and predictors of fluid resuscitation in patients with severe sepsis and septic shock. Crit Care Med. 2019;47:1582–90.

19. Lewis SR, et al. Colloids versus crystalloids for fluid resuscitation in critically ill people. Cochrane Database Syst Rev. 2018;8:CD000567.
20. De Backer D, et al. How can assessing hemodynamics help to assess volume status? Intensive Care Med. 2022;48:1482–94.
21. Vincent J-L, Pinsky MR. We should avoid the term 'fluid overload'. Crit Care. 2018;22:214.
22. Monnet X, Shi R, Teboul J-L. Prediction of fluid responsiveness. What's new? Ann Intensive Care. 2022;12:46.
23. Avni T, et al. Vasopressors for the treatment of septic shock: systematic review and meta-analysis. PLoS One. 2015;10:e0129305.
24. Gamper G, et al. Vasopressors for hypotensive shock. Cochrane Database Syst Rev. 2016;2:CD003709.
25. Levy B, Perez P, Perny J, Thivilier C, Gerard A. Comparison of norepinephrine-dobutamine to epinephrine for hemodynamics, lactate metabolism, and organ function variables in cardiogenic shock. A prospective, randomized pilot study. Crit Care Med. 2011;39:450–5.
26. Zimmer AJ, et al. Bloodstream infections in hematologic malignancy patients with fever and neutropenia: are empirical antibiotic therapies in the United States still effective? Open Forum Infect Dis. 2022;9:240.
27. Classen AY, et al. Primary prophylaxis of bacterial infections and Pneumocystis jirovecii pneumonia in patients with hematologic malignancies and solid tumors: 2020 updated guidelines of the Infectious Diseases Working Party of the German Society of Hematology and Medical Oncology (AGIHO/DGHO). Ann Hematol. 2021;100:1603–20.
28. De Waele JJ, Girardis M, Martin-Loeches I. Source control in the management of sepsis and septic shock. Intensive Care Med. 2022;48(12):1799–802. https://doi.org/10.1007/s00134-022-06852-5.
29. Timsit J-F, et al. Expert consensus-based clinical practice guidelines management of intravascular catheters in the intensive care unit. Ann Intensive Care. 2020;10:118.
30. Rearigh L, Stohs E, Freifeld A, Zimmer A. De-escalation of empiric broad spectrum antibiotics in hematopoietic stem cell transplant recipients with febrile neutropenia. Ann Hematol. 2020;99:1917–24.
31. Rygård SL, et al. Low-dose corticosteroids for adult patients with septic shock: a systematic review with meta-analysis and trial sequential analysis. Intensive Care Med. 2018;44:1003–16.
32. Badawi O, Waite MD, Fuhrman SA, Zuckerman IH. Association between intensive care unit-acquired dysglycemia and in-hospital mortality. Crit Care Med. 2012;40:3180–8.
33. Marik PE, Khangoora V, Rivera R, Hooper MH, Catravas J. Hydrocortisone, vitamin C, and thiamine for the treatment of severe sepsis and septic shock: a retrospective before-after study. Chest. 2017;151:1229–38.
34. McClave SA, Heyland DK. The physiologic response and associated clinical benefits from provision of early enteral nutrition. Nutr Clin Pract. 2009;24:305–15.

# Diffuse Alveolar Hemorrhage in Hematopoietic Stem Cell Transplantation

14

Zhenmei Zhang, Steve G. Peters, and Hemang Yadav

## Introduction

Diffuse alveolar hemorrhage (DAH) is the clinical syndrome in which bleeding occurs into the lung alveoli. Typically, this results in dyspnea and diffuse infiltrates on chest imaging, and it may cause frank hemoptysis in some patients. DAH can occur after both allogeneic and autologous hematopoietic stem cell transplantation (HSCT).

Although DAH is rare overall, it is seen as a complication of several systemic diseases. Since the mechanism of DAH development in these settings has been relatively better studied than DAH after HSCT, it is worthwhile discussing these conditions when considering post-HSCT DAH [1]. The vasculitides, in particular anti-neutrophil cytoplasmic antibody (ANCA)-associated vasculitis, as well as several systemic rheumatologic diseases such as anti-glomerular basement membrane disease, rheumatoid arthritis, and systemic lupus erythematosus, are associated with the development of DAH. The mechanism of action in these conditions appears to be pulmonary capillaritis [1–3]. Alveolar wall inflammation leads to disruption of the alveolar-capillary basement membrane barrier with resultant hemorrhage into the alveoli [4]. Inflammation is typically neutrophilic and centers around capillaries and small veins. Unlike pulmonary infections, where neutrophilic infiltration is intra-alveolar, infiltration is typically interstitial. Capillaritis often leads to fibrinoid necrosis of alveolar and vessel walls. Pulmonary capillaritis has also been reported as a reaction to certain drugs, including carbimazole, propylthiouracil, and hydralazine [5]. The second major category of DAH syndromes is that of bland hemorrhage, typically characterized by hemorrhage into the alveolar space without inflammation or alveolar damage. This is typically seen in patients on anticoagulation or in those with left ventricular failure [6]. The third major category of the DAH syndromes is associated with diffuse alveolar damage (DAD). This can occur with acute respiratory distress syndrome (ARDS), several drugs (e.g., cytotoxic chemotherapy, amiodarone), radiation therapy, and pulmonary infections [7].

Importantly, these categories aren't mutually exclusive, and a patient may develop DAH in the context of multiple histopathologic injuries. It is not unreasonable to consider the HSCT patient susceptible to bland hemorrhage from thrombocytopenia, diffuse alveolar damage due to infections and ARDS, and capillaritis due to medications.

Z. Zhang · S. G. Peters · H. Yadav (✉)
Division of Pulmonary and Critical Care Medicine, Mayo Clinic, Rochester, MN, USA
e-mail: yadav.hemang@mayo.edu



A. O. Soubani (ed.), *Pulmonary and Critical Care Considerations of Hematopoietic Stem Cell Transplantation*, https://doi.org/10.1007/978-3-031-28797-8_14

## Definition and Diagnosis

DAH after HSCT was first described in 1989 in a case series of 29 autologous HSCT patients [8]. Since then, multiple studies have furthered our understanding of this post-HSCT pulmonary complication.

The definition of DAH consists of three main criteria (Fig. 14.1). First, there needs to be evidence of diffuse lung involvement rather than focal disease, and this is typically demonstrated with bilateral pulmonary infiltrates on chest imaging. Second, there are some consequences of alveolar hemorrhage, typically hypoxemia and a new oxygen requirement. Third, there needs to be evidence of alveolar hemorrhage, usually requiring bronchoscopy with bronchoalveolar lavage (BAL). A fiberoptic bronchoscope is passed through the vocal cords and advanced to a single lung segment until it cannot be advanced further ("wedged"). This segment is typically chosen based upon (a) affected areas on radiographic imaging and (b) likelihood of a good return for BAL (often the right middle lobe or lingula). Serial aliquots of saline (typically 20cc) are instilled into this wedged segment, and the return is examined for evidence of hemorrhage. A sample is considered "progressively bloody" if subsequent aliquots are more hemorrhagic than the last (Fig. 14.2). Typically, at least 4–8 aliquots are instilled, and the fluid is sent for appropriate laboratory studies (Table 14.1). Most centers send BAL fluid for cytologic analysis for hemosiderin-laden macrophages. The cutoff for a "positive" BAL is 20% or more hemosiderin-laden macrophages [9].

A major limiting factor in prior DAH literature is its variable and inconsistent definition. Some studies require rigorous bronchoscopic confirmation of alveolar hemorrhage, whereas others diagnose DAH based on "clinician opinion," with or without bronchoscopic criteria. The latter is particularly unreliable given the clinical (respiratory failure), radiographic (diffuse bilateral infiltrates), and hematologic (declining hemoglobin) findings of DAH that are commonly seen in HSCT when patients are vulnerable to a range of pulmonary complications and often in

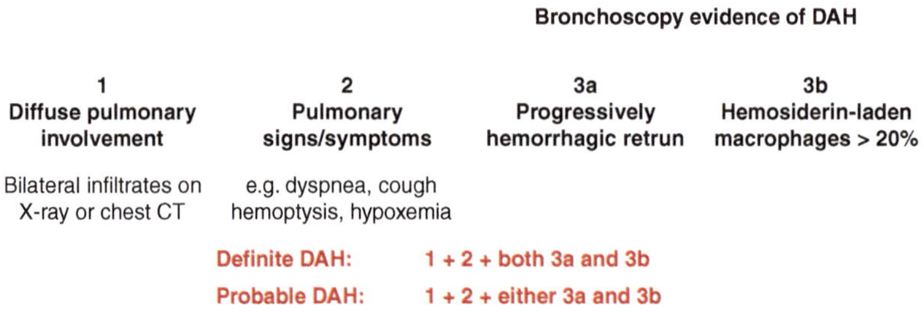


**Fig. 14.1** Diagnostic criteria for diffuse alveolar hemorrhage. *DAH* diffuse alveolar hemorrhage, *CT* computed tomography

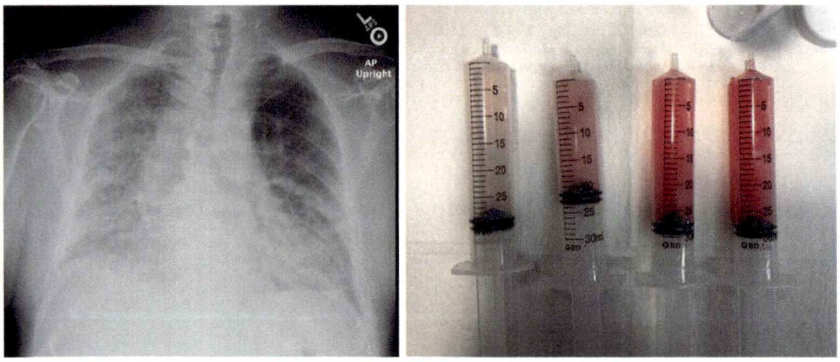

**Fig. 14.2** Radiographic and bronchoscopic features of diffuse alveolar hemorrhage. Left: characteristic chest X-ray showing diffuse bilateral pulmonary infiltrates. Right: Serial aliquots show a progressively hemorrhagic return. Hemosiderin-laden macrophages in this patient were 43%

**Table 14.1** Bronchoalveolar lavage testing for diffuse alveolar hemorrhage

| | |
|---|---|
| Non-infectious studies | Cell count and differential |
| | Cytology, including hemosiderin-laden macrophages |
| Viral studies | Influenza A/B and RSV PCR |
| | Respiratory viral culture |
| | Adenovirus PCR<br>SARS CoV-2 PCR<br>Cytomegalovirus PCR |
| Bacterial studies | Gram stain |
| | Nocardia stain |
| | Legionella PCR |
| | Legionella culture |
| | Aerobic bacterial culture |
| Fungal studies | Fungal smear |
| | Pneumocystis PCR |
| | Aspergillus antigen |
| | Fungal culture |
| Mycobacterial studies | Acid fast smear |
| | Mycobacteria culture |

need of transfusion support. Concise definitions as proposed in Fig. 14.1 may help to standardize DAH research.

Some studies include all patients with the DAH syndrome, while other studies only include those in whom an inciting event or infection is not identified. Importantly, most DAH studies are dated, from an era in which the evaluation for infection was often more technically limited than what occurs currently. For example, polymerase-chain reaction assays, now routine in the infectious evaluation of the immunocompromised transplant patient, were not available in many of these studies. As such, a report of "noninfectious DAH" may not always have been the case. Understanding that infectious evaluation is imperfect, the best option may be to consider DAH as an umbrella for the pulmonary syndrome, with subsequent stratification between infectious and noninfectious causes.

Radiographic abnormalities in DAH are nonspecific. Most patients have a mild interstitial or alveolar pattern on the chest radiograph at initial presentation, and bilateral lung involvement is more common than unilateral involvement. The most common finding on CT is bilateral ground glass opacities and a "crazy paving" pattern with middle or lower lobe predominance [7, 10].

The vast majority of DAH patients will be unable to perform pulmonary function testing due to the severity of their illness. However, in studies that have been completed, the presence of blood in the airways may lead to an increase in the measured diffusing capacity for carbon monoxide (DLCO) compared to baseline pulmonary function testing (typically performed before HSCT for all recipients) [11].

## Clinical Presentation and Time Course

The main clinical features of DAH are nonspecific, with dyspnea and cough being the most common [8]. Even in non-HSCT DAH syndromes, hemoptysis is not universal. In DAH after HSCT, hemoptysis is uncommon, only occurring in only 15% of the cases [8, 12, 13]. Patients typically progress to hypoxia and acute respiratory failure with less than 10% of patients on room air on initial presentation. Around 50% require invasive mechanical ventilation in recent reports [13].

Early studies of DAH noted that most patients presented within the first 30 days of HSCT, often coinciding with the phase of pre-engraftment thrombocytopenia and neutropenia, in which patients were also most susceptible to bland hemorrhage and infectious pneumonia [8, 13, 14]. More recently, there have been substantial improvements in peri-transplant outcomes. Improved understanding of the infectious syndromes after HSCT has led to guideline-based, standardized antibacterial and antifungal prophylaxis with significant reductions in post-HSCT infections [15]. There has also been a steady improvement in the management of critical care syndromes, with better treatment of sepsis, ARDS, and pneumonia [16]. With that, the median time to DAH diagnosis is now around 4 months after HSCT, and DAH can no longer be considered as only an early complication of HSCT [13].

## Incidence

As outlined above, there has been substantial inconsistency in prior studies regarding DAH definition, with not all studies including both infectious and noninfectious DAH and many including patients without bronchoscopic confirmation of DAH. As such, the reported incidence of DAH in these studies has ranged fairly widely from 1% to 16% [17–20]. In a large recent cohort study using a standardized definition of DAH (including both infectious and noninfectious cases), the incidence was 2.3% [13]. Consistent with most prior reports, the rate of DAH was higher in those undergoing allogeneic HSCT compared to autologous HSCT (7.2% versus 1.1%) [13, 18, 20].

## Risk Factors

Data regarding underlying risk factors for DAH are limited. Pre-HSCT cumulative cyclophosphamide dose, conditioning regimen, use of total body irradiation or thoracic radiation, delayed platelet engraftment, and age have been associated with increased risk of DAH in HSCT recipients [8, 21–23]. Patients with acute graft-versus-host disease are also more likely to develop DAH [24].

In those diagnosed with DAH, several factors are associated with worse survival [13, 22]. These include platelet count (OR 0.98, lower platelet count associated with worse outcomes), higher INR (OR 4.08), and the need for invasive mechanical ventilation (OR 8.2). The higher INR was associated with poorer outcomes despite median INR being relatively close to normal (1.3). As such, this may be a marker of severity of illness or nutritional deficit rather than coagulopathy. In line with this, correction of underlying coagulopathy has not been shown to change outcome [13, 22, 25]. Other risk factors associated with poor outcomes in DAH patients include delayed platelet engraftment and high D-dimer level, both of which may be indicators of other systemic illness [22].

Those diagnosed with DAH more than 30 days after HSCT are also more likely to have worse outcomes (OR for mortality: 7.06) [13]. This may reflect the fact that early DAH may be from treatable causes such as pneumonia, whereas later-onset DAH may be a form of noninfectious lung injury less amenable to treatment and reversal.

## Pathogenesis

As discussed above, the three histopathologic etiologies of alveolar hemorrhage syndromes are pulmonary capillaritis, bland hemorrhage, and diffuse alveolar damage [26]. Almost certainly, post-HSCT DAH is a combination of these different etiologies to varying degrees, likely driven predominantly by the latter two (bland hemorrhage and diffuse alveolar damage). Limited research has been done regarding the pathogenesis of DAH, and our understanding is largely limited to autopsy studies. Coagulopathy and severity of acute respiratory failure typically preclude transbronchoscopic or surgical lung biopsy.

In a 1989 study of 29 patients with DAH after autologous HSCT, autopsies were performed in 15 patients [8]. All 15 patients had evidence of diffuse alveolar damage. Other findings noted in patients included patchy hyaline membrane deposition within alveoli, fibroblast proliferation, and interalveolar connective tissue deposition. In a postmortem study of allogeneic HSCT recipients, 11 DAH cases were identified. Seven cases had DAD with the remaining having infectious pneumonia (bacterial, viral, or fungal) [27]. In a recent study of 99 DAH patients, seven deceased patients underwent autopsy with no cases of capillaritis, one case of bland alveolar hemorrhage, and four cases of DAD [13]. Taken together, these findings support the notion that the major histopathologic hallmarks of post-HSCT DAH are DAD and bland hemorrhage. DAD is often seen with ARDS, and one could consider DAH a phenotype of post-HSCT ARDS. It is unknown if there are specific pathophysiology features of DAD in this setting that are unique to the post-

HSCT setting, or whether it represents a result of one of the many types of lung injury HSCT patients may experience. Pretransplant exposures predisposing to DAD include chemotherapy and radiation therapy. Post-transplant exposures include pulmonary infections, aspiration, transfusion-associated acute lung injury, and graft versus host (GvH) disease [25, 28].

Capillaritis has typically not been reported in autopsy studies. This is important to consider given that the mainstay of specific pharmacologic therapy is high-dose corticosteroids, as inferred from the treatment of DAH associated with the ANCA vasculitis syndromes. However, one major limitation of autopsy studies is that they are often carried out long after the initial DAH episode, anywhere from 12 to 45 days from diagnosis, such that there may be an evolution of pulmonary pathology findings by the time of autopsy [8, 13, 27].

## Management and Treatment

The mainstay of DAH management is supportive care. To prevent the progression or worsening of ARDS in hospitalized patients, prompt empiric antimicrobial coverage is essential while infectious studies are pending. If a patient requires mechanical ventilation, early application of a lung-protective ventilation strategy is important in preventing the progression of respiratory failure. The ARDS Network trial showed lower tidal volume (now typically 4–6 cc/kg of ideal body weight), lower plateau pressure ($P_{plat}$) less than 25 mmHg, and adequate positive end-expiratory pressure (PEEP) greater than 5 mmHg were associated with lower mortality and a greater number of ventilator-free days [29]. However, the relationship between tidal volume, plateau pressure, and optimal PEEP is complex, and driving pressure ($P_{plat}$-PEEP) has been proposed as a surrogate for the effect of tidal volume on the remaining functional lung size. Driving pressure has been strongly associated with survival, and maintaining a driving pressure below 15 mmHg is an important part of lung-protective ventilation [30]. In mechanically ventilated patients with moderate-to-severe ARDS ($PaO_2/FiO_2$ ratio less than 150), patients may benefit from other lung-protective interventions, including neuromuscular blockade, especially if there is substantial ventilatory dyssynchrony [31, 32]. Dyssynchrony is where there is inappropriate timing between delivery of the mechanical breath and patient effort, resulting in the possibility of ventilator-induced lung injury. Other interventions that may be beneficial in ARDS patients are prone positioning [33] and fluid-restrictive resuscitation [34]. Adhering to these ARDS best practices is important in the supportive care of DAH patients, although there are limited data on mechanical ventilation strategies specific to this subset of patients.

In addition to supportive therapy, many patients receive high-dose corticosteroids, typically after infection has been excluded by microbiological studies of BAL fluid. The use of high-dose corticosteroids (≥1 g methylprednisone per day) was extrapolated from the treatment of alveolar hemorrhage in patients with ANCA vasculitis [35]. However, there is inconsistent evidence regarding the benefit of corticosteroids in patients with DAH after HSCT. Early small case series and retrospective studies suggested high-dose corticosteroids dramatically improved survival [36–38], but these results have not been replicated in more recent, larger cohorts [13, 22]. Additionally, higher doses of corticosteroid therapy (≥250 mg methylprednisolone per day) have been associated with worse outcomes than lower dose steroid therapy (<250 mg methylprednisolone per day), but the studies were limited either by an absence of confirmation by bronchoscopy or by a small sample size [13, 39]. In a recent cohort study of 92 allogeneic DAH patients, medium-dose corticosteroids (defined as methylprednisolone 10–20 mg/kg/day) had better 30-day survival than patients who received low-dose corticosteroids (methylprednisolone <10 mg/kg/day) or high-dose corticosteroids (methylprednisolone >20 mg/kg/day) [22]. However, these effects did not persist, and 60- and 100-day mortality was not different between the three groups. In summary, although moderate-dose corticosteroid therapy is considered standard of care for DAH patients once infection has been excluded, this practice is not clearly supported by evidence. There is an important unmet need to conduct randomized clinical trials to further investigate the optimal treatment for DAH in HSCT recipients. Our preferred approach is to exclude infection with bronchoscopy/BAL, allow culture data to adequately mature for at least 24 h, then administer 1–2 mg/kg of methylprednisone if cultures remain negative. Duration of therapy is determined on a case-by-case basis, but typically we would favor relatively short-course corticosteroids (3–7 days) over extended-duration steroids.

Other adjunctive therapies have also been trialed in HSCT patients with DAH, but there is a paucity of data regarding their effectiveness and safety. Aminocaproic acid (ACA) is an antifibrinolytic that inhibits plasmin and has been used in dental procedures, after biopsies, and in cardiac surgery to achieve hemostasis. In a case series of eight allogeneic HSCT patients who received ACA (1000 mg every 6 h) in addition to high-dose corticosteroids, survival was superior when compared to historical controls (100-day mortality of 44% versus 83%). However, in a larger cohort of 119 HSCT patients with DAH admitted to the intensive care unit, there was no difference in mortality between patients who received adjunctive ACA versus those who received high-dose steroids alone [39]. Tranexamic acid (TXA) is another antifibrinolytic that inhibits the conversion of plasminogen into plasmin. Intrapulmonary or nebulized TXA has been used for DAH of other etiologies, but rarely in HSCT recipients outside of two isolated case reports [40, 41]. Recombinant Factor VIIa, an approved agent for major bleeding in patients with hemophilia and successfully used in patients with acquired thrombocytopathies, has also been attempted in HSCT patients with DAH when conventional therapy with high-dose steroids and platelet transfusions proved ineffective [42, 43]. Although case reports showed improved clinical outcomes, a more recent larger retrospective cohort study failed to show benefit with recombinant factor VIIa [14, 44, 45]. Along with the other adjunctive therapies described, use of Factor VIIa in DAH is not routinely recommended [46, 47].

## Prognosis

DAH is associated with dramatically high morbidity and mortality. In historic studies, mortality associated with DAH was between 60% and 80%. Despite advances in post-transplant care and critical care delivery for HSCT recipients, contemporary studies show little change in overall survival. In a cohort of 99 DAH cases, in-hospital mortality was 56% and 90-day mortality was 64% [13]. In a cohort of 92 allogeneic HSCT patients who developed DAH, overall mortality was remarkably high: 91% at 90 days [22]. Both cohorts are the closest approximations to contemporary practice available. Although patients often present with acute respiratory failure, the most common causes of death are multi-organ failure and sepsis. Respiratory failure with active pulmonary hemorrhage accounts for less than 15% of the deaths [37].

## Research and Conclusions

Diffuse alveolar hemorrhage is an uncommon but devastating complication of HSCT. The underlying etiology is most likely a combination of diffuse alveolar damage (ARDS) and bland hemorrhage. The mainstay of therapy is supportive critical care. Corticosteroids (typically low dose: 1–2 mg/kg methylprednisone/day) can be considered after infection is excluded, but evidence for their efficacy is relatively scant. Prospective mechanistic studies and DAH clinical trials are needed to better guide management.

## References

1. Travis WD, Colby TV, Lombard C, Carpenter HA. A clinicopathologic study of 34 cases of diffuse pulmonary hemorrhage with lung biopsy confirmation. Am J Surg Pathol. 1990;14(12):1112–25.
2. Mark EJ, Ramirez JF. Pulmonary capillaritis and hemorrhage in patients with systemic vasculitis. Arch Pathol Lab Med. 1985;109(5):413–8.
3. Lazor R, Bigay-Game L, Cottin V, et al. Alveolar hemorrhage in anti-basement membrane antibody disease: a series of 28 cases. Medicine. 2007;86(3):181–93.
4. Lee AS, Specks U. Pulmonary capillaritis. Semin Respir Crit Care Med. 2004;25(5):547–55.

5. Radić M, Martinović Kaliterna D, Radić J. Drug-induced vasculitis: a clinical and pathological review. Neth J Med. 2012;70(1):12–7.
6. Bast A, Drent M. The role of vitamin K in the etiology of diffuse alveolar hemorrhage. Sarcoidosis Vasc Diffuse Lung Dis. 2019;36(3):251–2.
7. Spira D, Wirths S, Skowronski F, et al. Diffuse alveolar hemorrhage in patients with hematological malignancies: HRCT patterns of pulmonary involvement and disease course. Clin Imaging. 2013;37(4):680–6.
8. Robbins RA, Linder J, Stahl MG, et al. Diffuse alveolar hemorrhage in autologous bone marrow transplant recipients. Am J Med. 1989;87(5):511–8.
9. De Lassence A, Fleury-Feith J, Escudier E, Beaune J, Bernaudin JF, Cordonnier C, Alveolar hemorrhage. Diagnostic criteria and results in 194 immunocompromised hosts. Am J Respir Crit Care Med. 1995;151(1):157–63.
10. Worthy SA, Flint JD, Müller NL. Pulmonary complications after bone marrow transplantation: high-resolution CT and pathologic findings. Radiographics. 1997;17(6):1359–71.
11. Greening AP, Hughes JM. Serial estimations of carbon monoxide diffusing capacity in intrapulmonary haemorrhage. Clin Sci. 1981;60(5):507–12.
12. Snowden JA, Badoglio M, Labopin M, et al. Evolution, trends, outcomes, and economics of hematopoietic stem cell transplantation in severe autoimmune diseases. Blood Adv. 2017;1(27):2742–55.
13. Zhang Z, Wang C, Peters SG, et al. Epidemiology, risk factors, and outcomes of diffuse alveolar hemorrhage after hematopoietic stem cell transplantation. Chest. 2021;159(6):2325–33.
14. Gupta S, Jain A, Warneke CL, et al. Outcome of alveolar hemorrhage in hematopoietic stem cell transplant recipients. Bone Marrow Transplant. 2007;40(1):71–8.
15. Center for International B, Marrow Transplant R, National Marrow Donor P. Guidelines for preventing infectious complications among hematopoietic cell transplant recipients: a global perspective. Bone Marrow Transplant. 2009;44(8):453–558.
16. Meyer N, Harhay MO, Small DS, et al. Temporal trends in incidence, sepsis-related mortality, and hospital-based acute care after sepsis. Crit Care Med. 2018;46(3):354–60.
17. Capizzi SA, Kumar S, Huneke NE, et al. Peri-engraftment respiratory distress syndrome during autologous hematopoietic stem cell transplantation. Bone Marrow Transplant. 2001;27(12):1299–303.
18. Afessa B, Tefferi A, Litzow MR, Krowka MJ, Wylam ME, Peters SG. Diffuse alveolar hemorrhage in hematopoietic stem cell transplant recipients. Am J Respir Crit Care Med. 2002;166(5):641–5.
19. Huaringa AJ, Leyva FJ, Signes-Costa J, et al. Bronchoalveolar lavage in the diagnosis of pulmonary complications of bone marrow transplant patients. Bone Marrow Transplant. 2000;25(9):975–9.
20. Ho VT, Weller E, Lee SJ, Alyea EP, Antin JH, Soiffer RJ. Prognostic factors for early severe pulmonary complications after hematopoietic stem cell transplantation. Biol Blood Marrow Transplant. 2001;7(4):223–9.
21. Mo XD, Xu LP, Liu DH, et al. High-dose cyclophosphamide therapy associated with diffuse alveolar hemorrhage after allogeneic hematopoietic stem cell transplantation. Respiration. 2013;86(6):453–61.
22. Wu J, Fu HX, He Y, et al. Risk factors and outcomes of diffuse alveolar haemorrhage after allogeneic haematopoietic stem cell transplantation. Bone Marrow Transplant. 2021;56(9):2097–107.
23. Jules-Elysee K, Stover DE, Yahalom J, White DA, Gulati SC. Pulmonary complications in lymphoma patients treated with high-dose therapy autologous bone marrow transplantation. Am Rev Respir Dis. 1992;146(2):485–91.
24. Wojno KJ, Vogelsang GB, Beschorner WE, Santos GW. Pulmonary hemorrhage as a cause of death in allogeneic bone marrow recipients with severe acute graft-versus-host disease. Transplantation. 1994;57(1):88–92.
25. Srivastava A, Gottlieb D, Bradstock KF. Diffuse alveolar haemorrhage associated with microangiopathy after allogeneic bone marrow transplantation. Bone Marrow Transplant. 1995;15(6):863–7.
26. Lara AR, Schwarz MI. Diffuse alveolar hemorrhage. Chest. 2010;137(5):1164–71.
27. Agusti C, Ramirez J, Picado C, et al. Diffuse alveolar hemorrhage in allogeneic bone marrow transplantation. A postmortem study. Am J Respir Crit Care Med. 1995;151(4):1006–10.
28. Ferrara JL. Cytokines other than growth factors in bone marrow transplantation. Curr Opin Oncol. 1994;6(2):127–34.
29. Network TARDS. Ventilation with lower tidal volumes as compared with traditional tidal volumes for acute lung injury and the acute respiratory distress syndrome. N Engl J Med. 2000;342(18):1301–8.
30. Amato MBP, Meade MO, Slutsky AS, et al. Driving pressure and survival in the acute respiratory distress syndrome. N Engl J Med. 2015;372(8):747–55.
31. Papazian L, Forel J-M, Gacouin A, et al. Neuromuscular blockers in early acute respiratory distress syndrome. N Engl J Med. 2010;363(12):1107–16.
32. The National Heart L, and Blood Institute PETAL Clinical Trials Network. Early neuromuscular blockade in the acute respiratory distress syndrome. N Engl J Med. 2019;380(21):1997–2008.
33. Guérin C, Reignier J, Richard J-C, et al. Prone positioning in severe acute respiratory distress syndrome. N Engl J Med. 2013;368(23):2159–68.
34. Wiedemann HP, Wheeler AP, Bernard GR, et al. Comparison of two fluid-management strategies in acute lung injury. N Engl J Med. 2006;354(24):2564–75.
35. Levy JB, Turner AN, Rees AJ, Pusey CD. Long-term outcome of anti-glomerular basement membrane antibody disease treated with plasma exchange and immunosuppression. Ann Intern Med. 2001;134(11):1033–42.
36. Chao NJ, Duncan SR, Long GD, Horning SJ, Blume KG. Corticosteroid therapy for diffuse alveolar hem-

orrhage in autologous bone marrow transplant recipients. Ann Intern Med. 1991;114(2):145–6.
37. Metcalf JP, Rennard SI, Reed EC, et al. Corticosteroids as adjunctive therapy for diffuse alveolar hemorrhage associated with bone marrow transplantation. University of Nebraska Medical Center Bone Marrow Transplant Group. Am J Med. 1994;96(4):327–34.
38. Raptis A, Mavroudis D, Suffredini AF, et al. High-dose corticosteroid therapy for diffuse alveolar hemorrhage in allogeneic bone marrow stem cell transplant recipients. Bone Marrow Transplant. 1999;24(8):879–83.
39. Rathi NK, Tanner AR, Dinh A, et al. Low-, medium- and high-dose steroids with or without aminocaproic acid in adult hematopoietic SCT patients with diffuse alveolar hemorrhage. Bone Marrow Transplant. 2015;50(3):420–6.
40. Solomonov A, Fruchter O, Zuckerman T, Brenner B, Yigla M. Pulmonary hemorrhage: a novel mode of therapy. Respir Med. 2009;103(8):1196–200.
41. O'Neil ER, Schmees LR, Resendiz K, Justino H, Anders MM. Inhaled tranexamic acid as a novel treatment for pulmonary hemorrhage in critically ill pediatric patients: an observational study. Crit Care Explor. 2020;2(1):e0075.
42. Révész T, Arets B, Bierings M, van den Bos C, Duval E. Recombinant factor VIIa in severe uremic bleeding. Thromb Haemost. 1998;80(2):353.
43. Vidarsson B, Onundarson PT. Recombinant factor VIIa for bleeding in refractory thrombocytopenia. Thromb Haemost. 2000;83(4):634–5.
44. Hicks K, Peng D, Gajewski JL. Treatment of diffuse alveolar hemorrhage after allogeneic bone marrow transplant with recombinant factor VIIa. Bone Marrow Transplant. 2002;30(12):975–8.
45. Pastores SM, Papadopoulos E, Voigt L, Halpern NA. Diffuse alveolar hemorrhage after allogeneic hematopoietic stem-cell transplantation: treatment with recombinant factor VIIa. Chest. 2003;124(6):2400–3.
46. Pathak V, Kuhn J, Gabriel D, Barrow J, Jennette JC, Henke DC. Use of activated factor VII in patients with diffuse alveolar hemorrhage: a 10 years institutional experience. Lung. 2015;193(3):375–9.
47. Park JA. Treatment of diffuse alveolar hemorrhage: controlling inflammation and obtaining rapid and effective hemostasis. Int J Mol Sci. 2021;22(2):793.

# 15 Engraftment Syndrome and Peri-engraftment Respiratory Distress

Thomas R. Spitzer

## Introduction

Engraftment syndrome (ES) is a complication of hematopoietic stem cell transplantation (HSCT), occurring at the time of neutrophil recovery and mediated by a number of cellular interactions and proinflammatory cytokines [1–5]. First described in the setting of autologous HSCT and by the various terms engraftment syndrome, auto-aggression syndrome, and capillary leak syndrome, it has also been described in the setting of syngeneic and allogeneic HSCT [1–22]. While different criteria have been proposed for the definition of ES, the hallmark and most common features of the syndrome are fever and systemic vascular leak, resulting in organ dysfunction. The reported incidence of ES after HSCT has varied, widely from 7% to 48%, depending in large part on the criteria used to establish the diagnosis [6–22]. The pulmonary manifestations of ES are primarily those of noncardiogenic pulmonary edema due to the vascular leak. The differential diagnosis of these pulmonary complications is broad and will be addressed in this chapter.

## Definition of ES

ES has been described, mostly in the autologous HSCT setting, according to variable clinical manifestations occurring at the time of engraftment (neutrophil recovery to ≥500/ul). Two formal diagnostic criteria have been developed for ES. Spitzer developed criteria based on the clinical manifestations of ES, initially in the setting of nonmyeloablative HSCT and subsequently in a larger cohort of allogeneic HSCT recipients [1]. The criteria include major criteria (reflecting the frequency of noninfectious fever, pulmonary vascular leak, and, in the original cohort of patients, rash not attributable to graft versus host disease (GVHD)) and minor criteria emphasizing other organ injury that occurs due to ES.

The criteria by Maiolino et al. were developed in the setting of autologous HSCT and include fever as a major criterion and several minor criteria reflecting organ manifestations of vascular leak. In addition, diarrhea is included as a minor criterion [2].

Another important difference between the two criteria for ES is the time of onset: within 96 h of neutrophil recovery to ≥500/ul according to the Spitzer criteria, and within 24 h of neutrophil recovery according to the Maiolino criteria.

T. R. Spitzer (✉)
Department of Medicine, Massachusetts General Hospital, Boston, MA, USA
e-mail: tspitzer@mgh.harvard.edu



A. O. Soubani (ed.), *Pulmonary and Critical Care Considerations of Hematopoietic Stem Cell Transplantation*, https://doi.org/10.1007/978-3-031-28797-8_15

## Distinction of ES from Other Cytokine-Mediated Syndromes After HSCT

An inflammatory state exists universally after HSCT and may be due to conditioning therapy, infection, neutrophil expansion at the time of engraftment, or immune cellular interactions, including the initially T-cell-mediated complications of allogeneic HSCT (GVHD and graft rejection).

A diagnosis of ES requires the exclusion of non-ES causes of fever and other manifestations of inflammation and appropriate timing of the clinical manifestations (shown in Fig. 15.1) [23]. After autologous HSCT, the diagnosis is more straightforward and can be made with confidence if an infectious etiology has been excluded. After allogeneic HSCT, ES must be distinguished from immune-mediated transplant complications, notably GVHD and less commonly graft rejection. While it has been argued that ES after allogeneic HSCT is just an early manifestation of acute GVHD (or hyperacute GVHD when the syndrome occurs within the first 2 weeks after transplantation), the fact that it occurs after autologous HSCT, has different (albeit sometimes overlapping) clinical manifestations, and may resolve without or with minimal treatment, strengthens the argument that ES may occur independently of GVHD after allogeneic HSCT. It is not surprising that ES may be associated with a higher risk of acute GVHD given the proinflammatory cytokine environment that exists, potentially triggering the immune-mediated cascade that characterizes GVHD. Studies have reached different conclusions about whether the risk of GVHD is increased in patients who develop ES. A meta-analysis by Poonsombudlert et al. of 8 studies of ES after allogeneic HSCT showed a significantly increased risk of GVHD (a pooled OR of 2.76) in patients with ES [24]. Of note, in the analysis of ES after allogeneic HSCT by Omer et al. at our institution, the risk of early (within 28 days) acute GVHD but not the overall risk of acute or chronic GVHD was increased in 217 patients [20]. Of the 48 patients with ES, only 15 (31%) developed grade II-IV acute GVHD by day 180 post-transplant.

A cytokine-mediated syndrome was also described at our institution following combined bone marrow and kidney transplantation for tolerance induction in patients with end-stage renal

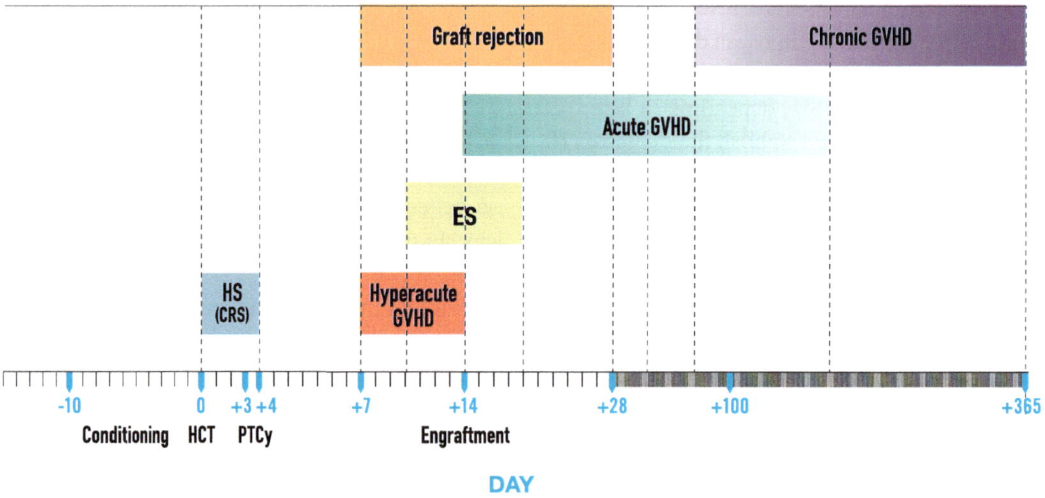


**Fig. 15.1** Timing of cytokine syndromes after hematopoietic stem cell transplantation. *CRS* cytokine release syndrome, *ES* engraftment syndrome, *GVHD* graft-versus-host disease, *HCT* hematopoietic stem cell transplantation, *HS* halo-storm, *PTCy* posttransplant cyclophosphamide. Originally published in: Spitzer, TR. Cytokine syndromes associated with hematopoietic cellular therapy. Adv Cell Gene Ther. 2021; 4:e98. https://doi.org/10.1002/acg2.98. Permission for use granted by John Wiley and Sons. Ltd

disease without an underlying malignancy [25]. The syndrome occurred 1–2 weeks post-transplant and was characterized by profound fluid retention and acute kidney injury. In an analysis of chimerism studies, it became apparent that the cytokine storm occurred in the setting of hematopoietic graft rejection. Pulmonary manifestations of this phenomenon, subsequently termed chimerism transition syndrome, were less prominent than the kidney injury. Similar cytokine-mediated manifestations have also been observed after hematopoietic graft rejection after nonmyeloablative HSCT [26].

The cytokine profile of engraftment syndrome has been studied, but the data are limited by the variable panel of cytokines that were measured, whether plasma or serum levels or cytokine mRNA were assessed, and the different timing of the measurements. Not surprisingly, a large number of proinflammatory cytokines have been found to be elevated in both GVHD and ES and include interleukin (IL)-1, IL-2, IL-6, IL-7, IL-8, IL-10, tumor necrosis factor-α, and interferon-γ [27–32]. Khandelwal reported cytokine levels in pediatric HSCT recipients with ES, isolated acute GVHD, or both [32]. Significantly higher levels of IL-1b and IL-2 were seen in patients with isolated ES. Levels of the anti-inflammatory cytokines IL-4 and IL-13 were also higher in patients with ES. While of interest and worthy of further study, cytokine levels are not a reliable way to distinguish cytokine-mediated syndromes after HSCT.

## Mechanism of the Pulmonary Manifestations of ES

The etiology of ES has not been fully elucidated but is likely the result of endothelial injury from chemoradiotherapy as conditioning for HSCT and the proinflammatory cytokine environment that occurs during neutrophil and other effector cell expansion and interaction during engraftment. The endothelial cell injury from conditioning therapy is a prerequisite for ES, as the spectrum of clinical manifestations doesn't occur after conventional chemotherapy followed by neutrophil recovery. The intensity of the conditioning regimen, especially with high-dose TBI regimens, has correlated with the incidence of ES in some series [7, 19]. Biomarkers of endothelial injury, including thrombomodulin and plasminogen activator type 1, have been shown to be elevated in capillary leak syndrome after allogeneic HSCT [33, 34]. The same endothelial injury that predisposes to other complications such as thrombotic microangiopathy and hepatic veno-occlusive disease may also be a triggering event in terms of initiating a cytokine cascade that, at the time of engraftment, culminates in ES. T-cell and other effector cell alloreactivity after allogeneic HSCT may contribute to the clinical manifestations of ES even in the absence of GVHD. Complement activation has also been shown to occur in ES and may exacerbate endothelial injury [35].

The resultant cytokine cascade, which involves elevated levels of multiple potentially targetable proinflammatory cytokines such as IL-1, IL-6, TNF-α and interferon-γ leads to further endothelial injury and systemic vascular leak. Thrombocytopenia may be a cause of alveolar hemorrhage in the context of pulmonary vascular endothelial injury and vascular leak.

## Pulmonary Manifestations of ES

The cardinal pulmonary manifestation of ES is noncardiogenic pulmonary edema. Clinically, dyspnea and hypoxemia, usually in the setting of significant volume overload and weight gain, occur, beginning as early as 96 h before engraftment. Examination of the lungs is typically remarkable for tachypnea, bilateral "wet" crackles, and the absence of signs of heart failure such as an S3 gallop and jugular venous distention. Radiologic findings include diffuse bilateral interstitial infiltrates and the absence of cephalization of vessels or cardiomegaly. Bilateral pleural effusions are common. CT scans may similarly show bilateral infiltrates, including ground glass opacities. Atypical radiologic findings may also occur, including multifocal consolidation.

While pulmonary edema is included in the criteria for ES, few series have detailed the nature of the pulmonary manifestations of ES or described the incidence of this complication (shown in Table 15.1). Including pulmonary infiltrates and/or hypoxemia, the incidence of pulmonary manifestations has ranged from 20% to 100% of the patients with ES. Two more recent series of ES after allogeneic HSCT using the Spitzer criteria or modified Spitzer criteria revealed that half of the patients had pulmonary edema [18, 19]. In the series by Omer et al., 52% of 48 patients with ES had pulmonary infiltrates consistent with ES, while Chang reported that 54% of 119 patients with ES had pulmonary edema.

Risk factors for the development of ES (although not necessarily for the pulmonary manifestations of ES) have varied widely according to the study. More aggressive preparative therapy (including regimens with myeloablative doses of total body irradiation), disease (higher incidence following autologous HSCT for breast cancer), a higher number of infused mononuclear or CD34+ progenitor cells, a faster time to neutrophil engraftment, and non-HLA matched related donors have been shown in some series to predict for ES [7, 9, 11, 12, 19].

In its most severe form, the pulmonary manifestations of ES can be severe and life-threatening. Shortly after the initial reports describing engraftment syndrome, Marin et al. reported two patients who developed respiratory failure requiring mechanical ventilation in association with ES [36]. Capizzi et al. coined the term "peri-engraftment respiratory distress syndrome" (PERDS) to describe the respiratory compromise that occurred in 19 of 416 (4.6%) patients who underwent autologous HSCT [37]. Six of the 19 patients had an alveolar hemorrhage. PERDS was believed to be contributory to 4 deaths. Early corticosteroid administration was effective in ameliorating the syndrome. Elbahlawan et al. described 30 patients among 1527 HSCT recipients (67% of whom underwent allogeneic HSCT) who developed acute respiratory failure due to engraftment, requiring mechanical ventilation [38]. Children who developed acute respiratory failure during engraftment had better intensive care unit survival rates than children who developed acute respiratory failure due to other etiologies.

**Table 15.1** Summary of the literature on engraftment syndrome including pulmonary involvement

| Author | Transplant type | Incidence of ES | Incidence of pulmonary manifestations of ES | Reference |
|---|---|---|---|---|
| Autologous | | | | |
| Ravoet | Auto | 6/61 (10%) | 6/6 (100%) with pulmonary infiltrates | [7] |
| Carreras | Auto | 43/328 (13%) | 16/43 (37%) pulmonary infiltrates<br>14/43 (33%) hypoxemia | [17] |
| Khan | Auto (breast Ca) | 33/85 (39%) | NS | [13] |
| Maiolino | Auto | 25/125 (20%) | 13/25 (56%) with pulmonary infiltrates | [2] |
| Edenfeld | Auto | 11/1589 (7%) | NS | [12] |
| Madero | Auto (Peds) | 30/156 (19%) | 20/30 (67%)<br>7/20 (35%) with ARDS/MV | [14] |
| Sheth | Auto | 46/178 (26%) | 5/46 (11%) hypoxemia<br>9/46 (20%) pulmonary infiltrates | [21] |
| Allogeneic | | | | |
| Gorak | Allo (NMA) | 15/149 (10%) | 15/15 (100%) with pulmonary infiltrates<br>13/15 (87%) with hypoxia | [15] |
| Schmid | Peds Allo (MAC) | 29/61 (48%) | 7/29 (24%) | [16] |
| Omer | Allo (RIC/MAC) | 48/217 (22%) | 25/48 (52%) | [20] |
| Chang | Allo (RIC/MAC) | 119/927 (13%) | 64/119 (54%) | [19] |
| Syngeneic | | | | |
| Koreth | Syn | 15/32 (47%) | NS | [18] |

*Auto* autologous, *Allo* allogeneic, *Syn* syngeneic, *Ca* cancer, *NMA* nonmyeloablative, *MAC* myeloablative conditioning, *RIC* reduced intensity conditioning, *Peds* pediatric, *NS* not stated

## Differential Diagnosis of Pulmonary ES

Because respiratory symptoms and signs usually occur in the context of neutropenia (or only recent neutrophil recovery), often with fever, and with chest X-ray and CT scans showing bilateral pulmonary infiltrates, the differential diagnosis is broad and can be broken down as follows:

### Infection

The risk of diffuse pneumonia and the offending organism(s) most likely to cause pneumonia vary according to the type of transplant (autologous vs allogeneic), infection history (particularly the CMV serostatus), and history of recent infection exposure. All transplant patients are at risk for Pneumocystis jirovecii pneumonia (PJP), but prophylaxis is standard of care, and early PJP is very uncommon. Cytomegalovirus pneumonia used to be a frequent cause of morbidity and mortality after allogeneic HSCT but is much less common now with viral monitoring and preemptive treatment of CMV infection [39]. It is most common in CMV-seropositive transplant recipients. When it does occur, it is usually later (after the first month) than when ES is first seen. Other infectious causes of diffuse pneumonia, especially occurring so early post-transplant, are uncommon.

### Diffuse Alveolar Hemorrhage (DAH)

DAH may occur after autologous or allogeneic HSCT and has a similar time of onset as ES (usually before day 30 post-transplant, at a median of about 2 weeks post-HSCT) [40]. Criteria for the diagnosis of DAH include diffuse alveolar injury, the absence of an infectious etiology, and, on bronchoscopy, progressive bloodier returns on bronchoalveolar lavage. The presumed etiology of DAH is similar to that of ES, namely endothelial injury initiated by conditioning therapy and cytokine release damaging further endothelial membrane, leading to vascular leak. Hemorrhage may occur because of severe thrombocytopenia and other coagulopathies. When considered in the differential diagnosis, bronchoscopy may be indicated as the treatment is different than that for ES (with DAH requiring higher doses of corticosteroids).

### Heart Failure

A cardiogenic cause of pulmonary edema should also be considered, particularly if the exam, radiologic findings, and/or serum biomarkers suggest a cardiac origin. Transient heart failure is common after HSCT [41]. As age and comorbidity eligibility boundaries have broadened significantly in the past 1-2 decades, some patients have a significant cardiac history coming into transplant. Many patients with hematologic malignancies may have received a significant cumulative anthracycline dose. Cardiac insults in the peri-transplant period may include high-dose cyclophosphamide, which is associated with a risk of myopericarditis, especially with doses of $\geq$120 mg/kg. Other conditioning regimens, including, for example, fludarabine or the combination of fludarabine and melphalan, can occasionally be cardiotoxic. [42].

There is a higher incidence of cardiac toxicity (as determined by serial transthoracic echocardiograms (TTEs), albeit mostly subclinical, than observed clinically in HSCT patients [43]. As opposed to cumulative, dose-related anthracycline-induced cardiomyopathy, most cardiac injury from preparative chemotherapy is largely reversible.

### GVHD

It is controversial whether acute GVHD of the lung occurs [44, 45]. While pneumonitis in association with other manifestations of acute GVHD has been described, and a pathologic exam has shown lymphocytic infiltrates in some cases, GVHD typically occurs later than ES. An exception is hyperacute GVHD, which occurs within the first 2 weeks after HSCT. More typical manifestations of GVHD, including rash (with consistent biopsy findings), gut involvement with vomiting and/or diarrhea, and cholestatic hepatopathy, are expected in that setting.

## Drug-Induced Pneumonitis

Some chemotherapy drugs may cause acute lung injury, which many present as diffuse pneumonitis [46, 47]. Carmustine (BCNU), which is included in many autologous HSCT regimens, typically causes delayed (after the first month) bilateral pneumonitis. Interstitial pneumonitis can also occasionally be caused by alkylating agents such as cyclophosphamide and melphalan. Busulfan may cause lung injury, but it is usually later than when ES occurs, and tends to be more insidious, sometimes with progression to pulmonary fibrosis. Low-dose methotrexate, commonly given for GVHD prophylaxis, rarely causes an idiosyncratic pneumonitis, often with pleural effusions.

## Idiopathic Pneumonia Syndrome (IPS)

IPS is an all-encompassing term to describe diffuse alveolar injury of noninfectious etiology after HSCT [48, 49]. The median time to diagnosis of IPS is about 2 months, and most definitions require that IPS occurs within the first 100 days post-HSCT. It has, however, been described from as early as 1 week to 1-year post-transplant. It occurs more frequently after allogeneic HSCT. Other risk factors include TBI-based preparative therapy and acute GVHD. Although it has been defined by the lack of an infectious origin, one study identified a possible infectious etiology in over half (56.5%) of the patients with a diagnosis of IPS when BAL specimen quantitative polymerase chain reaction testing for 28 pathogens was performed [50]. ES can be distinguished from IPS by its usually earlier onset and other findings, including volume overload.

## Diagnostic Evaluation

In the proper clinical setting, notably with volume overload and often with a noninfectious fever around the time of neutrophil engraftment, ES is the most likely cause of new-onset respiratory symptoms and signs. A chest X-ray should be obtained to evaluate for diffuse interstitial infiltrates. CT imaging is not necessary unless an infectious etiology is strongly suspected. A more invasive evaluation can be considered to evaluate for infection or DAH, as clinically indicated, or if there hasn't been a rapid response to treatment of ES with corticosteroids. A lung biopsy should be avoided when there is compelling evidence for a diagnosis of ES.

An evaluation for a cardiac etiology of pulmonary edema should include a careful exam with attention to signs of heart failure, a chest X-ray, and an NT-pro-B-Natriuretic Peptide (BNP) level. A TTE should be obtained according to clinical suspicion for heart failure.

A review of medications, particularly chemotherapy drugs, should be undertaken to determine if there is a convincing temporal relationship between the drug administration and lung injury.

## Treatment of ES

Treatment guidelines for ES are not well established given the variable practices reported in the literature and the lack of randomized controlled trials to guide treatment. ES does not always require treatment and may be self-resolving, as 29% and 21% of patients did not require therapy in the series of Omer et al. and Chang et al., respectively [19, 20]. ES is well known to be exquisitely sensitive to corticosteroids, which remain the initial therapy of choice when treatment is required. The recommended dose range of corticosteroids has been variable depending on the severity of the clinical manifestations of ES. For high fever unresponsive to other measures, for example, methylprednisolone (or prednisone equivalent) doses of 0.5 to 1.0 mg/kg/day are usually sufficient, and defervescence is expected within hours. For mild respiratory symptoms and signs, similar doses may be sufficient. For more severe symptoms and signs of respiratory distress (e.g., for $FiO_2$ requirements of ≥40%), higher doses of methyl-prednisolone in the range of 2–10 mg/kg/day may be effective in preempting acute respiratory failure and avoiding mechanical ventilation. Methylprednisolone doses up to 1000 mg/day may be used if there is concern for diffuse alveolar hemorrhage. Corticosteroids should be tapered as quickly as possible, usually over 3–7 days, given the usually rapid response to treatment and the desire to avoid the increased infection risk associated with corticosteroids.

For volume overload and pulmonary edema due to ES, loop diuretic therapy is usually indicated but must be undertaken with caution, particularly in patients on a calcineurin inhibitor (CNI) after allogeneic HSCT. ES is a state of intravascular volume depletion, and vigorous diuresis may cause or aggravate acute kidney injury caused in part by a CNI-induced reduction in renal blood flow.

Targeting specific proinflammatory cytokines is of theoretical value in ES but has not been well studied. As IL-6 levels have been found to be elevated in ES, tocilizumab has been proposed as a possible treatment for ES, given its effectiveness in treating cytokine release syndrome after immune effector cell therapy [51]. Given the rapid resolution of ES with corticosteroids in most cases of ES, tocilizumab might be considered in more severe presentations of the syndrome, such as in impending respiratory failure.

Etanercept, an inhibitor of TNF-α, has been of possible benefit in the treatment of IPS. Retrospective comparisons have suggested improvements in outcomes for IPS treated with etanercept [52]. A prospective, randomized, placebo-controlled trial, while underpowered, did not show an improved response rate with etanercept [53]. There is no evidence of the benefit of etanercept for ES.

Given the temporal overlap of ES and DAH and the higher risk of bleeding in the peri-engraftment period (prior to platelet recovery), maintenance of an adequate platelet count (at least 10,000/ul) is crucial. For patients with ongoing bleeding at other sites or suspicion of alveolar hemorrhage, higher platelet thresholds are likely necessary. Other coagulation abnormalities should also be corrected, as is feasible.

Confidence in a diagnosis or ES and exclusion of other causes of acute lung injury is important from a therapy standpoint for other reasons as well. Avoiding the empiric use of amphotericin B, for example, is desirable to avoid causing or exacerbating AKI. When PJP is in the differential diagnosis, avoiding the myelosuppressive effects of empiric high-dose co-trimoxazole is also desirable.

## Conclusions and Future Direction

ES and the pulmonary manifestations of ES are a result of endothelial injury from preparative therapy and a proinflammatory cytokine cascade occurring at the time of neutrophil engraftment after HSCT. Exclusion of other diagnoses that can present with similar clinical manifestations is paramount. Early diagnosis and treatment of ES, when indicated, is crucial, particularly when there is significant organ compromise. Early administration of corticosteroids is especially important in the management of noncardiogenic pulmonary edema due to ES, in order to avoid respiratory failure requiring mechanical ventilation. Additional investigation is warranted to determine the value of targeting specific cytokines, such as IL-6, with tocilizumab.

## References

1. Spitzer TR. Engraftment syndrome following hematopoietic stem cell transplantation. Bone Marrow Transplant. 2001;27:893–8982.
2. Maiolino A, Biasoli I, Lima J, Portugal AC, Pulcheri W, Nucci M. Engraftment syndrome following autologous hematopoietic stem cell transplantation: definition of diagnostic criteria. Bone Marrow Transplant. 2003;31:393–7.
3. Spitzer TR. Engraftment syndrome: double-edged sword of hematopoietic cell transplants. Bone Marrow Transplant. 2016;50:469–75.
4. Cornell RF, Hari P, Drobyski WR. Engraftment syndrome following autologous stem cell transplan-

tation-an update unifying the definition and management approach. Biol Blood Marrow Transplant. 2015;21:2061–8.
5. Grant A, Chapman LRM, Mitchell R, O'Brien TA. Engraftment syndrome following hematopoietic stem cell transplant: a review of the literature. Clin Transpl. 2020;34:13875. https://doi.org/10.1111/ctr.13875.
6. Lee C, Gingrich RD, Hohl RJ, Ajram KA. Engraftment syndrome in autologous bone marrow and peripheral stem cell transplantation. Bone Marrow Transplant. 1995;16:175–82.
7. Ravoet C, Feremans W, Husson B, Majois F, Kentos A, Lambermont M, et al. Clinical evidence for an engraftment syndrome associated with early and steep neutrophil recovery after autologous blood stem cell transplantation. Bone Marrow Transplant. 1996;18:943–7.
8. Cahill RA, Spitzer TR, Mazumder A. Marrow engraftment and clinical manifestations of capillary leak syndrome. Bone Marrow Transplant. 1996;18:177–84.
9. Moreb JS, Kubilis PS, Mullins DL, Myers L, Youngblood M, Hutcheson C. Increased frequency of autoaggression syndrome associated with autologous stem cell transplantation in breast cancer patients. Bone Marrow Transplant. 1997;19:101–6.
10. Nurnberger W, Willers R, Burcach S, Gobel U. Risk factors for capillary leakage syndrome after bone marrow transplantation. Ann Hematol. 1997;74:221–4.
11. de Arriba F, Corral J, Ayala F, Heras I, Moraleda JM, Osma MM, et al. Autoaggression syndrome resembling acute graft-versus-host disease grade IV after autologous peripheral blood stem cell transplantation for breast cancer. Bone Marrow Transplant. 1999;23:621–4.
12. Edenfield WJ, Moores LK, Goodwin G, Lee N. An engraftment syndrome in autologous stem cell transplantation related to mononuclear cell dose. Bone Marrow Transplant. 2000;25:405–9.
13. Khan SA, Gaa B, Pollock BH, Shea B, Reddy V, Wingard J, et al. Engraftment syndrome in breast cancer patients after stem cell transplantation is associated with poor long-term survival. Bone Marrow Transplant. 2001;7:433–8.
14. Madero L, Vincent MG, Sevilla J, Prudencio M, Rodriguez F, Diaz MA. Engraftment syndrome in children undergoing autologous peripheral blood progenitor cell transplantation. Bone Marrow Transplant. 2002;30:355–8.
15. Gorak E, Geller N, Srinivasan R, Espinoza-Delgado I, Donohue T, Barrett AJ, et al. Engraftment syndrome after nonmyeloablative allogeneic hematopoietic stem cell transplantation: incidence and effects on survival. Biol Blood Marrow Transplant. 2005;11:542–50.
16. Schmid I, Stachel D, Pagel P, Albert MH. Incidence, predisposing factors, and outcome of engraftment syndrome in pediatric allogeneic stem cell transplant recipients. Biol Blood Marrow Transplant. 2008;14:438–44.
17. Carreras E, Fernandez-Aviles F, Silva L, Guerrero M, Fernandez de Larrea C, Martinez C, et al. Engraftment syndrome after auto-SCT: analysis of diagnostic criteria and risk factors in a large series from a single center. Bone Marrow Transplant. 2010;45:1417–22.
18. Koreth J, Biernacki M, Aldridge J, Kim HT, Alyea EP, Armand P, et al. Syngeneic donor hematopoietic stem cell transplantation is associated with high rates of engraftment syndrome. Biol Blood Marrow Transplant. 2011;17:421–8.
19. Chang L, Frame D, Braun T, Gatza E, Hanauer DA, Zhao S, et al. Engraftment syndrome after allogeneic hematopoietic cell transplantation predicts poor outcomes. Biol Blood Marrow Transplant. 2014;20:1407–17.
20. Omer AK, Kim HT, Yalamarti B, McAfee S, Dey BR, Ballen KK, et al. Engraftment syndrome after allogeneic hematopoietic cell transplantation in adults. Am J Hematol. 2014;89:698–705.
21. Sheth V, Jain R, Gore A, Ghanekar A, Saikia T. Engraftment syndrome: clinical features and predictive factors in autologous stem cell transplant. Indian J Hematol Blood Transfus. 2018;34:448–53.
22. Liu Z, Zhang S, Horn B, Moreb JS. Postautologous stem cell transplantation engraftment syndrome: improved treatment and outcomes. Clin Transpl. 2020;34:12797. https://doi.org/10.1111/ctr.12797.
23. Spitzer TR. Cytokine syndromes associated with hematopoietic cellular therapy. Adv Cell Gene Ther. 2021;4:98. https://doi.org/10.1002/acg2.98.
24. Poonsombudlert K, Kewcharoen J, Prueksapraopong C, Limpruttidham. Engraftment syndrome and acute graft-versus-host disease: a meta-analysis. Hawaii J Health Soc Welf. 2020;1:194–201.
25. Farris AB, Taheri D, Kawai T, Fazlollahi L, Wong W, Tolkoff-Rubin N, et al. Acute renal endothelial injury during marrow recovery in a cohort of combined kidney and marrow allografts. Am J Transplant. 2011;11:1464–77.
26. Colby C, McAfee S, Sackstein R, Dey BR, Saidman S, Sachs DH, et al. Engraftment syndrome following non-myeloablative conditioning therapy and HLA-matched bone marrow transplantation for hematologic malignancy. Blood. 2000;96:520.
27. Antin J, Ferrara L. Cytokine dysregulation and acute graft versus host disease. Blood. 1992;80:2964–8.
28. Rabinowitz J, Petros WP, Stuart AR, Peters WP. Characterization of endogenous cytokine concentrations after high-dose chemotherapy with autologous bone marrow support. Blood. 1993;81:2452–9.
29. Takatsuka H, Takemoto Y, Yamada S, Wada H, Tamura S, Fujimori Y, et al. Complications after bone marrow transplantation are manifestations of systemic inflammatory response syndrome. Bone Marrow Transplant. 2000;26:419–26.
30. Deeg HJ. Cytokines in graft-versus-host-disease and the graft-versus-leukemia reaction. Int J Hematol. 2001;74:26–32.
31. Toubai T, Tanaka J, Paczesny S, Shono Y, Reddy P, Imamura M. Role of cytokines in the pathophysiol-

ogy of acute graft-versus-host disease (GVHD): are serum/plasma cytokines potential biomarkers for diagnosis of acute GVHD following allogeneic hematopoietic cell transplantation (alloHSCT)? Curr Stem Cell Res Ther. 2012;7:229–39.
32. Khandelwal P, Mellor-Heineke S, Rehman N, Lane A, Smiley K, Villanueva J, et al. Cytokine profile of engraftment syndromes in pediatric hematopoietic stem cell transplant recipients. Biol Blood Marrow Transplant. 2016;22:690–7.
33. Nurnberger W, Michelmann I, Burdach S, Gobel U. Endothelial dysfunction after bone marrow transplantation: increase of soluble thrombomodulin and PAI-1 in patients with multiple transplant-related complications. Ann Hematol. 1998;76:61–5.
34. Ikezoe T, Takeuchi A, Taniguchi A, Togitani K, Yokoyama A. Recombinant human soluble thrombomodulin counteracts capillary leakage associated with engraftment syndrome. Bone Marrow Transplant. 2011;46:616–8.
35. Salat C, Holler E, Schleuning M, Eisele B, Reinhardt B, Kolb H, et al. Levels of the terminal complement complex, C3a-desArg and C1-inhibitor in adult patients with capillary leak syndrome following bone marrow transplantation. Ann Hematol. 1995;71:271–4.
36. Marin D, Berrade J, Ferra C, et al. Engraftment syndrome and survival after respiratory failure post-bone marrow transplantation. Intensive Care Med. 1998;24:732–5.
37. Capizzi SA, Kumar S, Huneke NE. Peri-engraftment respiratory distress syndrome during autologous hematopoietic stem cell transplantation. Bone Marrow Transplant. 2001;27:1299–303.
38. Elbahlawan L, Morrison R, Li Y, Huang S, Cheng C, Avent Y, et al. Outcome of acute respiratory failure secondary to engraftment syndrome in children after hematopoietic stem cell transplant. Front Oncol. 2020. https://doi.org/10.3389/fonc.2020.584269.
39. Erard V, Guthrie KA, Seo Smith J, Huang ML, Chien J, et al. Reduced mortality of cytomegalovirus pneumonia after hematopoietic cell transplantation due to antiviral therapy and changes in transplantation practices. Clin Infect Dis. 2015;61:31–9.
40. Keklik F, Alrawi EB, Cao Q, Benjanyan N, Rashidi A, Lazaryan A, et al. Diffuse alveolar hemorrhage is most often fatal and is affected by graft source, conditioning regimen toxicity, and engraftment kinetics. Haematologica. 2018;103:2109–15.
41. Blaes A, Konety S, Hurley P. Cardiovascular complications of hematopoietic stem cell transplantation. Curr Treat Options Cardiovasc Med. 2016;18:25–34.
42. Morandi P, Ruffini PA, Benvenuto GM, Raimondi R, Fosser V. Cardiac toxicity of high-dose chemotherapy. Bone Marrow Transplant. 2005;35:323–34.
43. Kupari M, Volin L, Suokas A, Hekali P, Ruutu T. Cardiac involvement in bone marrow transplantation: serial changes in left ventricular size, mass and performance. J Intern Med. 1990;227:259–66.
44. Atkinson K, Turner J, Biggs JC, Dodds A, Concannon A. An acute pulmonary syndrome representing acute graft-versus-host disease involving the interstitium. Bone Marrow Transplant. 1991;8:231–4.
45. Cooke KR, Yanik G. Acute lung injury after allogeneic stem cell transplantation: is the lung a target of acute graft-versus-host disease? Bone Marrow Transplant. 2004;34:753–65.
46. Abid SH, Malhotra V, Perry MC. Radiation-induced and chemotherapy-induced pulmonary injury. Curr Opin Oncol. 2001;13:242–8.
47. Lane AA, Armand P, Feng Y, Neuberg DS, Abramson JS, Brown JR, et al. Risk factors for development of pneumonitis after high-dose chemotherapy with cyclophosphamide, BCNU and etoposide followed by autologous stem cell transplant. Leuk Lymphoma. 2012;53:1130–6.
48. Clark JG, Hansen JA, Hertz I, Parkman R, Jensen L, Peavy HH. Idiopathic pneumonia syndrome after bone marrow transplantation. Am Rev Respir Dis. 1993;147:1601–6.
49. Wenger DS, Triplette M, Crothers K, Cheng G-S, Hill JA, Milano F, et al. Incidence, risk factors and outcomes of idiopathic pneumonia syndrome after allogeneic hematopoietic cell transplantation. Biol Blood Marrow Transplant. 2020;26:413–20.
50. Seo S, Renaud C, Kuypers JM, Chiu CY, Huang M-L, Samayoa E, et al. Idiopathic pneumonia syndrome after hematopoietic cell transplantation: evidence of occult infectious etiologies. Blood. 2015;125:3789–97.
51. Kotch C, Barrett D, Teachey DT. Tocilizumab for the treatment of chimeric antigen receptor T cell-induced cytokine release syndrome. Expert Rev Clin Immunol. 2019;15:813–22.
52. Tizon R, Frey N, Heitjen DF, Tan KS, Goldstein SC, Hexner EO, et al. High-dose corticosteroids with or without etanercept for the treatment of idiopathic pneumonia syndrome after allo-SCT. Bone Marrow Transplant. 2012;47:1332–7.
53. Yanik GA, Horowitz MM, Weisdorf DJ, Logan BR, Ho VT. Randomized, double-blind, placebo-controlled trial of soluble tumor necrosis factor receptor: Enbrel (etanercept) for the treatment of idiopathic pneumonia syndrome after allogeneic stem cell transplantation: Blood and Marrow Transplant Clinical Trials Network protocol. Biol Blood Marrow Transplant. 2014;20:858–64.

# 16 Idiopathic Pneumonia Syndrome

Rachel N. Criner and Vivek N. Ahya

## Introduction

Idiopathic pneumonia syndrome (IPS) is an umbrella term for several forms of acute noninfectious diffuse lung injury that typically occurs within the first few months of hematopoietic stem cell transplantation (HSCT) [1, 2]. These conditions have overlapping clinical presentations, imaging characteristics, and histopathological findings and may be categorized by sites of primary lung injury: parenchymal injury—acute interstitial pneumonia (AIP), post-transplant acute respiratory distress syndrome (ARDS), vascular endothelial injury—diffuse alveolar hemorrhage (DAH), peri-engraftment respiratory distress syndrome (PERDS), and airway epithelial injury—cryptogenic organizing pneumonia (COP) (see Fig. 16.1). Although IPS is a heterogeneous syndrome, progression to respiratory failure is common, and it is associated with high mortality [1]. To better characterize and study this condition, the National Heart, Lung, and Blood Institute (NHLBI) established a formal definition in 1991, which described IPS as a clinical syndrome radiographically manifested as diffuse alveolar infiltrates in the absence of active pneumonia [2]. The IPS definition was further refined in 2010 by the American Thoracic Society to exclude cardiac and renal disease and iatrogenic fluid overload as potential causes of pulmonary infiltrates. IPS may develop after either autologous or allogeneic HSCT but has a higher incidence after allogeneic transplantation, highlighting the importance of both conditioning regimen toxicity and the alloimmune or graft-versus-host response in mediating lung injury [1].

R. N. Criner
Department of Thoracic Medicine and Surgery, Lewis Katz School of Medicine at Temple University, Philadelphia, USA
e-mail: rachel.criner@tuhs.temple.edu

V. N. Ahya (✉)
Division of Pulmonary, Allergy, and Critical Care, University of Pennsylvania Perelman School of Medicine, Philadelphia, PA, USA
e-mail: Vivek.Ahya@pennmedicine.upenn.edu



A. O. Soubani (ed.), *Pulmonary and Critical Care Considerations of Hematopoietic Stem Cell Transplantation*, https://doi.org/10.1007/978-3-031-28797-8_16

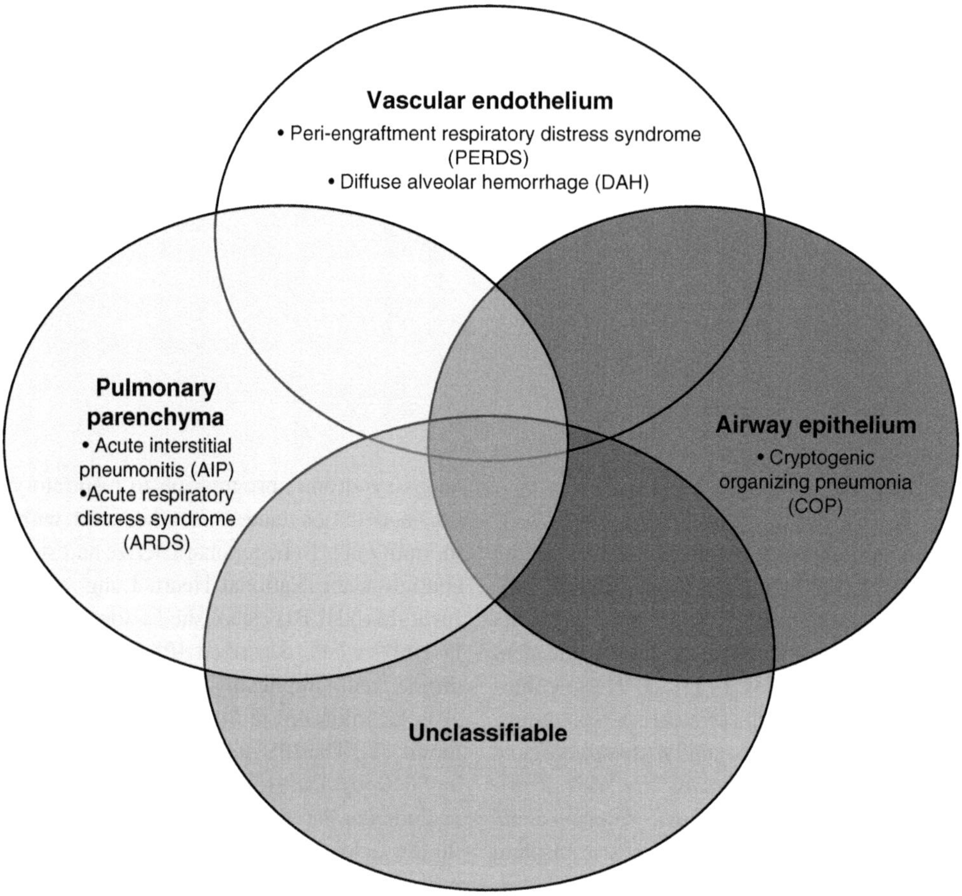


**Fig. 16.1** Idiopathic pneumonia syndrome causes a spectrum of disease presentations based on the major site of anatomical injury, as determined by bronchoscopy with bronchoalveolar lavage, computerized tomography of the chest, echocardiogram, angiography, and/or lung biopsy

## Incidence

The reported incidence of IPS varies greatly in the literature. A review of 12 studies published prior to the formal definition of IPS by the NHLBI in 1993 reported an incidence of 2–17% [3]. More recent single-center studies using the IPS consensus definition have reported a similar incidence, with a range of 3.7–21% [4–8]. The wide incidence range is likely due to differences in patient populations as well as the diversity and intensity of condition regimens. IPS typically occurs early after transplantation, with a median time of 25 days in a large single-center study and most cases developing within 100 days [4–6, 8, 9]. Late-onset IPS, i.e., after day 100 of HSCT, has been infrequently reported [10, 11].

## Risk Factors

### Conditioning Regimen

The type and intensity of the conditioning regimen administered before hematopoietic stem cell infusion is a major risk factor for IPS. Myeloablative or conventional conditioning regimens typically include high doses of chemotherapy with or without total body irradiation (TBI) to eradicate malignancy, while reduced-intensity or non-myeloablative regimens rely more heavily on immunologic mechanisms (i.e., graft-versus-tumor effects) [12, 13]. The application of myeloablative conditioning regimens is limited by organ toxicity and is generally not an option for older patients with comorbidities [12–14]. Not surprisingly, these high-dose conditioning regimens have been reported to increase the risk of IPS [4, 5, 14]. For example, a retrospective cohort analysis of 1100 allogeneic HSCT patients at Fred Hutchinson Cancer Research Center (FHCRC) in Seattle, WA, found that patients with conventional conditioning ($n$ = 917) had a significantly higher IPS incidence at 120 days compared to those receiving nonmyeloablative conditioning ($n$ = 183) (8.4% vs. 2.2%) [4]. However, in a more contemporary analysis from the same group, only conventional myeloablative regimens that included high-dose TBI (>12 Gy) were associated with an increased incidence of IPS compared to patients who had received non-myeloablative regimens or conventional regimens without TBI [6]. This finding was also seen in another study of 202 adults and children who underwent myeloablative conditioning with cyclophosphamide with or without fludarabine and subsequent TBI [7]. Those receiving a high TBI dose (>15 cGY/min) had an IPS incidence rate of 29% within 100 days of HSCT, compared to a 10% incidence in patients receiving low dose TBI (≤15 cGY/min) [7]. Fukuda et al. reported similar findings in patients greater than 40 years old, reporting that high TBI (≥12 Gy) was a significant risk factor for IPS, compared to those receiving non-TBI-based (0 Gy) conventional conditioning (16% vs. 5.8%). This trend was not consistently seen in patients 40 years of age or younger [4]. In another single study of only pediatric patients (ages 1–21), high-dose TBI (>15 Gy) was again associated with IPS [15]. In the future, conditioning regimen strategies employing three-dimensional image-guided intensity-modulated radiotherapy to reduce lung dose and exposure may potentially reduce IPS risk [16].

## Acute Graft-Versus-Host Disease

Among recipients of allogeneic HSCT, the presence of high grade acute graft-versus-host disease (aGVHD) has been significantly associated with IPS [4, 5, 17]. In a single-center cohort analysis of 369 adults who underwent allogeneic HSCT with conditioning regimens that included TBI and partial T-cell depletion, acute GVHD grade II or higher was identified as an independent risk factor for post-transplant pulmonary complications, including IPS [17]. Other reported risk factors for IPS include transplants from unrelated donors and an underlying diagnosis of acute leukemia or myelodysplastic syndrome. However, it is difficult to determine whether these truly represent independent risks or represent conditions associated with higher rates of aGVHD and/or increased intensity conditioning regimens [4, 5].

## Infections

Recently, in a study of pediatric patients who underwent pretransplant surveillance for respiratory viral infections, the detection of viral infection in the lower respiratory tract (bronchoalveolar lavage fluid) was identified on multivariate analysis as an independent risk factor for post-transplant IPS, albeit of borderline significance ($p$ = 0.06) [18]. The authors hypothesized that respiratory viral infections induced tissue damage and enhanced lung immunogenicity, thereby increasing the risk for alloimmune-mediated lung injury. Further studies are needed to evaluate this hypothesis, which will require close attention to ruling out progressive respiratory viral infection rather than IPS as the cause of lung injury.

## Pretransplant Pulmonary Function

The presence of pretransplant lung disease has been reported to increase the risk for post-transplant respiratory complications. In a recent single-center study, pulmonary function abnormalities, including reduced forced vital capacity (FVC), forced expiratory volume ($FEV_1$), and diffusion capacity (DLCO) were all associated with increased risk of post-transplant ARDS [19]. This finding has been observed in older studies as well. For example, in a comprehensive analysis of almost 3000 patients transplanted at the FHCRC, reductions in pulmonary function parameters were significantly associated with post-transplant respiratory failure and mortality. The investigators used these measurements to establish a pretransplant lung function score (LFS) calculated by incorporating the severity of decline in FEV1 and DLCO. The patients with the highest LFS ($FEV_1$ < 60% predicted and DLCO <60% predicted) had the lowest probability of survival. Notably, if this group received high-dose TBI as part of the conditioning regimen, mortality was extremely high [20]. In another investigation evaluating risk factors for non-relapse mortality after HSCT, severe pulmonary dysfunction before transplant, defined by the presence of dyspnea at rest, need for supplemental oxygen or DLCO, and/or $FEV_1 \leq 65\%$ predicted, was associated with an increased risk of mortality, especially for patients who had received conditioning with fludarabine and melphalan [21]. Thus, pre-HSCT pulmonary function measurements are important tools to assess risk for early post-transplant pulmonary complications and may inform decisions regarding the type of conditioning regimen to utilize. However, no single PFT parameter should be used alone to exclude transplantation as an option, but rather these studies should be incorporated into a more comprehensive assessment of the risks and benefits of the procedure [22].

## Pathophysiology

The pathophysiology of IPS is complex and incompletely understood. Insights from preclinical and translational studies have highlighted the pivotal role of the adaptive and innate immune systems [23, 24]. Murine models of IPS demonstrate significant injury in multiple lung compartments, including the alveolar, interstitial, bronchial, and vascular tissues [1]. These studies suggest that the conditioning regimen is directly toxic to the lung, and that injury is further amplified by the resulting immunologic responses that involve the release of pro-inflammatory cytokines and interaction of donor T lymphocytes with host antigen-presenting cells [25]. This alloimmune response activates T cells and induces the production of interleukin-2 (IL-2) and interferon-gamma (IFN-$\gamma$), resulting in the clonal expansion of activated T cells and macrophages. Activated macrophages secrete tumor necrosis factor-alpha (TNF-$\alpha$), a critical cytokine thought to have a prominent role in IPS pathogenesis [25]. Murine studies have shown that increasing levels of donor-derived TNF-$\alpha$ in bronchoalveolar lavage (BAL) fluid and lung tissue are associated with greater severity of lung injury and that the use of donor TNF-$\alpha$ knockout mice or administration of TNF-$\alpha$ neutralizing antibodies mitigates lung damage [26, 27].

Animal studies have also demonstrated that in addition to TNF-$\alpha$, BAL fluid also contains high levels of lipopolysaccharide (LPS) or endotoxin [28]. LPS is derived from the outer membrane of Gram-negative bacteria and is absorbed into the systemic circulation through the intestinal epithelia. LPS, through interactions with LPS-binding protein and cluster of differentiation 14 (CD14) is recognized by the innate immune system receptor, Toll-like receptor 4 (TLR4) [29]. This interaction ultimately activates innate immune responses and the production of TNF-$\alpha$ [29]. Murine studies have shown that transplantation with donor mice that are LPS-resistant have lower levels of TNF-$\alpha$ and LPS in BAL fluid and less severe IPS. These findings have supported the hypothesis that there is a "gut-liver-lung axis of inflammation," whereby gut injury through conditioning regimen toxicity or acute GVHD facilitates translocation of bacterial LPS into the systemic circulation to augment the pro-inflammatory cytokine storm and ultimately contribute to the development of both lung and hepatic injury [28]. Notably, in the clinical setting, patients with IPS have also been shown to have elevated TNF-$\alpha$, other pro-inflammatory cytokines, and components of the LPS pathway in BAL fluid [30]. Overall, these studies laid the foundation for human clinical trials of TNF-$\alpha$ – blockade in patients with IPS [9, 31].

## Clinical Presentation and Diagnostic Criteria

Patients with IPS present with the acute onset of cough, tachypnea, shortness of breath, with or without fever, hypoxemia, diffuse infiltrates on CXR, and often rapidly progress to respiratory failure [23]. Diagnosis of IPS requires evidence of diffuse alveolar injury without active lower respiratory tract infection and the exclusion of cardiac and renal dysfunction and iatrogenic volume overload as the causes of pulmonary disease (see Fig. 16.2) [1, 2].

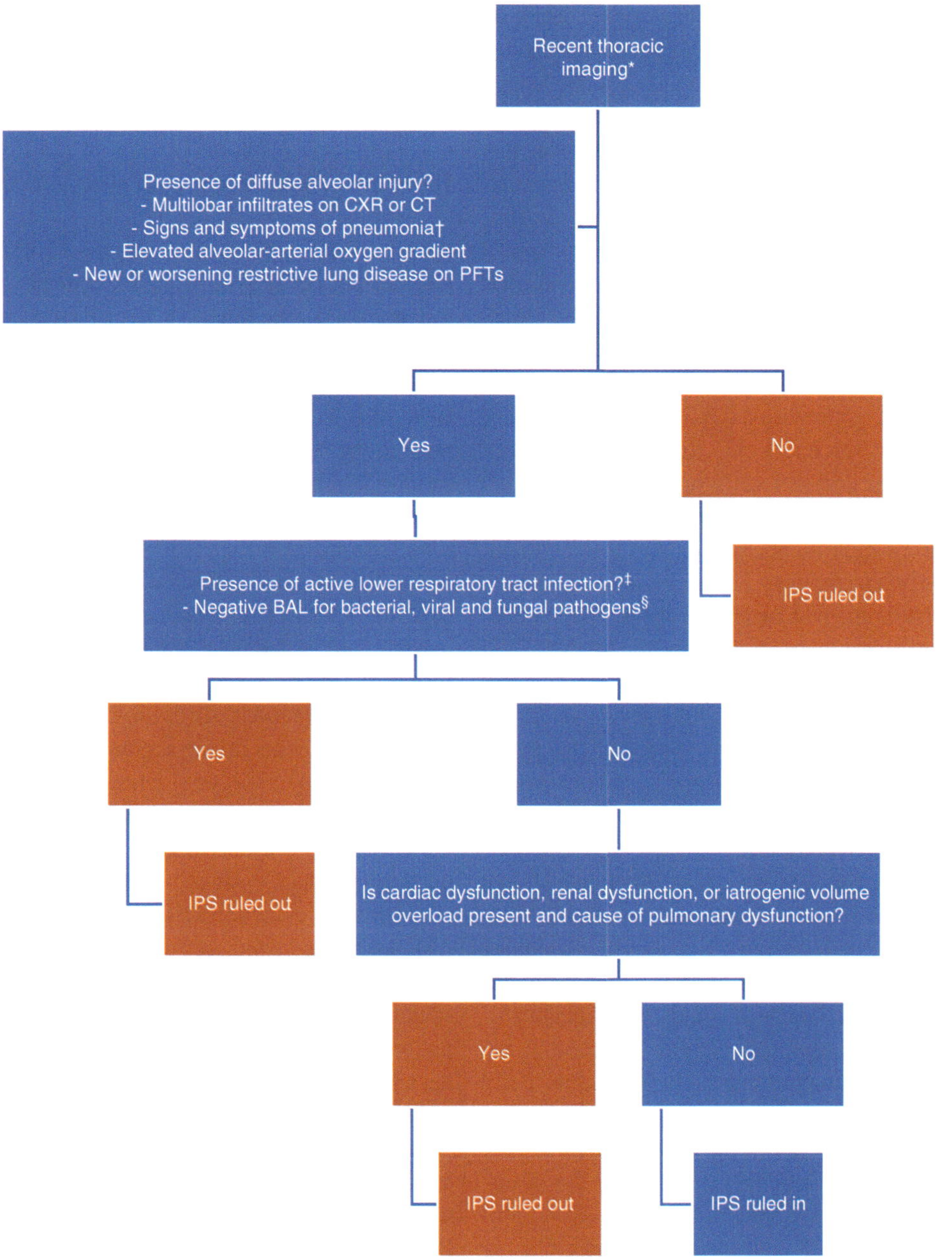


**Fig. 16.2** Diagnostic algorithm for Idiopathic Pneumonia Syndrome. *Idiopathic pneumonia syndrome typically occurs within 120 days after hematopoietic cell transplantation; IPS occurring after 120 days is considered late-onset. †Pneumonia signs and symptoms include cough, dyspnea, tachypnea, and/or rales. ‡Additional infectious testing to consider includes serum galactomannan enzyme-linked immunosorbent assay for *Aspergillus* species and polymerase chain reaction for human metapneumovirus, rhinovirus, coronavirus, human herpesvirus 6, *Chlamydia*, *Mycoplasma*, and *Aspergillus* species. A transbronchial biopsy can be considered for additional confirmation of the absence of infection. §If the pathogen is isolated but not clinically significant, IPS can still be considered. *HSCT* indicates hematopoietic stem cell transplantation, *CXR* chest X-ray, *CT* chest tomography, *PFTs* pulmonary function tests, *BAL* bronchoalveolar lavage, *CMV* cytomegalovirus, *RSV* respiratory syncytial virus, *HSV* herpes simplex virus, *VZV* varicella-zoster virus, *IPS* idiopathic pneumonia syndrome

Exclusion of active infection is confirmed with bronchoscopy and the absence of bacterial, fungal, and viral pathogens on BAL samples [1]. Quantitative polymerase chain reaction testing of BAL fluid for specific viral, fungal, and atypical infections and serum galactomannan enzyme-linked immunosorbent assay for *Aspergillus* species should be obtained, if available, as occult infection may have a clinical presentation similar to IPS. In a single-center study, 57% of patients initially diagnosed with IPS were subsequently found to have infections with human herpesvirus-6, human rhinovirus, cytomegalovirus, and *Aspergillus* species [1, 32]. Transbronchial biopsies may be considered for additional evaluation and/or confirmation of a noninfectious etiology but rarely identify information that alters clinical management and may be associated with excessive risk in the neutropenic or thrombocytopenic patient with respiratory failure [33, 34].

Radiographic imaging of patients with IPS typically demonstrates multilobar infiltrates; however, findings on initial presentation can be variable. One study of the imaging characteristics of patients with IPS demonstrated the following findings on computed tomography (CT): ground-glass opacities (93%), consolidation (21%), ground-glass opacities with consolidation (14%), and coarse reticulation (14%) [35]. Infiltrates were predominantly central (71%) and symmetric (71%) [35]. Although not part of the diagnosis, over 50% of cases had pleural effusions at the time of presentation [35]. In this same study group, follow-up CT imaging at more than 60 days after IPS resolution was predominated by coarse reticulation (71%), suggesting the development of a fibrotic process in IPS survivors [35].

There has been interest in identifying plasma biomarkers to aid in IPS diagnosis. Lipopolysaccharide-binding protein (LBP) has been identified as a potential diagnostic plasma biomarker, with one study showing a fivefold increase at the time of IPS diagnosis in a cohort of 24 adult and pediatric patients [36]. Other plasma biomarkers associated with IPS diagnosis include stimulation-2 (ST2), interleukin-6, and tumor necrosis factor receptor 1 [37]. At present, however, these plasma biomarkers have not undergone prospective validation. Further investigation is required to determine utility in the clinical setting.

## DAH and PERDS

As previously discussed, DAH and PERDS are two subtypes of IPS with distinct clinical presentations. DAH, like other forms of IPS, is characterized by the development of dyspnea, fever, diffuse infiltrates on CXR, and rapid development of respiratory failure. Hemoptysis may be present but is not a common finding. High resolution CT typically demonstrates diffuse ground glass opacities in the mid- to lower-lung zones, more prominent in the peri-hilar regions. Interlobular septal thickening is seen in some patients with DAH, creating a "crazy-paving" pattern [38]. DAH is distinguished from other forms of IPS by bronchoscopy. The finding of progressively bloody BAL fluid on sequential aliquots from several lung segments supports the diagnosis if infectious etiologies and cardiogenic pulmonary edema are excluded. The presence of more than 20% hemosiderin-laden macrophages on a cytological evaluation of BAL fluid adds confirmatory evidence [39]. A small post-mortem study, however, suggested that bronchoscopy may not have sufficient sensitivity or specificity for the diagnosis of DAH; 7 of 13 patients with hemorrhagic BAL fluid did not have histologic evidence of DAH, while 4 of 8 patients with DAH did not have hemorrhagic BAL fluid [40]. Although thrombocytopenia is almost always present, it does not appear to be more common in patients with DAH compared to other patients. However, delayed platelet engraftment resulting in prolonged thrombocytopenia may be a risk factor [41]. DAH, like other types of IPS, is seen after both autologous and allogeneic transplantation and occurs in 2 to 8% of HSCT recipients in contemporary studies [41, 42]. Most cases of DAH typically present in the first post-transplant month, often around the time of engraftment and neutrophil influx. Later presentations can occur and may be associated with a poorer prognosis [39].

PERDS is a type of IPS that develops around neutrophil engraftment and is the respiratory manifestation of a diffuse capillary leak disorder termed engraftment syndrome. This condition generally has a better prognosis than other types of IPS. The timing of acute lung injury (within 5 days of engraftment) and the presence of extrapulmonary manifestations of engraftment syndrome, such as fever in the absence of infection, erythrodermatous rash, fluid retention, and, in its fulminant form, multi-organ dysfunction and hemodynamic collapse, are consistent with the clinical diagnosis of PERDS [23, 43, 44].

## Management

The potential for rapidly progressive respiratory failure in IPS requires prompt and aggressive care. Supportive management includes the administration of supplemental oxygenation, non-invasive ventilation (NIV), and invasive mechanical ventilation (IMV). As respiratory failure requiring IMV is a poor prognostic factor, there has been interest in evaluating the role of NIV as a way to avert intubation. Most of the published studies demonstrating the benefit of NIV, however, have been in the broader population of immunocompromised patients and did not specifically evaluate patients with early post-HSCT respiratory failure [45]. Available data in this population suggests that while NIV support may be attempted and is not associated with poorer outcomes in most studies, a high percentage of patients progress to respiratory failure requiring IMV [46–50]. Invasive mechanical ventilation also has the advantage of safely permitting diagnostic bronchoscopy to evaluate for lower respiratory tract infection and subtypes of IPS such as DAH that may warrant specific interventions. Support with extracorporeal membrane oxygenation (ECMO) platforms may be considered but infection, thrombosis, and bleeding risks are extremely high in this heavily immunocompromised cytopenic patient population. In a recent meta-analysis, ECMO support for respiratory failure in patients who had undergone HSCT (all causes, not just IPS) had a pooled mortality rate of 84% [51–53].

### Corticosteroids

Treatment of IPS has generally targeted the inflammatory and immunologic mechanisms identified as having a central role in pathogenesis. Intermediate or high doses of corticosteroids are frequently administered to patients with IPS; however, data demonstrating their benefit are sparse. In patients with post-HSCT DAH, varying doses ranging from 30 mg of methylprednisolone per day to "pulse doses" of up to 1500 mg daily for several days have been reported, with several retrospective studies reporting better outcomes with treatment [23]. Notably, a non-randomized, single-center prospective study suggested benefit with lower doses (<250 mg/day), although mortality remained high [54]. The subset of IPS patients with PERDS is most likely to derive benefit from corticosteroids, especially if initiated early. Typically, patients with PERDS are treated with 0.5–1.5 mg/kg/day of IV methylprednisolone with tapering of the dosage after clinical response [55, 56].

### Antibiotics

Although absence of infection is necessary for the diagnosis of IPS, empiric administration of broad-spectrum antibiotics is often included in the treatment strategy for these heavily immunocompromised patients at high risk for rapidly progressive respiratory failure and death [1, 8].

### Etanercept

Over the last 20 years, etanercept, a soluble TNF-α binding protein, has been introduced as a potential therapeutic agent, based on preclinical and translational data highlighting the pivotal role of this cytokine in IPS pathogenesis [25]. Unfortunately, while preliminary outcomes after etanercept treatment were encouraging, more recent evidence suggests that longer-term survival is poor. A 2008 single-center study at the University of Michigan treated 15 IPS patients with etanercept in combination with corticosteroids, with the primary outcome of supplemental oxygen discontinuation during study treatment [9]. Etanercept was dosed at 0.4 mg/kg (maximum dose 25 mg) subcutaneously twice weekly for a maximum of 8 doses, and the corticosteroid dose was 2 mg/kg/day for 7 days with tapering then determined by the patient's physician [9]. Thirteen of the 15 patients (87%) had a reduction in oxygen requirement, and 10 of the 15 patients (67%) were completely weaned off supplemental oxygen within a median time of 7 days [9]. Early initiation of etanercept therapy was associated with a greater likelihood of clinical improvement [9]. A 2012 retrospective single-center study at the University of Pennsylvania compared the 28-day survival of IPS patients treated with high-dose corticosteroids only ($n = 22$) to those treated with a combination of high-dose corticosteroids and etanercept ($n = 17$) [8]. Corticosteroids were dosed at 1 g of methylprednisolone for 3 days with a 50% taper every 3 days until at 1 mg/kg/day with subsequent tapering based on clinical status. Etanercept was dosed at 25 mg subcutaneously twice a week for 4 weeks and initiated within 3 days of starting corticosteroids. The high-dose steroid-only group was transplanted a few years earlier than the steroid-etanercept combination group and thus had somewhat different conditioning and was more likely to have received bone marrow grafts rather than peripheral blood stem cell grafts [8]. The study found a significant 28-day survival advantage in the steroids plus etanercept group (88%), compared to the steroids only group (36%) ($p < 0.001$). However, long-term survival was low with only 18% of patients who received steroids plus etanercept surviving at 2 years [8]. Subsequently, a phase III, randomized, double-blind, placebo-controlled, multicenter trial of etanercept plus corticosteroids compared to a placebo plus corticosteroids was conducted. Unfortunately, enrollment ($n = 34$) was poor, and the study was discontinued early by the Data Safety Monitoring Board due to poor accrual [31]. The study found no significant difference in 4-week, 8-week, and 1-year overall survival (4-week: etanercept 69% vs. placebo 72%; 8-week: 63% vs. 61%; 1-year: 23% vs. 17%), or in supplemental oxygen discontinuation at 4 weeks ($p = 0.69$) [31]. In the absence of alternative therapies, corticosteroids and etanercept are often still administered, but the data supporting their use are limited. Of note, late-onset IPS, i.e., IPS that develops after 100 days from HSCT, may have a more favorable response to etanercept in combination with high-dose corticosteroids [10, 11]. A study of 23 HSCT patients who developed late-onset IPS reported that 43% ($n = 10$) had both resolution of pulmonary symptoms and supplemental oxygen use within 28 days of treatment initiation, while 12 of the remaining 13 patients had progressive hypoxemic respiratory failure and eventual death [11]. At the time of treatment initiation, the patients who had a complete response had a less severe lung injury and did not require NIV or IMV support [11]. Two-year survival in complete responders was significantly higher at 67% [11].

## Adjunctive Therapies: DAH

Adjunctive therapies that promote hemostasis have been explored for patients with DAH. The antifibrinolytic agent aminocaproic acid was not associated with improved outcomes in a retrospective analysis of 119 patients who received this agent in conjunction with corticosteroids [54]. In contrast, another study of only 14 patients reported that the 9 patients who received corticosteroids and aminocaproic acid had lower 100-day mortality [57]. Recombinant factor VIIa (rFVIIa) promotes thrombin generation at the site of tissue injury, and off-label uses of this agent administered systemically or via the intrapulmonary route have been tried in patients with DAH. At present, there are no randomized controlled trials evaluating the efficacy of this agent. Limited experience in the post-HSCT population with DAH suggests that systemic administration of rFVIIa is not associated with reduced mortality or ventilator-free days. Additionally, thromboembolic complications may be higher [58, 59]. Intrapulmonary installation of rFVIIa to facilitate direct exposure of the agent to sites of lung injury and reduce thrombosis risk has been reported to achieve hemostasis in small case series [60–62]. More rigorous studies are required to evaluate short-term benefits and their impact on longer-term outcomes.

## Lung Transplantation

Lung transplantation is generally not an option for patients due to the presence of recent malignancy and high risk for infection and bleeding, however, there is one recent report of a successful bilateral lung transplant procedure performed for IPS diagnosed 5 months after HSCT for a patient with myelodysplastic syndrome who had achieved bone marrow engraftment [63].

## Outcomes

Despite advances in critical care and treatment with immunomodulatory agents and other adjunctive therapies, mortality remains high for patients who develop IPS [3–5]. While studies have reported mortality rates as high as 87% within 120 days after transplantation, early outcomes may be improving [4, 5]. A recent retrospective single-center cohort study of 1829 adults who underwent allogeneic HSCT at FHCRC reported that 67 patients (3.7%) met the NHLBI criteria for IPS. The mortality rate was 46% at day 120. However, longer-term outcomes remained poor, with only 30% surviving for 1 year [6]. Outcomes were somewhat better in a 2019 single-center analysis of 202 patients transplanted at the University of Minnesota for the diagnosis of acute leukemia. In this study, 21% developed IPS with 60% surviving for 1 year [7]. IPS often progresses rapidly from onset to respiratory failure with death occurring within a few weeks to months [4–6, 8, 25]. The need for IMV in particular is strongly associated with poor outcomes and death [4, 6]. In the study mentioned above from the FHCRC, 59% of patients who required mechanical ventilation died by day 120; in contrast, the mortality rate at this time point was 35% for patients with IPS who did not require IMV. At 1 year, the mortality rate was 79% for patients requiring IMV vs. 57% for patients with IPS who did not need IMV [6]. The development of multi-organ dysfunction, especially renal and hepatic dysfunction, in patients with IPS may is an ominous sign [6].

## Conclusion

IPS remains a formidable problem and continues to be associated with poor outcomes. While preclinical studies have offered mechanistic insight, our understanding of this condition remains incomplete. With improvements in the delivery of critical care, short-term outcomes may be improving, but long-term survival generally remains poor. Initial optimism for treatment with immunomodulatory agents such as corticosteroids and etanercept has not been supported by outcomes reported in subsequent studies. There is a tremendous need for additional investigation to better understand mechanisms and develop novel approaches to prevent and treat this devastating complication. Unfortunately, at the time of this writing, there are no active U.S. clinical trials studying IPS.

## References


1. Panoskaltsis-Mortari A, Griese M, Madtes DK, Belperio JA, Haddad IY, Folz RJ, et al. An official American Thoracic Society Research statement: noninfectious lung injury after hematopoietic stem cell transplantation: idiopathic pneumonia syndrome. Am J Respir Crit Care Med. 2011;183(9):1262–79.
2. Clark JG, Hansen JA, Hertz MI, Parkman R, Jensen L, Peavy HH. NHLBI workshop summary. Idiopathic pneumonia syndrome after bone marrow transplantation. Am Rev Respir Dis. 1993;147(6 Pt 1):1601–6.
3. Afessa B, Litzow MR, Tefferi A. Bronchiolitis obliterans and other late onset non-infectious pulmonary complications in hematopoietic stem cell transplantation. Bone Marrow Transplant. 2001;28(5):425–34.
4. Fukuda T, Hackman RC, Guthrie KA, Sandmaier BM, Boeckh M, Maris MB, et al. Risks and outcomes of idiopathic pneumonia syndrome after nonmyeloablative and conventional conditioning regimens for allogeneic hematopoietic stem cell transplantation. Blood. 2003;102(8):2777–85.
5. Zhu KE, Hu JY, Zhang T, Chen J, Zhong J, Lu YH. Incidence, risks, and outcome of idiopathic pneumonia syndrome early after allogeneic hematopoietic stem cell transplantation. Eur J Haematol. 2008;81(6):461–6.
6. Wenger DS, Triplette M, Crothers K, Cheng GS, Hill JA, Milano F, et al. Incidence, risk factors, and outcomes of idiopathic pneumonia syndrome after allogeneic hematopoietic cell transplantation. Biol Blood Marrow Transplant. 2020;26(2):413–20.
7. Gao RW, Weisdorf DJ, DeFor TE, Ehler E, Dusenbery KE. Influence of total body irradiation dose rate on

idiopathic pneumonia syndrome in acute Leukemia patients undergoing allogeneic hematopoietic cell transplantation. Int J Radiat Oncol Biol Phys. 2019;103(1):180–9.
8. Tizon R, Frey N, Heitjan DF, Tan KS, Goldstein SC, Hexner EO, et al. High-dose corticosteroids with or without etanercept for the treatment of idiopathic pneumonia syndrome after Allo-SCT. Bone Marrow Transplant. 2012;47(10):1332–7.
9. Yanik GA, Ho VT, Levine JE, White ES, Braun T, Antin JH, et al. The impact of soluble tumor necrosis factor receptor etanercept on the treatment of idiopathic pneumonia syndrome after allogeneic hematopoietic stem cell transplantation. Blood. 2008;112(8):3073–81.
10. Tun HW, Wallace KH, Grinton SF, Khoor A, Burger CD. Etanercept therapy for late-onset idiopathic pneumonia syndrome after nonmyeloablative allogeneic hematopoietic stem cell transplantation. Transplant Proc. 2005;37(10):4492–6.
11. Thompson J, Yin Z, D'Souza A, Fenske T, Hamadani M, Hari P, et al. Etanercept and corticosteroid therapy for the treatment of late-onset idiopathic pneumonia syndrome. Biol Blood Marrow Transplant. 2017;23(11):1955–60.
12. Gyurkocza B, Sandmaier BM. Conditioning regimens for hematopoietic cell transplantation: one size does not fit all. Blood. 2014;124(3):344–53.
13. Pollack SM, O'Connor TP Jr, Hashash J, Tabbara IA. Nonmyeloablative and reduced-intensity conditioning for allogeneic hematopoietic stem cell transplantation: a clinical review. Am J Clin Oncol. 2009;32(6):618–28.
14. Nusair S, Breuer R, Shapira MY, Berkman N, Or R. Low incidence of pulmonary complications following nonmyeloablative stem cell transplantation. Eur Respir J. 2004;23(3):440–5.
15. Abugideiri M, Nanda RH, Butker C, Zhang C, Kim S, Chiang KY, et al. Factors influencing pulmonary toxicity in children undergoing allogeneic hematopoietic stem cell transplantation in the setting of Total body irradiation-based myeloablative conditioning. Int J Radiat Oncol Biol Phys. 2016;94(2):349–59.
16. Vogel J, Hui S, Hua CH, Dusenbery K, Rassiah P, Kalapurakal J, et al. Pulmonary toxicity after total body irradiation—critical review of the literature and recommendations for toxicity reporting. Front Oncol. 2021;11:708906.
17. Huisman C, van der Straaten HM, Canninga-van Dijk MR, Fijnheer R, Verdonck LF. Pulmonary complications after T-cell-depleted allogeneic stem cell transplantation: low incidence and strong association with acute graft-versus-host disease. Bone Marrow Transplant. 2006;38(8):561–6.
18. Versluys B, Bierings M, Murk JL, Wolfs T, Lindemans C, Vd Ent K, et al. Infection with a respiratory virus before hematopoietic cell transplantation is associated with alloimmune-mediated lung syndromes. J Allergy Clin Immunol. 2018;141(2):697–703.e8.
19. Herasevich S, Frank RD, Bo H, Alkhateeb H, Hogan WJ, Gajic O, et al. Pretransplant risk factors can predict development of acute respiratory distress syndrome after hematopoietic stem cell transplantation. Ann Am Thorac Soc. 2021;18(6):1004–12.
20. Parimon T, Madtes DK, Au DH, Clark JG, Chien JW. Pretransplant lung function, respiratory failure, and mortality after stem cell transplantation. Am J Respir Crit Care Med. 2005;172(3):384–90.
21. Fein JA, Shimoni A, Labopin M, Shem-Tov N, Yerushalmi R, Magen H, et al. The impact of individual comorbidities on non-relapse mortality following allogeneic hematopoietic stem cell transplantation. Leukemia. 2018;32(8):1787–94.
22. Chien JW, Sullivan KM. Carbon monoxide diffusion capacity: how low can you go for hematopoietic cell transplantation eligibility? Biol Blood Marrow Transplant. 2009;15(4):447–53.
23. Ahya VN. Noninfectious acute lung injury syndromes early after hematopoietic stem cell transplantation. Clin Chest Med. 2017;38(4):595–606.
24. Haider S, Durairajan N, Soubani AO. Noninfectious pulmonary complications of haematopoietic stem cell transplantation. Eur Respir Rev. 2020;29(156):190119.
25. Cooke KR, Yanik G. Acute lung injury after allogeneic stem cell transplantation: is the lung a target of acute graft-versus-host disease? Bone Marrow Transplant. 2004;34(9):753–65.
26. Hildebrandt GC, Olkiewicz KM, Corrion LA, Chang Y, Clouthier SG, Liu C, et al. Donor-derived TNF-alpha regulates pulmonary chemokine expression and the development of idiopathic pneumonia syndrome after allogeneic bone marrow transplantation. Blood. 2004;104(2):586–93.
27. Cooke KR, Hill GR, Gerbitz A, Kobzik L, Martin TR, Crawford JM, et al. Tumor necrosis factor-alpha neutralization reduces lung injury after experimental allogeneic bone marrow transplantation. Transplantation. 2000;70(2):272–9.
28. Cooke KR, Hill GR, Gerbitz A, Kobzik L, Martin TR, Crawford JM, et al. Hyporesponsiveness of donor cells to lipopolysaccharide stimulation reduces the severity of experimental idiopathic pneumonia syndrome: potential role for a gut-lung axis of inflammation. J Immunol. 2000;165(11):6612–9.
29. Zamyatina A, Heine H. Lipopolysaccharide recognition in the crossroads of TLR4 and Caspase-4/11 mediated inflammatory pathways. Front Immunol. 2020;11.
30. Clark JG, Madtes DK, Martin TR, Hackman RC, Farrand AL, Crawford SW. Idiopathic pneumonia after bone marrow transplantation: cytokine activation and lipopolysaccharide amplification in the bronchoalveolar compartment. Crit Care Med. 1999;27(9):1800–6.
31. Yanik GA, Horowitz MM, Weisdorf DJ, Logan BR, Ho VT, Soiffer RJ, et al. Randomized, double-blind, placebo-controlled trial of soluble tumor necrosis factor receptor: enbrel (etanercept) for the treatment

of idiopathic pneumonia syndrome after allogeneic stem cell transplantation: blood and marrow transplant clinical trials network protocol. Biol Blood Marrow Transplant. 2014;20(6):858–64.
32. Seo S, Renaud C, Kuypers JM, Chiu CY, Huang ML, Samayoa E, et al. Idiopathic pneumonia syndrome after hematopoietic cell transplantation: evidence of occult infectious etiologies. Blood. 2015;125(24):3789–97.
33. O'Dwyer DN, Duvall AS, Xia M, Hoffman TC, Bloye KS, Bulte CA, et al. Transbronchial biopsy in the management of pulmonary complications of hematopoietic stem cell transplantation. Bone Marrow Transplant. 2018;53(2):193–8.
34. Harris B, Lowy FD, Stover DE, Arcasoy SM. Diagnostic bronchoscopy in solid-organ and hematopoietic stem cell transplantation. Ann Am Thorac Soc. 2013;10(1):39–49.
35. Spira D, Faul C, Schaup V, Wirths S, Schulze M, Sauter A, et al. HRCT findings in idiopathic pneumonia syndrome with documentation of the disease course. Eur J Radiol. 2012;81(2):e147–52.
36. Schlatzer DM, Dazard J-E, Ewing RM, Ilchenko S, Tomcheko SE, Eid S, et al. Human biomarker discovery and predictive models for disease progression for idiopathic pneumonia syndrome following allogeneic stem cell transplantation. Mol Cell Proteomics. 2012;11(6):M111.015479–M111.
37. Seo S, Yu J, Jenkins IC, Leisenring WM, Steven-Ayers T, Kuypers JM, et al. Diagnostic and prognostic plasma biomarkers for idiopathic pneumonia syndrome after hematopoietic cell transplantation. Biol Blood Marrow Transplant. 2018;24(4):678–86.
38. Tanaka N, Kunihiro Y, Kobayashi T, Yujiri T, Kido S, Ueda K, et al. High-resolution CT findings of idiopathic pneumonia syndrome after haematopoietic stem cell transplantation: based on the updated concept of idiopathic pneumonia syndrome by the American Thoracic Society in 2011. Clin Radiol. 2016;71(10):953–9.
39. Afessa B, Tefferi A, Litzow MR, Peters SG. Outcome of diffuse alveolar hemorrhage in hematopoietic stem cell transplant recipients. Am J Respir Crit Care Med. 2002;166(10):1364–8.
40. Agustí C, Ramirez J, Picado C, Xaubet A, Carreras E, Ballester E, et al. Diffuse alveolar hemorrhage in allogeneic bone marrow transplantation. A postmortem study. Am J Respir Crit Care Med. 1995;151(4):1006–10.
41. Wu J, Fu H-X, He Y, Mo X-D, Liu X, Cai X, et al. Risk factors and outcomes of diffuse alveolar haemorrhage after allogeneic haematopoietic stem cell transplantation. Bone Marrow Transplant. 2021;56(9):2097–107.
42. Fan K, McArthur J, Morrison RR, Ghafoor S. Diffuse alveolar hemorrhage after pediatric hematopoietic stem cell transplantation. Front Oncol. 2020;10:1757.
43. Grant A, Chapman LR, Mitchell R, O'Brien TA. Engraftment syndrome following hematopoietic stem cell transplant: a review of the literature. Clin Transpl. 2020;34(6):e13875.
44. Wieruszewski PM, May HP, Peters SG, Gajic O, Hogan WJ, Dierkhising RA, et al. Characteristics and outcome of periengraftment respiratory distress syndrome after autologous hematopoietic cell transplant. Ann Am Thorac Soc. 2021;18(6):1013–9.
45. Hilbert G, Gruson D, Vargas F, Valentino R, Gbikpi-Benissan G, Dupon M, et al. Noninvasive ventilation in immunosuppressed patients with pulmonary infiltrates, fever, and acute respiratory failure. N Engl J Med. 2001;344(7):481–7.
46. Wermke M, Schiemanck S, Höffken G, Ehninger G, Bornhäuser M, Illmer T. Respiratory failure in patients undergoing allogeneic hematopoietic SCT—a randomized trial on early non-invasive ventilation based on standard care hematology wards. Bone Marrow Transplant. 2012;47(4):574–80.
47. Shen J, Hu Y, Zhao H, Xiao Z, Zhao L, Du A, et al. Risk factors of non-invasive ventilation failure in hematopoietic stem-cell transplantation patients with acute respiratory distress syndrome. Ther Adv Respir Dis. 2020;14:1753466620914220.
48. Mokart D, Granata A, Crocchiolo R, Sannini A, Chow-Chine L, Brun J-P, et al. Allogeneic hematopoietic stem cell transplantation after reduced intensity conditioning regimen: outcomes of patients admitted to intensive care unit. J Crit Care. 2015;30(5):1107–13.
49. Gristina GR, Antonelli M, Conti G, Ciarlone A, Rogante S, Rossi C, et al. Noninvasive versus invasive ventilation for acute respiratory failure in patients with hematologic malignancies: a 5-year multicenter observational survey. Crit Care Med. 2011;39(10):2232–9.
50. Tamburro RF, Cooke KR, Davies SM, Goldfarb S, Hagood JS, Srinivasan A, et al. Pulmonary complications of pediatric hematopoietic cell transplantation. A National Institutes of Health workshop summary. Ann Am Thorac Soc. 2021;18(3):381–94.
51. Pravin RR, Huang BX, Sultana R, Tan CW, Goh KJ, Chan M-Y, et al. Mortality trends of oncology and hematopoietic stem cell transplant patients supported on extracorporeal membrane oxygenation: a systematic review and meta-analysis. J Intensive Care Med. 2022;37(4):555–64.
52. Koinuma T, Nunomiya S, Wada M, Koyama K, Suzuki T. Concurrent treatment with a tumor necrosis factor-alpha inhibitor and veno-venous extracorporeal membrane oxygenation in a post-hematopoietic stem cell transplant patient with idiopathic pneumonia syndrome: a case report. J Intensive Care. 2014;2(1):48.
53. Liao WI, Tsai SH, Chiu SK. Successful use of extracorporeal membrane oxygenation in a hematopoietic stem cell transplant patient with idiopathic pneumonia syndrome. Respir Care. 2013;58(2):e6–10.
54. Rathi NK, Tanner AR, Dinh A, Dong W, Feng L, Ensor J, et al. Low-, medium- and high-dose steroids with or without aminocaproic acid in adult hematopoietic SCT patients with diffuse alveolar hemorrhage. Bone Marrow Transplant. 2015;50(3):420–6.
55. Cornell RF, Hari P, Drobyski WR. Engraftment syndrome after autologous stem cell transplanta-

tion: an update unifying the definition and management approach. Biol Blood Marrow Transplant. 2015;21(12):2061–8.
56. Capizzi S, Kumar S, Huneke N, Gertz M, Inwards D, Litzow M, et al. Peri-engraftment respiratory distress syndrome during autologous hematopoietic stem cell transplantation. Bone Marrow Transplant. 2001;27(12):1299–303.
57. Wanko SO, Broadwater G, Folz RJ, Chao NJ. Diffuse alveolar hemorrhage: retrospective review of clinical outcome in allogeneic transplant recipients treated with aminocaproic acid. Biol Blood Marrow Transplant. 2006;12(9):949–53.
58. Elinoff JM, Bagci U, Moriyama B, Dreiling JL, Foster B, Gormley NJ, et al. Recombinant human factor VIIa for alveolar hemorrhage following allogeneic stem cell transplantation. Biol Blood Marrow Transplant. 2014;20(7):969–78.
59. Simpson E, Lin Y, Stanworth S, Birchall J, Doree C, Hyde C. Recombinant factor VIIa for the prevention and treatment of bleeding in patients without haemophilia. Cochrane Database Syst Rev. 2012(3):CD005011.
60. Baker MS, Diab KJ, Carlos WG, Mathur P. Intrapulmonary recombinant factor VII as an effective treatment for diffuse alveolar Hemorrhage: a case series. J Bronchol Interv Pulmonol. 2016;23(3):255–8.
61. Heslet L, Nielsen JD, Nepper-Christensen S. Local pulmonary administration of factor VIIa (rFVIIa) in diffuse alveolar hemorrhage (DAH) - a review of a new treatment paradigm. Biologics. 2012;6:37–46.
62. Baker MS, Diab KJ, Carlos WG, Mathur P. Intrapulmonary recombinant factor VII as an effective treatment for diffuse alveolar hemorrhage: a case series. J Bronchol Interv Pulmonol. 2016;23(3):255–8.
63. Said SA, Okamoto T, Sakanoue I, Unai S, Budev M, Akindipe O, et al. Lung transplant for patient with idiopathic pneumonia syndrome. Ann Thorac Surg. 2020;110(2):e87–e9.

# Bronchiolitis Obliterans Syndrome 17

Louise Bondeelle and Anne Bergeron

## Introduction

In 1982, Roca et al. were the first to describe a patient with no previous pulmonary history who developed a progressive obstructive lung disease in the setting of skin and mucosal chronic graft-versus-host disease (GVHD) within one year after an allogeneic hematopoietic stem cell transplant (HSCT) and over the next 5 months following an acute respiratory episode, which eventually led to death from respiratory failure [1]. Lung histology showed obstruction of the small airways. The authors suggested that obliterative bronchiolitis/bronchiolitis obliterans (BO) should be included among the severe pulmonary complications of chronic GVHD (cGVHD) [1]. Since then, bronchiolitis obliterans has been recognized as the most common late-onset pulmonary complication after allogeneic HSCT and the only complication formally associated with chronic GVHD. While a histological diagnosis based on lung biopsy analysis was initially required for the diagnosis of BO, the histological criteria have been progressively replaced by respiratory functional criteria. The term bronchiolitis obliterans syndrome (BOS) now defines this pulmonary functional entity, while the term bronchiolitis obliterans (BO) defines the histological entity. Although the prognosis of this complication remains poor and there are still many unknowns about its pathophysiology and treatment [2], research in this area is active. BOS is also a dreaded complication after lung transplantation and is the most common form of graft rejection (Chronic Lung Allograft Dysfunction, CLAD). Posttransplant BOS is likely the final pathway of an uncontrolled alloimmune reaction. Post-lung transplantation BOS and post-HSCT BOS are usually compared both clinically and pathophysiologically. Nevertheless, the mode of onset and evolution of BOS, risk factors, and effects of treatments differ according to the type of transplant. If some pathophysiological mechanisms may be common, others are certainly different [2, 3]. A major issue is that lung cGVHD is part of a systemic disease, whereas CLAD is a purely pulmonary disease. These different points must make us vigilant about the translation of knowledge from one model to the next. In this chapter, we will focus on studies specifically obtained in post-HSCT BOS.

L. Bondeelle
Faculty of Medicine, University of Geneva, Geneva, Switzerland
e-mail: louise.bondeelle@unige.ch

A. Bergeron (✉)
Faculty of Medicine, University of Geneva, Geneva, Switzerland

Service de Pneumologie, Hôpitaux Universitaires de Genève, University of Geneva, Genève, Switzerland
e-mail: anne.bergeron@hcuge.ch



A. O. Soubani (ed.), *Pulmonary and Critical Care Considerations of Hematopoietic Stem Cell Transplantation*, https://doi.org/10.1007/978-3-031-28797-8_17

## Epidemiology

Epidemiological data have reported a wide range of prevalence or incidence of post-HSCT BOS depending on the study. This variability is related to several factors, including the consideration of BO and/or BOS, the biases of retrospective studies, which are in the majority, notably associated with the frequency of monitoring of pulmonary function testing (PFT), and the PFT criteria used for the diagnosis of BOS. Thus, the overall incidence of BOS varied from 2 to 26% of allogeneic HSCT recipients [4–14], being 10% at 36 months post-HSCT in the only prospective cohort [15]. The incidence was the highest in a subpopulation of patients who developed extrathoracic chronic GVHD [11, 12, 16]. BOS is usually diagnosed beyond the third month and within the first 2 years after HSCT, although it is infrequently diagnosed outside of these time frames [11–13, 15, 16]. In the only prospective cohort, BOS occurred with an observed median (IQR) time of 8.8 (2.9–19.7) months after Day 100 post-HSCT [15].

## Pathophysiology

The pathophysiology of BO is not well understood. The pathology of BO suggests that injury and inflammation of the airway epithelium and subepithelial structures lead to excessive fibroproliferation, which is due to aberrant tissue repair, including ineffective epithelial regeneration, in response to tissue injury [2]. BO is likely the result of multiple alloimmune and nonimmune epithelial aggressions, such as chemotherapy/radiotherapy conditioning, gastroesophageal reflux, or respiratory pathogens, notably community-acquired viruses. It was suggested that single nucleotide polymorphisms (SNPs) of genes that affect innate immunity pathways, such as bactericidal/permeability-increasing proteins or NOD2/CARD15, may result in an uncontrolled innate immune response in the recipient and lead to BO [17, 18].

Macrophages have been shown to be involved in the development of BO. In one mouse model, donor bone marrow was the source of CSF-1R$^{+}$ tissue-resident macrophages that were essential for the development of BO in dependence on both IL-17 and CSF-1/CSF-1R [19]. In human lung tissue of patients with post-HSCT BO, some data have suggested that donor-derived M1 macrophages may be involved in the pathogenesis of the early-stage region of BOS, whereas M2 macrophage polarization infiltrating late-stage regions of BOS might be involved in fibrosis [20].

B-cell signaling may also have a central role in the development of BOS. In a mouse model, donor B-cell alloantibody deposition and germinal center formation were shown to be required for the development of bronchiolitis obliterans [21]. In addition, high levels of CD19 + CD21$^{low}$ B cells and soluble B-cell-activating factor were found to be specific to HSCT recipients with BOS [22].

## Risk Factors

The concurrent presence of chronic extrathoracic GVHD and BOS found in all retrospective studies has led to the consideration of BOS as pulmonary cGVHD. The only prospective cohort published to date has clarified that the occurrence of chronic extrathoracic GVHD is also predictive of BOS [15].

In addition to cGVHD, many other factors associated with BOS have been proposed. Among these risk factors, smoking history and older age of the recipient, sex matching of donor/recipient, cytomegalovirus matching of donor/recipient, acute GVHD, and transplantation procedure (including both the characteristics of conditioning regimen and the stem cell source) were associated with BOS in some studies [7, 8, 12, 16, 23–25]. Specifically, with regard to the HSCT procedure, a busulfan-based conditioning regimen, unrelated transplants, and a peripheral blood stem cell source were associated with BOS [12, 24, 25]. Post-HSCT community-acquired respiratory virus-related infections were also identified as triggers for BOS [26, 27]. Different parameters of pretransplant lung function were also predictive of BOS in some retrospective studies but not in others. For example, while some studies found no association with pretransplant maximal expiratory flow at 50% and 25% of forced vital capacity <70% predicted [28], others found that pretransplant forced expiratory flow between 25% and 75% of maximum ($FEF_{25-75}$) was associated with an increased risk of BOS [29]. More interestingly, the trajectory of lung function in the first months after transplantation seemed to predict the occurrence of BOS. Thus, both an early decline in forced expiratory volume in one second (FEV1) and/or in FEF25–75 were recently associated with the development of BOS [10, 29].

The identification of these risk factors is not homogeneous in the different studies. The need to include a sufficient number of patients with BOS in retrospective studies for analysis requires the selection of a cohort of transplant patients over a long period of time during which transplant practices have changed, including stem cell sources and conditioning regimens, as well as the profile of transplant patients who notably become older over time [30]. Overall, these factors have influenced the incidence of chronic GVHD and, thus, probably that of BOS.

In the ALLOPULM prospective cohort, the use of peripheral blood stem cells and bronchial abnormalities on the computed tomography (CT) scan (including centrilobular micronodules, tree-in-bud pattern, and bronchial thickening) at Day 100 post-HSCT, as well as the occurrence of a lower respiratory tract infection between HSCT, and Day 100 and a 10% FEV1 decline from baseline to Day 100, were found to be predictive factors for BOS [15].

Conversely, other transplant characteristics, such as T-cell depletion with antithymocyte globulin administration or cord blood as the stem cell source, were identified as protective factors against BOS [14, 23, 25, 31].

## Diagnostic Criteria

Clinical signs of BOS are nonspecific and may include dyspnea and/or cough, wheezing, or repeated lung infections, or they may be diagnosed incidentally. Indeed, BOS often occurs in patients whose activity is limited by posttransplant fatigue and/or disabling extrathoracic GVHD, which limits the evaluation of exertional dyspnea. Lung auscultation may be normal or reveal wheezing, subcrepitant, or squeaks suggestive of a small airway obstruction.

The definitive diagnosis of BO is based on lung biopsy analysis. Transbronchial biopsies are not sensitive enough for the diagnosis of BO; thus, a surgical lung biopsy is usually necessary to identify the pathologic features of BO. These features include an obliterative bronchiolitis characterized by thickening of the bronchiolar wall via inflammatory fibrosis; this thickening is located between the epithelium and the smooth muscle, narrowing the airway lumen [2, 32] (Fig. 17.1).

Given the invasiveness of surgical lung biopsy, the diagnosis of BOS based on PFT is now endorsed [33–35] (Fig. 17.1). However, in addition to obliterative bronchiolitis, a spectrum of histological bronchiolar lesions has been described in patients with BOS, including the presence of more or less inflammation with or without fibrosis and bronchiolectasis [36, 37]. It is currently unknown whether these different histological aspects result from different pathophysiological mechanisms or if they are BO lesions at different stages.

Patients may have subclinical changes in pulmonary function before a diagnosis of BOS is made. Therefore, close PFT monitoring is necessary for the early diagnosis of BOS. Although the optimal frequency of PFT monitoring is not clearly defined, the NIH conference in 2015 proposed monitoring PFTs with at least limited spirometry every 3 months during the first 1 to 2 years, followed by additional PFTs in the setting of unexplained irreversible decline of FEV1 > 10% or active extrathoracic cGVHD [38]. However, real-world rates of PFT monitoring in HSCT recipients are far lower than recommended [39]. Even if PFTs are performed regularly, it is very difficult to capture the onset of respiratory function decline, which is often abrupt. To be more efficient, the use of handheld home spirometry is being evaluated. If the corre-

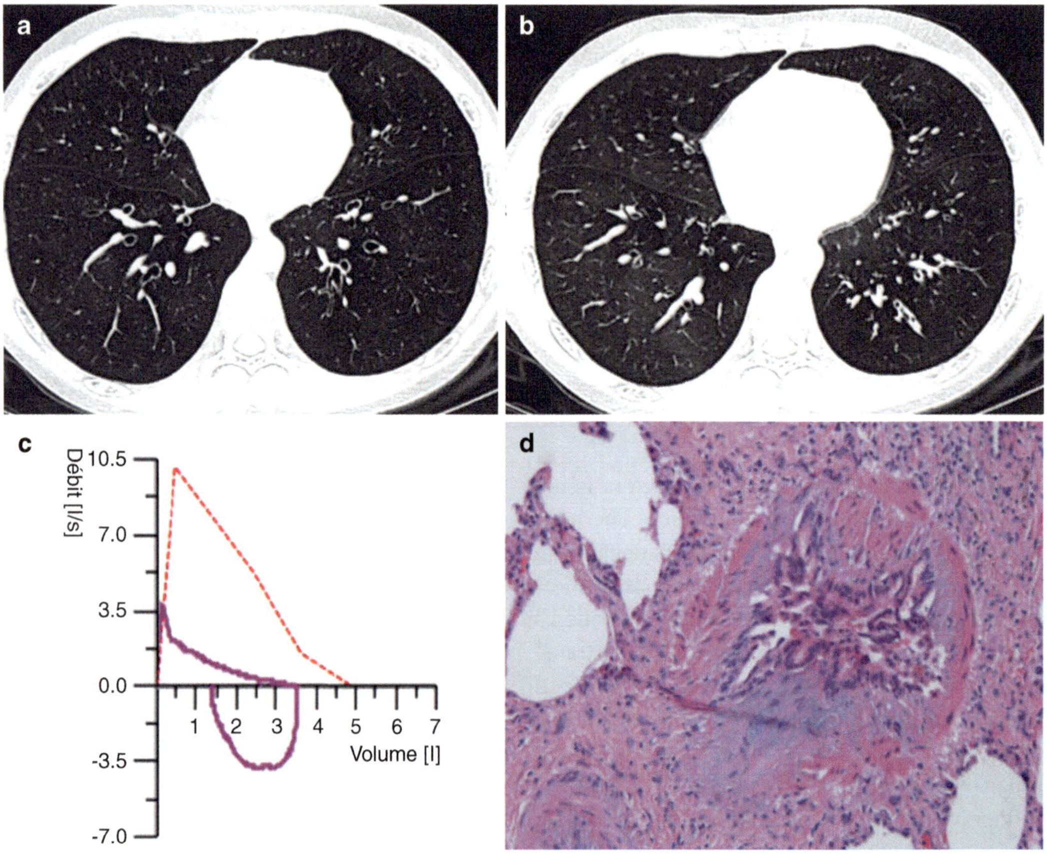


**Fig. 17.1** Diagnosis of bronchiolitis obliterans in allogeneic HSCT recipients. Inspiratory chest CT scan (**a**) showing heterogeneous lung parenchyma and air trapping on forced expiration (**b**). Flow-volume loop showing a severe obstructive ventilatory disorder (**c**). Lung biopsy showing constrictive bronchiolitis (**d**). (Courtesy Dr. V. Meignin)

lation with conventional spirometry is good, the problem of patient adherence remains, and the usefulness of this practice, which requires a specific health organization to monitor the data with close collaboration between HSCT physicians and pulmonologists, must be demonstrated in a large HSCT recipient population [40].

Thus, a diagnosis of BOS relies mainly on post-HSCT PFT demonstrating new onset airflow obstruction. The PFT criteria defining BOS have evolved since the first NIH consensus conference in 2005 [41], and the currently used criteria were published in 2015 [33]. A diagnosis of BOS requires at least one extrathoracic manifestation of chronic GVHD and a workup to rule out a respiratory infection. The functional diagnosis criteria for BOS are as follows [33]: FEV1/vital capacity (VC) < 0.7 or the fifth percentile of predicted (either forced VC or slow VC, whichever is greater), with an FEV1 < 75% of predicted with ≥10% decline over less than 2 years. FEV1 should not be corrected to >75% of that predicted with albuterol, and the patient must present with one of the two supporting features of BOS:

(a) Evidence of air trapping by PFTs as follows: residual volume (RV) > 120% of predicted or an RV/total lung capacity (TLC) ratio elevated outside the 90% confidence interval, or.
(b) Evidence of either air trapping, as determined by expiratory CT or small airway thickening, or bronchiectasis, as determined by high-resolution chest CT.

However, some studies analyzing PFTs of patients with biopsy-proven BO showed that these patients did not have all of the PFT diagnostic criteria as defined above [36, 42]. Indeed, these definitions mainly rely on the decrease in the FEV1/VC ratio, whereas a significant proportion of patients with BOS have a normal FEV1/VC ratio due to a concomitant decrease in FEV1 and VC [13, 15]; this was recently described as PRISm (preserved ratio impaired spirometry) in patients with chronic obstructive pulmonary disease (COPD) [43]. This PFT profile was recently identified in the 2020 Highly morbid forms report of the National Institutes of Health Consensus Development Project on Criteria for Clinical Trials in Chronic Graft-versus-Host Disease [35]. In the case of PRISm, it is essential to complete the measurement of all lung volumes to properly phenotype the ventilatory disorder as BOS and to rule out a restrictive ventilatory disorder in the case of a decrease in TLC, which would require different management.

Making an early diagnosis of BOS is the greatest challenge for reversing lung impairment and improving the morbidity and mortality of BOS. Unfortunately, despite the evolution of PFT criteria, it is likely that a decrease in the FEV1/VC ratio already reflects an advanced fixed stage of BOS, which includes the involvement of numerous bronchioles with irreversible fibrosis. Therefore, these criteria are likely inaccurate for diagnosing early forms of the disease. While most patients characterized by PRISm eventually develop a low FEV1/VC ratio in their follow-up [15], whether this PFT profile reflects an early stage of BOS should be investigated. However, rather than relying on a single post-HSCT lung function value measured at a given time, various data suggest the need to consider the evolution of post-HSCT lung function parameters in comparison with pretransplant values for diagnosing early BOS [9, 10, 15, 29, 44, 45].

In addition to PFT abnormalities, chest high-resolution CT scan features of airway disease as determined by centrilobular micronodules, bronchial wall thickening, bronchiectasis, or air trapping are part of the NIH diagnostic criteria for BOS [35] (Fig. 17.1). However, several points should be emphasized regarding the positioning of the chest CT scan in the diagnostic strategy of BOS. Contrary to PFT monitoring, which is cost-effective and safe, CT scans cannot be repeated in a systematic, sequential way. Rather, they are only performed when clinical or PFT abnormalities are found. A chest CT alone cannot make the diagnosis of BOS. The CT scan is indisputably indicated to eliminate a differential diagnosis of BOS at the time an alteration of PFT is diagnosed during the post-HSCT follow-up. Otherwise, the presence of bronchial abnormalities only confirms the PFT diagnosis of BOS without providing any further information [46]. It is still further recommended to perform expiratory cuts to facilitate the identification of air trapping [35]. However, the development of minimum-intensity projections (MinIP) applied to routine inspiratory cuts that allow the identification of mosaic attenuation and thus air trapping should make us reconsider this recommendation to protect patients from unnecessary irradiation [47]. It should also be noted that, in the ALLOPULM cohort, 23% and 34% of patients had significant air trapping before transplantation and at 100 days post-HSCT, respectively; the presence of this air trapping was not predictive of the occurrence of BOS. Conversely, the presence of bronchial abnormalities, i.e., centrilobular micronodules, tree-in-bud pattern, and bronchial thickening, 100 days after HSCT was associated with the subsequent occurrence of BOS [15]. New imaging techniques are being evaluated to diagnose BOS early. Nevertheless, they are still in the field of research. If these techniques, such as parametric response mapping, demonstrate their ability to diagnose BOS similarly to PFTs or qualitative radiologist assessment of CT scans, their positioning to diagnose BOS before PFTs and their routine superiority to chest CT scans will need to be demonstrated [48, 49].

## Management and Outcome

Regardless of the treatment instituted, the mortality of BOS is approximately 50% at 5 years in the most recent series [11, 13, 16, 50]. Au et al. found that BOS conferred a 1.6-fold increase in the risk for mortality after diagnosis [11]. The prognosis of BOS is even worse if the onset is early after HSCT, particularly within the first year [8, 13, 16, 51]. BOS-related deaths are frequently caused by respiratory failure and/or infection resulting from increased immunosuppression. The prognoses of BOS diagnosed with the 2015 NIH criteria and those of PRISm were found to be similar [13]. Lymphocytic bronchiolitis has a better prognosis than obliterative bronchiolitis [36].

Beyond the increased mortality in the HSCT recipient population, BOS is also associated with significant morbidity and increased health care requirements [52]. Although it is difficult to be definitive about the natural history of BOS due to the lack of continuous PFT monitoring, the $FEV_1$ trajectory in patients with BOS usually follows a more or less rapid and severe $FEV_1$ decline in the 6 months prior to diagnosis, followed by $FEV_1$ stabilization after diagnosis [15, 51, 53]. Once the BOS is installed, no means to restore respiratory function is currently available.

## Treatment

Because BOS is considered pulmonary cGVHD, systemic corticosteroids have been the standard treatment despite the lack of evidence for their efficacy and the numerous side effects [54]. Otherwise, a number of studies have assessed the effect of various drugs on overall cGVHD, but it is often difficult to find data focused on PFT parameters in these publications [55–65]. The definition of BOS response to treatment used by the NIH guidelines, which relies on a global modification of FEV1, lacks precision to assess the impact of treatment on lung function [66]. Nevertheless, in studies evaluating the overall effect of a treatment on overall cGVHD, lung cGVHD is the least accessible to treatment compared to cGVHD in other organs, with a poor effect regardless of the drug tested [59–62, 64]. This further confirms that the diagnostic criteria for BOS likely reflect a fixed process with poor accessibility to any immunosuppressive therapy.

Evidence-based for specific BOS treatment is limited (Table 17.1). Five prospective studies are available; of these, only two were randomized placebo-controlled studies. One reported the lack of efficacy of azithromycin on both FEV1 and the clinical symptoms in patients with late BOS [67], and the other reported the significant efficacy of inhaled budesonide/formoterol on FEV1 in patients with newly diagnosed moderate to severe BOS [69]. It was striking that, in the latter study, 25% of the patients in the placebo group had an improvement of 200 mL and 12% in FEV1, which provided insights into the natural course of the disease and reinforced the need for placebo-controlled studies [69]. The three other studies were open-label, single-arm studies. One study suggested a corticosteroid-sparing effect of the combination of fluticasone, azithromycin, and montelukast (FAM) in the treatment of new-onset BOS with no significant change in FEV1 [86]. Another study showed that a 6-month treatment with montelukast was associated with stable FEV1 in patients diagnosed with moderate to severe BOS, a median of 2 years before study enrollment [81]. Finally, the third study found that a 12-month course of pirfenidone was potentially efficacious in stabilizing the PFT decline in moderate to severe BOS diagnosed at a median of 3 years before inclusion in the trial [83].

In addition to these prospective studies, numerous retrospective studies with all the biases that are associated with this study design have reported the effect of different drugs on BOS (Table 17.1). The major issue in assessing the effect of a treatment on BOS lies in the choice of endpoints. Most of the studies conclude treatment efficacy when the FEV1 stabilizes. The recent better understanding of the natural course of BOS, which usually includes a plateau phase of FEV1 after a rapid decline, should provide a more critical perspective when reviewing these results to determine the actual effect of the intervention [15, 51]. Considering a significant improvement in FEV1 [69] or a change in the trajectory of FEV1 decline before and after the intervention (with the limitation of the timing of PFT performed before study entry), as suggested by the NIH consensus and that has been investigated in the most recent studies, is probably more appropriate than considering stabilization of FEV1 over the study period [66, 81, 83].

**Table 17.1** Clinical studies focused on post-HSCT BOS treatment strategies

| Treatment | Study design | Results | Reference |
|---|---|---|---|
| Alvelestat (MPH966), oral neutrophil elastase inhibitor | Prospective, open-label<br>(*n* = 34) | Ongoing | NCT02669251 |
| Azithromycin | Randomized, double-blinded, placebo-controlled<br>Case series | No change in FEV1<br>FEV1 improvement in 8/8 patients | Lam et al. [67]<br>Khalid et al. [68] |
| Bortezomib | Phase 2<br>Prospective, open-label<br>(*n* = 17) *The study was closed before the accrual goal of 20 evaluable patients was reached due to slow accrual* | Pending | NCT01163786 |
| Budesonide/formoterol | Retrospective<br>Randomized, double-blinded, placebo-controlled | FEV1 improvement in 7/7 patients<br>FEV1 improvement | Bergeron et al. [13]<br>Bergeron et al. [69] |
| Inhaled cyclosporine A | Prospective, open-label<br>(*n* = 10)<br>Prospective, open-labelq<br>(*n* = 8)<br>Phase II prospective, multicenter, single-blind, randomized | 5/10 FEV1 improvement, including 3 decrease in steroids<br>3/8 FEV1 improvement and 1/8 FEV1 stabilization<br>Ongoing | Purev et al. [70]<br>Gormley et al. [71]<br>*Extension Study: NCT01273207*<br>NCT04107675<br>BOSTON-4 |
| Extracorporeal photopheresis | Case series<br>Case series<br>Case series<br>Case control | PFT stabilization in 6/9 patients<br>FEV1 improvement in 10/12 patients<br>FEV1 stabilization at 3 months in 7/8 patients; FEV1 decline in 6/8 at 1 year<br>No change in FEV1; improvement in survival | Lucid et al. [72]<br>Del Fante et al. [73]<br>Brownback et al. [74]<br>Hefazi et al. [75] |
| Fluticasone | Retrospective<br>(*n* = 17) | FEV1 stabilization | Bashoura et al. [76] |
| High-dose steroids | Case series | FEV1 stabilization in 5/5 patients | Ratjen et al. [77] |
| | Case series | FEV1 improvement in 4/12 patients | Ehud Even-Or et al. [78] |
| Imatinib | Prospective, open-label | FEV1 improvement in 1/9 patients | Stadler et al. [79] |
| | Case series | FEV1 stabilization in 2/2 | Watanabe et al. |
| | Retrospective pediatric study<br>(*n* = 13) | FEV1 improvement in 10/13 | Faraci et al. [80] |
| Interferon gamma | Prospective open-label | Ongoing | NCT01639261 |
| Itacitinib, Selective JAK 1 Inhibitor | Phase I trial | Ongoing | NCT04239989 |
| Montelukast | Prospective, open-label<br>(*n* = 25) | 23/25 stability or improvement (<15% FEV1 decline) | Williams et al. [81] |

(continued)

**Table 17.1** (continued)

| Treatment | Study design | Results | Reference |
|---|---|---|---|
| Nintedanib | Case report<br>Multicenter Phase II Trial<br>Prospective, open-label<br>(*n* = 20) | FEV1 and FVC improvement<br>Ongoing | Tang et al. [82]<br>NCT03805477 |
| Pirfenidone | Phase 1<br>(*n* = 22) | Tolerability 59%<br>Stabilization of PFT and increase in PROs | Matthaiou et al. [83] |
| Rituximab | Case series | No response in 3/3 patients | Lorillon et al. [84] |
| | Case series | FEV1 improvement in 7/13 patients | Brownback et al. [74] |
| Ruxolitinib, JAK2 inhibitor | Retrospective<br>(*n* = 30)<br>Prospective, open-label<br>(*n* = 50)<br>Prospective, open-label<br>(*n* = 50)<br>Prospective, open-label<br>(*n* = 40) | FEV1 stabilization<br>Start in June 2022<br>Ongoing<br>Ongoing | Zhao et al. [85]<br>NCT05413356<br>NCT03674047<br>NCT04908735 |
| *Combination* | | | |
| Fluticasone plus azithromycin plus montelukast | Case control<br>(*n* = 8 cases)<br>Prospective open-label<br>(*n* = 36) | FEV1 stabilization<br>FEV1 stabilization despite reduction in steroids | Norman et al. [54]<br>Williams et al. [86] |
| Budesonide/formoterol plus N-acetylcysteine plus montelukast | Retrospective<br>(*n* = 61) | FEV1 improvement | Kim et al. [87] |
| Inhaled tiotropium plus Budesonide/formoterol | Retrospective<br>(*n* = 86) | FEV1 improvement in 41% of patients | Lim et al. [88] |
| *Non drug-related treatment* | | | |
| Rehabilitation | Case series | exercise tolerance and dyspnea improvement | Choi et al. [89] |
| Mesenchymal stem cells | Multicenter prospective cohort study | FEV1 improvement or steroid sparing in 35/49 patients | Chen et al. [90] |

*BOS* bronchiolitis obliterans syndrome, *FEV1* forced expiratory volume in 1 second, *HSTC* hematopoietic stem cell transplantation, *LONIPCs* late-onset noninfectious pulmonary complications, *LTx* lung transplantation, *PFT* pulmonary function test, *PROs* patient-reported outcomes

Currently, the development of a more effective treatment strategy for BOS is needed and should focus on patients with early-stage BOS, who are probably the most responsive to treatment. In addition to these limited treatment options, pulmonary rehabilitation may be an important adjunctive therapy for improving patients' quality of life [89].

Finally, lung transplantation has become a reasonable therapeutic option for selected allogeneic HSCT recipients with post-BOS chronic respiratory failure [91]. The selection criteria for consideration of a lung transplant remain to be better defined. Particular attention should be given to the risk of severe infections after lung transplantation, which seems to be higher in HSCT recipients than in other patient populations [92].

## BOS Prophylaxis

Given the current poor prognosis for BOS and the limited treatment options, prophylactic strategies should be investigated. In a double-blind placebo-controlled trial, administration of prophylactic azithromycin given for 2 years from the time of conditioning regimen resulted in worse airflow decline–free survival than placebo due to an increase in hematological relapse [93]; these findings required an early trial termination, and it has been the subject of an alert by the US and European drug agencies. Furthermore, azithromycin did not prevent the occurrence of BOS [93]. These results raised the question of a potentially harmful effect of azithromycin in the treatment of established BOS and, thus, later in the course of HSCT. A two-center exposed/unexposed study design actually found a higher prevalence of subsequent solid cancers but not hematological relapse in patients who received azithromycin for BOS compared to BOS not treated with azithromycin [94]. Another retrospective study found an association between azithromycin administration late after HSCT and hematologic relapse, but only in patients who received antithymocyte globulin [95]. In light of these data, if it is no longer acceptable to administer long-term azithromycin in the early period of HSCT, the use of azithromycin later for BOS must be carefully weighed against the benefit-risk balance, keeping in mind the low level of evidence of its efficacy for BOS.

## Conclusion

Although BOS has been identified for many years as pulmonary cGVHD, its prognosis has changed little. BOS remains the least sensitive form of GVHD to the various treatments tested. Recent data have shown that BOS is in fact a grouping of different entities and that the diagnostic criteria currently used must evolve to better detect the early phase of BOS. Current research is active in this field, which will likely be the key to better adapting treatments and improving the respiratory function of these patients. A better understanding of the pathophysiology of BOS should also open new therapeutic perspectives.

## References


1. Roca J, Grañeña A, Rodriguez-Roisin R, Alvarez P, Agusti-Vidal A, Rozman C. Fatal airway disease in an adult with chronic graft-versus-host disease. Thorax. 1982;37(1):77–8.
2. Barker AF, Bergeron A, Rom WN, Hertz MI. Obliterative bronchiolitis. N Engl J Med. 2014;370(19):1820–8.
3. Bos S, Beeckmans H, Vanstapel A, Sacreas A, Geudens V, Willems L, et al. Pulmonary graft-versus-host disease and chronic lung allograft dysfunction: two sides of the same coin? Lancet Respir Med. 2022;10:796.
4. Solh M, Arat M, Cao Q, Majhail NS, Weisdorf D. Late-onset noninfectious pulmonary complications in adult allogeneic hematopoietic cell transplant recipients. Transplantation. 2011;91(7):798–803.
5. Clark JG, Crawford SW, Madtes DK, Sullivan KM. Obstructive lung disease after allogeneic marrow transplantation. Clinical presentation and course. Ann Intern Med. 1989;111(5):368–76.
6. Chan CK, Hyland RH, Hutcheon MA, Minden MD, Alexander MA, Kossakowska AE, et al. Small-airways disease in recipients of allogeneic bone marrow transplants. An analysis of 11 cases and a review of the literature. Medicine (Baltimore). 1987;66(5):327–40.
7. Marras TK, Szalai JP, Chan CK, Lipton JH, Messner HA, Laupacis A. Pulmonary function abnormalities after allogeneic marrow transplantation: a systematic review and assessment of an existing predictive instrument. Bone Marrow Transplant. 2002;30(9):599–607.
8. Dudek AZ, Mahaseth H, DeFor TE, Weisdorf DJ. Bronchiolitis obliterans in chronic graft-versus-host disease: analysis of risk factors and treatment outcomes. Biol Blood Marrow Transplant. 2003;9(10):657–66.
9. Chien JW, Martin PJ, Gooley TA, Flowers ME, Heckbert SR, Nichols WG, et al. Airflow obstruction after myeloablative allogeneic hematopoietic stem cell transplantation. Am J Respir Crit Care Med. 2003;168(2):208–14.
10. Abedin S, Yanik GA, Braun T, Pawarode A, Magenau J, Goldstein SC, et al. Predictive value of bronchiolitis obliterans syndrome stage 0p in chronic graft-versus-host disease of the lung. Biol Blood Marrow Transplant. 2015;21(6):1127–31.
11. Au BK, Au MA, Chien JW. Bronchiolitis obliterans syndrome epidemiology after allogeneic hematopoietic cell transplantation. Biol Blood Marrow Transplant. 2011;17(7):1072–8.
12. Ditschkowski M, Elmaagacli AH, Koldehoff M, Gromke T, Trenschel R, Beelen DW. Bronchiolitis obliterans after allogeneic hematopoietic SCT: further insight—new perspectives? Bone Marrow Transplant. 2013;48(9):1224–9.
13. Bergeron A, Godet C, Chevret S, Lorillon G, Peffault de Latour R, de Revel T, et al. Bronchiolitis obliterans syndrome after allogeneic hematopoietic SCT:

phenotypes and prognosis. Bone Marrow Transplant. 2013;48(6):819–24.
14. Duque-Afonso J, Ihorst G, Wäsch R, Bertz H, Müller-Quernheim J, Finke J, et al. Identification of risk factors for bronchiolitis obliterans syndrome after reduced toxicity conditioning before hematopoietic cell transplantation. Bone Marrow Transplant. 2013;48(8):1098–103.
15. Bergeron A, Chevret S, Peffault de Latour R, Chagnon K, de Margerie-Mellon C, Rivière F, et al. Noninfectious lung complications after allogeneic haematopoietic stem cell transplantation. Eur Respir J. 2018;51(5):1702617.
16. Vieira AG, Funke VA, Nunes EC, Frare R, Pasquini R. Bronchiolitis obliterans in patients undergoing allogeneic hematopoietic SCT. Bone Marrow Transplant. 2014;49(6):812–7.
17. Touihri M, Torjeman L, Kaabi H, Chabaane M, Othman TB, Hmida S. Bronchiolitis obliterans after allogeneic hematopoietic stem cell transplantation: the effect of NOD2/CARD15 mutations in a Tunisian population. Hum Immunol. 2019;80(3):163–8.
18. Chien JW, Zhao LP, Hansen JA, Fan WH, Parimon T, Clark JG. Genetic variation in bactericidal/permeability-increasing protein influences the risk of developing rapid airflow decline after hematopoietic cell transplantation. Blood. 2006;107(5):2200–7.
19. Alexander KA, Flynn R, Lineburg KE, Kuns RD, Teal BE, Olver SD, et al. CSF-1-dependant donor-derived macrophages mediate chronic graft-versus-host disease. J Clin Invest. 2014;124(10):4266–80.
20. Kuroi T, Fujii N, Ichimura K, Seike K, Yamamoto A, Kambara Y, et al. Characterization of localized macrophages in bronchiolitis obliterans after allogeneic hematopoietic cell transplantation. Int J Hematol. 2021;114(6):701–8.
21. Flynn R, Du J, Veenstra RG, Reichenbach DK, Panoskaltsis-Mortari A, Taylor PA, et al. Increased T follicular helper cells and germinal center B cells are required for cGVHD and bronchiolitis obliterans. Blood. 2014;123(25):3988–98.
22. Kuzmina Z, Krenn K, Petkov V, Körmöczi U, Weigl R, Rottal A, et al. CD19(+)CD21(low) B cells and patients at risk for NIH-defined chronic graft-versus-host disease with bronchiolitis obliterans syndrome. Blood. 2013;121(10):1886–95.
23. Nakasone H, Kanda J, Yano S, Atsuta Y, Ago H, Fukuda T, et al. A case-control study of bronchiolitis obliterans syndrome following allogeneic hematopoietic stem cell transplantation. Transpl Int. 2013;26(6):631–9.
24. Santo Tomas LH, Loberiza FR Jr, Klein JP, Layde PM, Lipchik RJ, Rizzo JD, et al. Risk factors for bronchiolitis obliterans in allogeneic hematopoietic stem-cell transplantation for leukemia. Chest. 2005;128(1):153–61.
25. Gazourian L, Rogers AJ, Ibanga R, Weinhouse GL, Pinto-Plata V, Ritz J, et al. Factors associated with bronchiolitis obliterans syndrome and chronic graft-versus-host disease after allogeneic hematopoietic cell transplantation. Am J Hematol. 2014;89(4):404–9.
26. Erard V, Chien JW, Kim HW, Nichols WG, Flowers ME, Martin PJ, et al. Airflow decline after myeloablative allogeneic hematopoietic cell transplantation: the role of community respiratory viruses. J Infect Dis. 2006;193(12):1619–25.
27. Sheshadri A, Chemaly RF, Alousi AM, Shah PK, Rondon G, Bashoura L, et al. Pulmonary impairment after respiratory viral infections is associated with high mortality in allogeneic hematopoietic cell transplant recipients. Biol Blood Marrow Transplant. 2019;25(4):800–9.
28. Scheidl S, Zinke-Cerwenka W, Flick H, Gaal S, Avian A, Greinix H, et al. Whole-body lung function test-derived outcome predictors in allogeneic stem cell transplantation. Biol Blood Marrow Transplant. 2019;25(1):129–36.
29. Jamani K, He Q, Liu Y, Davis C, Hubbard J, Schoch G, et al. Early post-transplantation spirometry is associated with the development of bronchiolitis obliterans syndrome after allogeneic hematopoietic cell transplantation. Biol Blood Marrow Transplant. 2020;26(5):943–8.
30. Snowden JA, Sánchez-Ortega I, Corbacioglu S, Basak GW, Chabannon C, de la Camara R, et al. Indications for haematopoietic cell transplantation for haematological diseases, solid tumours and immune disorders: current practice in Europe, 2022. Bone Marrow Transplant. 2022;57:1217–39.
31. Dirou S, Malard F, Chambellan A, Chevallier P, Germaud P, Guillaume T, et al. Stable long-term pulmonary function after fludarabine, antithymocyte globulin and i.v. BU for reduced-intensity conditioning allogeneic SCT. Bone Marrow Transplant. 2014;49(5):622–7.
32. Yousem SA. The histological spectrum of pulmonary graft-versus-host disease in bone marrow transplant recipients. Hum Pathol. 1995;26(6):668–75.
33. Jagasia MH, Greinix HT, Arora M, Williams KM, Wolff D, Cowen EW, et al. National Institutes of Health Consensus Development Project on Criteria for Clinical Trials in Chronic Graft-versus-Host Disease: I. The 2014 Diagnosis and Staging Working Group report. Biol Blood Marrow Transplant. 2015;21(3):389–401.e1.
34. Shulman HM, Cardona DM, Greenson JK, Hingorani S, Horn T, Huber E, et al. NIH Consensus development project on criteria for clinical trials in chronic graft-versus-host disease: II. The 2014 Pathology Working Group Report. Biol Blood Marrow Transplant. 2015;21(4):589–603.
35. Wolff D, Radojcic V, Lafyatis R, Cinar R, Rosenstein RK, Cowen EW, et al. National Institutes of Health Consensus Development Project on Criteria for Clinical Trials in Chronic Graft-versus-Host Disease: IV. The 2020 Highly morbid forms report. Transplant Cell Ther. 2021;27(10):817–35.
36. Holbro A, Lehmann T, Girsberger S, Stern M, Gambazzi F, Lardinois D, et al. Lung histology predicts outcome of bronchiolitis obliterans syndrome after hematopoietic stem cell transplantation. Biol Blood Marrow Transplant. 2013;19(6):973–80.

37. Meignin V, Thivolet-Bejui F, Kambouchner M, Hussenet C, Bondeelle L, Mitchell A, et al. Lung histopathology of non-infectious pulmonary complications after allogeneic haematopoietic stem cell transplantation. Histopathology. 2018;73(5):832–42.
38. Carpenter PA, Kitko CL, Elad S, Flowers ME, Gea-Banacloche JC, Halter JP, et al. National Institutes of Health Consensus Development Project on Criteria for Clinical Trials in Chronic Graft-versus-Host Disease: V. The 2014 Ancillary Therapy and Supportive Care Working Group Report. Biol Blood Marrow Transplant. 2015;21(7):1167–87.
39. Sheshadri A, Sacks NC, Healey BE, Raza S, Boerner G, Huang HJ. Lung function monitoring after lung transplantation and allogeneic hematopoietic stem cell transplantation. Clin Ther. 2022;44:755.
40. Turner J, He Q, Baker K, Chung L, Lazarevic-Fogelquist A, Bethune D, et al. Home spirometry telemonitoring for early detection of bronchiolitis obliterans syndrome in patients with chronic graft-versus-host disease. Transplant Cell Ther. 2021;27(7):616.e1–6.
41. Filipovich AH, Weisdorf D, Pavletic S, Socie G, Wingard JR, Lee SJ, et al. National Institutes of Health consensus development project on criteria for clinical trials in chronic graft-versus-host disease: I. Diagnosis and staging working group report. Biol Blood Marrow Transplant. 2005;11(12):945–56.
42. Uhlving HH, Andersen CB, Christensen IJ, Gormsen M, Pedersen KD, Buchvald F, et al. Biopsy-verified bronchiolitis obliterans and other noninfectious lung pathologies after allogeneic hematopoietic stem cell transplantation. Biol Blood Marrow Transplant. 2015;21(3):531–8.
43. Wan ES, Balte P, Schwartz JE, Bhatt SP, Cassano PA, Couper D, et al. Association between preserved ratio impaired spirometry and clinical outcomes in US adults. JAMA. 2021;326(22):2287–98.
44. Thompson PA, Lim A, Panek-Hudson Y, Tacey M, Hijazi R, Ng AP, et al. Screening with spirometry is a useful predictor of later development of noninfectious pulmonary syndromes in patients undergoing allogeneic stem cell transplantation. Biol Blood Marrow Transplant. 2014;20(6):781–6.
45. Peha M. In: Med AJRC, editor. Detection of FEV1 decline preceding bronchiolitis obliterans syndrome diagnosis in allogeneic hematopoietic stem cell transplant recipients. San Francisco: ATS; 2022.
46. Myrdal OH, Aaløkken TM, Diep PP, Ruud E, Brinch L, Fosså K, et al. Late-onset, noninfectious pulmonary complications following allogeneic hematopoietic stem cell transplantation: a nationwide cohort study of long-term survivors. Respiration. 2022;101(6):544–52.
47. Zompatori M, Fasano L, Fabbri M, Maraldi F, Carvelli P, Laporta T, et al. Assessment of the severity of pulmonary emphysema by computed tomography. Monaldi Arch Chest Dis. 1997;52(2):147–54.
48. Sharifi H, Guenther ZD, Leung ANC, Johnston L, Lai YK, Hsu JL, et al. Head-to-head comparison of qualitative radiologist assessment with automated quantitative computed tomography analysis for bronchiolitis obliterans syndrome after hematopoietic cell transplantation. J Thorac Imaging. 2022;37(2):109–16.
49. Cheng GS, Selwa KE, Hatt C, Ram S, Fortuna AB, Guerriero M, et al. Multicenter evaluation of parametric response mapping as an indicator of bronchiolitis obliterans syndrome after hematopoietic stem cell transplantation. Am J Transplant. 2020;20(8):2198–205.
50. Pham J, Rangaswamy J, Avery S, Borg B, Martin C, Munsif M, et al. Updated prevalence, predictors and treatment outcomes for bronchiolitis obliterans syndrome after allogeneic stem cell transplantation. Respir Med. 2020;177:106286.
51. Cheng GS, Storer B, Chien JW, Jagasia M, Hubbard JJ, Burns L, et al. Lung function trajectory in bronchiolitis obliterans syndrome after allogeneic hematopoietic cell transplant. Ann Am Thorac Soc. 2016;13(11):1932–9.
52. Sacks NC, Healey BE, Raza S, Cyr PL, Boerner G, Sheshadri A. The economic burden of NIPC and BOS following allogeneic HSCT in patients with commercial insurance in the United States. Blood Adv. 2022;6(5):1566–76.
53. Kwok WC, Liang BM, Lui MMS, Tam TCC, Sim JPY, Tse EWC, et al. Rapid versus gradual lung function decline in bronchiolitis obliterans syndrome after haematopoietic stem cell transplantation is associated with survival outcome. Respirology. 2019;24(5):459–66.
54. Norman BC, Jacobsohn DA, Williams KM, Au BK, Au MA, Lee SJ, et al. Fluticasone, azithromycin and montelukast therapy in reducing corticosteroid exposure in bronchiolitis obliterans syndrome after allogeneic hematopoietic SCT: a case series of eight patients. Bone Marrow Transplant. 2011;46(10):1369–73.
55. Busca A, Locatelli F, Marmont F, Ceretto C, Falda M. Recombinant human soluble tumor necrosis factor receptor fusion protein as treatment for steroid refractory graft-versus-host disease following allogeneic hematopoietic stem cell transplantation. Am J Hematol. 2007;82(1):45–52.
56. Olivieri A, Locatelli F, Zecca M, Sanna A, Cimminiello M, Raimondi R, et al. Imatinib for refractory chronic graft-versus-host disease with fibrotic features. Blood. 2009;114(3):709–18.
57. Kim SJ, Lee JW, Jung CW, Min CK, Cho B, Shin HJ, et al. Weekly rituximab followed by monthly rituximab treatment for steroid-refractory chronic graft-versus-host disease: results from a prospective, multicenter, phase II study. Haematologica. 2010;95(11):1935–42.
58. Zeiser R, Burchert A, Lengerke C, Verbeek M, Maas-Bauer K, Metzelder SK, et al. Ruxolitinib in corticosteroid-refractory graft-versus-host disease after allogeneic stem cell transplantation: a multicenter survey. Leukemia. 2015;29(10):2062–8.
59. Zeiser R, Polverelli N, Ram R, Hashmi SK, Chakraverty R, Middeke JM, et al. Ruxolitinib for glucocorticoid-refractory chronic graft-versus-host disease. N Engl J Med. 2021;385(3):228–38.

60. Cutler C, Lee SJ, Arai S, Rotta M, Zoghi B, Lazaryan A, et al. Belumosudil for chronic graft-versus-host disease after 2 or more prior lines of therapy: the ROCKstar study. Blood. 2021;138(22):2278–89.
61. Miklos D, Cutler CS, Arora M, Waller EK, Jagasia M, Pusic I, et al. Ibrutinib for chronic graft-versus-host disease after failure of prior therapy. Blood. 2017;130(21):2243–50.
62. Doki N, Toyosaki M, Shiratori S, Osumi T, Okada M, Kawakita T, et al. An open-label, single-arm, multicenter study of ibrutinib in japanese patients with steroid-dependent/refractory chronic graft-versus-host disease. Transplant Cell Ther. 2021;27(10):867.e1–9.
63. Wertheimer T, Dohse M, Afram G, Weber D, Heidenreich M, Holler B, et al. Abatacept as salvage therapy in chronic graft-versus-host disease—a retrospective analysis. Ann Hematol. 2021;100(3):779–87.
64. Koshy AG, Kim HT, Stroopinsky D, Liegel JJ, Arnason JE, Ho VT, et al. Phase II clinical trial of abatacept for steroid-refractory chronic graft versus host disease. Blood. 2021;138(Supplement 1):264.
65. Lazaryan A, Lee S, Arora M, Kim J, Betts BC, Khimani F, et al. A phase 2 multicenter trial of ofatumumab and prednisone as initial therapy for chronic graft-versus-host disease. Blood Adv. 2022;6(1):259–69.
66. Lee SJ, Wolff D, Kitko C, Koreth J, Inamoto Y, Jagasia M, et al. Measuring therapeutic response in chronic graft-versus-host disease. National Institutes of Health consensus development project on criteria for clinical trials in chronic graft-versus-host disease: IV. The 2014 Response Criteria Working Group report. Biol Blood Marrow Transplant. 2015;21(6):984–99.
67. Lam DC, Lam B, Wong MK, Lu C, Au WY, Tse EW, et al. Effects of azithromycin in bronchiolitis obliterans syndrome after hematopoietic SCT—a randomized double-blinded placebo-controlled study. Bone Marrow Transplant. 2011;46(12):1551–6.
68. Khalid M, Al Saghir A, Saleemi S, Al Dammas S, Zeitouni M, Al Mobeireek A, et al. Azithromycin in bronchiolitis obliterans complicating bone marrow transplantation: a preliminary study. Eur Respir J. 2005;25(3):490–3.
69. Bergeron A, Chevret S, Chagnon K, Godet C, Bergot E, Peffault de Latour R, et al. Budesonide/Formoterol for bronchiolitis obliterans after hematopoietic stem cell transplantation. Am J Respir Crit Care Med. 2015;191(11):1242–9.
70. Purev E, Gormley N, Ramos C, Reger R, Tian X, Cho E, et al. Inhaled cyclosporine solution for the treatment of bronchiolitis obliterans following hematopoietic stem cell transplantation (HSCT) or lung transplantation. Biol Blood Marrow Transplant. 2015;21(2, Supplement):S347–S8.
71. Gormley N, Ramos C, Reger R, Tropea M, Tian X, Cho E, et al. Inhaled cyclosporine for the treatment of bronchiolitis obliterans following hematopoietic stem cell transplantation (HSCT) or lung transplantation. Blood. 2013;122(21):2057.
72. Lucid CE, Savani BN, Engelhardt BG, Shah P, Clifton C, Greenhut SL, et al. Extracorporeal photopheresis in patients with refractory bronchiolitis obliterans developing after allo-SCT. Bone Marrow Transplant. 2011;46(3):426–9.
73. Del Fante C, Perotti C. Extracorporeal photopheresis for bronchiolitis obliterans syndrome after allogeneic stem cell transplant: an emerging therapeutic approach? Transfus Apher Sci. 2017;56(1):17–9.
74. Brownback KR, Simpson SQ, Pitts LR, Polineni D, McGuirk JP, Ganguly S, et al. Effect of extracorporeal photopheresis on lung function decline for severe bronchiolitis obliterans syndrome following allogeneic stem cell transplantation. J Clin Apher. 2016;31(4):347–52.
75. Hefazi M, Langer KJ, Khera N, Adamski J, Roy V, Winters JL, et al. Extracorporeal photopheresis improves survival in hematopoietic cell transplant patients with bronchiolitis obliterans syndrome without significantly impacting measured pulmonary functions. Biol Blood Marrow Transplant. 2018;24(9):1906–13.
76. Bashoura L, Gupta S, Jain A, Couriel DR, Komanduri KV, Eapen GA, et al. Inhaled corticosteroids stabilize constrictive bronchiolitis after hematopoietic stem cell transplantation. Bone Marrow Transplant. 2008;41(1):63–7.
77. Ratjen F, Rjabko O, Kremens B. High-dose corticosteroid therapy for bronchiolitis obliterans after bone marrow transplantation in children. Bone Marrow Transplant. 2005;36(2):135–8.
78. Even-Or E, Ghandourah H, Ali M, Krueger J, Wall DA, Sweezey NB, et al. Efficacy of high dose steroids for bronchiolitis obliterans syndrome post pediatric hematopoietic stem cell transplantation. Biol Blood Marrow Transplant. 2017;23(3):S270.
79. Stadler M, Ahlborn R, Kamal H, Diedrich H, Buchholz S, Eder M, et al. Limited efficacy of imatinib in severe pulmonary chronic graft-versus-host disease. Blood. 2009;114(17):3718–9.
80. Faraci M, Ricci E, Bagnasco F, Pierri F, Giardino S, Girosi D, et al. Imatinib melylate as second-line treatment of bronchiolitis obliterans after allogeneic hematopoietic stem cell transplantation in children. Pediatr Pulmonol. 2020;55(3):631–7.
81. Williams KM, Pavletic SZ, Lee SJ, Martin PJ, Farthing DE, Hakim FT, et al. Prospective phase II trial of montelukast to treat bronchiolitis obliterans syndrome after hematopoietic cell transplantation and investigation into bronchiolitis obliterans syndrome pathogenesis. Transplant Cell Ther. 2022;28(5):264.e1–9.
82. Tang W, Yu T, Dong T, Liu T, Ji J. Nintedanib in bronchiolitis obliterans syndrome after allogeneic hematopoietic stem cell transplantation. Chest. 2020;158(3):e89–91.
83. Matthaiou EI, Sharifi H, O'Donnell C, Chiu W, Owyang C, Chatterjee P, et al. The safety and tolerability of pirfenidone for bronchiolitis obliterans syndrome after hematopoietic cell transplant (STOP-BOS) trial. Bone Marrow Transplant. 2022;57:1319.

84. Lorillon G, Robin M, Meignin V, Ribaud P, Lescoeur B, Gossot D, et al. Rituximab in bronchiolitis obliterans after haematopoietic stem cell transplantation. Eur Respir J. 2011;38(2):470–2.
85. Zhao Y, OuYang G, Shi J, Luo Y, Tan Y, Yu J, et al. Salvage therapy with low-dose ruxolitinib leads to a significant improvement in bronchiolitis obliterans syndrome in patients with cGVHD after allogeneic hematopoietic stem cell transplantation. Front Pharmacol. 2021;12:668825.
86. Williams KM, Cheng GS, Pusic I, Jagasia M, Burns L, Ho VT, et al. Fluticasone, azithromycin, and montelukast treatment for new-onset bronchiolitis obliterans syndrome after hematopoietic cell transplantation. Biol Blood Marrow Transplant. 2016;22(4):710–6.
87. Kim SW, Rhee CK, Kim YJ, Lee S, Kim HJ, Lee JW. Therapeutic effect of budesonide/formoterol, montelukast and N-acetylcysteine for bronchiolitis obliterans syndrome after hematopoietic stem cell transplantation. Respir Res. 2016;17(1):63.
88. Lim J, Silvia P, Kim HJ. Efficacy of inhaled tiotropium add-on to budesonide/formoterol in patients with bronchiolitis obliterans developing after hematopoietic stem cell transplantation. 2022. https://doi.org/10.21203/rs.3.rs-1678517/v1.
89. Choi HE, Lim SN, Lee JH, Park SH. Comprehensive pulmonary rehabilitation in patients with bronchiolitis obliterans syndrome: a case series. Respir Med Case Rep. 2020;31:101161.
90. Chen S, Zhao K, Lin R, Wang S, Fan Z, Huang F, et al. The efficacy of mesenchymal stem cells in bronchiolitis obliterans syndrome after allogeneic HSCT: a multicenter prospective cohort study. EBioMedicine. 2019;49:213–22.
91. Greer M, Berastegui C, Jaksch P, Benden C, Aubert J, Roux A, et al. Lung transplantation after allogeneic stem cell transplantation: a pan-European experience. Eur Respir J. 2018;51(2):1701330.
92. Riddell P, Vasudevan-Nampoothiri R, Ma J, Singer LG, Lipton JH, Juvet SC. Lung transplantation for late-onset non-infectious chronic pulmonary complications of allogeneic hematopoietic stem cell transplant. Respir Res. 2021;22(1):101.
93. Bergeron A, Chevret S, Granata A, Chevallier P, Vincent L, Huynh A, et al. Effect of azithromycin on airflow decline-free survival after allogeneic hematopoietic stem cell transplant: the ALLOZITHRO randomized clinical trial. JAMA. 2017;318(6):557–66.
94. Cheng GS, Bondeelle L, Gooley T, He Q, Jamani K, Krakow EF, et al. Azithromycin use and increased cancer risk among patients with bronchiolitis obliterans after hematopoietic cell transplantation. Biol Blood Marrow Transplant. 2020;26(2):392–400.
95. Sheshadri A, Saliba R, Patel B, Ahmed T, Bueno LC, Arain MH, et al. Azithromycin may increase hematologic relapse rates in matched unrelated donor hematopoietic cell transplant recipients who receive anti-thymocyte globulin, but not in most other recipients. Bone Marrow Transplant. 2021;56(3):745–8.

# 18 Late-Onset Interstitial Lung Disease Following Allogeneic Hematopoietic Stem Cell Transplantation

Frédéric Schlemmer, Louise Bondeelle, and Anne Bergeron

## Introduction

Currently, bronchiolitis obliterans (BO) is the only late-onset noninfectious pulmonary complication (LONIPC) after allogeneic hematopoietic stem cell transplantation (HSCT) to be formally recognized as pulmonary graft-versus-host disease (GVHD). However, other pulmonary manifestations have been described following HSCT. Late-onset interstitial lung diseases (ILD) following HSCT were first identified almost 30 years ago [1–6]. At that time, it was described as nonclassifiable interstitial pneumonia. The authors have already described these complications as a heterogeneous group of pulmonary processes with variable treatment efficacy and outcome. Later, post-allograft organizing pneumonia (OP) was identified [4, 7]. Finally, based on the evolution of knowledge in the field of idiopathic interstitial lung disease, post allograft ILD has been further specified as a wider group of diffuse interstitial pathologies [8–11]. Thus, according to the international consensus for idiopathic ILD [12], almost all types of ILD except usual interstitial pneumonia and desquamative interstitial pneumonia have been found after HSCT [10].

F. Schlemmer (✉)
Pulmonology Unit—Medical ICU, Assistance Publique-Hôpitaux de Paris, Henri Mondor University Hospitals, Créteil, France

Faculty of Medicine, Paris-Est Créteil University (UPEC), Créteil, France
e-mail: frederic.schlemmer@aphp.fr

L. Bondeelle
Faculty of Medicine, University of Geneva, Geneva, Switzerland

A. Bergeron
Faculty of Medicine, University of Geneva, Geneva, Switzerland

Service de Pneumologie, Hôpitaux Universitaires de Genève, Genève, Switzerland



A. O. Soubani (ed.), *Pulmonary and Critical Care Considerations of Hematopoietic Stem Cell Transplantation*, https://doi.org/10.1007/978-3-031-28797-8_18

Recently, ILD was further specified in the NIH criteria for pulmonary GVHD [13]. Nevertheless, the pathophysiology of post-HSCT ILDs is poorly understood. However, both the frequent histologic association with obliterative bronchiolitis and the clinical association with other manifestations of GVHD raise the question of whether these ILDs would be part of the spectrum of lung chronic GVHD. In any case, it is particularly important to differentiate ILD from BO because their management is different.

The diagnosis of bronchiolitis obliterans syndrome (BOS) is based on the occurrence of a new obstructive ventilatory disorder on pulmonary function testing [14]. Recently, another respiratory functional profile has been identified in the follow-up of some hematopoietic stem cell recipients: a restrictive syndrome, defined by reduced forced vital capacity (FVC) with preserved forced expiratory volume first second ($FEV_1$)/FVC ratio and reduced total lung capacity (TLC), usually with reduced diffusing capacity for carbon monoxide ($DL_{CO}$) [13]. The differentiation of the respiratory entities associated with this functional profile is in progress, but it is likely that ILDs are part of it [8, 15]. Such functional profiles have previously been described following lung transplantation, another alloimmunity situation. The comparison of the two conditions could make it possible to better phenotype the patients and better understand the pathophysiological mechanisms by taking into consideration the specificities of each [16, 17]. It is important to note that chronic lung GVHD is part of a systemic disease, whereas lung dysfunction after a lung transplant is a purely pulmonary disease.

## Epidemiology

In retrospective studies, ILDs accounted for 20 to 72% of LONIPCs [6, 18–23], with a 2-year cumulative incidence of 6% among 438 patients surviving more than 3 months after an allogeneic HSCT over a 12-year period [21]. A recent prospective observational single-center study of more than 200 of these patients found a 3-year cumulative incidence of 5% [9].

## Pathophysiology

The pathophysiological characteristics of late-onset post-HSCT ILDs are poorly known. No animal model exists to improve our knowledge of the pathogenesis of these entities. However, both the occurrence of post-HSCT ILD in patients receiving little or no immunosuppressive treatment and the efficacy of corticosteroids on ILD suggest an immunological process [15]. The strong association with extrathoracic chronic GVHD (cGVHD) further reinforces this hypothesis [7, 8, 15].

Late-onset ILDs include heterogeneous entities with mainly an inflammatory pattern: organizing pneumonia (OP), lymphoid interstitial pneumonia, eosinophilic pneumonia, diffuse alveolar damage (DAD), acute fibrinous organizing pneumonia (AFOP), and nonspecific interstitial pneumonia (NSIP) [7, 8, 10, 24–32]. More recently, pleuroparenchymal fibroelastosis (PPFE) was described as a noninflammatory ILD [10, 33–37]. Meignin et al. showed that almost all cases of ILD presented with the association of obliterative bronchiolitis [10], in accordance with former studies of post-allogeneic HSCT PPFE or NSIP, in which lesions of obliterative bronchiolitis were present in 70–100% of cases [33, 34].

## Spectrum of Post-HSCT Interstitial Lung Diseases

Diagnosis of specific ILDs is based on the initial presentation (acute versus chronic), a CT scan pattern, a histological pattern, and a functional respiratory profile.

### Organizing Pneumonia

OP is the most frequent ILD reported in studies of LONIPC [6, 8, 10, 20, 21, 23, 28, 38, 39] (Table 18.2). In a case-control study [7], the median time from HSCT to OP onset was 108 days (range: 5–2819 days). The clinical presentation was similar to that of cryptogenic OP,

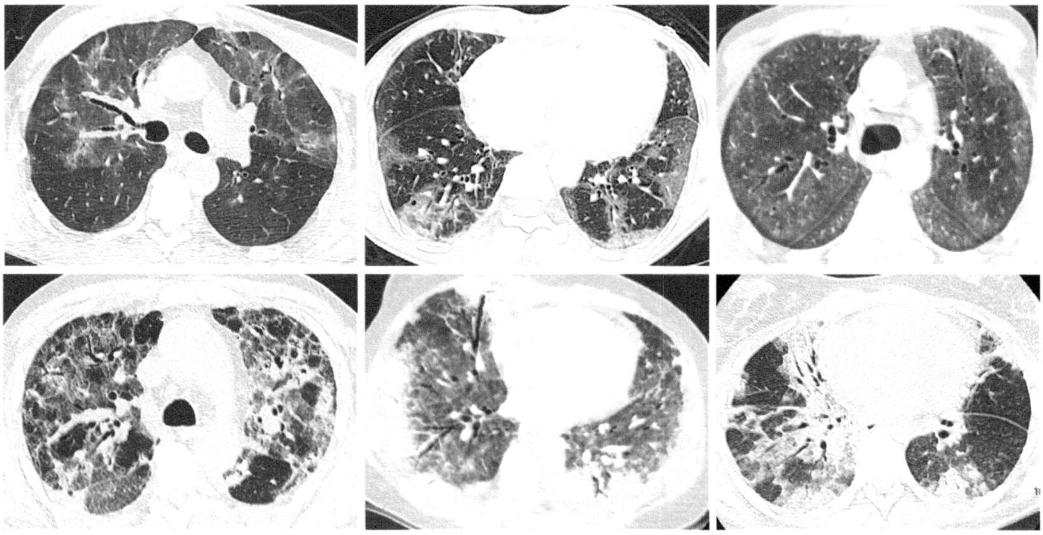

**Fig. 18.1** Chest CT images in late-onset noninfectious ILDs after allogeneic hematopoietic stem cell transplantation

mimicking unresolved or subacute infectious pneumonia with unspecific symptoms. On chest CT, alveolar consolidations most frequently have a predominant peri-bronchovascular or subpleural topography [40, 41] (Fig. 18.1), whereas the classical migratory character of COP is usually missing [7]. Pulmonary function tests most frequently reveal a restrictive lung defect [7]. OP is histologically defined by the characteristic presence of buds of granulation tissue within the distal airways and the alveoli, consisting of fibroblasts and myofibroblasts intermixed with loose connective matrix and associated with chronic interstitial inflammation. Several histopathological and clinical studies on LONIPCs highlighted the frequent overlap between interstitial pneumonia, including OPs, and bronchiolar lesions, suggestive of concomitant bronchiolitis obliterans in this specific context [10, 38, 39].

## Pleuroparenchymal Fibroelastosis

Among post-HSCT ILDs, PPFE was the most recently described [10, 33–37]. It is a rare idiopathic interstitial pneumonia that is histologically characterized by pleural and subpleural parenchymal thickening due to elastic fiber proliferation with minimal inflammation. It typically involves not only the upper lobes but also the medial and lower lung areas, either at diagnosis or systematically during follow-up [37]. A definite diagnosis of PPFE requires histological confirmation, but the presence of typical CT-scan findings has proven sufficient for the clinical diagnosis of PPFE after the exclusion of other lung diseases [42–45] (Fig. 18.2). The exact incidence of post-HSCT PPFE is difficult to assess since it usually occurs several years after transplantation, when many patients do not undergo a systematic long-term pulmonary follow-up. Its estimated prevalence ranges from 0.5 to 1.5%, with a median delay between HSCT and diagnosis of PPFE of around 9 years [37, 43, 44], much longer than for other ILDs [9]. In the largest series, including 15 cases, all met the radiological criteria for PPFE, and 7 were confirmed by lung histology. PFTs typically showed a severe restrictive lung defect. Less than half of the patients had cGVHD at the time of the PPFE diagnosis, while the study was in accordance with the possible role of previous chemotherapy with an alkylating agent and/or total body irradiation. Recurrent lower respiratory tract infections before diagnosis were frequent, as was its association with other LONIPCs (BO, OP, NSIP). PPFE was almost systematically progressive, with an overall poor prognosis [37].

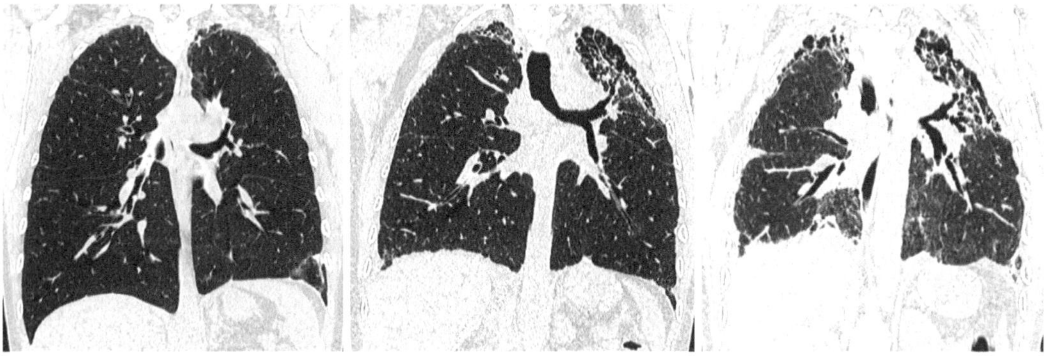

**Fig. 18.2** Sequential chest CT images in a patient with pleuroparenchymal fibroelastosis, obtained at 2 months, 3 years and 6 years, respectively, after allogeneic hematopoietic stem cell transplantation for angioimmunoblastic T-cell lymphoma. In the image on the left, a slight pleural thickening was already visible at the apex of the left lung, which then spread to the middle and lower parts of the lungs, as well as progression of lung fibrosis predominantly in the upper left lobe and the right apex, and global parenchymal retraction of both lungs

**Table 18.1** Histological and usual chest CT patterns of interstitial lung disease reported as late-onset noninfectious pulmonary complications of allogeneic hematological stem cell transplantation (adapted from [10])

| Pathological ILD entity | Usual chest CT pattern |
|---|---|
| Organizing pneumonia (OP) | AC (predominant peri-bronchovascular or subpleural topography is frequent, patchy or more diffuse) +/− GGO, nodular lesions, +/− traction bronchiectasis (fibrotic OP or possible association with DAD or fibrotic NSIP) |
| Nonspecific interstitial pneumonia (NSIP) | GGO (subpleural predominance or diffuse), reticulations, traction bronchiectasis |
| Diffuse alveolar damage (DAD) | GGO (frequently diffuse) +/− AC, traction bronchiectasis (rapidly progressive) |
| Acute fibrinous organizing pneumonia (AFOP) | Nodular lesions, AC, GGO |
| Acute eosinophilic pneumonia (AEP) | GGO, AC |
| Lymphoid interstitial pneumonia (LIP) | GGO +/− AC, reticulations, +/− traction bronchiectasis |
| Pleuroparenchymal fibroelastosis (PPFE) | Pleural thickening (upper lobes systematically involved, lower lobes initially preserved), reticulations (subpleural topography) +/− traction bronchiectasis (consider an associated ILD), reduced lung volume +/− pleural effusion |

*AC* alveolar consolidations, *GGO* ground glass opacities, *ILD* interstitial lung disease

## Other Noninfectious ILDs

As previously mentioned, other post-HSCT ILDs have been reported (Table 18.1) and are frequently associated with extra-pulmonary cGVHD. When applying the international consensus classification for idiopathic ILD [12, 46], NSIP and DAD look quite frequent on lung histology, LIP more rarely [4, 10]. NSIP is defined by diffuse alveolar wall thickening by uniform fibrosis, preserved alveolar architecture, and mild interstitial inflammation, without honeycombing or fibroblastic foci. DAD is the histopathological pattern of acute interstitial pneumonia, a clinical entity characterized by rapidly progressive respiratory failure and an overall poor prognosis. Histology reveals a diffuse involvement with uniform thickening of alveolar walls, edema, hyaline membranes, and interstitial acute inflammation at the exudative early phase, followed by loose organizing fibrosis mostly within alveolar septa and type II pneumocyte hyperplasia during the organizing phase, finally regressing or progressing to end-stage fibrosis. LIP Is defined by a dense interstitial lymphoid infiltrate with associated type II cell hyperplasia and a mild increase in alveolar macrophages [12].

Several cases of acute eosinophilic pneumonia (AEP) were reported, typically occurring during the first months following AHSCT in the context of GVHD flare, with fever, dyspnea, diffuse parenchymal opacities, and high blood eosinophilia [31, 32, 47]. BAL fluid analyses usually meet the diagnostic criteria for AEP (eosinophils >25% of nucleated BAL cells) in the absence of any other cause (infectious, drug, or specific). For the majority of reported cases, the diagnosis was confirmed by a lung biopsy (surgical or transbronchial) with a favorable outcome after corticosteroid therapy.

Acute fibrinous organizing pneumonia (AFOP), a rare and recently described histologic entity of acute lung injury, has also been reported in the context of HSCT [25–27]. AFOP cases occurred between 25 days and 11 months after HSCT. Clinical presentation usually includes fever, cough, and progressive dyspnea that may lead to acute respiratory failure. Chest CTs showed multifocal pulmonary nodules, ground glass opacities, and/or consolidations. Diagnosis relied on lung histology in all cases, revealing patchy, or more diffuse, prominent organizing intra-alveolar fibrin deposition characteristic of AFOP and occasionally associated with DAD lesions (without hyaline membranes) [25].

Sarcoidosis, systematically involving the lungs, has been rarely described in the context of both allogeneic and autologous HSCT. In a recent case series and literature review including 13 biopsy-proven cases diagnosed in HSCT recipients [48], sarcoidosis occurred after a median interval of 20 months (range: 3–30), more often in women and in patients of Caucasian ethnicity, with radiological lung lesions (not precisely described) and/or extrapulmonary involvement (e.g., skin and liver) in around two-thirds (none had lymph node involvement). A history of GVHD was found in only half of the cases (which do not support a potential link between the two diseases), with a response to steroids in all cases (around two-third) justifying it.

## Risk Factors

History of chest irradiation prior to HSCT and occurrence of early pneumonia (within 100 days) after HSCT were identified as being predictive of the development of LONIPCs [9]. In a recent retrospective study including 238 consecutive patients diagnosed with ILD ($n = 79$, 33%) or BOS ($n = 159$, 67%) after allogeneic HSCT, risk factors for both complications were compared [15]. Male sex was more frequently associated with BOS than with ILD (52% of males with BOS vs. 23% of males with ILD; $p < 0.0001$). HLA-matched 9/10 donors were more frequently observed in the BOS group than in the ILD group (20% vs. 5%), with significantly more female donor/male recipient mismatches among BOS patients. No difference in conditioning regimens was observed between the BOS and ILD groups, including total body irradiation. Prior thoracic irradiation and the absence of immunosuppressive treatment at the time of diagnosis were associated with an increased occurrence of ILD.

Risk factors based on other retrospective studies on OPs include female-to-male HSCT, HLA incompatibility, peripheral blood stem cell transplantation, conditioning regimens including total body irradiation and cyclophosphamide, and acute or chronic GVHD [7, 49], whereas busulfan-based myeloablative conditioning, fludarabine-based reduced-intensity conditioning, and in vivo T-cell ablation lowered the risk [49].

A history of sarcoidosis in graft donors was found occasionally, whereas HLA alleles known to be associated with sarcoidosis were very frequent [48].

## Diagnostic Criteria

Clinical signs of ILDs are nonspecific and may include dyspnea, cough, fever, extrathoracic symptoms related to ILDs, or be, very occasionally, diagnosed incidentally on follow-up PFTs. Clinical and/or biological autoimmunity features may occasionally be associated with ILD, with diagnosis criteria for systemic lupus erythematosus, primary Sjögren syndrome, polymyositis and anti-MDA5 syndrome, mixed connective tissue disease, or ANCA-associated vasculitis, in a few cases, which were associated with a poor outcome [24, 50, 51]. Lung auscultation may be either normal or reveal crackles suggestive of lung fibrosis.

Lung computed tomography (CT) reveals more or less extensive parenchymal lung lesions consisting of alveolar consolidations (AC) and/or ground glass opacities (GGO), whereas reticulations, septal thickening, bronchial thickening or dilatation, honeycombing, or air-leakage syndrome remain occasional [8]. Some radiological patterns may be suggestive of the underlying histopathology (Table 18.1). OP will be suspected in case of AC, typically peribronchial, subpleural, nodular, or patchy, with or without GGO [8, 40, 41]. Subpleural or more diffuse GGO, possibly associated with reticulations and signs of fibrosis (parenchymal retraction, fissural distortion, and/or traction bronchiectasis), may suggest NSIP but is also compatible with DAD or LIP, both of which have also been associated with the AC-predominant pattern [8, 12]. PPFE is usually suspected in case of pleural thickening with progressive parenchymal retraction, initially predominant in the upper regions of the lungs. Although the definite diagnosis of PPFE requires histological confirmation, the presence of typical radiologic findings on a CT scan has proven sufficient for the clinical diagnosis of PPFE after the exclusion of other lung diseases [42–45].

Like in non-HSCT settings, ILDs may have a broad spectrum of etiologies, including respiratory infections (opportunistic or not), that must be ruled out in the first place. After ruling out a pulmonary infection or in the absence of significant clinical or radiological improvement after an empirical or adapted antibiotic therapy, the integration of the patient's medical history and clinical presentation, lung imaging, biological and immunological tests, and BAL and noninvasive microbiological tests results may strengthen the hypothesis of an alternative diagnosis (Table 18.2). When performed in the absence of infection, BAL typically reveals a lymphocytic alveolitis in the large majority of cases [3, 7, 8, 52, 53], while a relative increase in neutrophil count may be noticed in one third of the cases, most frequently associated with a prominent increase in the lymphocyte count [8]. Furthermore, a significant increase of BAL eosinophils may be observed in a few cases [8], with acute or chronic eosinophilic pneumonia having been reported after HSCT [31, 32, 54]. To date, no correlation between BAL cytology and radiological features has been reported.

Given both the invasiveness of surgical lung biopsy and its minimal impact on patient care, the diagnosis of ILD should most of the time be

**Table 18.2** Diagnostic criteria for late-onset noninfectious interstitial lung disease[a] after allogeneic hematopoietic stem cell transplantation (adapted from [8])

| | |
|---|---|
| 1. | Presence of infiltrative parenchymal opacities (e.g., alveolar consolidations and/or ground-glass opacities) on chest CT<br>AND |
| 2. | No respiratory pathogens identification after consideration of all available microbiological techniques searching for bacteria, mycobacteria, viruses, fungi, and parasites, on respiratory (BAL and/or nasal aspirate/swab and/or sputum), blood and urine samples<br>AND/OR |
| 3. | No clinical or radiological improvements despite broad-spectrum antibiotic therapy<br>AND/OR |
| 4. | Clinical and radiological improvements after the initiation or increase of immunosuppressive therapy<br>AND/OR |
| 5. | No pathogen identification on a lung biopsy specimen (if performed[b]) and/or pathological lesions compatible with the suspicion of noninfectious post-allo HSCT ILD |

[a]A history of acute and/or chronic extrathoracic graft-versus-host disease and/or recent tapering or discontinuation of immunosuppressive therapy may be additional arguments for the diagnosis of late-onset noninfectious ILD
[b]After specific staining, consider metagenomic analysis

made without lung biopsy analysis. Progress in microbiological diagnostics applied to respiratory samples has significantly increased the performance of diagnosing infectious pneumonia. Nevertheless, if histological evidence is necessary and similar to what is done for ILDs in the non-HSCT context, transbronchial cryobiopsies might be an alternative to surgical lung biopsies for the diagnosis of post-HSCT ILDs [55].

## Management and Outcome

Overall prognosis of patients suffering from ILD after allogeneic HSCT was poor with a 39% estimated mortality in 2 years [8]. In a more recent retrospective study, the overall survival (OS) was 81% at 3 years and 71% at 5 years [15]. In this study, the OS of the patients suffering from ILD or BOS were compared; although OS did not differ between groups, the causes of death varied, with more cases of respiratory failure in the ILD group and more cases of infection in the BOS group [15]. Finally, hematological relapse may be more frequent in HSCT patients with ILD than in those with BOS [15].

Although no treatment guidelines are available, treatment with steroids showed some efficacy for the resolution or stabilization of ILDs [8], in contrast to BOS, where steroids have not proven their efficacy but only their numerous associated side effects [56]. However, there is a risk of relapse of ILD when decreasing the dose of steroids [7, 9, 15]. Regarding AFOP, response to steroids seems variable, while the TNF-α blocking agent Etanercept was reported as effective in one single case [27].

Lung transplantation is rarely performed in this setting due to concomitant extrapulmonary morbidity, excessive immunosuppression, and concerns about recurring malignancy being considered contraindications. A recent study assessed that no HSCT-specific factors influence outcome within a carefully selected patient cohort undergoing lung transplantation for LONIPCs [57].

The patient outcomes associated with PPFE were poor with a mortality rate of 47% and severe respiratory disability for the survivors [37]. Half of the patients were diagnosed with pneumothorax after a PPFE diagnosis. Pharmacological treatment showed poor response to antifibrotic drugs reported in a limited number of cases [37, 58]. Further studies are needed to determine the optimal therapeutic management of PPFE, including the specific treatment algorithm, the potential utility of positive pressure ventilation for patients with dyspnea and restrictive PFTs, and the place for lung transplantation. Lung transplantation could be an option in some cases, but contraindications are frequent enough that it remains preferentially proposed in cases of end-stage pulmonary fibrosis [59–61], most frequently related to PPFE in recent series [34, 62]. In the case of lung transplantation, optimal bilateral lung transplantation may be complicated by the absence of congruence between the size of the thoracic cavity and the graft due to the platythorax and related surgical concerns, whereas single transplantation has to be considered in the case of previous pleurodesis.

## Conclusion

Late-onset noninfectious ILDs constitute a rare complication of HSCT that might be, in some cases, related to a pulmonary localization of cGVHD. It would seem that ILDs are a heterogeneous group of disorders that cannot be summarized under a single entity. In cases of unresolved pneumonia or a restrictive lung defect during post-HSCT follow-up, an ILD should be suspected, and a systematic approach similar to the one used in any patient with an ILD should be proposed. Even if some specificities between BOS and ILD have recently been shown, the poor prognosis is the same. A better understanding of the pathophysiology of ILDs should also open new therapeutic perspectives. Their prevention, early recognition, and prompt management are mandatory to limit their impact on both the patient's functional and vital prognosis.

## References


1. Schwarer AP, Hughes JM, Trotman-Dickenson B, Krausz T, Goldman JM. A chronic pulmonary syndrome associated with graft-versus-host disease after allogeneic marrow transplantation. Transplantation. 1992;54(6):1002–8.
2. Kaplan EB, Pietra GG, August CS. Interstitial pneumonitis, pulmonary fibrosis, and chronic graft-versus-host disease. Bone Marrow Transplant. 1992;9(1):71–5.
3. Leblond V, Zouabi H, Sutton L, Guillon JM, Mayaud CM, Similowski T, et al. Late CD8+ lymphocytic alveolitis after allogeneic bone marrow transplantation and chronic graft-versus-host disease. Am J Respir Crit Care Med. 1994;150(4):1056–61.
4. Yousem SA. The histological spectrum of pulmonary graft-versus-host disease in bone marrow transplant recipients. Hum Pathol. 1995;26(6):668–75.
5. Soubani AO, Miller KB, Hassoun PM. Pulmonary complications of bone marrow transplantation. Chest. 1996;109(4):1066–77.
6. Palmas A, Tefferi A, Myers JL, Scott JP, Swensen SJ, Chen MG, et al. Late-onset noninfectious pulmonary complications after allogeneic bone marrow transplantation. Br J Haematol. 1998;100(4):680–7.
7. Freudenberger TD, Madtes DK, Curtis JR, Cummings P, Storer BE, Hackman RC. Association between acute and chronic graft-versus-host disease and bronchiolitis obliterans organizing pneumonia in recipients of hematopoietic stem cell transplants. Blood. 2003;102(10):3822–8.
8. Schlemmer F, Chevret S, Lorillon G, De Bazelaire C, Peffault de Latour R, Meignin V, et al. Late-onset noninfectious interstitial lung disease after allogeneic hematopoietic stem cell transplantation. Respir Med. 2014;108(10):1525–33.
9. Bergeron A, Chevret S, Peffault de Latour R, Chagnon K, de Margerie-Mellon C, Rivière F, et al. Noninfectious lung complications after allogeneic haematopoietic stem cell transplantation. Eur Respir J. 2018;51(5):1702617.
10. Meignin V, Thivolet-Bejui F, Kambouchner M, Hussenet C, Bondeelle L, Mitchell A, et al. Lung histopathology of non-infectious pulmonary complications after allogeneic haematopoietic stem cell transplantation. Histopathology. 2018;73(5):832–42.
11. Haider S, Durairajan N, Soubani AO. Noninfectious pulmonary complications of haematopoietic stem cell transplantation. Eur Respir Rev. 2020;29(156):190119.
12. Travis WD, Costabel U, Hansell DM, King TE, Lynch DA, Nicholson AG, et al. An official American Thoracic Society/European Respiràtory Society statement: update of the international multidisciplinary classification of the idiopathic interstitial pneumonias. Am J Respir Crit Care Med. 2013;188(6):733–48.
13. Wolff D, Radojcic V, Lafyatis R, Cinar R, Rosenstein RK, Cowen EW, et al. National Institutes of Health consensus development project on criteria for clinical trials in chronic graft-versus-host disease: IV. The 2020 highly morbid forms report. Transpl Cell Ther. 2021;27(10):817–35.
14. Jagasia MH, Greinix HT, Arora M, Williams KM, Wolff D, Cowen EW, et al. National Institutes of Health Consensus Development Project on Criteria for Clinical Trials in Chronic Graft-versus-Host Disease: I. The 2014 Diagnosis and Staging Working Group report. Biol Blood Marrow Transplant. 2015;21(3):389–401.e1.
15. Archer G, Berger I, Bondeelle L, de Margerie-Mellon C, Cassonnet S, de Latour RP, et al. Interstitial lung diseases after hematopoietic stem cell transplantation: new pattern of lung chronic graft-versus-host disease? Bone Marrow Transplant. 2022;29:1–7.
16. Pang Y, Charya AV, Keller MB, Sirajuddin A, Fu YP, Holtzman NG, et al. The ISHLT chronic lung allograft dysfunction consensus criteria are applicable to pulmonary chronic graft-versus-host disease. Blood Adv. 2022;6(14):4196–207.
17. Bos S, Beeckmans H, Vanstapel A, Sacreas A, Geudens V, Willems L, et al. Pulmonary graft-versus-host disease and chronic lung allograft dysfunction: two sides of the same coin? Lancet Respir Med. 2022;10(8):796–810.
18. Trisolini R, Stanzani M, Lazzari Agli L, Colangelo A, Bonifazi F, Falcioni S, et al. Delayed non-infectious lung disease in allogeneic bone marrow transplant recipients. Sarcoidosis Vasc Diffuse Lung Dis. 2001;18(1):75–84.
19. Sakaida E, Nakaseko C, Harima A, Yokota A, Cho R, Saito Y, et al. Late-onset noninfectious pulmonary complications after allogeneic stem cell transplantation are significantly associated with chronic graft-versus-host disease and with the graft-versus-leukemia effect. Blood. 2003;102(12):4236–42.
20. Patriarca F, Skert C, Sperotto A, Damiani D, Cerno M, Geromin A, et al. Incidence, outcome, and risk factors of late-onset noninfectious pulmonary complications after unrelated donor stem cell transplantation. Bone Marrow Transplant. 2004;33(7):751–8.
21. Patriarca F, Skert C, Bonifazi F, Sperotto A, Fili C, Stanzani M, et al. Effect on survival of the development of late-onset non-infectious pulmonary complications after stem cell transplantation. Haematologica. 2006;91(9):1268–72.
22. Nishio N, Yagasaki H, Takahashi Y, Muramatsu H, Hama A, Tanaka M, et al. Late-onset non-infectious pulmonary complications following allogeneic hematopoietic stem cell transplantation in children. Bone Marrow Transplant. 2009;44(5):303–8.
23. Ueda K, Watadani T, Maeda E, Ota S, Kataoka K, Seo S, et al. Outcome and treatment of late-onset noninfectious pulmonary complications after allogeneic haematopoietic SCT. Bone Marrow Transplant. 2010;45(12):1719–27.
24. Bergeron A, Bengoufa D, Feuillet S, Meignin V, Peffault de Latour R, Rybojad M, et al. The spectrum of lung involvement in collagen vascular-like diseases

following allogeneic hematopoietic stem cell transplantation: report of 6 cases and review of the literature. Medicine (Baltimore). 2011;90(2):146–57.
25. Nguyen LP, Ahdoot S, Sriratanaviriyakul N, Zhang Y, Stollenwerk N, Schivo M, et al. Acute fibrinous and organizing pneumonia associated with allogeneic hematopoietic stem cell transplant successfully treated with corticosteroids: a two-patient case series. J Investig Med High Impact Case Rep. 2016;4(2):2324709616643990.
26. Lee SM, Park JJ, Sung SH, Kim Y, Lee KE, Mun YC, et al. Acute fibrinous and organizing pneumonia following hematopoietic stem cell transplantation. Korean J Intern Med. 2009;24(2):156–9.
27. Simmons GL, Chung HM, McCarty JM, Toor AA, Farkas D, Miller K, et al. Treatment of acute fibrinous organizing pneumonia following hematopoietic cell transplantation with etanercept. Bone Marrow Transplant. 2017;52(1):141–3.
28. Jinta M, Ohashi K, Ohta T, Ieki R, Abe K, Kamata N, et al. Clinical features of allogeneic hematopoietic stem cell transplantation-associated organizing pneumonia. Bone Marrow Transplant. 2007;40(5):465–72.
29. Miyagawa-Hayashino A, Sonobe M, Kubo T, Yoshizawa A, Date H, Manabe T. Non-specific interstitial pneumonia as a manifestation of graft-versus-host disease following pediatric allogeneic hematopoietic stem cell transplantation. Pathol Int. 2010;60(2):137–42.
30. Wahla AS, Khan II, Loya A, Chin R. A new pattern of pulmonary graft vs host disease in a hematopoietic stem cell transplant patient. Clin Respir J. 2015;9(4):399–402.
31. Wagner T, Dhedin N, Philippe B, Rivaud E, Vernant JP, Couderc LJ. Acute eosinophilic pneumonia after allogeneic hematopoietic stem cell transplantation. Ann Hematol. 2006;85(3):202–3.
32. Yoshimi M, Nannya Y, Watanabe T, Asai T, Ichikawa M, Yamamoto G, et al. Acute eosinophilic pneumonia is a non-infectious lung complication after allogeneic hematopoietic stem cell transplantation. Int J Hematol. 2009;89(2):244–8.
33. von der Thüsen JH, Hansell DM, Tominaga M, Veys PA, Ashworth MT, Owens CM, et al. Pleuroparenchymal fibroelastosis in patients with pulmonary disease secondary to bone marrow transplantation. Mod Pathol. 2011;24(12):1633–9.
34. Takeuchi Y, Miyagawa-Hayashino A, Chen F, Kubo T, Handa T, Date H, et al. Pleuroparenchymal fibroelastosis and non-specific interstitial pneumonia: frequent pulmonary sequelae of haematopoietic stem cell transplantation. Histopathology. 2015;66(4):536–44.
35. Matsui T, Maeda T, Kida T, Fujita J, Tsuji H, Morii E, et al. Pleuroparenchymal fibroelastosis after allogeneic hematopoietic stem cell transplantation: important histological component of late-onset noninfectious pulmonary complication accompanied with recurrent pneumothorax. Int J Hematol. 2016;104(4):525–30.
36. Barisione G, Dominietto A, Bianchi R, Garlaschi A, Bacigalupo A, Stellino L, et al. Trajectory of lung function to pleuroparenchymal fibroelastosis late after haematopoietic stem-cell transplantation. Respir Med Case Rep. 2019;28:100915.
37. Bondeelle L, Gras J, Michonneau D, Houdouin V, Hermet E, Blin N, et al. Pleuroparenchymal fibroelastosis after allogeneic hematopoietic stem cell transplantation. Bone Marrow Transplant. 2020;55(5):982–6.
38. Uhlving HH, Andersen CB, Christensen IJ, Gormsen M, Pedersen KD, Buchvald F, et al. Biopsy-verified bronchiolitis obliterans and other noninfectious lung pathologies after allogeneic hematopoietic stem cell transplantation. Biol Blood Marrow Transplant. 2015;21(3):531–8.
39. Gazourian L, Spring L, Meserve E, Hwang D, Diaz AA, Ash SY, et al. Pulmonary clinicopathological correlation after allogeneic hematopoietic stem cell transplantation: an autopsy series. Biol Blood Marrow Transplant. 2017;23(10):1767–72.
40. Dodd JD, Müller NL. Bronchiolitis obliterans organizing pneumonia after bone marrow transplantation: high-resolution computed tomography findings in 4 patients. J Comput Assist Tomogr. 2005;29(4):540–3.
41. Pipavath SNJ, Chung JH, Chien JW, Godwin JD. Organizing pneumonia in recipients of hematopoietic stem cell transplantation: CT features in 16 patients. J Comput Assist Tomogr. 2012;36(4):431–6.
42. Reddy TL, Tominaga M, Hansell DM, von der Thusen J, Rassl D, Parfrey H, et al. Pleuroparenchymal fibroelastosis: a spectrum of histopathological and imaging phenotypes. Eur Respir J. 2012;40(2):377–85.
43. Mariani F, Gatti B, Rocca A, Bonifazi F, Cavazza A, Fanti S, et al. Pleuroparenchymal fibroelastosis: the prevalence of secondary forms in hematopoietic stem cell and lung transplantation recipients. Diagn Interv Radiol Ank Turk. 2016;22(5):400–6.
44. Namkoong H, Ishii M, Mori T, Sugiura H, Tasaka S, Sakurai M, et al. Clinical and radiological characteristics of patients with late-onset severe restrictive lung defect after hematopoietic stem cell transplantation. BMC Pulm Med. 2017;17(1):123.
45. Enomoto Y, Nakamura Y, Satake Y, Sumikawa H, Johkoh T, Colby TV, et al. Clinical diagnosis of idiopathic pleuroparenchymal fibroelastosis: a retrospective multicenter study. Respir Med. 2017;133:1–5.
46. American Thoracic Society, European Respiratory Society. American Thoracic Society/European Respiratory Society International Multidisciplinary Consensus Classification of the Idiopathic Interstitial Pneumonias. This joint statement of the American Thoracic Society (ATS), and the European Respiratory Society (ERS) was adopted by the ATS board of directors, June 2001 and by the ERS executive committee, June 2001. Am J Respir Crit Care Med. 2002;165(2):277–304.
47. Janin-Mercier A, Valade S, Boccon-Gibbod L, D'Agay MF, Bourges M, Devergie A, et al. Pulmonary

lesions following bone marrow graft. Study of 35 cases. Ann Pathol. 1985;5(3):183–94.
48. Wurm-Kuczera RI, Buentzel J, Koenig JFL, Legler T, Valk JJ, Hasenkamp J, et al. Sarcoidosis following hematopoietic stem cell transplantation: clinical characteristics and HLA associations. Front Immunol. 2021;12:746996.
49. Nakasone H, Onizuka M, Suzuki N, Fujii N, Taniguchi S, Kakihana K, et al. Pre-transplant risk factors for cryptogenic organizing pneumonia/bronchiolitis obliterans organizing pneumonia after hematopoietic cell transplantation. Bone Marrow Transplant. 2013;48(10):1317–23.
50. Lepelletier C, Bengoufa D, Lyes Z, de Masson A, Chasset F, Jachiet M, et al. Dermatopulmonary syndrome associated with anti-MDA5 antibodies after allogeneic hematopoietic stem cell transplantation. JAMA Dermatol. 2017;153(2):184–8.
51. Tamaki M, Matsumi S, Nakasone H, Nakamura Y, Kawamura M, Kawamura S, et al. Interstitial lung disease with anti-melanoma differentiation-associated gene 5 antibody after allogeneic hematopoietic stem cell transplantation. Bone Marrow Transplant. 2022;57(9):1382.
52. Brownback KR, Frey JW, Abhyankar S. Bronchoscopic features, associations, and outcomes of organizing pneumonia following allogeneic hematopoietic stem cell transplantation. Ann Hematol. 2019;98(9):2187–95.
53. Wolff D, Reichenberger F, Steiner B, Kahl C, Leithäuser M, Skibbe T, et al. Progressive interstitial fibrosis of the lung in sclerodermoid chronic graft-versus-host disease. Bone Marrow Transplant. 2002;29(4):357–60.
54. Richard C, Calavia J, Loyola I, Baró J, Cuadrado MA, Gómez-Casares MT, et al. Chronic eosinophilic pneumonia in a patient treated with allogeneic bone marrow transplantation. Med Clin (Barc). 1994;102(12):462–4.
55. Korevaar DA, Colella S, Fally M, Camuset J, Colby TV, Hagmeyer L, et al. European Respiratory Society guidelines on transbronchial lung cryobiopsy in the diagnosis of interstitial lung diseases. Eur Respir J. 2022;60(5):2200425.
56. Norman BC, Jacobsohn DA, Williams KM, Au BKC, Au MA, Lee SJ, et al. Fluticasone, azithromycin and montelukast therapy in reducing corticosteroid exposure in bronchiolitis obliterans syndrome after allogeneic hematopoietic SCT: a case series of eight patients. Bone Marrow Transplant. 2011;46(10):1369–73.
57. Greer M, Berastegui C, Jaksch P, Benden C, Aubert J, Roux A, et al. Lung transplantation after allogeneic stem cell transplantation: a pan-European experience. Eur Respir J. 2018;51(2):1701330.
58. Brownback KR, Pitts LR, Abhyankar S. Safety of nintedanib for treatment of fibrotic lung disease after allogeneic hematopoietic stem cell transplantation. Bone Marrow Transplant. 2018;53(9):1218–20.
59. Soubani AO, Kingah P, Alshabani K, Muma G, Haq A. Lung transplantation following hematopoietic stem cell transplantation: report of two cases and systematic review of literature. Clin Transpl. 2014;28(7):776–82.
60. Cheng GS, Edelman JD, Madtes DK, Martin PJ, Flowers MED. Outcomes of lung transplantation after allogeneic hematopoietic stem cell transplantation. Biol Blood Marrow Transplant. 2014;20(8):1169–75.
61. Kliman DS, Kotecha SR, Abelson DC, Snell GI, Glanville AR, Ma DDF. Favorable outcome of lung transplantation for severe pulmonary graft versus host disease: an Australian Multicenter case series. Transplantation. 2019;103(12):2602–7.
62. Riddell P, Vasudevan-Nampoothiri R, Ma J, Singer LG, Lipton JH, Juvet SC. Lung transplantation for late-onset non-infectious chronic pulmonary complications of allogeneic hematopoietic stem cell transplant. Respir Res. 2021;22(1):101.

# Other Noninfectious Pulmonary Complications

19

Aryan Shiari and Ayman O. Soubani

## Introduction

Hematopoietic stem-cell transplantation (HSCT) is a treatment modality for a growing number of hematologic and non-hematologic disorders. In HSCT patients, unhealthy native bone marrow cells are replaced by infusion of either autologous (patient's own cells) or allogeneic (donor stem cells), after administration of a short course of high-dose chemotherapy with or without radiation [1]. After HSCT, this subset of patients remains at risk for developing a variety of complications involving multiple organ systems. Of these complications, those involving the respiratory system are broadly categorized into infectious and noninfectious.

Noninfectious pulmonary complications are variable and dependent on the patient's time course post-HSCT. Major noninfectious complications include peri-engraftment respiratory distress syndrome, idiopathic pneumonia syndrome, diffuse alveolar hemorrhage, bronchiolitis obliterans syndrome, and interstitial lung disease, which have been covered in prior chapters.

Uncommon or less distinctive noninfectious complications covered in this chapter include pleural effusions, venous thromboembolism, pulmonary hypertension, thoracic air leak syndrome, post-transplant lymphoproliferative disorder (PTLD), pulmonary alveolar proteinosis (PAP), and the development of solid organ malignancies.

## Pleural Effusions

Pleural effusions are commonly encountered among patients who have undergone HSCT, with incidence rates reported as high as 9.9% within the first year and 11.8% within 5 years of allogeneic HSCT. Clinically significant pleural effusions in allogeneic HSCT patients have been noted to have a median onset of 40 days post-HSCT (range, 1–869) [2]. Incidence of pleural effusions in autologous HSCT remains unknown, and exact numbers have not been reliably demonstrated in current literature.

In allogeneic HSCT patients, a bi-modal distribution has been described for the formation of pleural effusion, consisting of early-onset occurring within 100 days and late-onset occurring after 100 days of transplantation.

A. Shiari · A. O. Soubani (✉)
Division of Pulmonary, Critical Care and Sleep Medicine, Wayne State University School of Medicine, Detroit, MI, USA
e-mail: asoubani@med.wayne.edu


A. O. Soubani (ed.), *Pulmonary and Critical Care Considerations of Hematopoietic Stem Cell Transplantation*, https://doi.org/10.1007/978-3-031-28797-8_19

Early-onset (less than 100 days) pleural effusions are frequently due to volume overload or infection etiologies. This coincides with the early onset reported time frames of fluid overload in allogeneic HSCT in the absence of other known transplant-related complications. Fluid overload was described in these studies as weight gain and edema requiring fluid removal with or without organ toxicity [3]. With regards to infections during the first 100 days post-HSCT, which include the pre-engraftment (0–30 days) and early post-engraftment phases (30–100 days), the most prevalent pathogens are bacterial and fungal species. These pathogens are also observed to cause secondary pleural effusions. Engraftment syndrome, malignant pleural effusion, new-onset congestive heart failure, and sinusoidal obstruction syndrome have also been cited as noninfectious causes of early-onset pleural effusions [2].

Late-onset (more than 100 days) pleural effusions can also be due to infections, including viral infections or volume overload; however, an increasing number of pleural effusions in this phase can be due to serositis-type chronic graft vs. host disease (GvHD) and cryptogenic organizing pneumonia, formerly called bronchiolitis obliterans organizing pneumonia or BOOP [2]. Suspicion for pleural effusion due to GvHD should be high in those who already have manifested GvHD in other organ systems, as pleural effusion is rarely noted as the first manifestation. Treatment typically involves escalating GvHD therapy after the exclusion of alternative etiologies.

Regardless of onset, Kaplan-Meier analysis of pleural effusions in the HSCT population has shown a statistically significant increase in mortality in patients with pleural effusions as compared to those without effusions (hazard ratio 1.49; 95%, CI, 1.09–2.04; $P = 0.011$). Furthermore, a significant association was found with a higher comorbidity index ($P = 0.03$) and the presence of GvHD ($P = 0.018$) in patients who developed pleural effusions. No significant association has been found between with race, disease risk index, HLA match, or donor type and the development of pleural effusion. Finally, pleural effusions in this subset of patients were associated with significantly inferior overall survival ($P < 0.001$) [2].

## Venous Thromboembolic Disease

Venous thromboembolism (VTE) is an established and increasingly recognized complication in the HSCT population. Multiple factors predispose HSCT patients to being at an increased risk for VTE compared to the general population. These factors include:

***Hematologic Malignancy***

Although VTE has historically been associated with solid organ malignancies, those with hematologic malignancies are also at an increased risk. VTE rates have been reported as high as 6% in patients with lymphoma, 10% in those with multiple myeloma (MM), and between 5% and 20% in those with acute leukemia [4–6]. Furthermore, in patients with newly diagnosed MM, incidence rates have been reported to increase by 14–26% if the immunomodulators used include thalidomide and dexamethasone. Additionally, use of lenalidomide with dexamethasone has also been associated with an increased risk of VTE as high as 75% [7, 8].

***Graft Vs Host Disease (GvHD)***

Both acute and chronic GvHD have been independently associated with the development of VTE. In patients who developed GvHD after their first VTE, 8% were found to have a subsequent VTE event. The most common organ involvements of GvHD in patients who developed VTE are the skin (65.9%), gastrointestinal (29.4%), ocular and oral (28.6%), and hepatic (21.4%) [9]. Increased VTE incidence due to GvHD in the HSCT population is postulated to be due to the known pro-inflammatory state of GvHD, which predisposes patients to thromboembolic events.

***Indwelling Vascular Catheters***

Central venous catheter placement as a means of vascular access is quite common for patients undergoing HSCT. Their use is variable, ranging from administration of chemotherapy, stem cell transfusion, nutritional support, plasmapheresis, extracorporeal photopheresis, and general administration of medication and fluids. Catheter-related thrombosis (CRT) is known to occur, with reported rates of ~12% in patients with hematologic malignancies and up to 8–21% in HSCT recipients [10]. CRT may be asymptomatic in up to 41% of patients, and common symptoms of discomfort, catheter malfunction, pain, and swelling may be absent. There is limited evidence that CRT results in increased rates of pulmonary embolism or mortality [11]. As a result, the cornerstone of therapy remains anticoagulation with low molecular weight heparin (LMWH) to prevent further extension of VTE, reduce VTE-related symptoms, and prevent embolization. For patients who have an ongoing need for catheters, anticoagulation should be continued without catheter removal as long as the access remains functional [12, 13]. Duration of therapy remains as per American College of Chest Physicians (ACCP) guidelines of 3 months or until the catheter is removed, whichever is longer [13]. Currently, the use of thromboprophylaxis for CRT remains controversial, and no official guidelines support prophylactic anticoagulation in this subset of patients to date.

***Cytotoxic Chemotherapy and Immune Modulators***

The use of cytotoxic chemotherapy agents and immune modulators have been linked to an increased risk of VTE. Risk factor for VTE in patients starting a new chemotherapy regimen as compared to the general population is two-to-six fold greater, with a reported mortality rate of 9% [14]. Cyclosporine, a commonly used immunosuppressive agent has been linked to increased incidence of thrombosis and endothelial cell perturbations. The hypothesized mechanism is through reduction in thrombomodulin activity of endothelial cells, and downregulation of the protein C anticoagulant pathway, increasing risk of thrombosis [15].

***Thrombocytopenia***

Majority of HSCT patients undergo a period of thrombocytopenia within 1–2 weeks of myeloablative therapy. Although thrombocytopenia itself is not a direct cause of VTE in the HSCT population, it is important to note that during the thrombocytopenic period this population is still susceptible to VTE events and low platelet count only confers partial protection. Prior studies have noted 60% of thrombotic events occurring with platelet counts less than $100 \times 10^9$/L, 34% of events occurred with a platelet count less than $50 \times 10^9$/L, and 13% occurred with a platelet count less than $20 \times 10^9$/L. Given low platelet count and concomitant risk of bleeding, mechanical thromboprophylaxis has been proposed using sequential pneumatic compression devices during thrombocytopenic periods, although balancing the risk of VTE and bleeding is challenging [16].

## VTE Prophylaxis and Treatment

A variety of well-established conditions observed in HSCT recipients, including an underlying diagnosis of multiple myeloma, GvHD, indwelling catheters, prolonged hospitalization, prior VTE, and the use of cytotoxic chemotherapy and immune modulators, have been associated with an increased risk of VTE. The presence of these conditions should prompt clinicians to perform risk stratifications of HSCT recipients, and the decision for thromboprophylaxis should be made with VTE vs. bleeding risk in mind. Providers should discuss with patients the benefits, harms, drug cost, and duration of prophylaxis.

Current indications for prophylaxis include patients with multiple myeloma following autologous HSCT and receiving immune modulatory drugs (lenalidomide, thalidomide, pomalidomide) and hospitalization or post-operative status in patients with platelet counts >50,000/μL. Patients with indwelling central venous catheters do not need routine prophylactic anticoagulation [17].

Prophylactic VTE regimens include aspirin for low-risk MM patients on immunomodulatory medications and LMWH (such as enoxaparin 40 mg SC daily) for higher-risk patients [17, 18].

The American Society of Clinical Oncology (ASCO) and National Comprehensive Cancer Network (NCCN) do not recommend the use of routine thromboprophylaxis in ambulating patients with known malignancy, which includes HSCT recipients [18, 19]. Furthermore, routine pharmacologic thromboprophylaxis should not be offered to patients admitted for the sole purpose of minor procedures or chemotherapy infusions, nor to patients undergoing stem cell/bone marrow transplantation procedures [18].

Patients with VTE who are not at an increased risk of bleeding and who platelet count >50,000/μL should be started on LMWH or unfractionated heparin. These patients may be continued on LMWH or switched to warfarin or one of the direct oral anticoagulants. There are no robust data or guidelines on which of the above options is recommended for HSCT patients. At this time, such a decision is made on an individual basis. The duration of anticoagulation is not studied in the HSCT patient population; however, based on patients with cancer diagnoses, it is suggested to continue treatment for 3–6 months or as long as the malignancy persists. For catheter-related thrombosis, the duration of treatment should be 3 months or as long as the catheter remains in place.

The use of inferior vena cava (IVC) filters should only be considered in patients whose anticoagulation is contraindicated or who developed VTE despite receiving chemical VTE prophylaxis. IVC filters should be retrieved and removed as soon as the contraindication to anticoagulation is resolved, as they pose a prothrombotic risk factor.

Until recently, limited risk-prediction models for VTE in HSCT survivors were available. The BMTSS-HiGHS2 risk model, utilizing a cohort of >2-year survivors of HSCT, analyzed 1751 recipients and found HSCT survivors have a 7.3-fold increased risk of VTE compared to siblings without a history of cancer. This finding is consistent with prior studies of HSCT recipients, which reported in increased risk of VTE (2.6-fold) compared to their siblings without cancer [20]. Risk was found to increase for at least 10 years post-HSCT. The BMTSS-HiGHS2 model discriminates between HSCT survivors with high and low risk of VTE by utilizing the following factors: history of stroke, chronic GvHD, hypertension, sex (male), and stem cell source (peripheral blood stem cells) [21].

Utilization of risk-prediction models such as the BMTSS-HiGHS2 in identifying high-risk HSCT recipients should be considered by clinicians to have informed decision-making discussions with this subset of patients, as they are at risk of not only VTE but also substantial bleeding complications while undergoing chemotherapy and in a thrombocytopenic state. In high-risk patients without thrombocytopenia and bleeding complications, a discussion regarding thromboprophylaxis may be considered given the absence of guidelines in this population subset.

## Pulmonary Hypertension

Pulmonary hypertension (PH) is defined as a mean pulmonary arterial pressure > 20 mmHg. PH is further classified into isolated precapillary PH (pulmonary artery wedge pressure ≤ 15 mmHg and pulmonary vascular resistance ≥3 WU), isolated post-capillary PH (pulmonary artery wedge pressure > 15 mmHg and pulmonary vascular resistance <3 WU) and combined pre- and postcapillary PH (pulmonary artery wedge pressure ≥ 15 mmHg and pulmonary vascular resistance ≥3 WU) [22].

Majority of the literature regarding PH in HSCT is derived from the pediatric population, and the median age of PH diagnosis after HSCT is 12.6 years (ranging from 1 month to 51 years) with 70% of patients having only pulmonary arteriole involvement and 23% of patients reporting pulmonary veno-occlusive disease (PVOD) [23].

PVOD is a rare type of PH with incidence rates of 0.1–0.2 cases per million [24]. PVOD is characterized by its preferential targeting of the pulmonary venules and subsequent obliteration by fibrous intimal thickening and patchy capillary proliferation. Similar to other types of PH, PVOD progression leads to increased pulmonary vascular resistance and subsequent right heart failure [24]. A triad of severe pulmonary arterial hypertension, radiographic evidence of pulmonary edema, and a normal pulmonary artery occlusion pressure have been classically attributed to the suspected presence of PVOD [25]. The lack of this triad, however, does not exclude PVOD. A definitive diagnosis of PVOD can only be made via surgical lung biopsy in order to determine the mechanism of vascular injury. The utility of surgical biopsy has been a topic of dispute given that treatment options are limited. Treatment of PVOD with various conventional pulmonary arterial hypertension therapies such as nitrates, calcium channel blockers, prostacyclins, and endothelin receptor antagonists has had limited success. Single and double lung transplantation remain the only therapeutic options shown to significantly prolong the lives of patients with PVOD. As a result, a biopsy should be considered in patients with clinical and radiographic features suggestive of the PVOD if the risk of surgical intervention is acceptable, as it can impact a patient's length of time awaiting transplant [26]. One-year mortality rates of PVOD patients have been reported as high as 70% [27], and the utility of lung transplantation is often diminished as wait times often exceed that of life expectancy in patients with PVOD. As a result, it is recommended that all patients with PVOD should be referred for transplantation at the time of diagnosis.

Bronchiolitis obliterans syndrome (BOS) and other forms of lung GvHD are major causes of morbidity and mortality in the post-HSCT population and have been linked to an increased risk of PH. In a retrospective analysis of 386 adult patients who developed BOS after HSCT, a 32.5% prevalence of PH was noted. It is uncertain whether PH develops in patients with BOS due to parenchymal changes or due to an associated vasculitis process [28]. Nevertheless, given the high prevalence of PH discovered in patients with BOS, there is growing expert recommendation that screening with transthoracic echocardiography should be considered in patients with BOS after HSCT [29].

There are currently no guidelines delineating alternative therapeutic approaches in PH management post-HSCT compared to the general PH population. Treatment approaches have been mainly reported in the pediatric population and were decided based on the clinical and hemodynamic status of patients at the time of diagnosis. In a study of 22 pediatric patients with diagnosed PH, vasoreactivity testing was initially used to identify responders for calcium channel blockers. Nonresponders were then either treated with monotherapy (phosphodiesterase-5 inhibitor (PDE5i) or endothelin receptor antagonist), oral dual therapy (PDE5i and endothelial receptor antagonist), or triple therapy with PDE5i, endothelial receptor antagonist, and prostanoids. In this study, all survivors were found to be weaned off pulmonary hypertension treatment after a median follow-up of 5 months utilizing the abovementioned treatment plan, while 7 patients died [30]. In adults, there have only been four reported cases of detailed management of PH after HSCT. In these cases, treatment options consist of PDE-5 inhibitors with inhaled and oral prostacyclin analogues, endothelin receptor antagonists with corticosteroid therapy, and more recently monotherapy with vasodilator therapy (tadalafil) [31–34]. All four patients were alive after treatment for a minimum of 29 months in post-treatment reported follow-up.

In summary, patients with pulmonary GvHD should be periodically monitored for evidence of PH by history, physical examination, and echocardiography. Early and accurate diagnosis followed by prompt treatment remains central to ensuring favorable outcomes. The management of PH in HSCT patients should follow guidelines

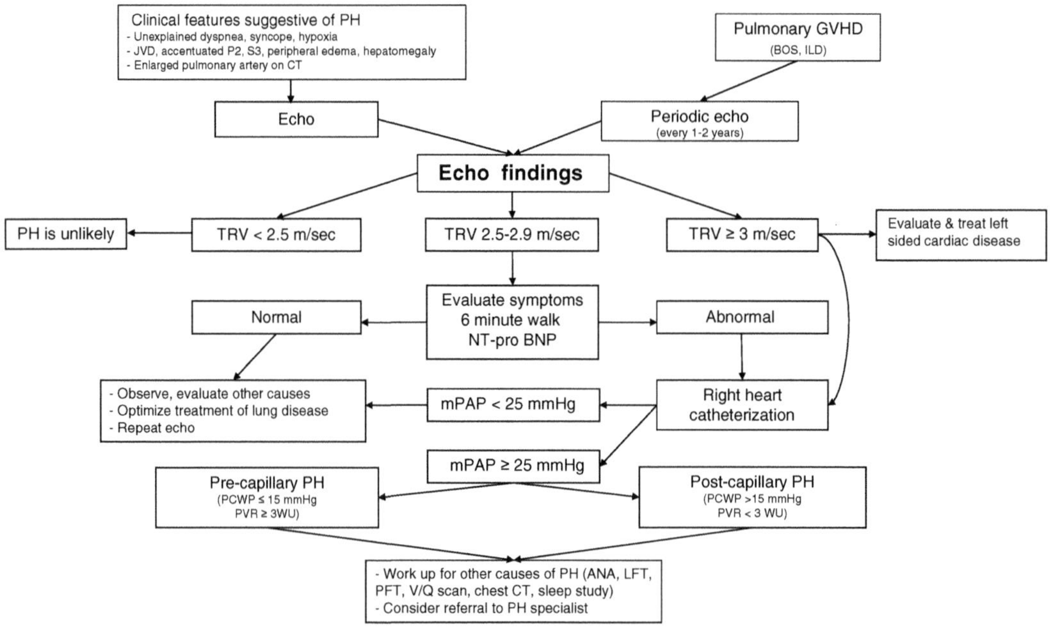


**Fig. 19.1** Suggested workup of patients with pulmonary hypertension following HSCT. *GvHD* graft vs. host disease, *BOS* bronchiolitis obliterans syndrome, *ILD* interstitial lung disease, *PH* pulmonary hypertension, *TRV* tricuspid regurgitant jet velocity, *PCWP* pulmonary capillary wedge pressure, *PVR* pulmonary vascular resistance, *WU* woods unit, *NT-pro-BNP* N-terminal-pro-brain natriuretic peptide, *mPAP* mean pulmonary artery pressure, *ANA* anti-nuclear antibody, *HIV* human immunodeficiency virus, *PFT* pulmonary function test, *LFTs* liver function tests, *V/Q scan* ventilation/perfusion scan

established in other patient populations, preferably by a PH specialist. Figure 19.1 provides a suggested approach to the evaluation of PH in a HSCT patient.

## Post-transplant Lymphoproliferative Disorder (PTLPD)

Post-transplant lymphoproliferative disorder (PTLD) is a less common complication of allogeneic HSCT and solid organ transplantation. PTLD is a heterogeneous group of lymphoproliferative diseases that have been associated with immunosuppression and Epstein-Barr virus (EBV) following transplantation. PTLD is broadly categorized into four main categories: early lesions (plasmocytic hyperplasia/infectious mononucleosis-like lesions), monomorphic-PTLD, polymorphic-PTLD, and classic Hodgkin lymphoma-like PTLD [35].

EBV is a common virus that typically causes infectious mononucleosis in the general population. As many as 90–95% of the general population will be infected with the EBV at some point during their lives. In the HSCT population, however, EBV can impart significant morbidity and mortality. During the first 6 months post transplantation where T-cell depletion is occurring, or during a period of intense immunosuppression for prevention or treatment of GvHD, EBV can have opportunistic expansion of EBV-transformed B-lymphocytes, resulting in PTLD. This proliferation is thought to be due to the reduced number of EBV-specific cytotoxic lymphocytes (CTLs) during these immunocompromised periods, resulting in uninhibited growth of EBV-infected cells. Despite many HSCT patients being positive for EBV, EBV-PTLD rates remain low in comparison to the total number of carriers, ranging from 1–17% [36–40]. This is because the proliferation of EBV-infected cells is enough in and of itself to result in PTLD. A second component is thought to be required. EBV-infected cells, unfathered during immunosuppression post-HSCT, must undergo errors in the B-cell replication cycle, resulting in a cell population that cannot exit the cell cycle and is also no longer inhibited by CTLs, finally resulting in PTLD [41].

Given the immunosuppressive state required for development of PTLD as noted above, it is not surprising that reported incidence has been largely (70%) within the first 6 months of HSCT, with only 4% of cases developing later than 12 months after HSCT [42]. PTLD can manifest in almost any organ system, however, thoracic involvement is most commonly encountered. Symptoms of pulmonary PTLD include fever, lymphadenopathy, cough, and dyspnea. Thoracic lymphadenopathy is the primary observed radiologic involvement, with enlarged lymph nodes commonly hypermetabolic on fluorodeoxyglucose positron emission tomography (FDG-PET) [43]. Parenchymal involvement is less frequently reported and manifests as nodules or masses. Extra-parenchymal disease is also observed, presenting as pleural effusion and less commonly as interstitial pneumonia.

EBV-associated pneumonia is a common differential diagnosis for PTLD in the HSCT population. Differentiation between the two remains challenging and often requires bronchoalveolar lavage (BAL) cytology along with surgical lung biopsy [44, 45]. A biopsy of lymphadenopathy, whether thoracic or in other organ systems, is ideal for PTLD diagnosis. This, however, is often unrealistic due to the critical nature of PTLD patients, and diagnosis is often made based on noninvasive approaches using quantitative EBV DNA titers combined with positron emission tomography–CT/CT imaging [46].

Treatment of PTLD typically involves the reduction of immunosuppressive regimen. Other therapies include the addition of rituximab, a CD20 monoclonal antibody, along with a reduction in immunosuppression [47–50]. Adoptive immunotherapy with EBV-specific cytotoxic T cells has also been proposed but isgenerally reserved for persistent diseases found to be refractory to initial therapy. This form of adoptive immunotherapy uses virus-specific T cells derived from HSCT donors or patient-derived normal T cells to combat PTLD. While initially proposed in 1994 for the treatment of PTLD [51], it has had limited use due to the generally low incidence of PTLD and the good therapeutic response of lowered immunosuppression.

Tabelecleucel, a cytotoxic lymphocyte activated against EBV, is currently the only FDA-approved treatment using adoptive immunotherapy for the treatment of rituximab-refractory EBV-PTLD. Currently, there are multiple clinical trials further evaluating the efficacy of Tabelecleucel in HSCT populations suffering from EBV-PTLD [52–56].

Clinical suspicion for PTLD post-HSCT should be high despite the low prevalence of disease, as delay in treatment results in rapid deterioration to multiorgan failure and death [57–59]. Mortality rate despite appropriate treatment remains high and has been reported at 2 years post-transplantation to be 42.5% in the allogeneic HSCT recipients and 15.4% in the autologous HSCT recipients [42, 60].

## Solid Malignancies

As HSCT outcomes have improved over the years, an increasing prevalence of chronic conditions and late complications are observed in long-term survivors. Of these late complications, the development of a secondary solid malignancy post-HSCT is rare but well-established in long-term survivors. Incidence rates are highest 3–5 years post-HSCT and have been observed in both autologous and allogeneic transplant survivors. Cumulative incidence ranges from 1.2 to 1.6% at 5 years, 2.2–6.1% at 10 years, and 3.8–14.9% at 15 years post-transplant [61]. Additional reported risk factors for the development of secondary solid malignancies are total body radiation, GvHD, immunosuppression related to GvHD, and association with viral infection [62, 63]. Second-stage solid malignancies in HSCT include skin cancers, melanoma, cancers of the oral cavity and salivary glands, the brain, liver, uterine cervix, thyroid, breast, bone, and connective tissue.

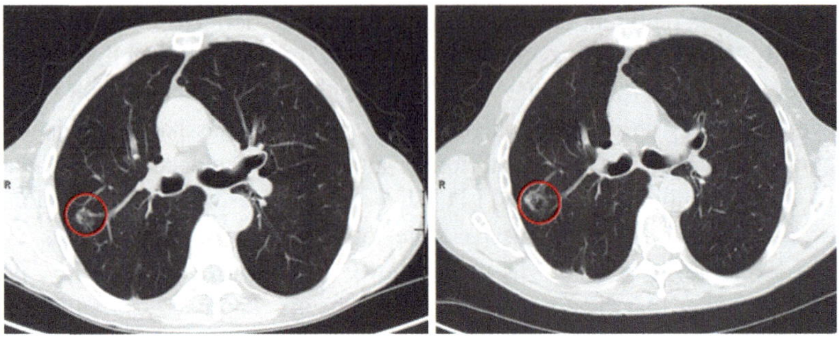


**Fig. 19.2** CT chest images of a patient with BOS following HSCT that show a small right upper lobe nodule (left panel) that increased in size a few months later (right panel). The patient was diagnosed with lung cancer and underwent a lobectomy

Standardized incidence ratios for the development of secondary lung cancer post-HSCT as compared to the general population have been reported to range from 0.7 to 2.6% [64–67]. Secondary lung cancer was found to be the most common site in allogeneic HSCT survivors who underwent treatment with high-dose busulfan and cyclophosphamide ($n = 11$, including 9 with non-small cell lung cancer among 66 patients with all solid cancers) [64] and occurred at a median of 4.5 years post transplantation (Fig. 19.2). Moreover, secondary lung malignancy was increased in older patients and in those with a prior history of tobacco use prior to HSCT (RR = 11.6, $P = 0.02$) [64]. As a result, patients who have undergone HSCT are recommended to undergo assessment for tobacco use and undergo subsequent smoking cessation counseling and treatment if indicated. Screening recommendations currently do not differ from the general population and adhere to the United States Preventative Task Force guidelines; offer low-dose computed tomography to adults aged 50–80 years who have at least a 20-pack-per-year smoking history and who currently smoke or have quit within the past 15 years. Screening is to be discontinued once a person has not smoked for 15 years, develops a health condition that substantially limits life expectancy, or lacks the ability or willingness to have curative lung surgery.

## Pulmonary Alveolar Proteinosis (PAP)

PAP is a rare, diffuse, and progressive pulmonary disease caused by the accumulation of lipoproteinaceous material, commonly surfactant phospholipids and surfactant apoproteins in the alveoli. The presence of surfactant in the alveoli is normal and essential to lung function for lowering surface tension, preventing atelectasis, and maintaining the air-water interface. Abnormal accumulation of surfactant, however, can impart significant morbidity and mortality by impairing normal gas exchange occurring at the level of the alveoli.

PAP has been broadly categorized into three categories: congenital, primary (autoimmune and hereditary), and secondary [68, 69]. Secondary PAP manifests similarly to primary PAP; however, it is caused by an underlying disease or toxic exposure. Reported secondary causes include chronic infections (human immunodeficiency virus, Nocardia, *Pneumocystis jirovecii*), hematologic disorders (myelodysplasia, leukemia, lymphoma), drug-induced conditions, including chemotherapy, dust inhalation (titanium, silica, aluminum, and others), lung transplantations, and HSCT. The pathophysiology of secondary PAP is currently not well understood. In secondary PAP, GM-CSF antibodies are not present, and it is not thought to be working through the same molecular pathways as primary PAP. Despite this, alveolar macrophages remain unable to maintain adequate surfactant homeostasis, through a currently poorly understood mechanism, although GM-CSF and macrophage function are thought to maintain a central role.

Reported incidence of PAP is limited. In a national survey of 43 HSCT centers, only 5 cases of adult-onset PAP after HSCT were identified between 2016 and 2019 [70]. This study remains the largest cohort of secondary PAP post-HSCT and only a scant few case reports are present to date [70–75]. The reported sample size is small ($n = 5$); however, two distinct time frames were observed for post-HSCT PAP. Early acute PAP occurring during the aplasia period ($n = 1$) and late onset progressive PAP, related to a highly suggested drug-induced macrophage dysfunction ($n = 4$) [70].

Diagnosis of PAP post-HSCT is challenging due to the absence of autoantibodies to GM-CSF, which are commonly found in primary diseases. A lung biopsy is deemed the gold standard for diagnosis; however, in the majority of cases, a biopsy is rarely required. Commonly positive PAS staining of intra- and extracellular material obtained by BAL is adequate for the diagnosis of PAP and negates the need for lung biopsy. Thoracic CT scan findings can also be highly suggestive of PAP in the correct clinical setting and should prompt clinicians to proceed with BAL. The most suggestive finding is that of the "crazy paving" pattern, which consists of groundglass opacities with superimposed interlobular septal thickening and intralobular septal thickening. Opacities are commonly in a geographical pattern, with the juxtaposition of healthy lung fields and opacities resulting in the characteristically reported presentation. Although nonspecific, a majority of patients with PAP demonstrate a "crazy paving" pattern on thoracic imaging, and the findings are highly suggestive of the disease [76–78]. The presence of pulmonary nodules or adenopathy is not commonly reported [79].

There is currently no specific therapy for secondary PAP, and thus far, treatment approaches have focused on treating the underlying condition. In the HSCT population, this has translated to either a second graft or the withdrawal of a suspected drug. Whole-lung lavage has also been the gold standard of therapy for PAP, and indications have varied based on institutional practices. Declining lung function, decreased oxygenation ($PaO_2$), worsening radiographic findings, and dyspnea with daily activities have been reported as indications for whole lung lavage [80]. Utilization of whole lung lavage has not been specifically ascribed to any category of PAP but is used for all types as it focuses on the physical removal of the accumulated proteinaceous material from the effective lung. Novel therapeutic options for PAP, including rituximab, inhaled GM-CSF, and plasmapheresis, are being considered; however, their use has thus far been limited to auto-immune variants of the disease [81–83].

## Thoracic Air-Leak Syndrome

Thoracic air-leak syndrome (TALS) refers to the presence of extra-alveolar air, which encompasses the conditions of spontaneous pneumomediastinum, pneumopericardium, subcutaneous emphysema, interstitial emphysema, and spontaneous pneumothorax (Fig. 19.3) [84]. Onset of TALS post-HSCT is approximately 425.9 ± 417.8 days (60–1825 days), with the most common manifestation being spontaneous pneumothorax [85]. TALS is thought to arise from the Macklin effect, which refers to three sequential pathophysiologic steps. First, trauma causes alveolar rupture, leading to dissection of air along the broncho-vascular sheath and finally spreading to the mediastinum [86]. Incidence of TALS is 0.83–2.3% [85, 87]. TALS occurs primarily in patients suffering from post-HSCT complications of cryptogenic organizing pneumonia (COP), bronchiolitis obliterans syndrome (BOS), and interstitial pneumonia. Risk factors for TALS are chronic GvHD, subsequent HSCT, age less than 38 years at transplant, male sex, and Tacrolimus-based GvHD prophylaxis [87].

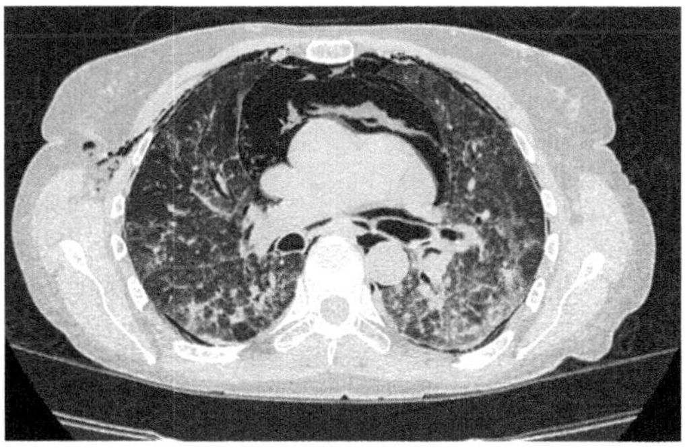

**Fig. 19.3** CT image of a patient with pulmonary fibrosis following HSCT showing pneumomediastium, small bilateral pneumothoraces, and subcutaneous emphysema consistent with thoracic air-leak syndrome

The presence of TALS in HSCT has a progressive course and can often be fatal, with mortality rates reported between 66% and 100% [85, 88–90]. Treatment for TALS largely depends on which type occurs and adheres to the standard treatment of the developed pathology. Persistent air leaks may require pleurodesis or pleurectomy.

Regardless of type, treatment response remains poor and largely focuses on supportive treatment of patients while awaiting spontaneous resolution after interventions with chest tube placement and oxygen therapy have been exhausted. A retrospective review of 18 patients with TALS found TALS persisted in 6 patients until death (33%), and of the 12 which resolved, the mean duration of air leak was not short, with 20.8 days (2–90 days) prior to recovery [85]. Of the 12 that recovered from TALS, only two survived, with 10 dying due to aggravation of pulmonary GvHD, concurrent pneumonia, and ultimately respiratory failure.

## References


1. Thomas ED, Lochte HL, Lu WC, Ferrebee JW. Intravenous infusion of bone marrow in patients receiving radiation and chemotherapy. N Engl J Med. 1957;257:491–6. https://doi.org/10.1056/nejm195709122571102.
2. Modi D, Jang H, Kim S, et al. Incidence, etiology, and outcome of pleural effusions in allogeneic hematopoietic stem cell transplantation. Am J Hematol. 2016;91:E341–7. https://doi.org/10.1002/ajh.24435.
3. Rondón G, Saliba RM, Chen J, et al. Impact of fluid overload as new toxicity category on hematopoietic stem cell transplantation outcomes. Biol Blood Marrow Transplant. 2017;23:2166–71. https://doi.org/10.1016/j.bbmt.2017.08.021.
4. Ottinger H, Belka C, Kozole G, et al. Deep venous thrombosis and pulmonary artery embolism in high-grade non Hodgkin's lymphoma: incidence, causes and prognostic relevance. Eur J Haematol. 2009;54:186–94. https://doi.org/10.1111/j.1600-0609.1995.tb00214.x.
5. Vu K, Luong NV, Hubbard J, et al. A retrospective study of venous thromboembolism in acute leukemia patients treated at the University of Texas MD Anderson Cancer Center. Cancer Med. 2015;4:27–35. https://doi.org/10.1002/CAM4.332.
6. Ku GH, White RH, Chew HK, et al. Venous thromboembolism in patients with acute leukemia: incidence, risk factors, and effect on survival. Blood. 2009;113:3911–7. https://doi.org/10.1182/blood-2008-08-175745.
7. Talamo GP, Ibrahim S, Claxton D, et al. Hypercoagulable states in patients with multiple myeloma can affect the thalidomide-associated venous thromboembolism. Blood Coagul Fibrinolysis. 2009;20:337–9. https://doi.org/10.1097/MBC.0B013E32832B27E6.
8. Kekre N, Connors JM. Venous thromboembolism incidence in hematologic malignancies. Blood Rev. 2019;33:24–32. https://doi.org/10.1016/j.blre.2018.06.002.
9. Kekre N, Kim HT, Ho VT, et al. Venous thromboembolism is associated with graft- versus -host disease and increased non-relapse mortality after allogeneic hematopoietic stem cell transplantation. Haematologica. 2017;102:1185–91. https://doi.org/10.3324/haematol.2017.164012.
10. Geerts W. Central venous catheter-related thrombosis. Hematology Am Soc Hematol Educ Program. 2014;2014:306–11. https://doi.org/10.1182/asheducation-2014.1.306.
11. Chopra V, Anand S, Hickner A, et al. Risk of venous thromboembolism associated with peripherally inserted central catheters: a systematic review and meta-analysis. Lancet. 2013;382:311–25. https://doi.org/10.1016/S0140-6736(13)60592-9.
12. Kucher N. Deep-vein thrombosis of the upper extremities. N Engl J Med. 2011;364:861–9. https://doi.org/10.1056/NEJMcp1008740.
13. Kearon C, Akl EA, Comerota AJ, et al. Antithrombotic therapy for VTE disease. Chest. 2012;141:e419S–96S. https://doi.org/10.1378/chest.11-2301.
14. Qureshi W, Ali Z, Amjad W, et al. Venous thromboembolism in cancer: an update of treatment and prevention in the era of newer anticoagulants. Front Cardiovasc Med. 2016;3:24. https://doi.org/10.3389/fcvm.2016.00024.
15. Garcia-Maldonado M, Kaufman CE, Comp PC. Decrease in endothelial cell-dependent protein c activation induced by thrombomodulin by treatment with cyclosporine. Transplantation. 1991;51:701–5. https://doi.org/10.1097/00007890-199103000-00030.
16. Gerber DE, Segal JB, Levy MY, et al. The incidence of and risk factors for venous thromboembolism (VTE) and bleeding among 1514 patients undergoing hematopoietic stem cell transplantation: implications for VTE prevention. Blood. 2008;112:504–10. https://doi.org/10.1182/blood-2007-10-117051.
17. Chaturvedi S, Neff A, Nagler A, et al. Venous thromboembolism in hematopoietic stem cell transplant recipients. Bone Marrow Transplant. 2016;51:473–8. https://doi.org/10.1038/bmt.2015.308.
18. Key NS, Khorana AA, Kuderer NM, et al. Venous thromboembolism prophylaxis and treatment in patients with cancer: ASCO clinical practice guide-

line update. J Clin Oncol. 2020;38:496–520. https://doi.org/10.1200/JCO.19.01461.
19. Streiff MB, Bockenstedt PL, Cataland SR, et al. Venous thromboembolic disease. J Natl Compr Cancer Netw. 2013;11:1402–29. https://doi.org/10.6004/JNCCN.2013.0163.
20. Gangaraju R, Chen Y, Hageman L, et al. Venous thromboembolism in autologous blood or marrow transplantation survivors: a report from the blood or marrow transplant survivor study. Biol Blood Marrow Transplant. 2019;25:2261–6. https://doi.org/10.1016/j.bbmt.2019.06.032.
21. Gangaraju R, Chen Y, Hageman L, et al. Late-occurring venous thromboembolism in allogeneic blood or marrow transplant survivors: a BMTSS-HiGHS2 risk model. Blood Adv. 2021;5:4102–11. https://doi.org/10.1182/bloodadvances.2021004341.
22. Simonneau G, Montani D, Celermajer DS, et al. Haemodynamic definitions and updated clinical classification of pulmonary hypertension. Eur Respir J. 2019;53:1801913. https://doi.org/10.1183/13993003.01913-2018.
23. Dandoy CE, Hirsch R, Chima R, et al. Pulmonary hypertension after hematopoietic stem cell transplantation. Biol Blood Marrow Transplant. 2013;19:1546–56. https://doi.org/10.1016/j.bbmt.2013.07.017.
24. Heath D, Segel N, Bishop J. Pulmonary veno-occlusive disease. Circulation. 1966;34:242–8. https://doi.org/10.1161/01.CIR.34.2.242.
25. Rambihar VS, Fallen EL, Cairns JA. Pulmonary veno-occlusive disease: antemortem diagnosis from roentgenographic and hemodynamic findings. Can Med Assoc J. 1979;120:1519–22.
26. Mandel J, Mark EJ, Hales CA. Pulmonary veno-occlusive disease. Am J Respir Crit Care Med. 2000;162:1964–73. https://doi.org/10.1164/ajrccm.162.5.9912045.
27. Holcomb BW Jr. Pulmonary veno-occlusive disease *. Chest J. 2000;118:1671. https://doi.org/10.1378/chest.118.6.1671.
28. Nathan SD, Shlobin OA, Ahmad S, et al. Pulmonary hypertension in patients with bronchiolitis obliterans syndrome listed for retransplantation. Am J Transplant. 2008;8:1506–11. https://doi.org/10.1111/j.1600-6143.2008.02277.x.
29. Pate A, Rotz S, Warren M, et al. Pulmonary hypertension associated with bronchiolitis obliterans after hematopoietic stem cell transplantation. Bone Marrow Transplant. 2016;51:310–2. https://doi.org/10.1038/bmt.2015.248.
30. Levy M, Moshous D, Szezepanski I, et al. Pulmonary hypertension after bone marrow transplantation in children. Eur Respir J. 2019;54:1900612. https://doi.org/10.1183/13993003.00612-2019.
31. Limsuwan A, Pakakasama S, Hongeng S. Reversible course of pulmonary arterial hypertension related to bone marrow transplantation. Heart Vessel. 2011;26:557–61. https://doi.org/10.1007/S00380-010-0100-6.
32. Grigg A, Buchanan M, Whitford H. Late-onset pulmonary arterial hypertension in association with graft-versus-host disease after allogeneic stem-cell transplantation. Am J Hematol. 2005;80:38–42. https://doi.org/10.1002/AJH.20373.
33. Tanaka TD, Ishizawar DC, Saito T, et al. Successful treatment of pulmonary hypertension following hematopoietic stem cell transplant with a single oral tadalafil: a case report. Pulm Circ. 2021;11:1–5. https://doi.org/10.1177/20458940211027791.
34. Nakaoka H, Sakata Y, Yamamoto M, et al. Pulmonary hypertension associated with bone marrow transplantation. J Cardiol Cases. 2010;2:e23–7. https://doi.org/10.1016/j.jccase.2010.01.008.
35. Bell D, Gaillard F. WHO classification of tumours of haematopoietic and lymphoid tissues. In: Radiopaedia.org. Radiopaedia.org; 2010. p 176–8, 171–5, 168–70, 150–1.
36. Al Hamed R, Bazarbachi AH, Mohty M. Epstein-Barr virus-related post-transplant lymphoproliferative disease (EBV-PTLD) in the setting of allogeneic stem cell transplantation: a comprehensive review from pathogenesis to forthcoming treatment modalities. Bone Marrow Transplant. 2020;55:25–39. https://doi.org/10.1038/s41409-019-0548-7.
37. Johansson J-E, Remberger M, Vl L, et al. Allogeneic haematopoietic stem-cell transplantation with reduced intensity conditioning for advanced stage Hodgkin's lymphoma in Sweden: high incidence of post transplant lymphoproliferative disorder. Bone Marrow Transplant. 2011;46:870–5. https://doi.org/10.1038/bmt.2010.238.
38. Hou H-AA, Yao M, Tang J-LL, et al. Poor outcome in post transplant lymphoproliferative disorder with pulmonary involvement after allogeneic hematopoietic SCT: 13 years' experience in a single institute. Bone Marrow Transplant. 2009;43:315–21. https://doi.org/10.1038/bmt.2008.325.
39. Buyck HCEE, Ball S, Junagade P, et al. Prior immunosuppressive therapy with antithymocyte globulin increases the risk of EBV-related lymphoproliferative disorder following Allo-SCT for acquired aplastic anaemia. Bone Marrow Transplant. 2009;43:813–6. https://doi.org/10.1038/bmt.2008.394.
40. Ocheni S, Kroeger N, Zabelina T, et al. EBV reactivation and post transplant lymphoproliferative disorders following allogeneic SCT. Bone Marrow Transplant. 2008;42:181–6. https://doi.org/10.1038/bmt.2008.150.
41. Compagno F, Basso S, Panigari A, et al. Management of PTLD after hematopoietic stem cell transplantation: immunological perspectives. Front Immunol. 2020;11:2252. https://doi.org/10.3389/fimmu.2020.567020.
42. Styczynski J, van der Velden W, Fox CP, et al. Management of Epstein-Barr virus infections and post-transplant lymphoproliferative disorders in patients after allogeneic hematopoietic stem cell transplantation: sixth European conference on infections in leukemia (ECIL-6) guidelines. Haematologica.

2016;101:803–11. https://doi.org/10.3324/haematol.2016.144428.
43. Yoon GY, Kim MY, Huh JR, et al. Posttransplant lymphoproliferative disorder of the thorax: CT and FDG-PET features in a single tertiary referral center. Medicine. 2015;94:e1274. https://doi.org/10.1097/MD.0000000000001274.
44. Liu Q, Fan Z, Luo X, et al. Epstein-Barr virus-associated pneumonia in patients with post-transplant lymphoproliferative disease after hematopoietic stem cell transplantation. Transpl Infect Dis. 2010;12:284–91. https://doi.org/10.1111/j.1399-3062.2010.00502.x.
45. Kunitomi A, Arima N, Ishikawa T. Epstein-Barr virus-associated post-transplant lymphoproliferative disorders presented as interstitial pneumonia; successful recovery with rituximab. Haematologica. 2007;92:e49–52. https://doi.org/10.3324/haematol.11142.
46. Fox CP, Burns D, Parker AN, et al. EBV-associated post-transplant lymphoproliferative disorder following in vivo T-cell-depleted allogeneic transplantation: clinical features, viral load correlates and prognostic factors in the rituximab era. Bone Marrow Transplant. 2014;49:280–6. https://doi.org/10.1038/bmt.2013.170.
47. Styczynski J, Gil L, Tridello G, et al. Response to rituximab-based therapy and risk factor analysis in Epstein Barr virus-related lymphoproliferative disorder after hematopoietic stem cell transplant in children and adults: a study from the infectious diseases working party of the European gro. Clin Infect Dis. 2013;57:794–802. https://doi.org/10.1093/cid/cit391.
48. Van Der Velden WJFM, Mori T, Stevens WBC, et al. Reduced PTLD-related mortality in patients experiencing EBV infection following allo-SCT after the introduction of a protocol incorporating pre-emptive rituximab. Bone Marrow Transplant. 2013;48:1465–71. https://doi.org/10.1038/bmt.2013.84.
49. Worth A, Conyers R, Cohen J, et al. Pre-emptive rituximab based on viraemia and T cell reconstitution: a highly effective strategy for the prevention of Epstein-Barr virus-associated lymphoproliferative disease following stem cell transplantation. Br J Haematol. 2011;155:377–85. https://doi.org/10.1111/j.1365-2141.2011.08855.x.
50. Ahmad I, Cau NV, Kwan J, et al. Preemptive management of epstein-barr virus reactivation after hematopoietic stem-cell transplantation. Transplantation. 2009;87:1240–5. https://doi.org/10.1097/TP.0b013e31819f1c49.
51. Papadopoulos EB, Ladanyi M, Emanuel D, et al. Infusions of donor leukocytes to treat Epstein-Barr virus-associated lymphoproliferative disorders after allogeneic bone marrow transplantation. N Engl J Med. 1994;330:1185–91. https://doi.org/10.1056/nejm199404283301703.
52. Prockop S, Reshef R, Tsai DE, et al. Long-term outcomes of subjects with Epstein-Barr virus-driven post-transplant lymphoproliferative disorder (EBV+PTLD) following solid organ (SOT) or allogeneic hematopoietic cell transplants (HCT) treated with Tabelecleucel on an expanded access program. Blood. 2019;134:4071. https://doi.org/10.1182/blood-2019-124904.
53. Prockop S, Hiremath M, Ye W, et al. A multicenter, open label, phase 3 study of Tabelecleucel for solid organ transplant subjects with Epstein-Barr virus-driven post-transplant lymphoproliferative disease (EBV+PTLD) after failure of rituximab or rituximab and chemotherapy. Blood. 2019;134:5326. https://doi.org/10.1182/blood-2019-129277.
54. Biotherapeutics A. Tabelecleucel for solid organ or allogeneic hematopoietic cell transplant participants with Epstein-Barr virus-associated post-transplant lymphoproliferative disease (EBV+ PTLD) after failure of rituximab or rituximab and chemotherapy. 2017. https://clinicaltrials.gov/ct2/show/NCT03394365. Accessed 3 Jan 2022.
55. Atara Biotherapeutics Tabelecleucel in combination with pembrolizumab in subjects with Epstein-Barr virus-associated nasopharyngeal carcinoma (EBV+ NPC)—full text view. ClinicalTrials.gov. https://clinicaltrials.gov/ct2/show/NCT03769467. Accessed 3 Jan 2022.
56. Prockop S, Gamelin L, Dinavahi R, et al. Overall survival by best overall response with tabelecleucel in patients with Epstein-Barr virus-driven post-transplant lymphoproliferative disease following solid organ or allogeneic hematopoietic cell transplant. Blood. 2021;138:887. https://doi.org/10.1182/blood-2021-147226.
57. Xuan L, Jiang X, Sun J, et al. Spectrum of epstein-barr virus-associated diseases in recipients of allogeneic hematopoietic stem cell transplantation. Transplantation. 2013;96:560–6. https://doi.org/10.1097/TP.0b013e31829d38af.
58. Reddy N, Rezvani K, Barrett AJ, Savani BN. Strategies to prevent EBV reactivation and posttransplant lymphoproliferative disorders (PTLD) after allogeneic stem cell transplantation in high-risk patients. Biol Blood Marrow Transplant. 2011;17:591–7. https://doi.org/10.1016/j.bbmt.2010.08.007.
59. Styczynski J, Einsele H, Gil L, Ljungman P. Outcome of treatment of Epstein-Barr virus-related post-transplant lymphoproliferative disorder in hematopoietic stem cell recipients: a comprehensive review of reported cases. Transpl Infect Dis. 2009;11:383–92. https://doi.org/10.1111/j.1399-3062.2009.00411.x.
60. Fujimoto A, Hiramoto N, Yamasaki S, et al. Risk factors and predictive scoring system for post-transplant lymphoproliferative disorder after hematopoietic stem cell transplantation. Biol Blood

Marrow Transplant. 2019;25:1441–9. https://doi.org/10.1016/J.BBMT.2019.02.016.
61. Danylesko I, Shimoni A. Second malignancies after hematopoietic stem cell transplantation. Curr Treat Options in Oncol. 2018;19:9. https://doi.org/10.1007/s11864-018-0528-y.
62. Tichelli A. Secondary neoplasia (other than PTLPS). Cham: Springer; 2019.
63. Chow EJ, Cushing-Haugen KL, Cheng G-S, et al. Morbidity and mortality differences between hematopoietic cell transplantation survivors and other cancer survivors. J Clin Oncol. 2017;35:306–13. https://doi.org/10.1200/JCO.2016.68.8457.
64. Majhail NS, Brazauskas R, Douglas Rizzo J, et al. Secondary solid cancers after allogeneic hematopoietic cell transplantation using busulfan-cyclophosphamide conditioning. Blood. 2011;117:316–22. https://doi.org/10.1182/blood-2010-07-294629.
65. Baker KS, DeFor TE, Burns LJ, et al. New malignancies after blood or marrow stem-cell transplantation in children and adults: incidence and risk factors. J Clin Oncol. 2003;21:1352–8. https://doi.org/10.1200/JCO.2003.05.108.
66. Rizzo JD, Curtis RE, Socié G, et al. Solid cancers after allogeneic hematopoietic cell transplantation. Blood. 2009;113:1175–83. https://doi.org/10.1182/blood-2008-05-158782.
67. Curtis RE, Rowlings PA, Deeg HJ, et al. Solid cancers after bone marrow transplantation. N Engl J Med. 1997;336:897–904. https://doi.org/10.1056/nejm199703273361301.
68. Suzuki T, Trapnell BC. Pulmonary alveolar proteinosis syndrome. Clin Chest Med. 2016;37:431–40. https://doi.org/10.1016/j.ccm.2016.04.006.
69. Carey B, Trapnell BC. The molecular basis of pulmonary alveolar proteinosis. Clin Immunol. 2010;135:223–35.
70. Salvator H, Tcherakian C, Maillard N, et al. Pulmonary alveolar proteinosis after allogeneic hematopoietic stem-cell transplantation in adults. Chest. 2021;160:1783–8. https://doi.org/10.1016/j.chest.2021.05.056.
71. Pidala J, Khalil F, Fernandez H. Pulmonary alveolar proteinosis following allogeneic hematopoietic cell transplantation. Bone Marrow Transplant. 2011;4611(46):1480–3. https://doi.org/10.1038/bmt.2010.321.
72. Lawi D, Dubruc E, Gonzalez M, et al. Secondary pulmonary alveolar proteinosis treated by lung transplant: a case report. Respir Med Case Rep. 2020;30:101108. https://doi.org/10.1016/j.rmcr.2020.101108.
73. Ansari M, Rougemont AL, Le Deist F, et al. Secondary pulmonary alveolar proteinosis after unrelated cord blood hematopoietic cell transplantation. Pediatr Transplant. 2012;16:E146. https://doi.org/10.1111/j.1399-3046.2011.01487.x.
74. Cordonnier C, Fleury-Feith J, Escudier E, et al. Secondary alveolar proteinosis is a reversible cause of respiratory failure in leukemic patients. Am J Respir Crit Care Med. 1994;149:788–94. https://doi.org/10.1164/AJRCCM.149.3.8118651.
75. Salvator H, Tcherakian C, Maillard N, et al. Pulmonary alveolar Proteinosis after allogeneic hematopoietic stem-cell transplantation in adults: a French Société francophone de Greffe de Moelle et Thérapie Cellulaire survey. Chest. 2021;160:1783–8. https://doi.org/10.1016/j.chest.2021.05.056.
76. Murch CR, Carr DH. Computed tomography appearances of pulmonary alveolar proteinosis. Clin Radiol. 1989;40:240–3. https://doi.org/10.1016/S0009-9260(89)80180-1.
77. Maimon N, Heimer D. Clinical images: the crazy-paving pattern on computed tomography. CMAJ. 2010;182:1545. https://doi.org/10.1503/cmaj.091422.
78. Chang HL. The crazy-paving sign. Radiology. 2007;243:905–6. https://doi.org/10.1148/radiol.2433041835.
79. Holbert JM, Costello P, Li W, et al. CT features of pulmonary alveolar proteinosis. Am J Roentgenol. 2001;176:1287–94. https://doi.org/10.2214/ajr.176.5.1761287.
80. Campo I, Luisetti M, Griese M, et al. Whole lung lavage therapy for pulmonary alveolar proteinosis: a global survey of current practices and procedures. Orphanet J Rare Dis. 2016;11:115. https://doi.org/10.1186/s13023-016-0497-9.
81. Tazawa R, Trapnell BC, Inoue Y, et al. Inhaled granulocyte/macrophage-Colony stimulating factor as therapy for pulmonary alveolar proteinosis. Am J Respir Crit Care Med. 2010;181:1345–54. https://doi.org/10.1164/rccm.200906-0978OC.
82. Luisetti M, Rodi G, Perotti C, et al. Plasmapheresis for treatment of pulmonary alveolar proteinosis. Eur Respir J. 2009;33:1220–2. https://doi.org/10.1183/09031936.00097508.
83. Kavuru MS, Malur A, Marshall I, et al. An open-label trial of rituximab therapy in pulmonary alveolar proteinosis. Eur Respir J. 2011;38:1361–7. https://doi.org/10.1183/09031936.00197710.
84. Franquet T, Rodríguez S, Hernández JM, et al. Air-leak syndromes in hematopoietic stem cell transplant recipients with chronic GVHD: high-resolution CT findings. J Thorac Imaging. 2007;22:335–40. https://doi.org/10.1097/RTI.0b013e3180cab6cf.
85. Moon MH, Sa YJ, Do CK, et al. Thoracic air-leak syndromes in hematopoietic stem cell transplant recipients with graft-versus-host disease: a possible sign for poor response to treatment and poor prognosis. J Korean Med Sci. 2010;25:658. https://doi.org/10.3346/jkms.2010.25.5.658.
86. Macklin TM, Macklin C. Malignant interstitial emphysema of the lungs and mediastinum as an important occult complication in many respiratory

diseases and other conditions. Medicine (Baltimore). 1944;23:281.
87. Sakai R, Kanamori H, Nakaseko C, et al. Air-leak syndrome following Allo-SCT in adult patients: report from the Kanto study group for cell therapy in Japan. Bone Marrow Transplant. 2011;46:379–84. https://doi.org/10.1038/bmt.2010.129.
88. Vogel M, Brodoefel H, Bethge W, et al. Spontaneous thoracic air-leakage syndrome in patients following allogeneic hematopoietic stem cell transplantation: causes, CT-follow up and patient outcome. Eur J Radiol. 2006;60:392–7. https://doi.org/10.1016/j.ejrad.2006.07.013.
89. Chakravorty I, Oldfield WLG, Gómez CMH. Rapidly progressive bronchiolitis obliterans Organising pneumonia presenting with pneumothorax, persistent air leak, acute respiratory distress syndrome and multi-organ dysfunction: a case report. J Med Case Rep. 2008;2:145. https://doi.org/10.1186/1752-1947-2-145.
90. Philit F, Wiesendanger T, Archimbaud E, et al. Post-transplant obstructive lung disease ('bronchiolitis obliterans'): a clinical comparative study of bone marrow and lung transplant patients. Eur Respir J. 1995;8:551–8. https://doi.org/10.1183/09031936.95.08040551.

# Pulmonary Rehabilitation in Hematopoietic Stem Cell Transplantation Patients

20

Shinichiro Morishita, Ryohei Jinbo, and Ryuichi Kasahara

## Introduction

Hematopoietic stem cell transplantation (HSCT) is a therapy that restores the immunopoietic function of hematopoietic stem cells (HSCs) damaged by aggressive chemotherapy with/without radiation therapy to eliminate an underlying disease by replacing them with HSCs previously harvested from the patient's own or another person's peripheral blood, bone marrow, or umbilical cord blood [1]. The main risks associated with this treatment modality are the development of infection and graft-versus-host disease (GVHD) [2]. Pulmonary complications after HSCT affect 45–60% of recipients [3, 4]. It is estimated that about 30% of patients who undergo HSCT die from pulmonary complications [5], and in patients on ventilators after autologous HSCT (auto-HSCT), the mortality rate exceeds 60% [6]. Pulmonary complications after HSCT can be infectious or noninfectious and include peri-engraftment respiratory distress syndrome (PERDS), idiopathic pneumonia syndrome (IPS), bronchiolitis obliterans syndrome (BOS), bacterial, fungal, and viral pneumonia, among others [7]. The timing of the onset of these symptoms varies from the pre/peri-HSCT phases (the first 30 days), the early post-HSCT phase (30–100 days), and the late post-HSCT phase (after 100 days) [7], and requires long-term management. Based on the wheel gear model, Wasserman et al. reported that exercise tolerance is associated with the lungs, heart, muscles, and mitochondria based on their role in tissue oxygen transport [8]. Most of the cardiopulmonary problems associated with HSCT are related to reduced aerobic capacity and performance status due to a lack of physical activity

S. Morishita (✉)
Department of Physical Therapy, School of Health Sciences, Fukushima Medical University, Fukushima, Japan
e-mail: morishit@fmu.ac.jp

R. Jinbo · R. Kasahara
Department of Rehabilitation, Kita-Fukushima Medical Center, Fukushima, Japan
e-mail: reha-jinbo@jinsenkai.or.jp; reha-ryu@jinsenkai.or.jp



A. O. Soubani (ed.), *Pulmonary and Critical Care Considerations of Hematopoietic Stem Cell Transplantation*, https://doi.org/10.1007/978-3-031-28797-8_20

[9]. Fatigue is also a result of anemia and the reduced oxygen levels in tissues that accompany anemia [10]. In our report, allogeneic hematopoietic stem cell transplantation (allo-HSCT) patients have decreased physical function and quality of life (QOL) 6–7 weeks after HSCT compared to before HSCT [11, 12]. In addition to GVHD and infections, decreased physical functioning, especially high levels of fatigue, adversely affected patients' QOL [11–13]. Thus, rehabilitation is important because pulmonary complications and the deterioration of cardiopulmonary and physical functions after HSCT can cause an increase in patients' activities of daily living (ADL), QOL, and mortality. In this chapter, we will discuss respiratory rehabilitation for patients with HSCT.

## Respiratory and Physical Functions of HSCT Patients

As mentioned earlier, there is a relationship between respiratory function and physical function in HSCT patients [9], and in order to describe the respiratory rehabilitation of HSCT patients, it is necessary to know about respiratory function and physical function. In this article, we will divide them into the pre-HSCT phase, peri-HSCT phase, early post-HSCT phase, and late post-HSCT phase.

### The Pre-HSCT Phase

In our previous study, 110 allo-HSCT patients reported a significant decrease in muscle strength, exercise capacity, and QOL compared to sex- and age-matched healthy subjects before HSCT [14]. In addition, 83 of 164 (50.6%) allo-HSCT patients experienced sarcopenia before allo-HSCT, and these patients experienced decreased muscle strength and increased fatigue after surgery compared to patients without sarcopenia. Patients with sarcopenia showed significantly lower scores on health-related QOL for physical function, body pain, and vitality than patients without sarcopenia [15].

According to another report, factors significantly associated with decreased leg extensor strength after allo-HSCT include leg extensor strength before HSCT, grade of acute GVHD, age, and the time interval between pre- and post-assessment in 88 patients who underwent allo-HSCT. After allo-HSCT, patients' leg extensor strength and peak $VO_2$ were significantly decreased [16].

In another study of 56 patients who underwent HSCT with either a sibling or an unrelated donor, maximal inspiratory muscle strength (PImax) fell below 80% and 60% of the predicted values in 42% and 18% of patients, respectively. Moreover, maximal expiratory muscle strength (PEmax) fell below 80% and 60% of the predicted values in 89% and 80% of patients, respectively. Grip strength of the dominant hand fell below 80% and 60% of the predicted values in 39% and 15% of patients, respectively, and the 6-min walk test (6MWT) fell below 80% and 60% of the predicted values in 58% and 9.6% of patients, respectively. The diffusing capacity of the lungs for carbon monoxide (DLCO) in lung function was significantly correlated with 6MWT [17].

As mentioned earlier, in exercise physiology, exercise tolerance is determined by cardiopulmonary function, muscle oxidative function, and hemoglobin levels. In our study, we found that changes in hemoglobin parameters of the tibialis anterior muscle in 16 patients before allo-HSCT were different from those in 21 age-matched healthy subjects. In healthy subjects, there was a correlation between muscle strength and hemoglobin dynamics, but this correlation was not observed in patients before allo-HSCT. It has been suggested that hemoglobin dynamics during and after exercise differ between patients with malignant hematopoietic diseases and healthy subjects [18].

Acute respiratory distress syndrome (ARDS) affects 5% of patients after HSCT, with a mortality rate of over 60% [19]. In a previous study, 164 patients who developed ARDS after HSCT had decreased pre-transplant forced ventilation (FVC), forced expiratory volume (FEV1), and diffusion capacity compared to 492 patients who did not develop ARDS after HSCT [20].

In another study of 629 patients undergoing auto-HSCT, among those treated with BEAM (carmustine, etoposide, cytarabine, melphalan), hemoglobin-corrected CO diffusing capacity (DLCOcSB) ≤60% of the predicted value and Karnofsky Performance Status (KPS) of ≤80% were associated with lower overall survival (OS). In patients who received high-dose melphalan, DLCOcSB ≤60% of the predicted value was associated with decreased OS, and KPS of 80% or less was associated with a DLCOcSB of 60% or less of the predicted value. Patients with DLCOcSB ≤60% of their predicted value were more likely to experience nonrecurrent death, including pulmonary death [21].

Thus, a significant proportion of patients had impaired respiratory and physical functions before undergoing HSCT. In addition, various factors, such as sarcopenia and decreased respiratory function before HSCT, affect the changes in physical function after HSCT and the morbidity and mortality of pulmonary complications. There may be a need to improve respiratory and physical functions before HSCT.

## The Peri-and Early Post-HSCT Phases

Allo-HSCT patients receive high-dose chemotherapy, total-body irradiation, and the donation of hematopoietic cells from human leukocyte antigen (HLA)-matched or mismatched donors. These patients are hospitalized in a single-bed isolation room for a period of 4–6 weeks, as the severely decreased bone marrow function increases the patient's risk of bleeding, infection, and anemia and results in weakness, fatigue, shortness of breath, and insomnia [22, 23]. In addition, patients with allo-HSCT often receive a large number of corticosteroids to prevent acute GVHD. In our study, the number of corticosteroid doses was significantly correlated with a decline in grip strength and knee extensor strength in 113 allo-HSCT patients [24].

In a previous study, 30 allo-HSCT patients showed a significant decrease in balance function when tested using the Timed Up and Go test after transplantation and a decrease in the total trajectory length of the center of pressure using the body sway test. In addition, balance function was significantly correlated with grip strength and knee extensor strength [25]. Another study of 23 patients with allo-HSCT and 21 patients with auto-HSCT showed that the patients' two-minute walk test (2MWT) and grip strength results were significantly worse after transplantation. According to the study, these significant differences correspond to decreased aerobic conditioning before and after physical stress, decreased functional and gait performance, decreased muscle strength and spinal flexibility, and decreased function in activities of daily living (ADLs) after HSCT [26].

Another report showed a significant decrease in 6MWT and grip strength at 6 weeks after allo-HSCT compared to 2 weeks before in 86 allo-HSCT patients and a significant decrease in upper limb muscle mass and trunk muscle mass after allo-HSCT [27]. Similarly, another study reported that 64 allo-HSCT patients had a significant decrease in grip strength and 6MWT score at discharge [28].

Another study examined exercise tolerance, pulmonary function, and muscle strength before and after HSCT in 34 patients with HSCT and found that exercise tolerance, respiratory function, and grip strength were significantly decreased after HSCT. There was no significant difference in exercise tolerance and pulmonary function according to the type of HSCT. Allo-HSCT had a significantly greater decrease in lower extremity muscle strength [29].

There is also a sex difference in QOL after allo-HSCT. In 64 allo-HSCT patients, a significant gender and time interaction was observed for hand strength and muscle mass, with males having a much greater decline in both categories than females [28]. Our study showed that in 100 patients (66 men and 34 women) who underwent allo-HSCT, women had significantly lower physical function and general health scores on health-related QOL tests than men after allo-HSCT [11]. Thus, male allo-HSCT patients tend to have greater amounts of reduced muscle strength, and female allo-HSCT patients tend to have lower QOL.

Fatigue is also one of the common side effects of HSCT. In one study ($n = 17$), seven patients with allo-HSCT and 10 patients with auto-HSCT showed both a significant increase in fatigue and a decrease in physical activity after high-dose chemotherapy and HSCT. In addition, during the acute phase after HSCT, there was an increase in symptoms experienced by patients, including fatigue, pain, nausea and vomiting, sleep disturbances, anorexia, and diarrhea [30].

The percentage of daily activity performed at an intensity greater than 3.0 metabolic equivalents (METs) has been shown to increase significantly after allo-HSCT in 30 patients. Daily activity time performed at intensities of 1.6–2.9 METs was significantly correlated with knee extensor strength only. The total number of steps per day and the percentage of activities performed with 1.6–2.9 METs and ≥ 3.0 METs were positively correlated with 6MWT. In addition, the physical function and general health subscales of health-related QOL were found to be positively correlated with activity on days exceeding 3.0 METs [31]. For patients with allo-HSCT, it may be important to assess physical activity prior to HSCT and to increase the level and intensity of physical activity to prevent a subsequent decline in physical function.

One study showed that both allo-HSCT patients ($n = 11$) and auto-HSCT patients ($n = 11$) with low peak $VO_2$ had higher symptom burden and poorer QOL in the early post-HSCT phase [32].

In another study, we investigated the differences in muscle oxygen consumption and blood flow to skeletal muscle, as well as the differences in fatigue levels, before and after allo-HSCT in 25 male patients. Muscle oxygen consumption, as indicated by changes in deoxyhemoglobin, and blood flow to skeletal muscle, as indicated by changes in total hemoglobin, were significantly lower after allo-HSCT than before allo-HSCT. Furthermore, there may be a relationship between malaise and decreased muscle oxygen consumption after allo-HSCT [33]. We also investigated the possible involvement of impaired skeletal muscle oxygenation in the decline of exercise capacity during early recovery in patients with allo-HSCT. The rate of decrease in muscle oxygen-hemoglobin saturation ($SmO_2$), shown as an index of skeletal muscle oxygenation, was significantly lower in 18 patients after allo-HSCT. Moreover, $SmO_2$ during and after exercise was also associated with 6MWT [34].

We also investigated the relationship between exercise tolerance, muscle oxidative metabolism, and cardiopulmonary function in post-allo-HSCT patients in a sterile isolation room. The results showed that muscle consumption and oxygen extraction were decreased after allo-HSCT compared to before allo-HSCT, and exercise tolerance was decreased after allo-HSCT. Exercise tolerance was associated with lung function, muscle oxygen consumption, and muscle oxygen extraction [35].

Physical function and QOL were also compared among 126 allo-HSCT patients (HLA-haploidentical donor [HID] group, $n = 100$; other donor group, $n = 26$) who received HSCT from HLA-matched siblings, matched unrelated donors, and unrelated cord blood donors. After HSCT, the haploid donor group showed significantly greater improvement in the General Health Subscale and Mental Component Summary of Quality of Life compared to the other donor groups. However, the haplotype donor group showed a significantly greater decrease in hand grip strength and knee extensor strength after HSCT compared to the other donor groups [12]. Based on these results, the type of donor may affect the QOL and physical function of HSCT recipients.

One study investigated the relationship between GVHD and physical function in 40 patients with allo-HSCT. Allo-HSCT patients showed 6% muscle weakness at 1 month after HSCT, whereas acute GVHD patients showed 12% muscle weakness in the same period [36].

In a study of physical function and QOL before allo-HSCT in 30 patients, grip strength and 6MWT score were significantly lower than before allo-HSCT, both at discharge and 1 year after allo-HSCT. However, both returned to their pre-HSCT levels within a year after HSCT. Similarly, QOL scores returned to pre-HSCT levels within 1 year after HSCT [37].

Thus, in the early phase after HSCT, respiratory and physical functions were decreased and were also associated with factors that inhibit exercise, such as increased fatigue and decreased muscle oxygen metabolism function. In addition, the type of donor and acute GVHD also affect physical function and other factors. We believe that it is highly beneficial to reduce functional decline through rehabilitation while taking into account the above-mentioned factors.

## The Late Post-HSCT Phase

A previous report compared dyspnea, exercise tolerance, physical activity level, and QOL in daily life in 80 patients who had undergone allo-HSCT (more than 100 days after allo-HSCT) and 60 age- and sex-matched healthy subjects. Energy expenditure, 6MWT, time spent doing physical activity, steps, mean metabolic equivalents, global health status, and the functional and social functioning subitems of the European Organization for Research and Treatment of Cancer Quality of Life Questionnaire (EORTC QLQ) were significantly lower in allogeneic transplant recipients compared to healthy controls. Dyspnea score, time spent lying down, sleep duration, EORTC QLQ symptoms, and fatigue subscales were significantly higher in allogeneic transplant patients compared to healthy controls. Patients with allo-HSCT had significantly lower dyspnea, exercise tolerance, physical activity level, and QOL in their daily lives after allo-HSCT [38]. In another study, the prevalence of respiratory and skeletal muscle weakness after HSCT was investigated in 44 patients who underwent HSCT with either a sibling or an unrelated donor. PImax fell below 80% of the predicted value in 52% of patients and below 60% of the predicted value in 20% of patients. PEmax fell below 80% of the predicted value in 88% of patients and below 60% of the predicted value in 74% of patients. Grip strength decreased to <80% of the predicted value in 75% of patients and to <60% of the predicted value in 47% of patients after HSCT. Analysis of the paired measurements obtained before and after HSCT also showed a significant decrease in both PImax and PEmax [39]. In one report, exercise tolerance, pulmonary function, and QOL of 103 survivors after HSCT were below their predicted values. When the subjects were classified into two groups according to their physical activity level (moderate/low activity and high activity) and compared, the more active subjects showed better results in exercise tolerance, pulmonary function, and QOL [40]. In another report, the effects of severe fatigue on pulmonary function, blood levels, dyspnea, respiratory muscle strength, peripheral muscle strength, exercise tolerance, depression, and QOL in 24 patients undergoing allo-HSCT were investigated. Compared to the 25 non-severely fatigued individuals, the severely fatigued individuals had significantly higher symptom QOL subscale and depression scores, as well as significantly lower peripheral muscle strength, global health status, and functional QOL subscale scores. Blood levels, lung function, dyspnea, and respiratory muscle strength were comparable between the two groups. In addition, 42.4% of the variance in severe fatigue was explained by symptom QOL—subscale scores and corticosteroid use after allo-HSCT. Although pulmonary and respiratory functions do not differ by degree of fatigue, patients with severe fatigue have more impairments in peripheral muscle strength, QOL, exercise tolerance, and depression. Furthermore, decreased QOL and the use of corticosteroids after allo-HSCT were suggested to be the most important predictors of severe fatigue [41].

Chronic graft-versus-host disease (cGVHD) is the most common long-term complication after allo-HSCT, affecting approximately 50% of patients [42]. A previous report investigated the relationship between 2MWT, grip strength, degree of involvement of specific organs (National Institutes of Health GVHD scale), KPS, and subjective well-being in 121 patients with cGVHD after allo-HSCT and found that fascial and pulmonary (FEV1) involvement, 2MWT, and subjective well-being were most strongly associated with KPS [43]. In another report, the knee extensor strength and 6MWT score of 162 patients with cGVHD recovered to near pre-allo-HSCT levels 12 months after undergoing allo-HSCT. High doses of glucocorticoids and cGVHD were associated with delayed recovery in body mass index (BMI), grip strength, knee extensor strength, and time spent standing on one leg. Pulmonary GVHD and high-dose glucocorticoids had a negative impact on the 6MWT score. Multivariate analysis revealed that cGVHD and glucocorticoids were independent risk factors for lower BMI and delayed muscle recovery, respectively [44]. In addition, a report investigating factors associated with fatigue in 263 patients with moderate to severe cGVHD showed that low activity and the presence of pulmonary, muscle, and joint symptoms were associated with fatigue, although there was no association with cGVHD severity [45].

GVHD of the lung is complicated by Bronchiolitis Obliterans Syndrome (BOS) [46]. BOS is irreversible, with varying degrees of progression and a mortality rate of up to 60% [47]. If medical therapy is unsuccessful, lung transplantation may be an option for eligible candidates [48]. One study examined the long-term outcomes and associated changes in physical function of 15 patients who underwent lung transplantation for late-onset noninfectious pulmonary complications (LONIPC) after allo-HSCT, including BOS. Two years after lung transplantation, dyspnea scores and performance status improved, but did not fully recover. Knee extensor strength and 6MWT scores showed poor results up to 3 months after implantation but improved over 2 years. The distance of 6MWT improved to almost the level of a healthy person. Recovery of exercise tolerance was associated with recovery of percent vital capacity (%VC) and knee extensor strength from 3 months to 2 years after lung transplantation. Furthermore, flattening of the thorax, a characteristic of LONIPC patients, was closely associated with %VC at 2 years after transplantation [49].

Thus, even in the late phase after HSCT, respiratory and physical functions are declining and may be associated with pulmonary complications, suggesting the need for long-term follow-up of respiratory and physical functions in order to maintain QOL.

## Rehabilitation of HSCT Patients

There are various reports that have examined the effects of rehabilitation on HSCT patients. As mentioned above, cardiopulmonary function in HSCT patients is not only affected by pulmonary complications but also associated with reduced aerobic capacity and performance status due to a lack of physical activity [9]. Therefore, in addition to rehabilitation of cardiopulmonary function, rehabilitation of physical function is also important.

## Exercise Therapy for Patients with HSCT

Combined with aerobic and strength training, physical exercise has been shown to have a significant positive effect on exercise tolerance (oxygen consumption and expiratory minute ventilation), muscle strength, and QOL (physical functioning level) in acute myeloid leukemia patients receiving high-dose chemotherapy with myeloablative chemotherapy and auto-HSCT for malignant hematologic diseases or solid tumors. Significant positive effects have been shown in exercise tolerance, muscle strength, and QOL in patients with acute myeloid leukemia receiving high-dose chemotherapy with HSCT. Patients in the training group required less antiemetic medication and experienced significantly less fatigue [50]. Physical exercise was also suggested to have beneficial effects in patients undergoing chemotherapy before HSCT.

A systematic review and meta-analysis of 11 randomized controlled trials (RCTs), which included patients undergoing either allo-HSCT or auto-HSCT ($n$ = 734), showed that physical exercise, which includes aerobic exercise, resistance training, and relaxing stretching exercises, may have positive effects on the physiological, psychological, and psychosocial health of allo-HSCT patients. Physical exercise during hospitalization has been shown to improve QOL and reduce fatigue in HSCT patients at discharge. The study suggested significant positive effects on QOL, fatigue, psychological well-being and distress, and physical functioning [51]. Another systematic review that includes eight studies in HSCT ($n = 472$) showed that physical exercise had a statistically significant and moderately favorable effect on cardiopulmonary function, lower extremity muscle strength, and fatigue. Patients who underwent allo-HSCT and auto-HSCT had small but significant positive effects on upper extremity muscle strength and overall QOL, as well as physical, emotional, and cognitive functioning [52]. In one RCT investigating the effects of aerobic exercise in 64 allo-HSCT and auto-HSCT patients, a physical exercise regimen that combined aerobic endurance training with ADL training using a bicycle ergometer had a significant positive effect on the training group in terms of muscular strength, endurance, pulmonary function, and QOL compared to the control group [53]. Similarly, a moderate exercise program was shown to increase endurance performance, muscle strength, fatigue levels, and emotional state without posing any additional risk in 47 allo-HSCT patients [54]. Another RCT in patients with allo-HSCT ($n = 100$) showed that regular light-intensity exercise, including walking or cycling, led to significant improvements in physical performance and in perceived physical and emotional status during recovery [55].

In 42 patients who underwent allo-HSCT, a combined physical exercise regimen had significant effects on aerobic capacity ($VO_2$max) and muscle strength (chest press, leg extension, right elbow flexion, right knee extension, and functional performance by the stair test). In addition, the physical exercise group had significantly less severe diarrhea and days of total parenteral nutrition after treatment [56]. Similarly, a structured physical exercise program of 4–6 weeks was shown to significantly improve treatment-related symptoms in a study of 42 HSCT patients [57]. In another study, the effects of endurance and resistance training sessions conducted at home before admission, during inpatient care, and for 6–8 weeks after discharge on physical function were examined in 105 HSCT patients. The physical exercise group showed significant improvements in fatigue scores, physical fitness, physical function, and overall quality of life [58].

The effectiveness of an outpatient physical exercise program for HSCT patients has also been evaluated. All patients were randomly assigned to a supervised physical education program ($n = 64$) or a usual care control group ($n = 67$). A 12-week outpatient program that included both aerobic and strength exercises was shown to improve the physical performance of allo-HSCT patients after the intervention. However, body composition, level of physical activity in daily life, fatigue, and QOL did not show improvement [59]. In another non-RCT study, the effectiveness of physical exercise was investigated without a control group, and 12 patients who followed a 12-week individualized mild aerobic exercise program showed significant improvement in fatigue after allo-HSCT [60]. A 6-week physical exercise program that included active exercise, muscle stretching, and walking on a treadmill resulted in significantly higher muscle strength in the nine allo-HSCT patients compared to the nine allo-HSCT patients in the control group [61].

In summary, physical exercise appears to have several beneficial effects on patients who have undergone HSCT, including a positive impact on physical and mental recovery before and after HSCT and the potential to accelerate the recovery of health and function in patients after HSCT [55]. Even light aerobic exercise has been shown to have beneficial effects on physical and mental recovery. Therefore, patients undergoing HSCT should engage in physical exercise to maintain physical function before, during, and after hospitalization and discharge. Physical exercise includes resistance training, aerobic exercise, and relaxation stretching and should be tailored to the patient's condition (Fig. 20.1). Further high-quality research is needed to determine the optimal exercise intervention method for HSCT patients.

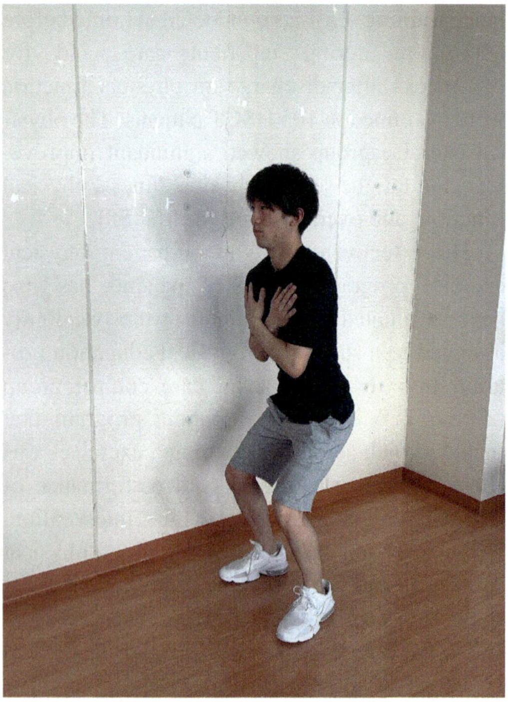

**Fig. 20.1** Resistance training (squats)

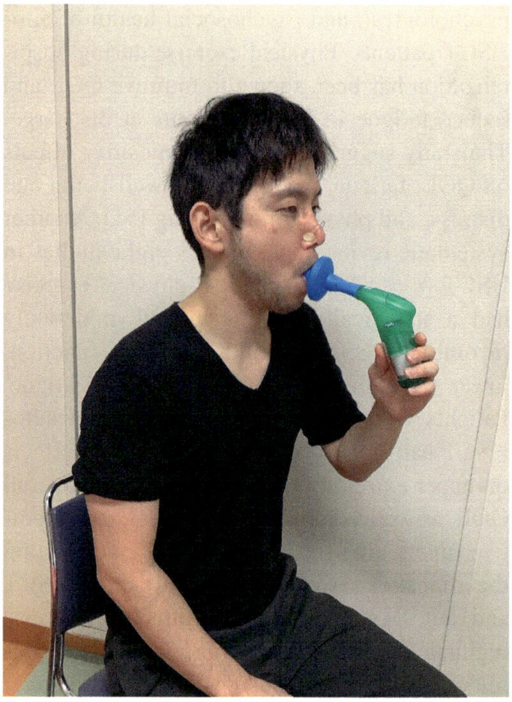

**Fig. 20.2** Inspiratory muscle training

## Respiratory Muscle Training for HSCT Patients

A limited number of studies on patients with HSCT have shown impaired inspiratory and expiratory muscle function and impaired functional motor skills before and after HSCT [17, 39]. Various studies have shown that weakness in the respiratory muscles is associated with decreased exercise capacity [62, 63]. There have been several reports on the effects of respiratory physiotherapy and respiratory muscle training on patients with HSCT.

A previous study examined the effects of respiratory physiotherapy in the early phase of 39 patients with HSCT. The treatment group underwent diaphragm autoreceptor stimulation, respiratory training, incentive spirometry, inspiratory muscle training (IMT), bronchial hygiene, and cough stimulation. The control group underwent an incentive spirometry-only protocol. There were significant differences between the two groups in tidal volume (TV) on day two after HSCT and in maximal inspiratory pressure (MIP), maximal expiratory pressure (MEP), and TV on day seven after HSCT. The results suggest that respiratory physiotherapy may contribute to the improvement of ventilation and respiratory muscle strength [64]. In another study, the impact of IMT on early transplant-related outcomes was investigated in 38 patients with allo-HSCT. Patients were assigned to a treatment group (40% of MIPs) or a control group (5% of MIPs) and received IMT (Fig. 20.2) for 6 weeks. The results showed significant improvements in exercise tolerance, respiratory muscle strength, depression, and the modified Borg scale in the treatment group compared to the control group [65]. One study examined the safety, feasibility, and preliminary efficacy of IMT in 31 hospitalized patients undergoing HSCT. Patients were randomly assigned to either the conventional physical rehabilitation group (control group) or the conventional physical rehabilitation plus IMT (IMT group). IMT was performed at 40% of maximal inspiratory pressure (MIP), five times a week, with each session lasting 10–20 min. The recruitment rate was 100%, the adherence rate was 91%, and the withdrawal rate on IMT was 13%. Two events were observed in a total of 126 IMT sessions (1.5%). MIP was significantly higher in the IMT group. When comparing the control and IMT groups, a trend toward negative outcomes was observed in the control group, including the need for oxygen therapy (18% vs. 6%), bleeding (12% vs. 6%), dyspnea (25% vs. 13%), and acute pulmonary edema (6% vs. 0%). The results suggest that IMT is safe, feasible, and improves inspiratory muscle strength in hospitalized patients undergoing HSCT [66].

Thus, respiratory physiotherapy and inspiratory muscle training can be safely implemented for HSCT patients and may have a positive impact on physical and respiratory functions.

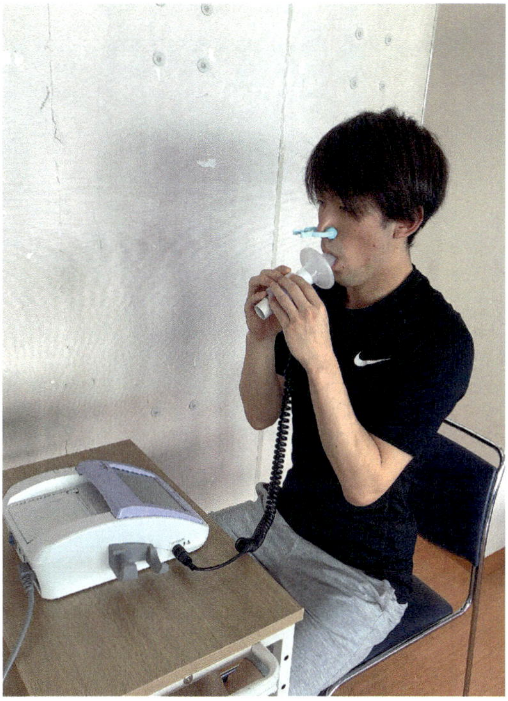

**Fig. 20.3** Evaluation of respiratory function using a spirometer

## Respiratory Rehabilitation of HSCT Patients with Pulmonary Complications

Respiratory rehabilitation has become a standard treatment for chronic obstructive pulmonary disease, a common lung disease [67]. Rehabilitation includes evaluation of respiratory function using a spirometer (Fig. 20.3), physical functions such as grip strength (Fig. 20.4) and exercise tolerance (Fig. 20.5), as well as ADL. Thereafter, stretching (Fig. 20.6), breathing training (Fig. 20.7), muscle strength training (Fig. 20.8a, b), aerobic exercise (Fig. 20.9), and ADL training (Fig. 20.10) are performed according to the general condition of the patient.

As mentioned above, one of the most challenging manifestations of chronic pulmonary GVHD is BOS, which is characterized clinically by obstructive airflow obstruction and pathologically by circumferential fibrous scar tissue targeting small airways. BOS is rare, difficult to diagnose, and associated with a high mortality rate [46, 47, 68]. As for treatment, the U.S. National Institutes of Health (NIH) Consensus Statement on cGVHD

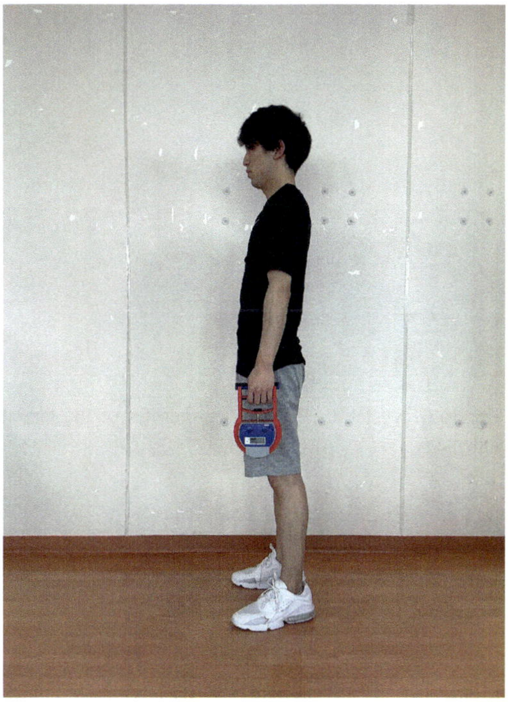

**Fig. 20.4** Evaluation of grip strength

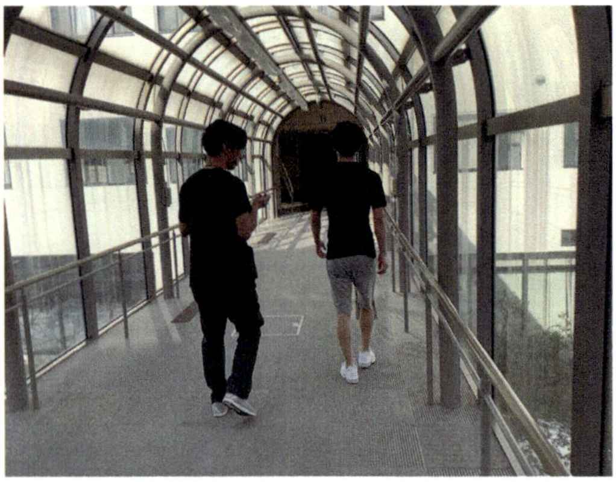

**Fig. 20.5** Assessment of exercise tolerance (6MWT)

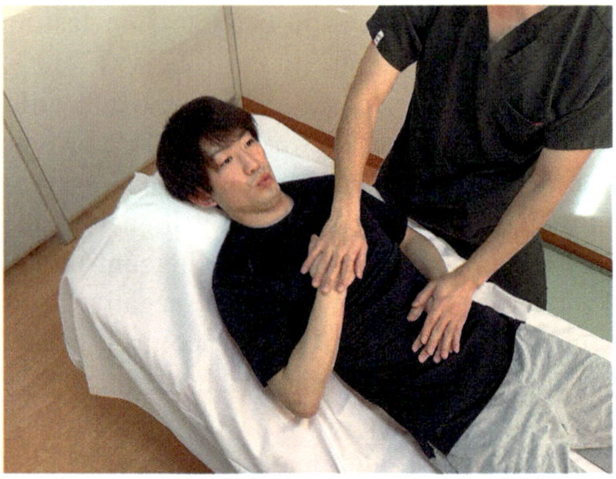

**Fig. 20.7** Abdominal breathing training

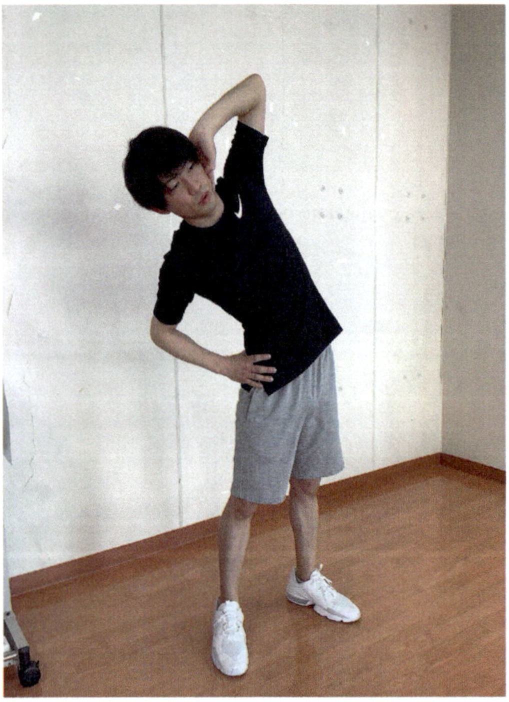

**Fig. 20.6** Stretch the respiratory muscles of the lateral abdomen

recommends pulmonary rehabilitation for patients with BOS, but few studies have examined this treatment [69].

In a previous report, 11 patients with BOS underwent a rehabilitation program of 24 sessions over 8 weeks. Specifically, the subjects were instructed on nutrition, medication, and oxygen safety, as well as pursed lip breathing, other breathing techniques, and the use and precautions of metered dose inhalers. In addition, strength training for upper and lower limbs using free weights and weight machines and cardiovascular exercises such as those using recumbent bikes and treadmills were performed. After the rehabilitation program, the 6MWT score and physical function score were significantly improved compared with those before the rehabilitation program [70].

Similarly, in another report, the detailed progress of a respiratory rehabilitation program for four patients with BOS was presented. Respiratory rehabilitation for patients with BOS was suggested to be beneficial for exercise tolerance and dyspnea [71].

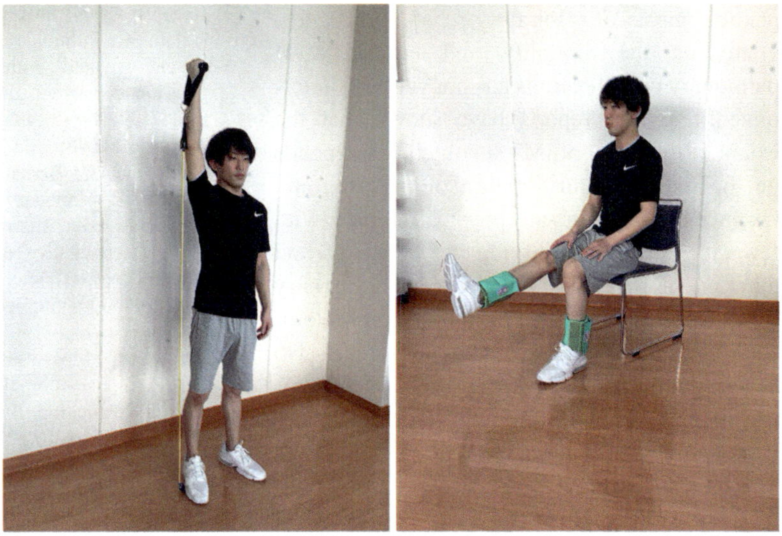

**Fig. 20.8** (**a**) Upper extremity muscle strength training. (**b**) Lower extremity muscle strength training

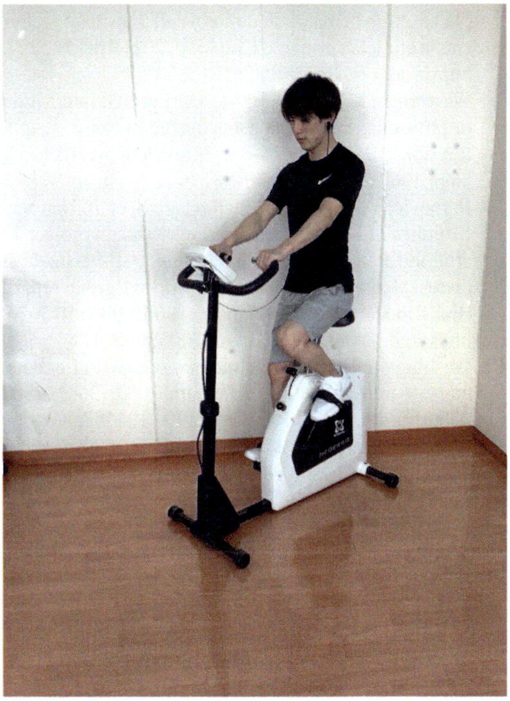

**Fig. 20.9** Aerobic exercise (Bicycle Ergometer)

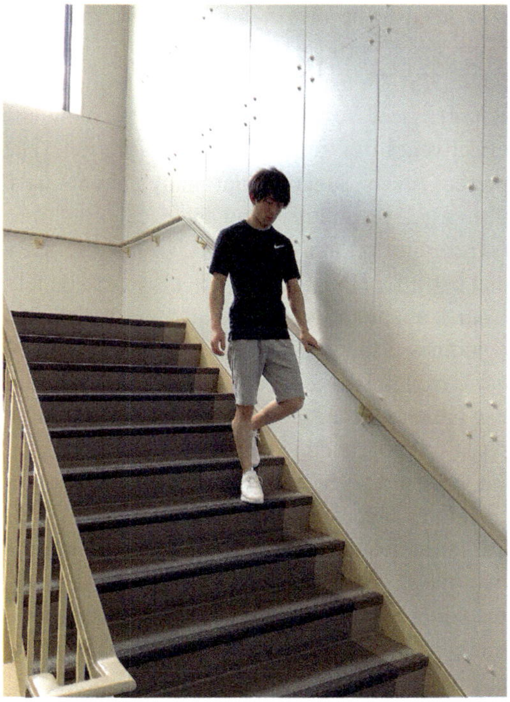

**Fig. 20.10** ADL training (stair climbing)

## Conclusions

Respiratory rehabilitation programs that combine respiratory muscle training and physical exercise are necessary to prevent or improve the decline of respiratory function and physical function in patients who have undergone HSCT. In the case of pulmonary complications, multidisciplinary respiratory rehabilitation is required. Future studies are needed that include patients who have undergone HSCT. For example, the impact of respiratory rehabilitation programs on the mortality and morbidity of pulmonary complications has not yet been determined. Previous reports have shown that the extent of the effect of IMT on outcomes depends on the intensity and duration of the program. Given that IMT is a safe physical therapy with few side effects, modifying the intensity and duration of IMT may help prevent pulmonary complications and reduce mortality from pulmonary complications. Patients with HSCT also experience fatigue due to a variety of factors, causing a decline in physical function. Cardiopulmonary exercise stress testing is the gold standard method for examining factors contributing to fatigue, but there are few reports in HSCT patients. Additionally, the impact of exercise training and psychosocial support on fatigue may need to be investigated. Finally, there are very few reports of rehabilitation for patients with HSCT and pulmonary complications. Reports need to be accumulated to show the effectiveness of respiratory rehabilitation. The present review suggests that many patients have decreased respiratory and physical functions before, during, and after HSCT and that early and late after HSCT, these patients would benefit from a respiratory rehabilitation program that combines respiratory muscle training and physical exercise. Therefore, clinicians should encourage patients to engage in physical exercise at all phases before and after HSCT, and physical exercise should be incorporated into the conditioning and recovery plans of all HSCT patients. Furthermore, since respiratory rehabilitation may be a means to improve survival rates, including prevention of pulmonary complications, it should be actively introduced, studied, and reported.

## References


1. Barriga F, Ramírez P, Wietstruck A, Rojas N. Hematopoietic stem cell transplantation: clinical use and perspectives. Biol Res. 2012;45(3):307–16. https://doi.org/10.4067/S0716-97602012000300012.
2. Smith LA, Wright-Kanuth MS. Complications and risks in hematopoietic stem cell transplant patients. Clin Lab Sci. 2001;14(2):118–24.
3. Jules-Elysee K, Stover DE, Yahalom J, White DA, Gulati SC. Pulmonary complications in lymphoma patients treated with high-dose therapy autologous bone marrow transplantation. Am Rev Respir Dis. 1992;146(2):485–91. https://doi.org/10.1164/ajrccm/146.2.485.
4. Cordonnier C, Bernaudin JF, Bierling P, Huet Y, Vernant JP. Pulmonary complications occurring after allogeneic bone marrow transplantation. A study of 130 consecutive transplanted patients. Cancer. 1986;58(5):1047–54. https://doi.org/10.1002/1097-0142(19860901)58:5<1047::aid-cncr2820580512>3.0.co;2-y.
5. Wah TM, Moss HA, Robertson RJ, Barnard DL. Pulmonary complications following bone marrow transplantation. Br J Radiol. 2003;76(906):373–9. https://doi.org/10.1259/bjr/66835905.
6. Shorr AF, Moores LK, Edenfield WJ, Christie RJ, Fitzpatrick TM. Mechanical ventilation in hematopoietic stem cell transplantation: can we effectively predict outcomes? Chest. 1999;116(4):1012–8. https://doi.org/10.1378/chest.116.4.1012.
7. Astashchanka A, Ryan J, Lin E, et al. Pulmonary complications in hematopoietic stem cell transplant recipients-a clinician primer. J Clin Med. 2021;10(15):3227. https://doi.org/10.3390/jcm10153227.
8. Wasserman K, Van Kessel AL, Burton GG. Interaction of physiological mechanisms during exercise. J Appl Physiol. 1967;22(1):71–85. https://doi.org/10.1152/jappl.1967.22.1.71.
9. Filipovich AH, Weisdorf D, Pavletic S, et al. National Institutes of Health consensus development project on criteria for clinical trials in chronic graft-versus-host disease: I. diagnosis and staging working group report. Biol Blood Marrow Transplant. 2005;11(12):945–56. https://doi.org/10.1016/j.bbmt.2005.09.004.
10. Washington RL. Cardiopulmonary sequelae after bone marrow transplantation. J Pediatr. 2000;136(3):280–2. https://doi.org/10.1067/mpd.2000.104387.
11. Morishita S, Kaida K, Yamauchi S, et al. Gender differences in health-related quality of life, physical function and psychological status among patients in the early phase following allogeneic haematopoietic stem cell transplantation. Psychooncology. 2013;22(5):1159–66. https://doi.org/10.1002/pon.3128.
12. Morishita S, Kaida K, Yamauchi S, et al. Early-phase differences in health-related quality of life, psychological status, and physical function between human leucocyte antigen-haploidentical and other allogeneic haematopoietic stem cell transplantation recipients. Eur J Oncol Nurs. 2015;19(5):443–50. https://doi.org/10.1016/j.ejon.2015.02.002.
13. Wiskemann J, Huber G. Physical exercise as adjuvant therapy for patients undergoing hematopoietic stem cell transplantation. Bone Marrow Transplant. 2008;41(4):321–9. https://doi.org/10.1038/sj.bmt.1705917.
14. Morishita S, Kaida K, Ikegame K, et al. Impaired physiological function and health-related QOL in patients before hematopoietic stem-cell transplanta-

tion. Support Care Cancer. 2012;20(4):821–9. https://doi.org/10.1007/s00520-011-1156-2.
15. Morishita S, Kaida K, Tanaka T, et al. Prevalence of sarcopenia and relevance of body composition, physiological function, fatigue, and health-related quality of life in patients before allogeneic hematopoietic stem cell transplantation. Support Care Cancer. 2012;20(12):3161–8. https://doi.org/10.1007/s00520-012-1460-5.
16. Ishikawa A, Otaka Y, Kamisako M, et al. Factors affecting lower limb muscle strength and cardiopulmonary fitness after allogeneic hematopoietic stem cell transplantation. Support Care Cancer. 2019;27(5):1793–800. https://doi.org/10.1007/s00520-018-4433-5.
17. White AC, Terrin N, Miller KB, Ryan HF. Impaired respiratory and skeletal muscle strength in patients prior to hematopoietic stem-cell transplantation. Chest. 2005;128(1):145–52. https://doi.org/10.1378/chest.128.1.145.
18. Wakasugi T, Morishita S, Kaida K, et al. Hemoglobin dynamics in the skeletal muscle of patients with malignant hematopoietic disease. Adv Exp Med Biol. 2018;1072:287–91. https://doi.org/10.1007/978-3-319-91287-5_46.
19. Yadav H, Nolan ME, Bohman JK, et al. Epidemiology of acute respiratory distress syndrome following hematopoietic stem cell transplantation. Crit Care Med. 2016;44(6):1082–90. https://doi.org/10.1097/CCM.0000000000001617.
20. Herasevich S, Frank RD, Bo H, et al. Pretransplant risk factors can predict development of acute respiratory distress syndrome after hematopoietic stem cell transplantation. Ann Am Thorac Soc. 2021;18(6):1004–12. https://doi.org/10.1513/AnnalsATS.202004-336OC.
21. Duque-Afonso J, Ewald S, Ihorst G, et al. The impact of pulmonary function in patients undergoing autologous stem cell transplantation. Blood Adv. 2021;5:4327. https://doi.org/10.1182/bloodadvances.2021004863.
22. Morishita S, Kaida K, Setogawa K, et al. Safety and feasibility of physical therapy in cytopenic patients during allogeneic haematopoietic stem cell transplantation. Eur J Cancer Care (Engl). 2013;22(3):289–99. https://doi.org/10.1111/ecc.12027.
23. Jarden M, Hovgaard D, Boesen E, Quist M, Adamsen L. Pilot study of a multimodal intervention: mixed-type exercise and psychoeducation in patients undergoing allogeneic stem cell transplantation. Bone Marrow Transplant. 2007;40(8):793–800. https://doi.org/10.1038/sj.bmt.1705807.
24. Morishita S, Kaida K, Yamauchi S, et al. Relationship between corticosteroid dose and declines in physical function among allogeneic hematopoietic stem cell transplantation patients. Support Care Cancer. 2013;21(8):2161–9. https://doi.org/10.1007/s00520-013-1778-7.
25. Morishita S, Kaida K, Aoki O, et al. Balance function in patients who had undergone allogeneic hematopoietic stem cell transplantation. Gait Posture. 2015;42(3):406–8. https://doi.org/10.1016/j.gaitpost.2015.07.011.
26. de Souza CV, Miranda EC, Garcia C, Aranha FJ, de Souza CA, Vigorito AC. Functional evaluation indicates physical losses after hematopoietic stem cell transplantation. Rev Bras Hematol Hemoter. 2012;34(5):345–51. https://doi.org/10.5581/1516-8484.20120090.
27. Takekiyo T, Dozono K, Mitsuishi T, et al. Effect of exercise therapy on muscle mass and physical functioning in patients undergoing allogeneic hematopoietic stem cell transplantation. Support Care Cancer. 2015;23(4):985–92. https://doi.org/10.1007/s00520-014-2425-7.
28. Takekiyo T, Dozono K, Nara S, et al. Gender differences in physical function and muscle mass change in patients undergoing allogeneic hematopoietic stem cell transplantation. Bone Marrow Transplant. 2017;52(10):1460–2. https://doi.org/10.1038/bmt.2017.156.
29. Silva TC, Silva PO, Morais DS, et al. Functional capacity, lung function, and muscle strength in patients undergoing hematopoietic stem cell transplantation: a prospective cohort study. Hematol Oncol Stem Cell Ther. 2021;14(2):126–33. https://doi.org/10.1016/j.hemonc.2020.08.004.
30. Danaher EH, Ferrans C, Verlen E, et al. Fatigue and physical activity in patients undergoing hematopoietic stem cell transplant. Oncol Nurs Forum. 2006;33(3):614–24. https://doi.org/10.1188/06.ONF.614-624.
31. Morishita S, Kaida K, Yamauchi S, et al. Relationship of physical activity with physical function and health-related quality of life in patients having undergone allogeneic haematopoietic stem-cell transplantation Eur J Cancer Care (Engl). 2017;26(4). https://doi.org/10.1111/ecc.12669.
32. Wood WA, Deal AM, Reeve BB, et al. Cardiopulmonary fitness in patients undergoing hematopoietic SCT: a pilot study. Bone Marrow Transplant. 2013;48(10):1342–9. https://doi.org/10.1038/bmt.2013.58.
33. Morishita S, Wakasugi T, Kaida K, et al. Fatigue, muscle oxygen consumption and blood flow to the skeletal muscle after allogeneic hematopoietic stem cell transplantation. Adv Exp Med Biol. 2018;1072:293–8. https://doi.org/10.1007/978-3-319-91287-5_47.
34. Wakasugi T, Morishita S, Kaida K, et al. Impaired skeletal muscle oxygenation following allogeneic hematopoietic stem cell transplantation is associated with exercise capacity. Support Care Cancer. 2018;26(7):2149–60. https://doi.org/10.1007/s00520-017-4036-6.
35. Wakasugi T, Morishita S, Kaida K, Ikegame K, Uchiyama Y, Domen K. Correction to: muscle oxygen extraction and lung function are related to exercise tolerance after allogeneic hematopoietic stem cell transplantation. Support Care Cancer. 2021;29(10):6049. https://doi.org/10.1007/s00520-021-06225-6.

36. Kramer M, Heussner P, Herzberg PY, et al. Validation of the grip test and human activity profile for evaluation of physical performance during the intermediate phase after allogeneic hematopoietic stem cell transplantation. Support Care Cancer. 2013;21(4):1121–9. https://doi.org/10.1007/s00520-012-1634-1.
37. Takekiyo T, Dozono K, Mitsuishi T, et al. Recovery of physical function and quality of life in patients undergoing hematopoietic stem cell transplantation: a 1-year follow-up. Bone Marrow Transplant. 2016;51(8):1127–30. https://doi.org/10.1038/bmt.2016.58.
38. Boşnak Güçlü M, Barğı G, Sucak GT. Impairments in dyspnea, exercise capacity, physical activity and quality of life of allogeneic hematopoietic stem cell transplantation survivors compared with healthy individuals: a cross sectional study. Physiother Theory Pract. 2021;37(1):52–63. https://doi.org/10.1080/09593985.2019.1594473.
39. Kovalszki A, Schumaker GL, Klein A, Terrin N, White AC. Reduced respiratory and skeletal muscle strength in survivors of sibling or unrelated donor hematopoietic stem cell transplantation. Bone Marrow Transplant. 2008;41(11):965–9. https://doi.org/10.1038/bmt.2008.15.
40. Penna GB, da Silva TC, Aparecida Paz A, Ziegler B. Functional capacity, pulmonary function, and quality of life in hematopoietic stem cell transplantation survivors. Support Care Cancer. 2021;29(7):4015–21. https://doi.org/10.1007/s00520-020-05947-3.
41. Barğı G, Boşnak Güçlü M, Türköz Sucak AG. Differences in pulmonary and extra-pulmonary characteristics in severely versus non-severely fatigued recipients of allogeneic hematopoietic stem cell transplantation: a cross-sectional, comparative study. Hematology. 2019;24(1):112–22. https://doi.org/10.1080/10245332.2018.1526441.
42. Gillis TA, Donovan ES. Rehabilitation following bone marrow transplantation. Cancer. 2001;92(4 Suppl):998–1007. https://doi.org/10.1002/1097-0142(20010815)92:4+<998::aid-cncr1412>3.0.co;2-k.
43. Andrews C, Smith S, Kennel M, Schilling S, Kalpakjian C. The association of performance status and disease severity in patients with chronic graft-vs-host disease. Arch Phys Med Rehabil. 2019;100(4):606–12. https://doi.org/10.1016/j.apmr.2018.04.034.
44. Hayakawa J, Miyamura D, Kimura SI, et al. Negative impact of chronic graft-versus-host disease and glucocorticoid on the recovery of physical function after allogeneic hematopoietic stem cell transplantation. Bone Marrow Transplant. 2019;54(7):994–1003. https://doi.org/10.1038/s41409-018-0365-4.
45. Im A, Mitchell SA, Steinberg SM, et al. Prevalence and determinants of fatigue in patients with moderate to severe chronic GvHD. Bone Marrow Transplant. 2016;51(5):705–12. https://doi.org/10.1038/bmt.2015.320.
46. Krowka MJ, Rosenow EC, Hoagland HC. Pulmonary complications of bone marrow transplantation. Chest. 1985;87(2):237–46. https://doi.org/10.1378/chest.87.2.237.
47. Yoshihara S, Yanik G, Cooke KR, Mineishi S. Bronchiolitis obliterans syndrome (BOS), bronchiolitis obliterans organizing pneumonia (BOOP), and other late-onset noninfectious pulmonary complications following allogeneic hematopoietic stem cell transplantation. Biol Blood Marrow Transplant. 2007;13(7):749–59. https://doi.org/10.1016/j.bbmt.2007.05.001.
48. Soubani AO, Uberti JP. Bronchiolitis obliterans following haematopoietic stem cell transplantation. Eur Respir J. 2007;29(5):1007–19. https://doi.org/10.1183/09031936.00052806.
49. Hamada R, Oshima Y, Sato S, et al. Physical function after lung transplantation for late-onset noninfectious pulmonary complications after allogeneic hematopoietic stem cell transplantation. Support Care Cancer. 2021;29(9):5447–54. https://doi.org/10.1007/s00520-021-06118-8.
50. Oechsle K, Aslan Z, Suesse Y, Jensen W, Bokemeyer C, de Wit M. Multimodal exercise training during myeloablative chemotherapy: a prospective randomized pilot trial. Support Care Cancer. 2014;22(1):63–9. https://doi.org/10.1007/s00520-013-1927-z.
51. van Haren IE, Timmerman H, Potting CM, Blijlevens NM, Staal JB, Nijhuis-van der Sanden MW. Physical exercise for patients undergoing hematopoietic stem cell transplantation: systematic review and meta-analyses of randomized controlled trials. Phys Ther. 2013;93(4):514–28. https://doi.org/10.2522/ptj.20120181.
52. Persoon S, Kersten MJ, van der Weiden K, et al. Effects of exercise in patients treated with stem cell transplantation for a hematologic malignancy: a systematic review and meta-analysis. Cancer Treat Rev. 2013;39(6):682–90. https://doi.org/10.1016/j.ctrv.2013.01.001.
53. Baumann FT, Kraut L, Schüle K, Bloch W, Fauser AA. A controlled randomized study examining the effects of exercise therapy on patients undergoing haematopoietic stem cell transplantation. Bone Marrow Transplant. 2010;45(2):355–62. https://doi.org/10.1038/bmt.2009.163.
54. Baumann FT, Zopf EM, Nykamp E, et al. Physical activity for patients undergoing an allogeneic hematopoietic stem cell transplantation: benefits of a moderate exercise intervention. Eur J Haematol. 2011;87(2):148–56. https://doi.org/10.1111/j.1600-0609.2011.01640.x.
55. DeFor TE, Burns LJ, Gold EM, Weisdorf DJ. A randomized trial of the effect of a walking regimen on the functional status of 100 adult allogeneic donor hematopoietic cell transplant patients. Biol Blood Marrow Transplant. 2007;13(8):948–55. https://doi.org/10.1016/j.bbmt.2007.04.008.
56. Jarden M, Baadsgaard MT, Hovgaard DJ, Boesen E, Adamsen L. A randomized trial on the effect of a multimodal intervention on physical capacity, functional performance and quality of life in adult patients undergoing allogeneic SCT. Bone

Marrow Transplant. 2009;43(9):725–37. https://doi.org/10.1038/bmt.2009.27.
57. Jarden M, Nelausen K, Hovgaard D, Boesen E, Adamsen L. The effect of a multimodal intervention on treatment-related symptoms in patients undergoing hematopoietic stem cell transplantation: a randomized controlled trial. J Pain Symptom Manag. 2009;38(2):174–90. https://doi.org/10.1016/j.jpainsymman.2008.09.005.
58. Wiskemann J, Dreger P, Schwerdtfeger R, et al. Effects of a partly self-administered exercise program before, during, and after allogeneic stem cell transplantation. Blood. 2011;117(9):2604–13. https://doi.org/10.1182/blood-2010-09-306308.
59. Knols RH, de Bruin ED, Uebelhart D, et al. Effects of an outpatient physical exercise program on hematopoietic stem-cell transplantation recipients: a randomized clinical trial. Bone Marrow Transplant. 2011;46(9):1245–55. https://doi.org/10.1038/bmt.2010.288.
60. Carlson LE, Smith D, Russell J, Fibich C, Whittaker T. Individualized exercise program for the treatment of severe fatigue in patients after allogeneic hematopoietic stem-cell transplant: a pilot study. Bone Marrow Transplant. 2006;37(10):945–54. https://doi.org/10.1038/sj.bmt.1705343.
61. Mello M, Tanaka C, Dulley FL. Effects of an exercise program on muscle performance in patients undergoing allogeneic bone marrow transplantation. Bone Marrow Transplant. 2003;32(7):723–8. https://doi.org/10.1038/sj.bmt.1704227.
62. Dimeo FC, Tilmann MH, Bertz H, Kanz L, Mertelsmann R, Keul J. Aerobic exercise in the rehabilitation of cancer patients after high dose chemotherapy and autologous peripheral stem cell transplantation. Cancer. 1997;79(9):1717–22.
63. Teasell R, Dittmer DK. Complications of immobilization and bed rest. Part 2: other complications. Can Fam Physician. 1993;39(1440–2):1445–6.
64. Bom EA, de Souza CV, Thiesen RA, Miranda EC, de Souza CA. Evaluation of respiratory conditions in early phase of hematopoietic stem cell transplantation. Rev Bras Hematol Hemoter. 2012;34(3):188–92. https://doi.org/10.5581/1516-8484.20120047.
65. Barğı G, Güçlü MB, Arıbaş Z, Akı Ş, Sucak GT. Inspiratory muscle training in allogeneic hematopoietic stem cell transplantation recipients: a randomized controlled trial. Support Care Cancer. 2016;24(2):647–59. https://doi.org/10.1007/s00520-015-2825-3.
66. de Almeida LB, Trevizan PF, Laterza MC, Hallack Neto AE, Perrone ACAS, Martinez DG. Safety and feasibility of inspiratory muscle training for hospitalized patients undergoing hematopoietic stem cell transplantation: a randomized controlled study. Support Care Cancer. 2020;28(8):3627–35. https://doi.org/10.1007/s00520-019-05209-x.
67. Alharbi MG, Kalra HS, Suri M, et al. Pulmonary rehabilitation in management of chronic obstructive pulmonary disease. Cureus. 2021;13(10):e18414. https://doi.org/10.7759/cureus.18414.
68. Au BK, Au MA, Chien JW. Bronchiolitis obliterans syndrome epidemiology after allogeneic hematopoietic cell transplantation. Biol Blood Marrow Transplant. 2011;17(7):1072–8. https://doi.org/10.1016/j.bbmt.2010.11.018.
69. Couriel D, Carpenter PA, Cutler C, et al. Ancillary therapy and supportive care of chronic graft-versus-host disease: national institutes of health consensus development project on criteria for clinical trials in chronic graft-versus-host disease: V. ancillary therapy and supportive care working group report. Biol Blood Marrow Transplant. 2006;12(4):375–96. https://doi.org/10.1016/j.bbmt.2006.02.003.
70. Tran J, Norder EE, Diaz PT, et al. Pulmonary rehabilitation for bronchiolitis obliterans syndrome after hematopoietic stem cell transplantation. Biol Blood Marrow Transplant. 2012;18(8):1250–4. https://doi.org/10.1016/j.bbmt.2012.01.017.
71. Choi HE, Lim SN, Lee JH, Park SH. Comprehensive pulmonary rehabilitation in patients with bronchiolitis obliterans syndrome: a case series. Respir Med Case Rep. 2020;31:101161. https://doi.org/10.1016/j.rmcr.2020.101161.

# 21 Pulmonary Complications of Common Hematopoietic Stem Cell Transplantation Therapies

Kyle R. Brownback

## Introduction

Drug toxicities of the respiratory system have long complicated the treatment of hematologic malignancies with chemotherapeutic agents, with the first report occurring in 1961 [1]. Due to the high risks of mortality and morbidity associated with these malignancies, an increased risk for toxicities involving the lungs has long been tolerated, making these complications not uncommon [2].

Many aspects have contributed to making these toxicities difficult to define and recognize in the hematopoietic stem cell transplantation (HSCT) patient population. To begin with, patients undergoing HSCT typically have many comorbidities and are profoundly immunosuppressed, leading to a higher risk for respiratory infections and difficulty in differentiating between pulmonary infection and pulmonary toxicity (Table 21.1). In many situations, patients are treated with both antimicrobials and corticosteroids, thereby making establishing a definitive diagnosis challenging.

Most toxicities associated with therapies used in HSCT are not reproducible in animal models. Additionally, the toxicities that have been associated with medications do not occur in all or even most patients who receive the drug at therapeutic doses, and the association between pharmacogenetics, drug metabolism, and patient factors leads to variable phenotypic expression of toxicity. Furthermore, the actual incidence of toxicity associated with these drugs is likely underreported, as it is estimated that under 5% of drug-induced pulmonary diseases are formally reported to the Food and Drug Administration [3].

K. R. Brownback (✉)
Division of Pulmonary, Critical Care and Sleep Medicine, University of Kansas School of Medicine, Kansas City, KS, USA
e-mail: kbrownback@kumc.edu



A. O. Soubani (ed.), *Pulmonary and Critical Care Considerations of Hematopoietic Stem Cell Transplantation*, https://doi.org/10.1007/978-3-031-28797-8_21

**Table 21.1** Conditioning regimens used in practice

| | | Dosing of agents |
|---|---|---|
| *Myeloablative regimens* | Cy/TBI | Cyclophosphamide 120 mg/kg administered over 2 days<br>TBI 12–14 Gy administered over 4 days |
| | Bu4/Cy | Busulfan 10–12 mg/kg administered over 4 days<br>Cyclophosphamide 120 mg/kg administered over 2 days |
| | Flu/Bu4 | Fludarabine 120–180 mg/m$^2$ administered over 4 days<br>Busulfan 16 mg/kg orally administered over 4 days |
| | BEAM | BCNU 300 mg/m$^2$ administered over 1 day<br>Etoposide 400–800 mg/m$^2$ administered over 4 days<br>Cytarabine 800–1600 mg/m$^2$ administered over 4 days<br>Melphalan 140 mg/m$^2$ administered over 1 day |
| | Melphalan | Melphalan 200 mg/m$^2$ administered over 1 day |
| *Nonmyeloablative regimens* | Flu/TBI | Fludarabine 90 mg/m$^2$ administered over 3 days<br>Low-dose TBI (2 Gy) administered on the day of graft infusion |
| | Flu/Mel | Fludarabine 125–150 mg/m$^2$ administered over 5 days<br>Melphalan 140 mg/m$^2$ administered over 2 days |
| | Flu/Bu2 | Fludarabine 150–160 mg/m$^2$ administered over 4–5 days<br>Busulfan 8–10 mg/kg administered orally over 2–3 days |
| | Flu/Cy | Fludarabine 150–180 mg/m$^2$ administered over 5–6 days<br>Cyclophosphamide 120/140 mg/kg administered over 2 days |
| | Flu/Bu/TT | Fludarabine 150 mg/m$^2$ administered over 3 days<br>Busulfan 8 mg/kg administered over 3 days<br>Thiotepa 5–10 mg/m$^2$ administered over 1–2 days |

Source: Gratwohl A, Carreras E. Principles of Conditioning. In: ESH-EBMT Handbook on Haematopoietic Stem Cell Transplantation 2012, sixth edition, Apperley J, Carreras E, Gluckman E, Masszi T (Eds), European School of Haematology, Paris 2012

## Mechanisms of Toxicity

The pathogenesis of lung injury associated with the use of chemotherapies or agents used in management of complications of HSCT is poorly understood. This is in part due to inability to have an accurate animal model of disease toxicity for the agents utilized during the HSCT process. Mechanisms of pulmonary injury that have been recognized previously related to antineoplastic agents include oxidative injury and direct cytotoxic effect of the agents on pneumocytes [4].

With regard to oxidative lung injury, this has been most heavily studied in bleomycin-induced lung injury. In this model, free oxygen radicals are produced by bleomycin-Fe complex oxidation and are subsequently activated by leukocytes [5]. The importance of free radicals in the pathogenesis of bleomycin lung toxicity is shown by the prevention of lung injury with the use of amifostine, a cytoprotective adjuvant that scavenges free radicals, in rats [6]. Additionally, high inspired oxygen levels may have an association with increased risk of pulmonary toxicity associated with bleomycin use [7].

Direct toxicity to the pneumocytes and the alveolar capillary endothelium is likely responsible for most pulmonary toxicities seen in the HSCT population. This toxicity can lead to subsequent release of inflammatory cytokines that can potentiate the inflammation and lead to capillary leak in some scenarios. Unchecked inflammation can progress to fibrosis if not recognized promptly.

## Conditioning Agents

### Busulfan

Busulfan is an alkylating agent that is used as a component of various conditioning regimens before HSCT. These regimens can include the myeloablative regimens of intravenous busulfan with cyclophosphamide (Bu4/Cy) and busulfan with fludarabine administered over 4 days (Bu4/

Flu). Busulfan is also part of the reduced intensity conditioning (RIC) regimens involving fludarabine and oral busulfan (Flu/Bu2) [8].

Busulfan can cause toxicity as soon as 4 weeks following the administration of the drug until over 1 year later [9], with an incidence of approximately 3–6% [10–13]. Risk factors for developing toxicity related to busulfan are still unclear, though the addition of total body irradiation or other alkylating agents may promote pulmonary toxicity [14]. The precise mechanism by which pulmonary toxicity occurs due to busulfan is not known. Pathologic specimens have displayed evidence of alveolitis with progression to interstitial edema and fibrosis [15]. Symptoms may be mild, including dyspnea and cough, but can progress to acute respiratory failure in some cases.

Specific manifestations of pulmonary toxicity caused by busulfan may include acute lung injury, organizing pneumonia, chronic fibrosis, and alveolar hemorrhage. Alveolar proteinosis has also been described as a manifestation of busulfan pulmonary toxicity when used in prolonged treatment of chronic leukemias [16, 17]. Determining that busulfan is the causative agent of lung injury can be particularly challenging, as during this time frame, there are several possible causes of respiratory failure, including cytomegalovirus pneumonitis, idiopathic pneumonia syndrome, bronchiolitis obliterans syndrome, and alveolar hemorrhage. Imaging findings associated with busulfan-induced lung injury can include fibrosis, ground-glass opacities, and consolidation (Fig. 21.1) [18]. Bronchoscopy with alveolar lavage is typically performed to exclude infectious etiologies, including cytomegalovirus, as the cause of respiratory decline. Findings on alveolar lavage that have been attributed to busulfan toxicity include neutrophilia, lymphocytosis, and alveolar hemorrhage [15, 19].

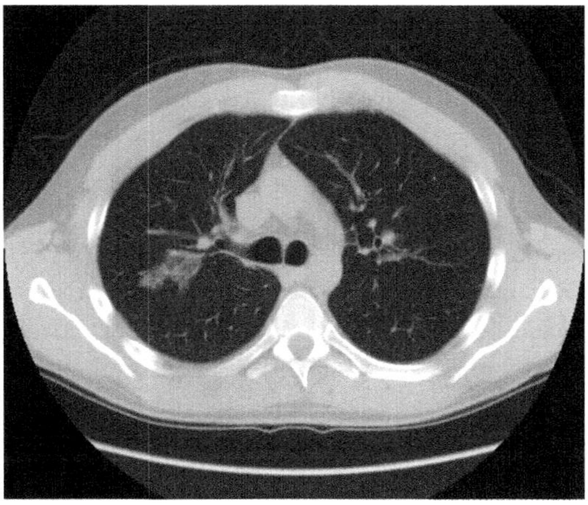

**Fig. 21.1** CT imaging of a patient diagnosed with organizing pneumonia associated with busulfan use, revealing alveolar infiltrates and a negative infectious evaluation

Typical treatments for busulfan pulmonary toxicity involve supportive care, utilization of supplemental oxygen when necessary, and avoidance of future pulmonary toxicity from other medications. No controlled studies have evaluated the use of corticosteroids or other steroid-sparing agents, though anecdotal reports do suggest some improvement in conditions that are typically steroid responsive, such as organizing pneumonia [20]. The use of corticosteroids should be considered in cases of acute respiratory failure due to drug toxicity or organizing pneumonia, with doses ranging from 1 mg/kg of prednisone equivalent daily upwards to 1 gm of methylprednisolone in cases of profound hypoxemic respiratory failure.

Outcomes following busulfan pulmonary toxicity are variable. In a case series following the use of busulfan and cyclophosphamide prior to allogeneic HSCT, a decrease in lung volumes and diffusion capacity was found in the months following HSCT, though this did resolve after a 5-year period of follow-up [9, 21]. Acute toxicity related to busulfan can be associated with a high incidence of death, especially when manifested as alveolar hemorrhage [14]. Larger-scale reports of outcomes following acute toxicity related to busulfan use in HSCT are not available.

## Carmustine

Carmustine, along with lomustine and fotemustine, forms a class of nitrosourea agents, which are used in the treatment of certain lymphomas, melanomas, and brain tumors. Carmustine is also used as a conditioning agent and is combined with etoposide, cytarabine, and melphalan to form BEAM myeloablative conditioning prior to HSCT in patients with history of lymphoma [8]. Nitrosoureas have been associated with the development of both acute interstitial pneumonitis and late-onset pulmonary fibrosis [22].

Nitrosoureas can cause acute interstitial pneumonitis in approximately 10% of patients [23]. Risk factors for developing pulmonary toxicity include receiving total doses greater than 1500 mg/m$^2$, prior history of lung disease, concurrent radiation, and use of cyclophosphamide [24–26]. Patients with acute pulmonary toxicity related to carmustine typically present with dyspnea that may progress to fulminant respiratory failure, with bilateral infiltrates on imaging (Fig. 21.2). The histopathology commonly reveals interstitial inflammation and hyaline membrane formation [27]. Diagnosis is made on clinical history and exclusion of infectious causes of acute lung injury. Treatment involves stopping carmustine at the earliest sign of pulmonary toxicity; pulmonary function testing is used for monitoring patients receiving carmustine to aid in early detection of pulmonary toxicity [28]. Corticosteroids may be employed in severe, early-onset disease [29].

Fibrotic changes associated with carmustine may develop many years after its use, with a predilection for involving the upper lobes [30]. There is an association between receiving carmustine at a young age and risk of subsequent lung fibrosis [31]. Carmustine toxicity is also associated with pleuroparenchymal fibroelastosis [32] and pneumothorax [25]. Diagnosis is based off of clinical history and imaging findings; lung biopsy is typically not required. No effective treatments have been identified for late-onset pulmonary fibrosis due to nitrosoureas, and lung function progressively declines in this condition [33].

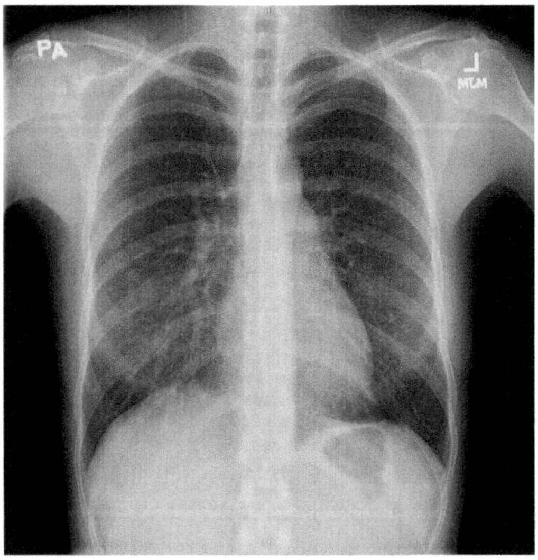


**Fig. 21.2** Chest X-ray imaging of a patient with carmustine pneumonitis, showing bilateral interstitial pneumonitis

The use of carmustine in conditioning regimens prior to HSCT has been associated with increased risk of developing idiopathic pneumonia syndrome (IPS) [34, 35], a heterogeneous condition of noninfectious lung injury and respiratory failure that occurs in the first 120 days following HSCT [36]. IPS is diagnosed by multi-lobar pulmonary opacities on chest imaging with hypoxemia and without infectious etiologies identified as a potential cause [37]. Treatment used in this situation involves corticosteroids that may be combined with anti-tumor necrosis factor (TNF) agents such as etanercept [38, 39].

## Cyclophosphamide

Cyclophosphamide is an alkylating agent that is used in the treatment of many autoimmune conditions and used in combination with chemotherapies in the treatment of a wide spectrum of malignancies. Cyclophosphamide is a component of myeloablative conditioning regimens prior to HSCT, including being administered intravenously over 2 days with total body irradiation (Cy/TBI) and in combination with intravenous busulfan (Bu4/Cy). Cyclophosphamide is also a component of Flu/Cy, an RIC regimen that also includes fludarabine [8].

Pulmonary toxicity caused by cyclophosphamide is quite rare, with an incidence of less than 1% reported [40]. Pathologically, cyclophosphamide is known to cause hyperplasia of type II pneumocytes, edema, and fibrosis [41]. Risk factors for the development of pulmonary toxicity after cyclophosphamide administration include concomitant radiation therapy, use of other agents known to cause pulmonary toxicity (amiodarone, busulfan), and exposure to high $FiO_2$ [42–45]. There may be a dose response with increase in incidence of pulmonary toxicity with higher doses of cyclophosphamide [43].

Cyclophosphamide pulmonary toxicity typically occurs in two different patterns: an early-onset pneumonitis that begins several months after receiving therapy and a late-onset toxicity with fibrosis that occurs many months to years later [46]. Early-onset cyclophosphamide toxicity typically presents 1–6 months after receiving the drug, with symptoms including dyspnea, cough, and fever, though in some cases, the patient may not have symptoms and only radiographic abnormalities [41]. Radiographic patterns that have been described include ground-glass, reticular, or nodular opacities. These abnormalities may favor the periphery of the lung [46].

In contrast, late-onset pulmonary toxicity due to cyclophosphamide typically occurs 6 months to several years after receiving the medication and is associated with fibrosis and diffuse reticular and nodular opacities (Fig. 21.3) [47, 48]. It can also be associated with pleural thickening and associated pleural-parenchymal fibroelastosis [32]. This condition can lead to the development of pneumothoraxes [49]. Mortality may exceed 60% in this toxicity [46].

Early-onset pulmonary toxicity due to cyclophosphamide is generally reversible and often improves with drug discontinuation alone [46]. Glucocorticoids have been used in the treatment of patients with severe presentations including acute respiratory failure, though the optimal dose and duration are not known [50]. Most patients recover from this condition, though death has been reported [41].

In late-onset pneumonitis, no treatments have been identified today that slow the progression of disease. Steroids are generally thought to be ineffective in this state. Though it has not been reported in this condition, consideration should be made toward the use of antifibrotics such as nintedanib in the treatment of progressive fibrosing lung disease, based on data showing benefit of nintedanib in similar clinical situations [51].

## Fludarabine

Fludarabine is a purine nucleoside analogue that is used in the treatment of a variety of conditions, including chronic lymphocytic leukemia and non-Hodgkin's lymphoma [52]. It is also combined with busulfan and given over 4 days in the myeloablative conditioning regimen Flu/Bu4 and is a component of multiple RIC regimens when combined with melphalan (Flu/Mel), oral busulfan (Flu/Bu2), cyclophosphamide (Flu/Cy), and total body irradiation (Flu/TBI) [8].

Pulmonary toxicity has been reported to occur in 8.6% of patients receiving fludarabine and is most common in patients with a prior history of chronic lymphocytic leukemia [53]. Onset of symptoms ranged from 3 days to after the seventh treatment cycle with the agent in the

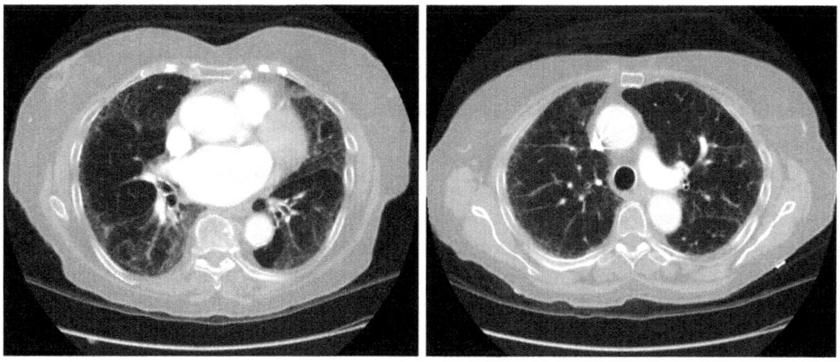

**Fig. 21.3** CT imaging of a patient with pulmonary fibrosis following cyclophosphamide treatment

largest case series. Symptoms may include cough and dyspnea, with chest imaging revealing mixed alveolar and interstitial infiltrates (Fig. 21.4.)

Because these patients treated with fludarabine are at risk for opportunistic infections [54], bronchoscopy with alveolar lavage is typically performed to exclude infectious etiologies. Alveolar lavage has been shown to have increased cellularity without a specific cell differential being seen, and lung biopsy specimens have shown interstitial inflammation and fibrosis [53].

In patients who are symptomatic related to fludarabine-pulmonary toxicity after drug withdrawal or completion, corticosteroids are used as a standard treatment. Excellent responses have been reported with resolution of symptoms being a common outcome [55–57]. Rechallenge with fludarabine after toxicity has been associated with recurrence of respiratory symptoms [53]. The reports of toxicity associated with fludarabine use have not occurred when fludarabine is used as part of the conditioning regimen before HSCT, and caution should be made when extrapolating the currently available clinical data into those clinical scenarios.

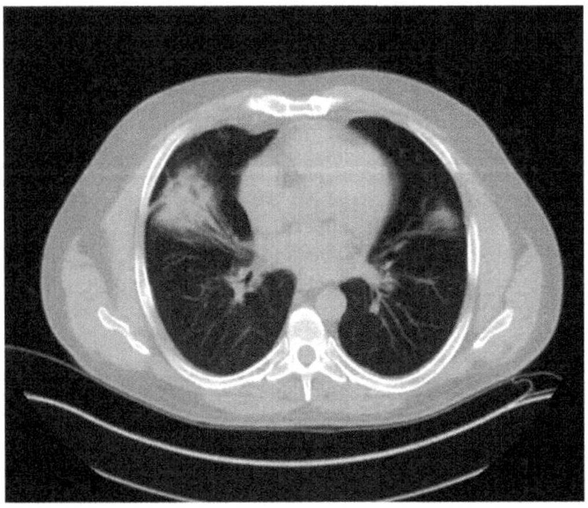

**Fig. 21.4** CT imaging of a patient showing alveolar infiltrates consistent with organizing pneumonia. The patient had received a fludarabine conditioning regimen and had no systemic manifestations of GVHD. The patient had no infectious etiologies identified on bronchoalveolar lavage (BAL) fluid testing and had subsequent improvement in symptoms and infiltrates after treatment with corticosteroids

## Cytarabine

Cytarabine is a cytotoxic agent used to induce remission in acute leukemias and is combined with carmustine, etoposide, and melphalan to form the BEAM conditioning regimen prior to HSCT [8]. Cytarabine has been associated with causing noncardiogenic pulmonary edema that occurs in the first 3 weeks after induction therapy [58, 59], though incidence is thought to be much lower based on recent data [60]. Drug discontinuation along with supportive care with oxygen and diuresis is utilized in treatment. The role of glucocorticoids for treatment is unknown and likely unnecessary. Outcomes are typically good with resolution of symptoms with treatment, though mortality has been reported [59].

## Etoposide

Etoposide is a podophyllotoxin, which is most used in the treatment of bronchogenic carcinoma. It is also a part of the BEAM conditioning regimen and may be combined with carmustine and cyclophosphamide for CBV regimen, which is used as a conditioning regimen for patients with various lymphomas [8]. Cases of pulmonary toxicity are very rare, and when reported, it has occurred after prolonged use of oral etoposide [61, 62]. Diagnosis is typically made by exclusion of infectious etiologies or radiation toxicity, and treatment with corticosteroids has been reported as being effective [63].

## Melphalan

Melphalan is an alkylating agent that is used in the treatment of multiple myeloma as a preparative regimen prior to autologous HSCT. Melphalan is combined with carmustine, etoposide, and cytarabine for BEAM regimen and is paired with fludarabine for the RIC regimen Flu/Mel [8]. Melphalan has a rare association with causing pulmonary toxicity, typically interstitial pneumonitis and fibrosis [64–66]. Pathologic evaluation of patients with pulmonary toxicity due to melphalan may reveal alveolar epithelial cell proliferation and interstitial fibrosis [67]. Reports have described favorable responses to drug discontinuation and treatment with corticosteroids [64].

## Total Body Irradiation

Total body irradiation (TBI) has been a standard component of many regimens prior to HSCT since its inception [68]. It is currently used in combination with cyclophosphamide in a myeloablative conditioning regimen and is combined with fludarabine in a lower dose in a non-myeloablative preparatory regimen [8]. Comparisons of TBI-containing preparative regimens to non-radiation-containing preparative regimens, such as Bu/Cy or BEAM, prior to HSCT have revealed no differences in treatment-related survival, graft-versus-host disease (GVHD), or overall survival [69, 70].

TBI regimens typically fractionate the dose of radiation administered over several days to decrease toxicity and improve tolerability [71]. Randomized trials have shown that doses above 15 Gy TBI may reduce risk of relapse, but at the expense of higher toxicity [72]. Toxicities associated with TBI include mucositis, infertility, and lung toxicity. Risk factors for the development of pulmonary complications associated with TBI include older age, increased dose rate, cytomegalovirus infection, single-fraction TBI, and abnormal pre-transplant pulmonary function testing (PFT) [73].

The manifestations of pulmonary toxicity related to TBI are highly variable. On one end of the spectrum, many patients who receive TBI may experience an asymptomatic decline in lung function following HSCT [74]. On the other end of the spectrum, it can include widespread alveolar injury progressing to fibrosis and irreversible lung injury and death, as is seen with radiation injury associated with solid tumors [75]. Additionally, the use of TBI with increased lung dose is associated with higher risk for development of IPS following HSCT [73].

IPS is a clinical syndrome that typically occurs within 4 months of HSCT and is a syndrome of diffuse lung injury without any identifiable infectious etiologies as a causative pathogen [37]. One of the most commonly associated risk factors for the development of IPS is receipt of higher intensity TBI [43].

Pulmonary toxicity following TBI is quite common, occurring in approximately 10–45% of recipients [76]. Fortunately, the majority of cases are relatively mild, with grades 1 and 2 toxicity reported in 64.9% of cases [77]. Manifestations of pulmonary toxicity of TBI include pneumonia, bronchial obstruction, dyspnea, pleural effusion, and acute respiratory distress syndrome (ARDS) [76].

Radiographic manifestations of pulmonary toxicity of TBI are highly variable, as is seen in other forms of radiation-induced lung injury [78]. Diagnosis is made based on time frame of development of respiratory symptoms, appropriate radiographic findings, and the exclusion of infectious etiologies, which sometimes requires bronchoscopy and alveolar lavage. Alveolar lavage fluid can display lymphocytosis in radiation toxicity [79]. Treatment of radiation pneumonitis is largely supportive, with a role for glucocorticoids in severe and symptomatic disease [80].

## Granulocyte Colony-Stimulating Factor

Granulocyte colony-stimulating factor (GCSF) is a bone marrow stimulant that produces an increase in serum granulocyte counts. Both GCSF and granulocyte-macrophage colony-stimulating factor (GM-CSF) are commonly used following both autologous and allogeneic HSCT, as they reduce time for neutrophil engraftment [81]. The use of GCSF or GM-CSF has not been associated with increased risk of development of GVHD [82].

When used following HSCT, neither GCSF nor GM-CSF has been associated with any notable toxicity [83, 84]. Multiple case reports have described pulmonary toxicity associated with GCSF use, with a proposed mechanism of action involving increased inflammatory mediators associated with neutrophil infiltration [85, 86]. These cases manifest as diffuse pneumonitis and

ARDS associated with GCSF use [87, 88]. Corticosteroids have been reported as being useful in the treatment of these toxicities.

## Medications Used in the Treatment of Graft-Versus-Host Disease

### Calcineurin Inhibitors

Cyclosporine and tacrolimus are distinct calcineurin inhibitors that are used in a variety of conditions, including in combination with methotrexate for prophylaxis against acute GVHD, with wide variations in regimens from various institutions [89]. These medications are typically given for 3–6 months following HSCT and gradually tapered. These drugs have also been employed in the treatment of chronic GVHD [90].

The use of calcineurin inhibitors is associated with increased risk of infection and reduction in neutrophil activity against fungal infections [91]. In patients undergoing solid-organ transplantation, the use of calcineurin inhibitors has been associated with an increased risk of various viral infections [92]. There is very limited evidence of associations between calcineurin inhibitor use and risk of interstitial pneumonitis or noninfectious lung toxicity.

### Rituximab

Rituximab is an anti-CD20 monoclonal antibody, first used in the treatment of non-Hodgkin's lymphoma. Its use has expanded to include many other hematologic malignancies, rheumatologic conditions, and GVHD. When used in the treatment of GVHD, rituximab is dosed 375 mg/$m^2$ weekly for 4 weeks and has been associated with clinical responses in up to 86% of patients [93]. Rituximab has also been shown to allow for reductions in doses of glucocorticoids and aid in stabilizing lung function in bronchiolitis obliterans associated with GVHD [94, 95].

Rituximab is known to cause infusion-related toxicity, including fevers, rigors, and bronchospasm in up to half of patients treated [96]. Rituximab has also been reported to cause interstitial lung disease in several case reports and series [97, 98]. Lung toxicity related to rituximab is suspected to be related to the release of cytokines including TNF-α. Histologic patterns reported as manifestations of rituximab-induced lung disease include organizing pneumonia, interstitial pneumonitis, and diffuse alveolar damage [99]. The majority of cases of pulmonary toxicity associated with rituximab use were seen in patients with lymphoma, with a mean onset of symptoms of 30 days from the most recent rituximab infusion. Treatments include rituximab discontinuation and use of corticosteroids, with mixed results.

### Ruxolitinib

Ruxolitinib is a Janus kinase (JAK) 1/2 inhibitor that was initially approved for the treatment of myelofibrosis. Its use has expanded to other conditions, including polycythemia vera, both acute and chronic GVHD, and many other areas under investigation. Ruxolitinib has been found to be highly effective in the management of patients with both acute and chronic GVHD [100, 101], with superior clinical response rates and ability to reduce steroid dose, including in patients with bronchiolitis obliterans syndrome [102].

Most toxicities associated with ruxolitinib include cytopenias, hepatic dysfunction, and increased risk of infections. Ruxolitinib has been implicated as exacerbating pulmonary arterial hypertension in a single case report [103], though a different case series reports improvement in pulmonary hemodynamics with the use of this medication [104]. Single case reports have implicated ruxolitinib as a potential cause of ARDS and pleural effusions [105, 106]. There have also been reports of ARDS and respiratory symptoms developing after withdrawal of ruxolitinib [107, 108].

### Sirolimus

Sirolimus is an immunosuppressant that is a mechanistic target of rapamycin kinase (mTOR) inhibitor. It inhibits activation of T and B cells and has been used in the treatment of lymphangioleiomyomatosis to prevent organ transplant rejection and as a coating-agent in drug-eluting stents. Sirolimus has been used in the treatment of chronic GVHD, with an overall reported response rate of 63% [109].

Pulmonary toxicities have been reported extensively associated with sirolimus use, with typical manifestations including interstitial pneumonitis, organizing pneumonia, and alveolar hemorrhage [110, 111]. The mechanism of action is unclear, and the typical presentation is highly variable. Drug discontinuation is largely effective in resolving toxicity, though steroids may be used in more severe cases [112].

## Ibrutinib

Ibrutinib is a drug that binds to Bruton's tyrosine kinase and inhibits B-cell proliferation. It has been used to treat chronic lymphocytic leukemia, mantle cell lymphoma, and Waldenstrom's macroglobulinemia. In a study involving patients with chronic GVHD with an inadequate response to corticosteroids, ibrutinib was found to have a response rate of 67% [113]. There was a decrease in median daily corticosteroid dose in responders and improvements seen in all organ systems involved.

Adverse respiratory events noted in trials of ibrutinib in the treatment of GVHD include pneumonia, upper respiratory tract infection, and respiratory failure [113, 114]. Pneumonitis has been reported and associated with ibrutinib use in patients with chronic lymphocytic leukemia, with resolution of infiltrates and symptoms with drug discontinuation and steroid use [115]. Given the overall common use of ibrutinib in patients with hematologic malignancies, the low incidence of reported toxicity is likely related to a low overall prevalence of pulmonary inflammation associated with the use of ibrutinib.

## Belumosudil

Belumosudil is a selective inhibitor of Rho-associated coiled-coil-containing protein kinase 2 (ROCK2), which has been shown to have an overall response rate of 74–77% in patients with chronic GVHD who had received two to five prior lines of therapy [116]. Adverse respiratory events noted in clinical trials included pneumonia and upper respiratory tract infections; there were no reported noninfectious pulmonary toxicities noted.

## Conclusion

Drug toxicities are common following HSCT, and many of the agents utilized regularly as part of conditioning regimens and in the treatment of chronic GVHD can cause various forms of pulmonary toxicity. Clinicians should have a high index of suspicion for these various drug toxicities, as early recognition, drug withdrawal, and treatment with corticosteroids may lead to reversibility of the toxicities. There is generally no specific testing that can confirm a diagnosis of drug-induced pulmonary toxicity, so diagnosis must be made based on clinical factors and exclusion of infectious etiologies, which often requires imaging studies and bronchoscopy with alveolar lavage.

## References

1. Oliner H, Schwartz R, Rubio F, Dameshek W. Interstitial pulmonary fibrosis following busulfan therapy. Am J Med. 1961;31:134–9.
2. Rosenow EC 3rd, Limper AH. Drug-induced pulmonary disease. Semin Respir Infect. 1995;10(2):86–95.
3. Nebeker JR, Barach P, Samore MH. Clarifying adverse drug events: a clinician's guide to terminology, documentation, and reporting. Ann Intern Med. 2004;140(10):795–801.
4. Vahid B, Marik PE. Pulmonary complications of novel antineoplastic agents for solid tumors. Chest. 2008;133(2):528–38.
5. Sleijfer S. Bleomycin-induced pneumonitis. Chest. 2001;120(2):617–24.
6. Nici L, Calabresi P. Amifostine modulation of bleomycin-induced lung injury in rodents. Semin Oncol. 1999;26(2 Suppl 7):28–33.
7. Ingrassia TS 3rd, Ryu JH, Trastek VF, Rosenow EC 3rd. Oxygen-exacerbated bleomycin pulmonary toxicity. Mayo Clin Proc. 1991;66(2):173–8.
8. Gratwohl A, Mohty M, Apperley J. The EBMT: history, present, and future. In: Carreras E, Dufour C,

Mohty M, Kroger N, editors. The EBMT handbook: hematopoietic stem cell transplantation and cellular therapies. Cham: Springer; 2019. p. 11–7.

9. Lund MB, Brinch L, Kongerud J, Boe J. Lung function 5 yrs after allogeneic bone marrow transplantation conditioned with busulphan and cyclophosphamide. Eur Respir J. 2004;23(6):901–5.
10. Bredeson C, LeRademacher J, Kato K, Dipersio JF, Agura E, Devine SM, et al. Prospective cohort study comparing intravenous busulfan to total body irradiation in hematopoietic cell transplantation. Blood. 2013;122(24):3871–8.
11. Copelan EA, Hamilton BK, Avalos B, Ahn KW, Bolwell BJ, Zhu X, et al. Better leukemia-free and overall survival in AML in first remission following cyclophosphamide in combination with busulfan compared with TBI. Blood. 2013;122(24):3863–70.
12. Fernandez HF, Tran HT, Albrecht F, Lennon S, Caldera H, Goodman MS. Evaluation of safety and pharmacokinetics of administering intravenous busulfan in a twice-daily or daily schedule to patients with advanced hematologic malignant disease undergoing stem cell transplantation. Biol Blood Marrow Transplant. 2002;8(9):486–92.
13. Ringden O, Remberger M, Ruutu T, Nikoskelainen J, Volin L, Vindelov L, et al. Increased risk of chronic graft-versus-host disease, obstructive bronchiolitis, and alopecia with busulfan versus total body irradiation: long-term results of a randomized trial in allogeneic marrow recipients with leukemia. Nordic Bone Marrow Transplantation Group. Blood. 1999;93(7):2196–201.
14. Crilley P, Topolsky D, Styler MJ, Bernstein E, Resnick K, Mullaney R, et al. Extramedullary toxicity of a conditioning regimen containing busulphan, cyclophosphamide and etoposide in 84 patients undergoing autologous and allogenic bone marrow transplantation. Bone Marrow Transplant. 1995;15(3):361–5.
15. Vergnon JM, Boucheron S, Riffat J, Guy C, Blanc P, Emonot A. Interstitial pneumopathies caused by busulfan. Histologic, developmental and bronchoalveolar lavage analysis of 3 cases. Rev Med Interne. 1988;9(4):377–83.
16. Aymard JP, Gyger M, Lavallee R, Legresley LP, Desy M. A case of pulmonary alveolar proteinosis complicating chronic myelogenous leukemia. A peculiar pathologic aspect of busulfan lung? Cancer. 1984;53(4):954–6.
17. Watanabe K, Sueishi K, Tanaka K, Nagata N, Hirose N, Shigematsu N, et al. Pulmonary alveolar proteinosis and disseminated atypical mycobacteriosis in a patient with busulfan lung. Acta Pathol Jpn. 1990;40(1):63–6.
18. Padley SP, Adler B, Hansell DM, Muller NL. High-resolution computed tomography of drug-induced lung disease. Clin Radiol. 1992;46(4):232–6.
19. Worth L, Tran H, Petropoulos D, Culbert S, Mullen C, Roberts W, et al. Hematopoietic stem cell transplantation for childhood myeloid malignancies after high-dose thiotepa, busulfan and cyclophosphamide. Bone Marrow Transplant. 1999;24(9):947–52.
20. Cleverley JR, Screaton NJ, Hiorns MP, Flint JD, Muller NL. Drug-induced lung disease: high-resolution CT and histological findings. Clin Radiol. 2002;57(4):292–9.
21. Lund MB, Kongerud J, Brinch L, Evensen SA, Boe J. Decreased lung function in one year survivors of allogeneic bone marrow transplantation conditioned with high-dose busulphan and cyclophosphamide. Eur Respir J. 1995;8(8):1269–74.
22. Massin F, Coudert B, Foucher P, Lombard JN, Reybet-Degat O, Jeannin L, et al. Nitrosourea-induced lung diseases. Rev Mal Respir. 1992;9(6):575–82.
23. Weinstein AS, Diener-West M, Nelson DF, Pakuris E. Pulmonary toxicity of carmustine in patients treated for malignant glioma. Cancer Treat Rep. 1986;70(8):943–6.
24. Aronin PA, Mahaley MS Jr, Rudnick SA, Dudka L, Donohue JF, Selker RG, et al. Prediction of BCNU pulmonary toxicity in patients with malignant gliomas: an assessment of risk factors. N Engl J Med. 1980;303(4):183–8.
25. Durant JR, Norgard MJ, Murad TM, Bartolucci AA, Langford KH. Pulmonary toxicity associated with bischloroethylnitrosourea (BCNU). Ann Intern Med. 1979;90(2):191–4.
26. Smith AC. The pulmonary toxicity of nitrosoureas. Pharmacol Ther. 1989;41(3):443–60.
27. Mitsudo SM, Greenwald ES, Banerji B, Koss LG. BCNU (1,3-bis-(2-chloroethyl)-1-nitrosurea) lung. Drug-induced pulmonary changes. Cancer. 1984;54(4):751–5.
28. Kalaycioglu M, Kavuru M, Tuason L, Bolwell B. Empiric prednisone therapy for pulmonary toxic reaction after high-dose chemotherapy containing carmustine (BCNU). Chest. 1995;107(2):482–7.
29. Cao TM, Negrin RS, Stockerl-Goldstein KE, Johnston LJ, Shizuru JA, Taylor TL, et al. Pulmonary toxicity syndrome in breast cancer patients undergoing BCNU-containing high-dose chemotherapy and autologous hematopoietic cell transplantation. Biol Blood Marrow Transplant. 2000;6(4):387–94.
30. O'Driscoll BR, Hasleton PS, Taylor PM, Poulter LW, Gattameneni HR, Woodcock AA. Active lung fibrosis up to 17 years after chemotherapy with carmustine (BCNU) in childhood. N Engl J Med. 1990;323(6):378–82.
31. O'Driscoll BR, Kalra S, Gattamaneni HR, Woodcock AA. Late carmustine lung fibrosis. Age at treatment may influence severity and survival. Chest. 1995;107(5):1355–7.
32. Beynat-Mouterde C, Beltramo G, Lezmi G, Pernet D, Camus C, Fanton A, et al. Pleuroparenchymal fibroelastosis as a late complication of chemotherapy agents. Eur Respir J. 2014;44(2):523–7.
33. Lohani S, O'Driscoll BR, Woodcock AA. 25-year study of lung fibrosis following carmustine therapy for brain tumor in childhood. Chest. 2004;126(3):1007.

34. Chen YB, Lane AA, Logan B, Zhu X, Akpek G, Aljurf M, et al. Impact of conditioning regimen on outcomes for patients with lymphoma undergoing high-dose therapy with autologous hematopoietic cell transplantation. Biol Blood Marrow Transplant. 2015;21(6):1046–53.
35. Rubio C, Hill ME, Milan S, O'Brien ME, Cunningham D. Idiopathic pneumonia syndrome after high-dose chemotherapy for relapsed Hodgkin's disease. Br J Cancer. 1997;75(7):1044–8.
36. Ahya VN. Noninfectious acute lung injury syndromes early after hematopoietic stem cell transplantation. Clin Chest Med. 2017;38(4):595–606.
37. Wenger DS, Triplette M, Crothers K, Cheng GS, Hill JA, Milano F, et al. Incidence, risk factors, and outcomes of idiopathic pneumonia syndrome after allogeneic hematopoietic cell transplantation. Biol Blood Marrow Transplant. 2020;26(2):413–20.
38. Tizon R, Frey N, Heitjan DF, Tan KS, Goldstein SC, Hexner EO, et al. High-dose corticosteroids with or without etanercept for the treatment of idiopathic pneumonia syndrome after allo-SCT. Bone Marrow Transplant. 2012;47(10):1332–7.
39. Yanik GA, Ho VT, Levine JE, White ES, Braun T, Antin JH, et al. The impact of soluble tumor necrosis factor receptor etanercept on the treatment of idiopathic pneumonia syndrome after allogeneic hematopoietic stem cell transplantation. Blood. 2008;112(8):3073–81.
40. Twohig KJ, Matthay RA. Pulmonary effects of cytotoxic agents other than bleomycin. Clin Chest Med. 1990;11(1):31–54.
41. Segura A, Yuste A, Cercos A, Lopez-Tendero P, Girones R, Perez-Fidalgo JA, et al. Pulmonary fibrosis induced by cyclophosphamide. Ann Pharmacother. 2001;35(7–8):894–7.
42. Spector JI, Zimbler H, Ross JS. Early-onset cyclophosphamide-induced interstitial pneumonitis. JAMA. 1979;242(26):2852–4.
43. Sampath S, Schultheiss TE, Wong J. Dose response and factors related to interstitial pneumonitis after bone marrow transplant. Int J Radiat Oncol Biol Phys. 2005;63(3):876–84.
44. Gupta S, Mahipal A. Fatal pulmonary toxicity after a single dose of cyclophosphamide. Pharmacotherapy. 2007;27(4):616–8.
45. Bhagat R, Sporn TA, Long GD, Folz RJ. Amiodarone and cyclophosphamide: potential for enhanced lung toxicity. Bone Marrow Transplant. 2001;27(10):1109–11.
46. Malik SW, Myers JL, DeRemee RA, Specks U. Lung toxicity associated with cyclophosphamide use. Two distinct patterns. Am J Respir Crit Care Med. 1996;154(6 Pt 1):1851–6.
47. Tsukamoto N, Matsukuma K, Matsuyama T, Kashimura M, Kamura T, Uchino H, et al. Cyclophosphamide-induced interstitial pneumonitis in a patient with ovarian carcinoma. Gynecol Oncol. 1984;17(1):41–51.
48. Abdel Karim FW, Ayash RE, Allam C, Salem PA. Pulmonary fibrosis after prolonged treatment with low-dose cyclophosphamide. A case report. Oncology. 1983;40(3):174–6.
49. Hamada K, Nagai S, Kitaichi M, Jin G, Shigematsu M, Nagao T, et al. Cyclophosphamide-induced late-onset lung disease. Intern Med. 2003;42(1):82–7.
50. Mark GJ, Lehimgar-Zadeh A, Ragsdale BD. Cyclophosphamide pneumonitis. Thorax. 1978;33(1):89–93.
51. Wells AU, Flaherty KR, Brown KK, Inoue Y, Devaraj A, Richeldi L, et al. Nintedanib in patients with progressive fibrosing interstitial lung diseases-subgroup analyses by interstitial lung disease diagnosis in the INBUILD trial: a randomised, double-blind, placebo-controlled, parallel-group trial. Lancet Respir Med. 2020;8(5):453–60.
52. Rai KR, Peterson BL, Appelbaum FR, Kolitz J, Elias L, Shepherd L, et al. Fludarabine compared with chlorambucil as primary therapy for chronic lymphocytic leukemia. N Engl J Med. 2000;343(24):1750–7.
53. Helman DL Jr, Byrd JC, Ales NC, Shorr AF. Fludarabine-related pulmonary toxicity: a distinct clinical entity in chronic lymphoproliferative syndromes. Chest. 2002;122(3):785–90.
54. Anaissie EJ, Kontoyiannis DP, O'Brien S, Kantarjian H, Robertson L, Lerner S, et al. Infections in patients with chronic lymphocytic leukemia treated with fludarabine. Ann Intern Med. 1998;129(7):559–66.
55. Kane GC, McMichael AJ, Patrick H, Erslev AJ. Pulmonary toxicity and acute respiratory failure associated with fludarabine monophosphate. Respir Med. 1992;86(3):261–3.
56. Levin M, Aziz M, Opitz L. Steroid-responsive interstitial pneumonitis after fludarabine therapy. Chest. 1997;111(5):1472–3.
57. Stoica GS, Greenberg HE, Rossoff LJ. Corticosteroid responsive fludarabine pulmonary toxicity. Am J Clin Oncol. 2002;25(4):340–1.
58. Andersson BS, Luna MA, Yee C, Hui KK, Keating MJ, McCredie KB. Fatal pulmonary failure complicating high-dose cytosine arabinoside therapy in acute leukemia. Cancer. 1990;65(5):1079–84.
59. Forghieri F, Luppi M, Morselli M, Potenza L. Cytarabine-related lung infiltrates on high resolution computerized tomography: a possible complication with benign outcome in leukemic patients. Haematologica. 2007;92(9):e85–90.
60. Moore JO, George SL, Dodge RK, Amrein PC, Powell BL, Kolitz JE, et al. Sequential multiagent chemotherapy is not superior to high-dose cytarabine alone as postremission intensification therapy for acute myeloid leukemia in adults under 60 years of age: cancer and leukemia group B study 9222. Blood. 2005;105(9):3420–7.
61. Hatakeyama S, Tachibana A, Morita M, Suzuki K, Okano H. Etoposide-induced pneumonitis. Nihon Kyobu Shikkan Gakkai Zasshi. 1997;35(2):210–4.

62. Dajczman E, Srolovitz H, Kreisman H, Frank H. Fatal pulmonary toxicity following oral etoposide therapy. Lung Cancer. 1995;12(1–2):81–6.
63. Gurjal A, An T, Valdivieso M, Kalemkerian GP. Etoposide-induced pulmonary toxicity. Lung Cancer. 1999;26(2):109–12.
64. Akasheh MS, Freytes CO, Vesole DH. Melphalan-associated pulmonary toxicity following high-dose therapy with autologous hematopoietic stem cell transplantation. Bone Marrow Transplant. 2000;26(10):1107–9.
65. Goucher G, Rowland V, Hawkins J. Melphalan-induced pulmonary interstitial fibrosis. Chest. 1980;77(6):805–6.
66. Westerfield BT, Michalski JP, McCombs C, Light RW. Reversible melphalan-induced lung damage. Am J Med. 1980;68(5):767–71.
67. Taetle R, Dickman PS, Feldman PS. Pulmonary histopathologic changes associated with melphalan therapy. Cancer. 1978;42(3):1239–45.
68. Buckner CD, Epstein RB, Rudolph RH, Clift RA, Storb R, Thomas ED. Allogeneic marrow engraftment following whole body irradiation in a patient with leukemia. Blood. 1970;35(6):741–50.
69. Hartman AR, Williams SF, Dillon JJ. Survival, disease-free survival and adverse effects of conditioning for allogeneic bone marrow transplantation with busulfan/cyclophosphamide vs total body irradiation: a meta-analysis. Bone Marrow Transplant. 1998;22(5):439–43.
70. Liu HW, Seftel MD, Rubinger M, Szwajcer D, Demers A, Nugent Z, et al. Total body irradiation compared with BEAM: Long-term outcomes of peripheral blood autologous stem cell transplantation for non-Hodgkin's lymphoma. Int J Radiat Oncol Biol Phys. 2010;78(2):513–20.
71. Shank B, Chu FC, Dinsmore R, Kapoor N, Kirkpatrick D, Teitelbaum H, et al. Hyperfractionated total body irradiation for bone marrow transplantation. Results in seventy leukemia patients with allogeneic transplants. Int J Radiat Oncol Biol Phys. 1983;9(11):1607–11.
72. Clift RA, Buckner CD, Appelbaum FR, Bearman SI, Petersen FB, Fisher LD, et al. Allogeneic marrow transplantation in patients with acute myeloid leukemia in first remission: a randomized trial of two irradiation regimens. Blood. 1990;76(9):1867–71.
73. Vogel J, Hui S, Hua CH, Dusenbery K, Rassiah P, Kalapurakal J, et al. Pulmonary toxicity after Total body irradiation-critical review of the literature and recommendations for toxicity reporting. Front Oncol. 2021;11:708906.
74. Gopal R, Ha CS, Tucker SL, Khouri IF, Giralt SA, Gajewski JL, et al. Comparison of two total body irradiation fractionation regimens with respect to acute and late pulmonary toxicity. Cancer. 2001;92(7):1949–58.
75. McDonald S, Rubin P, Phillips TL, Marks LB. Injury to the lung from cancer therapy: clinical syndromes, measurable endpoints, and potential scoring systems. Int J Radiat Oncol Biol Phys. 1995;31(5):1187–203.
76. Oertel M, Kittel C, Martel J, Mikesch JH, Glashoerster M, Stelljes M, et al. Pulmonary toxicity after Total body irradiation-An underrated complication? Estimation of risk via normal tissue complication probability calculations and correlation with clinical data. Cancers (Basel). 2021;13(12):2946.
77. Oertel M, Martel J, Mikesch JH, Scobioala S, Reicherts C, Kroger K, et al. The burden of survivorship on hematological patients-Long-term analysis of toxicities after Total body irradiation and allogeneic stem cell transplantation. Cancers (Basel). 2021;13(22):5640.
78. Choi YW, Munden RF, Erasmus JJ, Park KJ, Chung WK, Jeon SC, et al. Effects of radiation therapy on the lung: radiologic appearances and differential diagnosis. Radiographics. 2004;24(4):985–97. discussion 98.
79. Roberts CM, Foulcher E, Zaunders JJ, Bryant DH, Freund J, Cairns D, et al. Radiation pneumonitis: a possible lymphocyte-mediated hypersensitivity reaction. Ann Intern Med. 1993;118(9):696–700.
80. Bledsoe TJ, Nath SK, Decker RH. Radiation pneumonitis. Clin Chest Med. 2017;38(2):201–8.
81. Smith TJ, Bohlke K, Lyman GH, Carson KR, Crawford J, Cross SJ, et al. Recommendations for the use of WBC growth factors: American society of clinical oncology clinical practice guideline update. J Clin Oncol. 2015;33(28):3199–212.
82. Ho VT, Mirza NQ, Junco DD, Okamura T, Przepiorka D. The effect of hematopoietic growth factors on the risk of graft-vs-host disease after allogeneic hematopoietic stem cell transplantation: a meta-analysis. Bone Marrow Transplant. 2003;32(8):771–5.
83. Nemunaitis J, Rosenfeld CS, Ash R, Freedman MH, Deeg HJ, Appelbaum F, et al. Phase III randomized, double-blind placebo-controlled trial of rhGM-CSF following allogeneic bone marrow transplantation. Bone Marrow Transplant. 1995;15(6):949–54.
84. Nademanee A, Sniecinski I, Schmidt GM, Dagis AC, O'Donnell MR, Snyder DS, et al. High-dose therapy followed by autologous peripheral-blood stem-cell transplantation for patients with Hodgkin's disease and non-Hodgkin's lymphoma using unprimed and granulocyte colony-stimulating factor-mobilized peripheral-blood stem cells. J Clin Oncol. 1994;12(10):2176–86.
85. Yokose N, Ogata K, Tamura H, An E, Nakamura K, Kamikubo K, et al. Pulmonary toxicity after granulocyte colony-stimulating factor-combined chemotherapy for non-Hodgkin's lymphoma. Br J Cancer. 1998;77(12):2286–90.
86. Karlin L, Darmon M, Thiery G, Ciroldi M, de Miranda S, Lefebvre A, et al. Respiratory status deterioration during G-CSF-induced neutropenia recovery. Bone Marrow Transplant. 2005;36(3):245–50.
87. Aggarwal A, Baker CS, Evans TW, Haslam PL. G-CSF and IL-8 but not GM-CSF corre-

late with severity of pulmonary neutrophilia in acute respiratory distress syndrome. Eur Respir J. 2000;15(5):895–901.
88. Shalata W, Waichenberg L, Massalha I, Dudnik Y, Rouvinov K, Yakobson A. Pulmonary toxicity following administration of granulocyte colony-stimulating factor during chemotherapy for breast cancer: a case report and literature review. Anti-Cancer Drugs. 2021;32(10):1142–5.
89. Ruutu T, van Biezen A, Hertenstein B, Henseler A, Garderet L, Passweg J, et al. Prophylaxis and treatment of GVHD after allogeneic haematopoietic SCT: a survey of centre strategies by the European Group for blood and marrow transplantation. Bone Marrow Transplant. 2012;47(11):1459–64.
90. Koc S, Leisenring W, Flowers ME, Anasetti C, Deeg HJ, Nash RA, et al. Therapy for chronic graft-versus-host disease: a randomized trial comparing cyclosporine plus prednisone versus prednisone alone. Blood. 2002;100(1):48–51.
91. Imbert S, Bresler P, Boissonnas A, Gauthier L, Souchet L, Uzunov M, et al. Calcineurin inhibitors impair neutrophil activity against aspergillus fumigatus in allogeneic hematopoietic stem cell transplant recipients. J Allergy Clin Immunol. 2016;138(3):860–8.
92. Mallat SG, Tanios BY, Itani HS, Lotfi T, McMullan C, Gabardi S, et al. CMV and BKPyV infections in renal transplant recipients receiving an mTOR inhibitor-based regimen versus a CNI-based regimen: a systematic review and meta-analysis of randomized, controlled trials. Clin J Am Soc Nephrol. 2017;12(8):1321–36.
93. Kim SJ, Lee JW, Jung CW, Min CK, Cho B, Shin HJ, et al. Weekly rituximab followed by monthly rituximab treatment for steroid-refractory chronic graft-versus-host disease: results from a prospective, multicenter, phase II study. Haematologica. 2010;95(11):1935–42.
94. Brownback KR, Thomas LA, McGuirk JP, Ganguly S, Streiler C, Abhyankar S. Effect of rituximab on pulmonary function in bronchiolitis obliterans syndrome due to graft-versus-host-disease. Lung. 2017;195(6):781–8.
95. Cutler C, Miklos D, Kim HT, Treister N, Woo SB, Bienfang D, et al. Rituximab for steroid-refractory chronic graft-versus-host disease. Blood. 2006;108(2):756–62.
96. Bienvenu J, Chvetzoff R, Salles G, Balter C, Tilly H, Herbrecht R, et al. Tumor necrosis factor alpha release is a major biological event associated with rituximab treatment. Hematol J. 2001;2(6):378–84.
97. Naqibullah M, Shaker SB, Bach KS, Bendstrup E. Rituximab-induced interstitial lung disease: five case reports. Eur Clin Respir J. 2015;2:2.
98. Wagner SA, Mehta AC, Laber DA. Rituximab-induced interstitial lung disease. Am J Hematol. 2007;82(10):916–9.
99. Hadjinicolaou AV, Nisar MK, Parfrey H, Chilvers ER, Ostor AJ. Non-infectious pulmonary toxicity of rituximab: a systematic review. Rheumatology (Oxford). 2012;51(4):653–62.
100. Zeiser R, Polverelli N, Ram R, Hashmi SK, Chakraverty R, Middeke JM, et al. Ruxolitinib for glucocorticoid-refractory chronic graft-versus-host disease. N Engl J Med. 2021;385(3):228–38.
101. Zeiser R, von Bubnoff N, Butler J, Mohty M, Niederwieser D, Or R, et al. Ruxolitinib for glucocorticoid-refractory acute graft-versus-host disease. N Engl J Med. 2020;382(19):1800–10.
102. Streiler C, Shaikh F, Davis C, Abhyankar S, Brownback KR. Ruxolitinib is an effective steroid sparing agent in bronchiolitis obliterans due to chronic graft-versus-host-disease. Bone Marrow Transplant. 2020;55(6):1194–6.
103. Low AT, Howard L, Harrison C, Tulloh RM. Pulmonary arterial hypertension exacerbated by ruxolitinib. Haematologica. 2015;100(6):e244–5.
104. Tabarroki A, Lindner DJ, Visconte V, Zhang L, Rogers HJ, Parker Y, et al. Ruxolitinib leads to improvement of pulmonary hypertension in patients with myelofibrosis. Leukemia. 2014;28(7):1486–93.
105. Ayli M, Ozcan M, Cengiz SG. Ruxolitinib treatment in a patient with primary myelofibrosis resistant to conventional therapies and splenectomy: a case report. Turk J Haematol. 2015;32(2):180–3.
106. Kerget B, Araz O, Ucar EY, Akgun M, Saglam L. Acute respiratory distress syndrome; a rare complication caused by usage of ruxolitinib. Respir Med Case Rep. 2017;22:243–5.
107. Beauverd Y, Samii K. Acute respiratory distress syndrome in a patient with primary myelofibrosis after ruxolitinib treatment discontinuation. Int J Hematol. 2014;100(5):498–501.
108. Tefferi A, Pardanani A. Serious adverse events during ruxolitinib treatment discontinuation in patients with myelofibrosis. Mayo Clin Proc. 2011;86(12):1188–91.
109. Couriel DR, Saliba R, Escalon MP, Hsu Y, Ghosh S, Ippoliti C, et al. Sirolimus in combination with tacrolimus and corticosteroids for the treatment of resistant chronic graft-versus-host disease. Br J Haematol. 2005;130(3):409–17.
110. Chhajed PN, Dickenmann M, Bubendorf L, Mayr M, Steiger J, Tamm M. Patterns of pulmonary complications associated with sirolimus. Respiration. 2006;73(3):367–74.
111. Pham PT, Pham PC, Danovitch GM, Ross DJ, Gritsch HA, Kendrick EA, et al. Sirolimus-associated pulmonary toxicity. Transplantation. 2004;77(8):1215–20.
112. Errasti P, Izquierdo D, Martin P, Errasti M, Slon F, Romero A, et al. Pneumonitis associated with mammalian target of rapamycin inhibitors in renal transplant recipients: a single-center experience. Transplant Proc. 2010;42(8):3053–4.

113. Miklos D, Cutler CS, Arora M, Waller EK, Jagasia M, Pusic I, et al. Ibrutinib for chronic graft-versus-host disease after failure of prior therapy. Blood. 2017;130(21):2243–50.
114. Chin KK, Kim HT, Inyang EA, Ho V, Koreth J, Romee R, et al. Ibrutinib in steroid-refractory chronic graft-versus-host disease, a single-center experience. Transplant Cell Ther. 2021;27:990.e1.
115. Mato AR, Islam P, Daniel C, Strelec L, Kaye AH, Brooks S, et al. Ibrutinib-induced pneumonitis in patients with chronic lymphocytic leukemia. Blood. 2016;127(8):1064–7.
116. Cutler C, Lee SJ, Arai S, Rotta M, Zoghi B, Lazaryan A, et al. Belumosudil for chronic graft-versus-host disease after 2 or more prior lines of therapy: the ROCKstar study. Blood. 2021;138(22):2278–89.

# Sleep Disturbances in Hematopoietic Stem Cell Transplantation

22

Chithra Poongkunran, Diwakar D. Balachandran, Lara Bashoura, and Saadia A. Faiz

## Introduction

Individuals undergoing hematopoietic stem cell transplantation (HSCT) may experience significant sleep disruption before, during, and after their HSCT [1–3]. As in other types of cancer, studies suggest rates of sleep disturbance are substantially higher than the general population, and sleep problems can persist years after HSCT [4].

Sleep disruption can contribute to symptom burden, increased fatigue, and reduced quality of life (QOL). Sleep is a restorative biological process essential for maintaining health, healing, and emotional well-being, and loss of sleep is detrimental on many levels. Clinical studies indicate that sleep disruption has been associated with worse all-cause mortality [5]. Sleep deficit can affect multiple organ systems including immune function, physical function and coordination, cognitive performance, and metabolism [6].

C. Poongkunran
Divisions of Critical Care, Pulmonary and Sleep Medicine, McGovern Medical School at UTHealth, Houston, TX, USA
e-mail: Chithra.Poongkunran@uth.tmc.edu

D. D. Balachandran · L. Bashoura · S. A. Faiz (✉)
Department of Pulmonary Medicine, The University of Texas MD Anderson Cancer Center, Houston, TX, USA
e-mail: dbalachandran@mdanderson.org; lbashoura@mdanderson.org; safaiz@mdanderson.org

A growing body of evidence links sleep pathology to physiologically significant sequelae as it relates to cancer, both in terms of diagnosis, treatment, and outcomes [7]. Sleep disturbance is associated with greater fatigue and reduced QOL in HSCT, but it is seldom addressed by healthcare providers [3, 8, 9]. Furthermore, there is a paucity of data on sleep and hematologic malignancies, especially in those undergoing HSCT. The focus of this chapter is to highlight sleep disturbances in cancer patients, to summarize the medical literature about sleep in HSCT patients, and to describe screening, diagnostic, and therapeutic interventions to improve sleep.

## Sleep Disorders and Cancer

Sleep-related issues may emerge at any time during the continuum of cancer care, and sleep disturbance is a prominent concern in cancer patients. Problems with sleep are reported in 30 to 87% of cancer patients, and these encompass a variety of sleep-related issues including difficulty falling asleep, staying asleep, multiple awakenings during the night or earlier than intended, and/or nonrestorative sleep [10]. Some patients may have preexisting or a predisposition to developing sleep issues prior to cancer diagnosis. For example, somatic symptoms such as pain, breathing disorders, hormonal dysregulation, underlying medical conditions, or alcohol use can all



A. O. Soubani (ed.), *Pulmonary and Critical Care Considerations of Hematopoietic Stem Cell Transplantation*, https://doi.org/10.1007/978-3-031-28797-8_22

disrupt sleep. Psychiatric conditions, especially anxiety or depression, poor sleep hygiene, and psychosocial factors can also negatively impact sleep [11]. After diagnosis of cancer, side effects from therapies, anxiety or mood disorders, pain and financial stressors can all develop and contribute to sleep disruption, and these may persist into cancer survivorship.

## Insomnia

The most prevalent sleep-related issues identified in outpatient cancer patients in a large cross-sectional survey included insomnia, fatigue, leg restlessness, and excessive sleepiness [12]. A prospective study in cancer patients undergoing chemotherapy, of which 14% had a hematologic malignancy, found a high prevalence of insomnia, and rates for the cohort were nearly three times higher than rates in the general population [13]. Risk factors for insomnia are categorized into predisposing (anxiety, predisposition to rumination, age, female sex), precipitating (acute triggers, i.e., traumatic life event, medical or psychiatric diagnosis), and perpetuating factors (behavior develops to compensate for sleep loss) [10, 14].

Evaluation with clinical history, surveys, and sleep diaries can confirm the diagnosis. Several self-reported measures of sleep have been validated in cancer patients including the Insomnia Severity Index, Pittsburgh Sleep Quality Index (PSQI), and General Sleep Disturbances Questionnaire [15–17]. Sleep diaries also provide valuable information on sleep patterns, and they are inexpensive and readily available [18]. The diary is a simple 24-h log of sleep pattern kept over 7–14 days recording sleep/wake times, daytime napping, intake of medications, subjective sleep quality, and response to interventions. Diagnostic criteria for insomnia as a sleep disorder include difficulty initiating or maintaining sleep or earlier awakening than desired despite adequate opportunity and circumstances to sleep; significant functional impairment of daily activities; sleep disturbance occurs at least three nights a week for at least 3 months (chronic); symptoms are not better explained by another primary sleep disorder [1].

Treatment of insomnia centers around psychological intervention, specifically cognitive behavioral therapy (CBT), which targets maladaptive sleep behaviors and dysfunctional beliefs about sleep [10, 19]. Although many patients may use sleep aids, they can build up a tolerance to these medications, and their use can lead to potentially harmful pharmacological interactions [20]. The use of pharmacotherapy per the American Academy of Sleep Medicine (AASM) should be short- or intermediate-acting benzodiazepine receptor agonists or ramelteon, a melatonin receptor agonist [19]. No studies have specifically evaluated CBT or pharmacotherapy for insomnia in HSCT patients.

## Sleep-Related Breathing Disorders

Sleep-related breathing disorders include sleep apnea which may be obstructive (OSA) or central (CSA) and sleep-related hypoventilation. Definitions and polysomnographic criteria are established by the AASM [21]. The incidence of OSA in the adult population of the United States is estimated to be 4% in men and 2% in women. Risk factors for OSA include age, male gender, postmenopausal women, obesity, and craniofacial and upper airway abnormalities, and diabetes, congestive heart failure, kidney disease, and treatment-refractory hypertension are also concomitant [22, 23].

In cancer patients, those with head and neck cancer have an increased risk of OSA related to architectural distortion from the tumor and subsequent therapies [24]. Both animal models and population-based studies have demonstrated intermittent hypoxia and sleep fragmentation, both hallmarks of OSA, may enhance the proliferative and invasive properties of solid tumors [25]. Opioid therapy, often used for pain in cancer patients, can also result in OSA, CSA, and sleep-related hypoventilation [26]. Cardiac arrhythmia, depressed systolic function, pulmonary vascular disease, and pulmonary conditions may also lead to sleep-disordered breathing.

Weight gain related to corticosteroid therapy, hormonal changes resulting in early menopause, or underlying cardiac or pulmonary dysfunction places HSCT patients at risk for sleep-disordered breathing as well. Evaluation with nocturnal oximetry, home sleep testing, or polysomnography can diagnose the underlying sleep disorder. Treatment may include supplemental oxygen, positive airway pressure therapy, optimization of underlying cardiac or pulmonary condition, oral appliances, weight loss, alteration of sleep position, and adjustment of sedating medications.

## Movement Disorders

Movement disorders such as restless legs syndrome (RLS) or periodic limb movement disorder (PLMD) can also disrupt sleep, and they are typically diagnosed by clinical history but can be confirmed with polysomnography or actigraphy [27]. RLS is a common sensorimotor disorder characterized by uncomfortable and unpleasant sensation in the legs that are relieved by movement.

Evaluation for underlying metabolic abnormalities and review of medications are indicated prior to consideration of pharmacotherapy. Patients should be counseled to avoid certain antidepressants including citalopram, paroxetine, amitriptyline, mirtazapine, and tramadol, and substances such as caffeine that can aggravate the RLS symptoms [27]. In patients with mild and/or intermittent symptoms, non-pharmacological measures such as mental alerting activities, exercise, pneumatic compression devices, and applied heat may be sufficient for symptom relief [28]. In the context of patients with RLS symptoms requiring treatment, choosing the most appropriate intervention requires an individualized approach including patient-related symptoms, comorbidities relating to RLS, side effect profile, augmentation risks, and patient preferences.

In cancer patients, symptoms related to RLS or PLMD may overlap with neuropathy, and chemotherapy-related neuropathy from therapy regimens including platinum compounds, taxanes, vinca alkaloids, proteasome inhibitors, or thalidomide-based agents has been described [29].

## Circadian Rhythm Disorder

Circadian rhythms are endogenous, genetically based, physiological patterns that modulate biological functions on an approximately 24-h cycle including body temperature, cortisol, melatonin, and growth hormone secretions and rapid eye movement (REM) sleep [30]. Dysregulation of circadian rhythms can increase susceptibility to multiple diseases, particularly malignancy. There are multiple factors that can affect the sleep-wake cycle in cancer patients. Zeitgebers are cues that help to maintain alignment within the day, and the most potent zeitgeber includes the environmental light-dark cycle [31]. Feeding, activity, and social interactions are other nonphotic zeitgebers and clearly can be affected in HSCT patients who may take time off from work, isolate to avoid infection, and alter their daily routines [32].

Actigraphy may help confirm the diagnosis of a circadian rhythm disorder. It is an alternative objective method of estimating sleep by measuring gross motor movement continuously over periods of time, and it consists of a small, noninvasive piezoelectric monitor that is worn on the wrist to detect and record motion. Specialized software transforms the detected movements into electrical activity and identifies sleep versus waking using algorithms validated against polysomnography [33]. Actigraphy has been found to be a reliable and valid tool in patients with suspected circadian sleep-wake rhythm disorders. In patients who cannot reliably complete sleep logs, it can be used as a substitute in addition to self-reported sleep parameters. Actigraphs are relatively inexpensive and can be worn at home or in the hospital for several days or weeks. Actigraphy-derived metrics include time in bed, total sleep time, sleep onset latency, sleep efficiency, wake after sleep onset, wake episodes (also referred to as number of awakenings), number of sleep periods, light intensity, and activity counts. Treatment of circadian rhythm disorders includes light therapy to improve daytime alertness and entrain circadian rhythms. Other multimodality therapies including exercise, movement, yoga, and pharmacotherapy are undergoing investigation [30].

## Cancer-Related Fatigue (CRF)

CRF is one of the most prevalent and distressing symptoms in cancer patients. It is characterized by the following: (1) persistent physical, emotional, and/or cognitive tiredness or exhaustion related to cancer or cancer treatment; (2) not attributable to recent activity; and (3) it interferes with daytime functioning [30]. It may occur before, during, or after cancer diagnosis [34, 35]. The pathophysiology of CRF is complex and is postulated to result from a cascade of events resulting in pro-inflammatory cytokine production with resultant metabolic and/or endocrine dysregulation with disruption to circadian rhythm along with other sequelae [36]. Other underlying metabolic etiologies (anemia, hormonal dysfunction) must be excluded, and evaluation for both sleep disruption and sleep disorders is recommended. Often symptoms from CRF may be dismissed and attributed to disease, but if undiagnosed, then it can negatively impact clinical course and quality of life. Treatment for CRF can be multi-modality and includes exercise, sleep hygiene, correction of any metabolic abnormalities, and wake-promoting agents [34].

## Symptom Clusters

Symptom clusters denote an array of multiple co-occurring symptoms in patients with cancer with a temporal association as well as shared underlying mechanism or outcome [37]. Pain, fatigue, depression, anxiety, and sleep disturbance are common symptom clusters, and these clusters along with additional symptoms (dyspnea, nausea/vomiting) may vary based on the underlying cancer (Fig. 22.1). Depression and anxiety are

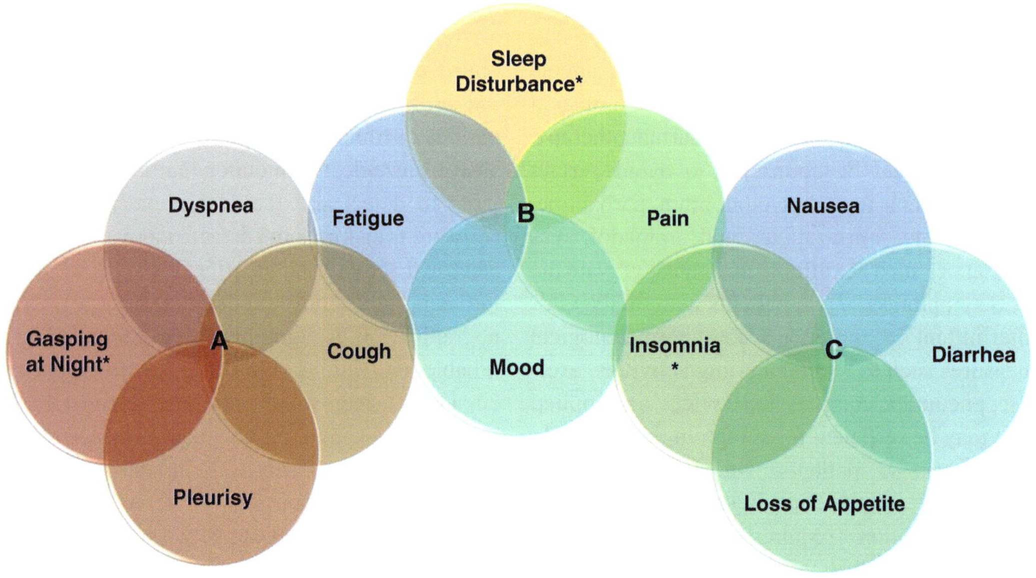


**Fig. 22.1** Symptom clusters. Symptom clusters may vary based on the cancer, and in those with hematopoietic stem cell transplantation (HSCT), symptoms will reflect their disease course, infectious and noninfectious complications, and organs affected by graft-versus-host disease (GVHD). For example, those with pulmonary GVHD may develop a respiratory (**a**) symptom cluster. This could potentially coexist with a psychoneurological (**b**) symptom cluster. Depending on the clinical scenario and timing, symptom clusters can change. Gastrointestinal (**c**) symptom clusters may also exist or overlap at various points in time during HSCT. Note that sleep disturbances (*) can vary from insomnia to excessive daytime sleepiness to nocturnal awakenings to signs and symptoms of sleep-disordered breathing (gasping for air, snoring arousals, witnessed apneas)

associated with sleep dysfunction, and depression, anxiety, sleep disruption, and fatigue can worsen cognitive dysfunction [38]. A review of 33 papers on QOL before and after HSCT identified fatigue, dyspnea, and insomnia as prominent and persistent symptoms [39]. Two other studies noted that in patients prior to undergoing HSCT, fatigue was the most prominent symptom followed by anxiety [40, 41]. Evaluation of symptoms in a longitudinal study of allogeneic HSCT over 5 years concluded fatigue should have priority in symptom management followed by interventions to address dyspnea and loss of appetite [42]. In HSCT, symptom clusters may vary based on disease course, infectious and noninfectious complications, and organs affected by graft-versus-host disease (GVHD). Further evaluation of symptom clusters in the HSCT cohort is needed.

## Sleep Disturbances Before, During, and After HSCT

HSCT has revolutionized treatment for numerous hematologic cancers and certain nonmalignant conditions, and the number of global HSCT over the years continues to grow especially with the allogeneic haploidentical cohort [43]. In addition to treatment of their underlying condition prior to HSCT, the transplant timeline consists of therapy with a conditioning regimen followed by engraftment and subsequently immune reconstitution [38]. Autologous HSCT collects stem cells from the patient, whereas allogeneic HSCT obtains them from a donor. There are many aspects to HSCT that can contribute to symptom burden as well as sleep disruption (Fig. 22.2). Although the conditioning regimen depends on the underlying disease, comorbid condition, performance status, and risk of graft rejection, both myeloablative and nonmyeloablative eradicate marrow cells, and each may have acute and chronic toxicities. The transplant procedure also includes hospitalization for close monitoring and engraftment prior to discharge. In the post-transplant period, patients are susceptible to post-transplant sequelae including infectious complications, autoimmune phenomena, chemotherapy toxicities, and end-organ dysfunction, and these may engender the need for additional therapies and interventions [44]. Estimates of sleep disruption for all phases of HSCT are concerning, and they include 32% in the pre-transplant period, 75%

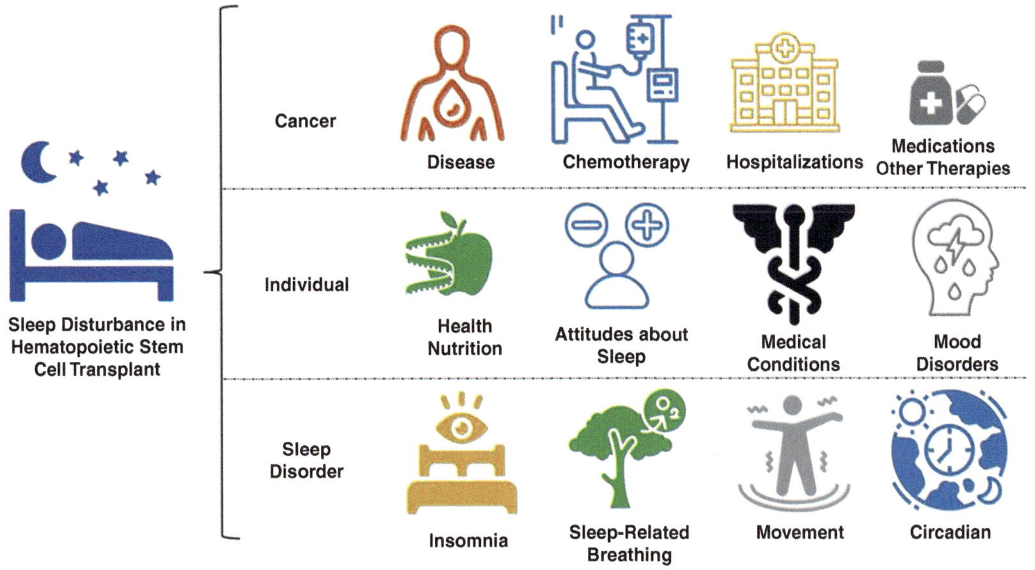


**Fig. 22.2** Factors affecting sleep disturbance in hematopoietic stem cell transplant. Many factors can contribute to sleep disturbance including cancer-related issues, individual predispositions, and underlying sleep disorder

during hospitalization for transplant, and up to 43% in the post-transplant period [2, 3]. Despite a high prevalence of sleep disruption and significant concern among HSCT recipients, relatively little research is available to characterize sleep disruption in this population [8]. The cumulative effect of prior therapies, transplant and its preparation, and potential complications can all significantly impact sleep.

## Acute Transplant Period

The acute transplant period would include the time after HSCT when the patient is hospitalized and before 100 days post-HSCT. The conditioning regimens are of variable intensity and toxicity, and these may be altered based on the underlying malignancy, patient comorbidities, performance status, and risk of graft rejection. Regardless, the time for conditioning and engraftment is an intense time, and it renders the patient vulnerable to a host of medical complications.

Sleep disruption during hospitalization is well established, and it can affect sleep-wake patterns both during the hospital stay and after discharge [45]. In a single center retrospective study of 69 patients, Boonstra and associates used the Insomnia Severity Index on the 14th day of hospitalization in a cohort of both autologous and allogeneic HSCT to evaluate for insomnia as a sleep disorder and as a symptom [2]. They found a prevalence rate of clinically significant insomnia (26%) and insomnia as a symptom in 74%. The most frequently reported factors contributing to sleep disruption were bathroom use and staff interruptions [2].

Encouraging comprehensive strategies to mitigate sleep disruption in hospitalized patients is paramount, and these interventions to raise awareness include education of healthcare providers and clustered care [46, 47]. Sharda and investigators evaluated the need for vital sign monitoring in a cohort of 20 patients post-HSCT, and they concluded vital sign monitoring during the night may not be needed for HSCT with low-risk profiles and could lead to improved sleep and health. Thus, in addition to environmental intervention to improve sleep, patient-based intervention may also be helpful.

Poor sleep quality and fatigue also contribute substantially to the symptom experience of patients during their HSCT trajectory, particularly during early recovery. In a longitudinal single center study of 50 patients with either autologous or allogeneic HSCT, Risher and colleagues used PSQI, sleep diaries, and QOL measures as follows: shortly before admission, daily during their hospital stay, shortly before discharge, and after transplant (day 80 to 120) [3]. They reported a prevalence of sleep disturbances of 32% before admission, 77% during the hospital stay, and 28% after discharge. Difficulty in maintaining sleep during the inpatient phase was reported in 82% and attributed to disturbing noises and the need to use the bathroom frequently. Sleep problems were significantly worse during the hospital stay compared to other measurement points ($p < 0.001$), and sleep difficulties in receiving allogeneic HSCT were less pronounced during admission and worse during the inpatient setting compared to autologous HSCT. Interestingly, they noted disrupted sleep was most pronounced during the phase of transplantation and engraftment or aplasia. The phase of aplasia is known as a time of strong physical and emotional distress, and their findings correspond to results from Anderson and associates where 39% described sleep disturbances as moderate or severe [48]. In contrast, others have demonstrated the pinnacle of sleep distress was at the time of the conditioning regimen. Specifically, in another prospective longitudinal single center study of 76 patients, investigators used the Symptom Distress Scale (SDS) and Medical Outcomes Short Form 36 Health Survey (SF-36, version 1), and data were gathered at four time points: baseline before conditioning regimen, day 0, day 30, and day 100 after HSCT [8]. At the time of the conditioning regimen, the report of insomnia was the highest (32%) as well as the SDS score. Interestingly, the authors described symptom clusters of fatigue, appearance change, and worry at baseline, and fatigue, insomnia, and bowel changes at days 0 and 30.

The post-hospital syndrome involves recovery from hospitalization including recuperation from the acute illness as well as rebound from the physiologic disruption created by the hospital environment [49]. During the hospital stay, patients are frequently deprived of sleep and less active, and along with medications, interventions, and lack of natural light, these contribute to dysregulation of their normal circadian rhythms. Hospitalized patients have polysomnographic evidence of sleep architectural changes with reductions in total sleep time, rapid eye movement (REM) sleep, and slow wave (delta, N3) sleep [49]. The first 100 days post-transplant are challenging. Side effects from conditioning regimen (mucositis, enteritis, nausea, and vomiting), potentially delirium and acute GVHD, can all disrupt sleep and contribute to symptom burden. Poor sleep quality may also result from frequent awakenings, pain, and administration of medications including corticosteroids and/or diuretics, and these all disrupt usual sleep patterns [50–52]. It appears that increases in sleep disruption are generally transient, and they return to pre-HSCT levels by day 100 [3, 48]. Patients receiving both allogeneic and autologous HSCT demonstrate similar levels of sleep disruption, but the timeline is variable.

## Post-transplant

Post-transplant patients can develop late-onset sleep problems due to perpetuation of previous maladaptive sleep behaviors, persistence, or exacerbation of chronic GVHD, residual impact from prior therapies, development of other medical or psychiatric issues, and/or disease-related sequelae. The overall prevalence of any sleep problems following the acute transplant period (after 100 days) ranges from 14 to 51% [53–55]. When compared to healthy individuals, sleep has been shown to be significantly worse among HSCT survivors, but the evidence is mixed [4, 56–58]. A study of 172 patients from five centers 43.5 months (mean) post-HSCT used both questionnaire and telephone interview to assess sleep and energy level problems and integrated the PSQI at the time of follow-up [59]. While the majority reported mild energy or sleep issues, 15 to 20% showed moderate to severe problems in these areas, and the presence of current sleep problems was associated with older age at the time of HSCT, receipt of total body irradiation during pre-HSCT conditioning, and female gender. Furthermore, most of the evidence regarding sleep disruption among HSCT recipients comes from single-item questions incorporated into QOL questionnaires, and these often fail to capture the complexity of sleep issues and/or confirm a sleep disorder. Similar to other data on sleep and HSCT, these are limited by small sample sizes and heterogeneous cohorts.

There has been only one study that has examined the prevalence of sleep disorders after transplant. Specifically, they evaluated 61 patients in a retrospective cohort study of individuals following allogeneic HSCT 1 to 10 years prior [60]. A structured survey with questions about sleep quality, sleep disturbances, and parasomnias was used, and they identified a prevalence of 26.2% with sleep disorders with 23% insomnia (95% CI 12.44–33.56), followed by 3.2% hypersomnia (95% CI 0–7.28). Factors associated with increased risk of developing sleep disorder included female sex with an adjusted relative risk (RR) of 2.37 (95% CI 1.0–5.7) and conditioning regimen with busulfan and cyclophosphamide RR 3.74 (95% CI 1.1–12.6) [60]. Overall, the data to date suggest that the prevalence and severity of sleep disruption remain relatively constant over time after a transient peak during the acute transplant period.

## Special Considerations

GVHD can manifest in multiple sites including the skin, mouth, eyes, gastrointestinal tract, lungs, joints, and genital tract. Both acute and chronic GVHD can contribute to symptom burden and adversely impact QOL [61]. Infection is also a major cause of morbidity and mortality among transplant recipients. Sequelae from high-dose immunosuppressive therapies (including corticosteroids), repeat hospitalizations, and multiple antimicrobial agents can all further exacerbate sleep disturbances. In addition, up to one-third of patients undergoing HSCT can have pulmonary complications, and these are associated with significant morbidity and mortality [62]. Both infectious and noninfectious pulmonary sequelae can impact sleep. Since respiratory symptoms are often present during the day, sleep-related breathing disorders may emerge with sleep. In those with idiopathic pneumonia syndrome, bronchiolitis obliterans, and pulmonary vascular disease, sleep-related hypoventilation may arise due to pulmonary pathology. Corticosteroid and/or bronchodilator therapies can also precipitate or exacerbate insomnia.

## Conclusion

Sleep is an extremely important component in the care of HSCT patients. Even in those with no sleep issues, the process of HSCT may lead to the development of sleep dysfunction. During HSCT, sleep disruption was increased during the first 100 days, with greatest disruption seen during the conditioning regimen and at the time of white blood cell count nadir. Similar to other cancer cohorts, insomnia is the most common sleep disorder in HSCT based on the limited literature available. Efforts to minimize sleep disturbances in the hospital during conditioning and engraftment are warranted. Education of patients, caregivers, and healthcare providers on sleep hygiene, sleep health, and signs and symptoms of sleep disorders is needed. As data accrue regarding the impact of sleep disruption and underlying sleep disorders in cancer, attention to sleep health from both the patient and healthcare providers is paramount. Further studies in HSCT patients using standardized surveys and assessments for sleep, longitudinal evaluation, and multicenter prospective trials are needed.

**Conflicts of Interest** The authors declare that no conflicts of interest exist.

**Funding** This research is supported in part by the National Institutes of Health through MD Anderson's Cancer Center Support Grant (CA016672).

## References

1. Jim HS, Evans B, Jeong JM, Gonzalez BD, Johnston L, Nelson AM, et al. Sleep disruption in hematopoietic cell transplantation recipients: prevalence, severity, and clinical management. Biol Blood Marrow Transplant. 2014;20(10):1465–84.
2. Boonstra L, Harden K, Jarvis S, Palmer S, Kavanaugh-Carveth P, Barnett J, et al. Sleep disturbance in hospitalized recipients of stem cell transplantation. Clin J Oncol Nurs. 2011;15(3):271–6.
3. Rischer J, Scherwath A, Zander AR, Koch U, Schulz-Kindermann F. Sleep disturbances and emotional distress in the acute course of hematopoietic stem cell transplantation. Bone Marrow Transplant. 2009;44(2):121–8.
4. Andrykowski MA, Bishop MM, Hahn EA, Cella DF, Beaumont JL, Brady MJ, et al. Long-term health-related quality of life, growth, and spiritual well-being after hematopoietic stem-cell transplantation. J Clin Oncol. 2005;23(3):599–608.
5. Cappuccio FP, D'Elia L, Strazzullo P, Miller MA. Sleep duration and all-cause mortality: a systematic review and meta-analysis of prospective studies. Sleep. 2010;33(5):585–92.
6. Hastings M, O'Neill JS, Maywood ES. Circadian clocks: regulators of endocrine and metabolic rhythms. J Endocrinol. 2007;195(2):187–98.
7. Sateia MJ, Lang BJ. Sleep and cancer: recent developments. Curr Oncol Rep. 2008;10(4):309–18.
8. Bevans MF, Mitchell SA, Marden S. The symptom experience in the first 100 days following allogeneic hematopoietic stem cell transplantation (HSCT). Support Care Cancer. 2008;16(11):1243–54.
9. Lee SJ, Joffe S, Kim HT, Socie G, Gilman AL, Wingard JR, et al. Physicians' attitudes about quality-of-life issues in hematopoietic stem cell transplantation. Blood. 2004;104(7):2194–200.
10. Palesh O, Peppone L, Innominato PF, Janelsins M, Jeong M, Sprod L, et al. Prevalence, putative mechanisms, and current management of sleep problems during chemotherapy for cancer. Nat Sci Sleep. 2012;4:151–62.
11. Strik H, Cassel W, Teepker M, Schulte T, Riera-Knorrenschild J, Koehler U, et al. Why do our cancer patients sleep so badly? Sleep disorders in cancer patients: a frequent symptom with multiple causes. Oncol Res Treat. 2021;44(9):469–75.
12. Davidson JR, MacLean AW, Brundage MD, Schulze K. Sleep disturbance in cancer patients. Soc Sci Med. 2002;54(9):1309–21.
13. Palesh OG, Roscoe JA, Mustian KM, Roth T, Savard J, Ancoli-Israel S, et al. Prevalence, demographics, and psychological associations of sleep disruption in patients with cancer: University of Rochester Cancer Center-Community Clinical Oncology Program. J Clin Oncol. 2010;28(2):292–8.
14. Savard J, Villa J, Ivers H, Simard S, Morin CM. Prevalence, natural course, and risk factors of insomnia comorbid with cancer over a 2-month period. J Clin Oncol. 2009;27(31):5233–9.

15. Buysse DJ, Reynolds CF 3rd, Monk TH, Berman SR, Kupfer DJ. The Pittsburgh sleep quality index: a new instrument for psychiatric practice and research. Psychiatry Res. 1989;28(2):193–213.
16. Van Onselen C, Paul SM, Lee K, Dunn L, Aouizerat BE, West C, et al. Trajectories of sleep disturbance and daytime sleepiness in women before and after surgery for breast cancer. J Pain Symptom Manag. 2013;45(2):244–60.
17. Savard MH, Savard J, Simard S, Ivers H. Empirical validation of the insomnia severity index in cancer patients. Psychooncology. 2005;14(6):429–41.
18. Carney CE, Buysse DJ, Ancoli-Israel S, Edinger JD, Krystal AD, Lichstein KL, et al. The consensus sleep diary: standardizing prospective sleep self-monitoring. Sleep. 2012;35(2):287–302.
19. Schutte-Rodin S, Broch L, Buysse D, Dorsey C, Sateia M. Clinical guideline for the evaluation and management of chronic insomnia in adults. J Clin Sleep Med. 2008;4(5):487–504.
20. Riechelmann RP, Tannock IF, Wang L, Saad ED, Taback NA, Krzyzanowska MK. Potential drug interactions and duplicate prescriptions among cancer patients. J Natl Cancer Inst. 2007;99(8):592–600.
21. Berry RB, Budhiraja R, Gottlieb DJ, Gozal D, Iber C, Kapur VK, et al. Rules for scoring respiratory events in sleep: update of the 2007 AASM manual for the scoring of sleep and associated events. Deliberations of the sleep apnea definitions task force of the American Academy of Sleep Medicine. J Clin Sleep Med. 2012;8(5):597–619.
22. Young T, Skatrud J, Peppard PE. Risk factors for obstructive sleep apnea in adults. JAMA. 2004;291(16):2013–6.
23. Epstein LJ, Kristo D, Strollo PJ Jr, Friedman N, Malhotra A, Patil SP, et al. Clinical guideline for the evaluation, management and long-term care of obstructive sleep apnea in adults. J Clin Sleep Med. 2009;5(3):263–76.
24. Faiz SA, Balachandran D, Hessel AC, Lei X, Beadle BM, William WN Jr, et al. Sleep-related breathing disorders in patients with tumors in the head and neck region. Oncologist. 2014;19(11):1200–6.
25. Gozal D, Farre R, Nieto FJ. Putative links between sleep apnea and cancer: from hypotheses to evolving evidence. Chest. 2015;148(5):1140–7.
26. Van Ryswyk E, Antic NA. Opioids and sleep-disordered breathing. Chest. 2016;150(4):934–44.
27. Aurora RN, Kristo DA, Bista SR, Rowley JA, Zak RS, Casey KR, et al. The treatment of restless legs syndrome and periodic limb movement disorder in adults—an update for 2012: practice parameters with an evidence-based systematic review and meta-analyses: an American Academy of Sleep Medicine Clinical Practice Guideline. Sleep. 2012;35(8):1039–62.
28. Lettieri CJ, Eliasson AH. Pneumatic compression devices are an effective therapy for restless legs syndrome: a prospective, randomized, double-blinded, sham-controlled trial. Chest. 2009;135(1):74–80.
29. St Germain DC, O'Mara AM, Robinson JL, Torres AD, Minasian LM. Chemotherapy-induced peripheral neuropathy: identifying the research gaps and associated changes to clinical trial design. Cancer. 2020;126(20):4602–13.
30. Balachandran DD, Miller MA, Faiz SA, Yennurajalingam S, Innominato PF. Evaluation and management of sleep and circadian rhythm disturbance in cancer. Curr Treat Options in Oncol. 2021;22(9):81.
31. Quante M, Mariani S, Weng J, Marinac CR, Kaplan ER, Rueschman M, et al. Zeitgebers and their association with rest-activity patterns. Chronobiol Int. 2019;36(2):203–13.
32. Roscoe JA, Morrow GR, Hickok JT, Bushunow P, Matteson S, Rakita D, et al. Temporal interrelationships among fatigue, circadian rhythm and depression in breast cancer patients undergoing chemotherapy treatment. Support Care Cancer. 2002;10(4):329–36.
33. Ancoli-Israel S, Martin JL, Blackwell T, Buenaver L, Liu L, Meltzer LJ, et al. The SBSM guide to actigraphy monitoring: clinical and research applications. Behav Sleep Med. 2015;13(Suppl 1):S4–S38.
34. Charalambous A, Berger AM, Matthews E, Balachandran DD, Papastavrou E, Palesh O. Cancer-related fatigue and sleep deficiency in cancer care continuum: concepts, assessment, clusters, and management. Support Care Cancer. 2019;27(7):2747–53.
35. Wu IHC, Balachandran DD, Faiz SA, Bashoura L, Escalante CP, Manzullo EF. Characteristics of cancer-related fatigue and concomitant sleep disturbance in cancer patients. J Pain Symptom Manag. 2022;63(1):e1–8.
36. Saligan LN, Olson K, Filler K, Larkin D, Cramp F, Yennurajalingam S, et al. The biology of cancer-related fatigue: a review of the literature. Support Care Cancer. 2015;23(8):2461–78.
37. Miaskowski C, Barsevick A, Berger A, Casagrande R, Grady PA, Jacobsen P, et al. Advancing symptom science through symptom cluster research: expert panel proceedings and recommendations. J Natl Cancer Inst. 2017;109(4):djw253.
38. Harrison RA, Sharafeldin N, Rexer JL, Streck B, Petersen M, Henneghan AM, et al. Neurocognitive impairment after hematopoietic stem cell transplant for hematologic malignancies: phenotype and mechanisms. Oncologist. 2021;26(11):e2021–e33.
39. Grulke N, Albani C, Bailer H. Quality of life in patients before and after haematopoietic stem cell transplantation measured with the European Organization for Research and Treatment of cancer (EORTC) quality of life Core questionnaire QLQ-C30. Bone Marrow Transplant. 2012;47(4):473–82.
40. Larsen J, Nordstrom G, Bjorkstrand B, Ljungman P, Gardulf A. Symptom distress, functional status and health-related quality of life before high-dose chemotherapy with stem-cell transplantation. Eur J Cancer Care (Engl). 2003;12(1):71–80.
41. Sherman AC, Simonton S, Latif U, Spohn R, Tricot G. Psychosocial adjustment and quality of life among

multiple myeloma patients undergoing evaluation for autologous stem cell transplantation. Bone Marrow Transplant. 2004;33(9):955–62.
42. Esser P, Kuba K, Scherwath A, Johansen C, Schwinn A, Schirmer L, et al. Stability and priority of symptoms and symptom clusters among allogeneic HSCT patients within a 5-year longitudinal study. J Pain Symptom Manag. 2017;54(4):493–500.
43. Niederwieser D, Baldomero H, Szer J, Gratwohl M, Aljurf M, Atsuta Y, et al. Hematopoietic stem cell transplantation activity worldwide in 2012 and a SWOT analysis of the worldwide network for blood and marrow transplantation group including the global survey. Bone Marrow Transplant. 2016;51(6):778–85.
44. Socie G, Mary JY, Esperou H, Robert DV, Aractingi S, Ribaud P, et al. Health and functional status of adult recipients 1 year after allogeneic haematopoietic stem cell transplantation. Br J Haematol. 2001;113(1):194–201.
45. Milani RV, Bober RM, Lavie CJ, Wilt JK, Milani AR, White CJ. Reducing hospital toxicity: impact on patient outcomes. Am J Med. 2018;131(8):961–6.
46. Auriemma CL, Greysen SR. Nudging providers to improve sleep for hospitalized patients. J Hosp Med. 2019;14(1):65–6.
47. Arora VM, Machado N, Anderson SL, Desai N, Marsack W, Blossomgame S, et al. Effectiveness of SIESTA on objective and subjective metrics of nighttime hospital sleep disruptors. J Hosp Med. 2019;14(1):38–41.
48. Anderson KO, Giralt SA, Mendoza TR, Brown JO, Neumann JL, Mobley GM, et al. Symptom burden in patients undergoing autologous stem-cell transplantation. Bone Marrow Transplant. 2007;39(12):759–66.
49. Krumholz HM. Post-hospital syndrome—an acquired, transient condition of generalized risk. N Engl J Med. 2013;368(2):100–2.
50. Larsen J, Nordstrom G, Ljungman P, Gardulf A. Symptom occurrence, symptom intensity, and symptom distress in patients undergoing high-dose chemotherapy with stem-cell transplantation. Cancer Nurs. 2004;27(1):55–64.
51. Hacker ED, Ferrans CE. Quality of life immediately after peripheral blood stem cell transplantation. Cancer Nurs. 2003;26(4):312–22.
52. Hacker ED, Fink AM, Peters T, Park C, Fantuzzi G, Rondelli D. Persistent fatigue in hematopoietic stem cell transplantation survivors. Cancer Nurs. 2017;40(3):174–83.
53. Mosher CE, DuHamel KN, Rini C, Corner G, Lam J, Redd WH. Quality of life concerns and depression among hematopoietic stem cell transplant survivors. Support Care Cancer. 2011;19(9):1357–65.
54. Worel N, Biener D, Kalhs P, Mitterbauer M, Keil F, Schulenburg A, et al. Long-term outcome and quality of life of patients who are alive and in complete remission more than two years after allogeneic and syngeneic stem cell transplantation. Bone Marrow Transplant. 2002;30(9):619–26.
55. Syrjala KL, Langer SL, Abrams JR, Storer BE, Martin PJ. Late effects of hematopoietic cell transplantation among 10-year adult survivors compared with case-matched controls. J Clin Oncol. 2005;23(27):6596–606.
56. Pallua S, Giesinger J, Oberguggenberger A, Kemmler G, Nachbaur D, Clausen J, et al. Impact of GvHD on quality of life in long-term survivors of haematopoietic transplantation. Bone Marrow Transplant. 2010;45(10):1534–9.
57. Bieri S, Roosnek E, Helg C, Verholen F, Robert D, Chapuis B, et al. Quality of life and social integration after allogeneic hematopoietic SCT. Bone Marrow Transplant. 2008;42(12):819–27.
58. Bishop MM, Beaumont JL, Hahn EA, Cella D, Andrykowski MA, Brady MJ, et al. Late effects of cancer and hematopoietic stem-cell transplantation on spouses or partners compared with survivors and survivor-matched controls. J Clin Oncol. 2007;25(11):1403–11.
59. Andrykowski MA, Carpenter JS, Greiner CB, Altmaier EM, Burish TG, Antin JH, et al. Energy level and sleep quality following bone marrow transplantation. Bone Marrow Transplant. 1997;20(8):669–79.
60. Faulhaber GA, Furlanetto TW, Astigarraga CC, Moser Filho HL, Paludo AP, Silla LM. Association of busulfan and cyclophosphamide conditioning with sleep disorders after hematopoietic stem cell transplantation. Acta Haematol. 2010;124(2):125–8.
61. Kurosawa S, Oshima K, Yamaguchi T, Yanagisawa A, Fukuda T, Kanamori H, et al. Quality of life after allogeneic hematopoietic cell transplantation according to affected organ and severity of chronic graft-versus-host disease. Biol Blood Marrow Transplant. 2017;23(10):1749–58.
62. Haider S, Durairajan N, Soubani AO. Noninfectious pulmonary complications of haematopoietic stem cell transplantation. Eur Respir Rev. 2020;29(156):190119.

# Lung Transplantation for Hematopoietic Stem Cell Transplant Patients

**23**

Shruti Gadre and Lauryn Benninger

## Lung Transplantation After Hematopoietic Stem Cell Transplantation

Hematopoietic stem cell transplantation (HSCT) is widely applied in the treatment of malignant, hematologic, autoimmune, and genetic diseases. Over the last 30 years, early mortality after allogeneic stem cell transplantation has declined, with a consequent increase in long-term morbidity [1]. Pulmonary complications, both infectious and noninfectious, occur in up to 60% of HSCT. Specific complications tend to occur within well-defined time periods. The timing and intensity of cytoreductive therapies, the pattern of immune reconstitution that follows, and the use of prophylactic strategies for infectious agents influence the duration of these intervals. Noninfectious pulmonary complications include entities such as acute lung injury syndromes (e.g., idiopathic pneumonia syndrome or diffuse alveolar hemorrhage), interstitial pneumonitis, pulmonary fibrosis, organizing pneumonia, and chronic airway disease in the form of bronchiolitis obliterans (Table 23.1). Lung transplantation is a viable option for selected individuals who develop end-stage lung disease following hematopoietic stem cell transplantation and has the potential to provide both quality of life and survival benefits [2–5]. Presently, only 1% of lung transplants are performed for bronchiolitis obliterans unrelated to previous lung transplant. Of those, cases related to HSCT represent only a subset [6, 7]. Over the last three decades, there has been a growing number of published data describing lung transplantation in patients who have undergone HSCT for various hematologic diseases; however, this literature is limited to case reports and case series.

**Table 23.1** Indications for lung transplantation in hematopoietic stem cell transplant patients

| *Noninfectious pulmonary complications after HSCT as indications for lung transplantation* |
|---|
| Bronchiolitis obliterans syndrome |
| Idiopathic pneumonia syndrome |
| Diffuse alveolar hemorrhage |
| Interstitial pneumonitis |
| Pulmonary fibrosis |
| Organizing pneumonia |

In 1992, Calhoun and colleagues published the first case report of a single lung transplant in a 25-old-year woman who developed severe pulmonary fibrosis following bone marrow transplantation [8]. Lung transplantation has also been described as a potential therapeutic option for patients with idiopathic pneumonia syndrome (IPS) who have failed medical therapy. Said and colleagues described a case of successful lung transplantation in a 44-year-old woman who

S. Gadre (✉) · L. Benninger
Department of Pulmonary and Critical Care Medicine, Respiratory Institute, Cleveland Clinic, Cleveland, OH, USA
e-mail: gadres@ccf.org; benninl3@ccf.org



A. O. Soubani (ed.), *Pulmonary and Critical Care Considerations of Hematopoietic Stem Cell Transplantation*, https://doi.org/10.1007/978-3-031-28797-8_23

developed IPS 5 months after HSCT for myelodysplastic syndrome. Despite aggressive medical management, the patient required intubation and extracorporeal membrane oxygenation while awaiting recovery. Her condition continued to deteriorate, and she ultimately underwent a double lung transplant with uneventful recovery [9].

Another rare indication for LTx after HSCT is Wiskott-Aldrich syndrome, a rare X-linked disorder characterized by immunodeficiency, eczema, and thrombocytopenia. Ueda and colleagues reported a case of a patient with Wiskott-Aldrich syndrome who underwent an HSCT at 1 year of age but subsequently developed severe pulmonary complications. The patient then underwent a single living donor lobar lung transplantation at 13 years of age without complications [10].

## Lung Transplant Referral, Evaluation, and Timing of Transplant

The optimal timing for referral and evaluation for LTx in this patient population is not well defined in the literature and will vary across transplant institutions. Decisions regarding referral and evaluation need to be extrapolated from the current knowledge of common indications for lung transplant employing the International Society for Heart and Lung Transplantation (ISHLT) consensus guidelines [11, 12]. As HSCT recipients remain at risk of recurrence of their original malignancies, the ISHLT guidelines recommend hematologic malignancy within the past 2 years and conservatively within the past 5 years as a contraindication to lung transplantation [11, 13]. Therefore, patients are considered acceptable candidates for a lung transplantation if the time interval between HSCT and lung transplantation is more than 5 years if HSCT was performed for malignant disease. However, based on published data, post-lung transplant recurrence of malignancy only affects 2% to 7% of HSCT recipients [14, 15]. In a case series of 64 patients, Soubani and colleagues reported the median time between HSCT and LTx was 52.3 months (range: 6–240 months). There was no significant difference in outcomes between patients undergoing transplant before or after 60 months of HSCT, as long as they did not have a malignancy at the time of transplantation [14]. Al-Adra and colleagues recommended a 2-year wait time for individuals with prior history of hematological malignancies prior to proceeding with solid organ transplantation [16]. All-cause 1-year mortality was reported to be increased in patients who underwent lung transplantation <2 years post-HSCT in a large case series of 105 patients from Europe (HR 7.5, 95% CI 2.3–23.8; $p = 0.001$) [17]. Therefore, patients may be candidates even if the time interval between HSCT and LTx is less than 5 years, more specifically when the interval is more than 2 years, and the risk of relapse is determined to be less than 20–30% [5]. Unfortunately, the most recent updated consensus document for the selection of lung transplant candidates from the ISHLT does not specifically address this cohort of patients [12].

Given this rare indication for LTx, as well as the complicated nature of the transplant process, referral should begin before the demand for transplant becomes critical. Early referral allows ample time for introduction and education regarding the concept of LTx as well as its requirements, potential complications, and anticipated outcomes. It also allows for further time to modify any hurdles to LTx such as nutritional status, physical deconditioning, other medical comorbidities, or lack of social support [11, 12].

A comprehensive evaluation for LTx includes a full assessment of the lung disease and its severity, anatomy, additional medical or surgical comorbidities and ensuing complications, nutritional status, degree of frailty and physical conditioning, as well as psychosocial circumstances. Every effort should be made to complete a full evaluation prior to proceeding with LTx listing. However, occasionally, an abrupt decline in function prompts a referral at a time that is less than ideal, and these individuals should complete as much of a full evaluation as possible, similar to other candidates. Referral of candidates requiring life-sustaining support, such as mechanical ventilation (MV) and/or extracorporeal life support (ECLS), as a bridge to transplant may be considered in highly selected patients and at centers with expertise in this area [3].

Individuals who develop end-stage lung disease after HSCT are considered to be at high risk owing to the need for additional immunosuppression after LTx and the presumed abnormal baseline immunology [2]. Given this, attention is recommended to encompass additional investigation into the extrapulmonary systemic manifestations of graft-versus-host disease, cellular and humoral immune dysfunction, hepatic and renal dysfunction, as well as esophageal disease [2, 13, 16]. Infectious complications and colonization with resistant organisms remain to be an issue for HSCT recipients and need to be thoroughly vetted prior to proceeding with LTx [2, 13]. Some patients may experience ABO blood type changes following HSCT [5]. The need for multiple transfusions can increase the likelihood of human leukocyte antigens (HLA) sensitization. High frequency of immunoglobulin replacement with recent infusions complicates serological testing for viral infections such as cytomegalovirus. Immunological response to pretransplant vaccination can also be impaired. Complications of previous intensive chemotherapy and radiotherapy along with graft-versus-host disease (GVHD) in non-pulmonary organs may lead to difficulties in surgical approaches and deficiencies in bone marrow reserve, which require consideration.

Most individuals requiring consideration for LTx after HSCT are younger in age; some of the larger case series report a mean age of 22–24 years old [2, 14, 18]. Most individuals receive bilateral lung transplant (76%) versus single/lobar transplantation (24%) [14]. The decision to transplant one or both lungs is primarily dependent on the underlying disease, but additional factors including patient age, functional status, presence of pulmonary hypertension, and center-specific preferences play a role. Single lung transplantation allows for more efficient utilization of a limited donor pool and is better tolerated by frail patients but theoretically provides less functional reserve than bilateral lung transplantation in the setting of allograft dysfunction. Bilateral lung transplantation is performed for patients with suppurative lung diseases to eliminate the risk of infection of the allograft from the infected native lung.

Given organ scarcity, consideration is given regarding the utilization of cadaveric vs. living-donor lobar lung transplantation (LDLLT), particularly in Japan. In a case series of 62 patients who underwent LTx after HSCT in six centers in Japan, 17 patients underwent cadaveric LTx, whereas 45 underwent LDLLT with acceptable outcomes [2].

Lung transplantation has evolved to represent the therapy of choice for a growing number of patients with end-stage lung disease after HSCT. Decisions about patient selection, timing of listing, and choice of procedure are critically important steps in optimizing the outcome of LTx. The criteria for consideration and listing for LTx after HSCT vary across transplant centers. Specific recommendations are not available and need to be extrapolated from the current knowledge of common indications for lung transplant with special regard to challenges in an HSCT recipient. Ideal candidates should have a prolonged malignancy-free survival (at least 2 years) after HSCT, minimal chronic GVHD with limited extra thoracic disease, normal engraftment, normal immune function, and normal nutritional status.

## Post-transplant Considerations

### Perioperative Issues

Lung transplantation in patients with a previous history of HSCT should be undertaken with careful planning and preparedness for the tumultuous perioperative course that may follow. Recipients undergoing LTx after HSCT typically need mechanical circulatory support via either cardiopulmonary bypass (CPB) or extracorporeal membrane oxygenation (ECMO). There is a tendency to have the lung parenchyma densely adherent to the chest wall as radiation pneumonitis can stimulate densely adherent lung tissue with underlying fibrosis. The degree of lung injury leads to the need for bypass, which, in conjunction with the dense adhesions, contributes to bleeding, and patients may need a temporary open chest.

Primary graft dysfunction (PGD) is a form of acute lung injury that occurs after lung transplantation [19]. PGD is characterized by hypoxemia and alveolar infiltrates in the allograft consistent with edema that develops within 72 h of lung transplantation and is graded from 0 to 3 based on $PaO_2$ to $FiO_2$ ratio. The incidence of severe PGD Grade 3 at a single time point has been reported to be between 7.9% and 25% in lung transplant recipients (LTRs) [20, 21]. Severe PGD has been associated with longer hospital length of stay, longer duration of mechanical ventilation, and higher 90-day mortality than those with lower-grade PGD [20, 21]. The incidence and outcomes of PGD are similar in LTx after HSCT. In a study of 62 LTRs after HSCT from Japan, severe primary graft dysfunction occurred in nine (4.5%) patients. In two patients, this resulted in early death 1 month after lung transplantation [2].

Not surprisingly, the overall post-transplant hospital length of stay for HSCT patients is longer compared to LTx for other indications. Hence, patients selected for LTx after HSCT should include clinically stable patients without active infection. Additionally, there needs to be a focus on preoperative optimization of nutrition in anticipation of a prolonged recovery and extensive patient counseling to ensure commitment to undertake the inherent risk of LTx in the background of HSCT.

## Immunosuppression

All lung transplant recipients receive immunosuppression with a calcineurin inhibitor (either tacrolimus or cyclosporine), corticosteroids, and a cell cycle inhibitor (either azathioprine or mycophenolate mofetil). In LTx after HSCT, induction immunosuppression with antithymocyte globulin is not routinely administered due to the increased infectious risk. Basiliximab (day 0 and day 4) may be administered if the initiation of calcineurin inhibitor is delayed. Patients receive methylprednisone 1gm intravenously at the time of surgery followed by a tapering dose of prednisone, based on institutional protocols. Calcineurin inhibitors are administered based on monitored levels. Tacrolimus target levels are typically 12 to 14 mg/dL in the first year and 10 to 12 mg/dL thereafter; and cyclosporine target levels are 250–300 mg/dL for first year post-transplant and 200–250 mg/dL thereafter. Immunosuppressive regimens in LTx after HSCT are comparable; however, institutional protocols may vary. Moreover, there is a focus on lowering immunosuppression post-LTx due to the elevated infection risk and pretransplant exposure to immunosuppression in LTRs with previous HSCT.

Kliman and colleagues studied LTRs after HSCT at two large Australian LTx centers. Eighteen patients (ages 10–64 years; median, 29.6 years) underwent bilateral LTx between 2002 and 2017 after having previously undergone an HSCT. Most patients undergoing evaluation for lung transplantation were on immunosuppressive agents (0–3 agents) at the time of referral. Prednisolone and cyclosporine were the most common agents with mycophenolate, tacrolimus, and extracorporeal photopheresis also used. The most common post-LTx immunosuppression regimens were prednisone, tacrolimus, and mycophenolate (33% of patients) and prednisone and tacrolimus (22% of patients). Five patients (28%) received basiliximab postoperatively [22].

Chen and colleagues showed that in patients who received lobar transplantation from the same donor, postoperative immunosuppression was able to be reduced significantly. In a retrospective review of 19 patients who underwent living donor lobar LTx after HSCT in Japan, eight patients had the same living donor for both LTx and HSCT. Trough levels of calcineurin inhibitors were maintained at a lower level throughout the postoperative period. Moreover, three patients were carefully tapered off immunosuppression. There was no significant difference in the infectious complications or the frequency of acute rejection between the two groups. Fifteen patients (79%) suffered from graft-versus-host disease at sites other than the lung, such as the skin and liver [23].

With the aim of reducing complications of LTx after HSCT, a retrospective Japanese study of 22 patients suggested improved survival when a lower dose of prednisone (<0.42 mg/kg/d) is used compared with higher doses [24]. Similar experience has been reported by the Australian group where less intense immunosuppressive regimens have been effective and well tolerated in LTx patients following HSCT [22]. Recurrence of GVHD in both the transplanted lung and other organs appears to be low. Further research is needed in this area to optimize the post-LTx immunosuppression for patients with a prior history of HSCT.

## Prophylaxis

Patients undergoing LTx after HSCT require prophylaxis against opportunistic infections. This typically consists of lifelong prophylaxis against *Pneumocystis jirovecii* with trimethoprim/sulfamethoxazole, inhaled pentamidine, atovaquone, or dapsone. Patients also receive antifungal prophylaxis with an azole antifungal for at least 3 months post-transplantation. Cytomegalovirus (CMV) prophylaxis, with ganciclovir 5 mg/kg IV OD, is commenced at the time of transplant and changed to valganciclovir 900 mg OD, based on renal function once enteral medications can be tolerated. CMV prophylaxis continued for 9 months in CMV IgG donor positive/recipient negative cases (CMV D+/R−), 6–9 months in CMV IgG D+/R+ cases, and 6–9 months in CMV IgG D−/R+ cases. CMV IgG D−/R− cases do not receive CMV prophylaxis but receive acyclovir for herpes simplex virus (HSV) prophylaxis instead. Following discontinuation of prophylaxis, serum CMV PCR is monitored weekly for 1 month. Additional perioperative antibiotic prophylaxis can be considered based on history of previous colonization. LTRs after HSCT remain at risk for late-onset CMV disease, and therefore, longer duration of CMV prophylaxis should be considered.

## Infections

LTx recipients after HSCT are at increased risk of infectious complications secondary to interruption of mucosal barriers associated with graft-versus-host disease (GVHD), hypogammaglobulinemia, prolonged immunosuppressive therapy, and colonization by resistant bacteria [14]. Opportunistic infections are common after lung transplantation, most commonly aspergillus and cytomegalovirus infections. Therapeutic antifungals and antivirals are often needed, and immunoglobulin replacement for hypogammaglobulinemia should be considered. Infectious complications can be severe and may lead to mortality.

Data from a retrospective multicenter pediatric survey on behalf of the European Society for Blood and Marrow Transplantation (EBMT) reported on 12 LTRs following HSCT in childhood [21]. Infectious complications occurred in five (42%) of LTRs. Two patients died 5 years and 10 years after LTx due to infection and underlying primary immunodeficiency [25]. In the largest study of lung transplantation after HSCT, sepsis accounted for 41% of deaths during follow-up. The authors identified the timing of allo-HSCT (within 2 years of LTx) and bridging to LTx (mechanical ventilation or extracorporeal life support) as risk factors for early sepsis-related mortality [17]. Similarly, Brockmann and colleagues reported that infectious complications were a major cause of mortality among 101 LTRs after HSCT; causes included aspergillosis, CMV encephalitis, and pneumocystis jiroveci pneumonia (PJP) pneumonitis [26].

Pneumatosis intestinalis is a rare complication following LTx after HSCT. The possible causes of pneumatosis intestinalis include CMV infection, *Clostridium difficile* colitis, long-term immunosuppression administered for pulmonary GVHD, and intense immunosuppression after LTx. It has been postulated that inflammation caused by infection destroys bowel mucosa, allowing invasion of gas producing bacteria or air itself. Corticosteroids independently appear to significantly increase the risk of development of pneumatosis intestinalis after HSCT. Corticosteroids may induce atrophy of the Peyer's patches, resulting in defects in the bowel mucosa and subsequent migration of gas or air into the submucosal and subserosal regions. Conservative therapy should be considered for the treatment of pneumatosis intestinalis developing after LTx [27].

The optimal approach for translating knowledge regarding potential immunodeficiency and resultant infection risk into post-transplant management is not clear-cut. It might be argued that a less intensive immunosuppressive regimen should be provided to LTRs after the previous HSCT. However, the complexity of the pathobiology and the impact of individualized factors in the pathogenesis of these deficits make a "one-size-fits-all" strategy inappropriate for this cohort. These patients commonly experience humoral immune deficiencies, as evidenced by the high proportion of patients requiring immunoglobulin replacement and low rates of donor-specific antibody development post-LTx. However, T-cell-mediated acute cellular rejection remains an ongoing concern. Strategies to optimize post-LTx outcomes in allo-HSCT recipients include prolonged CMV prophylaxis, preemptive antimicrobial therapy, monitoring for immunoglobulin deficiency, and, in appropriate cases, careful reduction of maintenance immunosuppression compared to standard regimens.

## Acute Rejection

Despite significant progress in the field of transplant immunology, acute rejection remains a frequent complication after lung transplantation [28]. Almost 30% of LTRs experience at least one episode of acute cellular rejection (ACR) during the first year after transplant. Acute cellular rejection and lymphocytic bronchiolitis have well-defined histopathologic diagnostic criteria and grading. Acute allograft rejection has been classically described based on the immunobiology and histopathologic features of T-cell-dependent (cellular) allo-immunity against the donor antigens expressed in the lung allograft. The diagnosis of acute rejection is made based on the presence of perivascular and interstitial mononuclear infiltrate in lung tissue [29]. Antibody-mediated rejection occurs due to humoral immunity-mediated production of donor-specific antibodies, targeted toward donor lung antigens, that create a propagating cycle of tissue injury and destruction [30].

It has been suggested that allogeneic HSCT increases risk of rejection after LTx because of the number of immunocompetent leukocytes present in the donor lung [26]. In a study of 62 LTRs after HSCT from Japan, there was a high incidence of acute rejection. Forty episodes of acute rejection occurred in 33 patients [2]. In the systematic review of 101 LTx after HSCT, Brockmann and colleagues reported rejection episodes in 19% of patients, and rejection was the cause of mortality in 6% of patients [26]. Koenecke and colleagues described outcomes of LTRs after HSCT within 107 European Group for Blood and Marrow transplantation member centers. Four out of the 12 patients had episodes of graft rejection after LTx. This led to respiratory failure and death in one patient and retransplantation in another patient. The rejection episodes were successfully treated with immunosuppressive therapy in the remaining two patients [25].

On the other hand, data regarding the incidence of antibody-mediated rejection in LTx after HSCT is sparse. The incidence of donor-specific antibodies in LTRs with a previous HSCT has been described to be low in association with immunodeficiency and hypogammaglobulinemia. Additional research is needed to better understand the risk of acute cellular and antibody-mediated rejection in LTRs with a history of HSCT.

## Chronic Lung Allograft Dysfunction

Chronic lung allograft dysfunction (CLAD) is the overarching term encompassing all forms of chronic lung dysfunction post-transplant. CLAD is defined as a substantial and persistent decline (>20%) in measured forced expiratory volume in 1 s (FEV1) from baseline. The baseline value is computed as the mean of the best two postoperative FEV1 measurements (taken >3 weeks apart). CLAD can present either as a restrictive pattern or an obstructive pattern, bronchiolitis obliterans syndrome (BOS), defined by the persistent decline in forced expiratory volume in 1 s (FEV1) and/or forced vital capacity (FVC) <80% of baseline post-transplant testing for >3 weeks [31].

In a multicenter case series describing the Australian experience of LTx after HSCT, CLAD developed in three out of 18 patients (17%) at 20, 25, and 75 months, respectively. One of the patients developed pulmonary graft failure and required a second LTx 40 months after the initial LTx. He survived up to 46 months following his second LTx before dying from recurrent CLAD and graft failure [22]. In a systematic review of LTx after HSCT, the reported recurrence of BOS after LTx in the HSCT population was higher at 32% and is comparable to the other indications for LTx [14].

## Malignancy

Relapse of underlying malignancy after LTx in HSCT is another major concern. Based on the available data, 2.5% of patients had a relapse of the primary hematologic malignancy, and 4.5% developed new malignancy (primarily skin and lymphoma) after lung transplantation [14]. Chen-Yoshikawa and colleagues reported recurrence of malignancy in four out of 62 (6.5%) LTRs after HSCT, and three patients eventually died. The development of recurrence of hematologic malignancy was significantly associated with a shorter interval between HSCT and lung transplantation. In the same cohort, one patient died of post-transplant lymphoproliferative disorder 7 months after transplantation [2].

## Mortality

For patients with end-stage lung disease, LTx can prolong life substantially; however, the survival statistics for lung transplant recipients still significantly lag behind other solid organ transplant recipients. There are limited data regarding the long-term outcomes in patients undergoing a LTx after HSCT. In a report of 13 LTRs following HSCT, the 1-year (90%) and 5-year (75%) survival did not differ from matched lung transplant controls (85% and 68%, respectively) [32]. In another series of nine patients, survival at 1 year and 5 years was 89% and 37%, respectively, which was lower than expected for other lung transplant recipients (49% at 5 years) [18]. In a retrospective single center cohort study at the Toronto General Hospital between 2003 and 2019, Riddell and colleagues assessed post-transplant outcomes of 19 adults who underwent double LTx after HSCT. The post-transplant survival was 50% at 5 years. Survival to 1 year was similar to matched control, but survival conditional of 1-year survival was lower in the allo-HSCT cohort. An increased risk of death due to infection was identified in the allo-HSCT cohort compared to matched controls [33].

## Health-Related Quality of Life

Lung transplantation after HSCT can improve survival in patients with pulmonary complications after HSCT. Similarly, improvement in health-related quality of life (HRQOL) after LTx is another important post-transplant outcome. Hamada and colleagues reported that the physical function and HRQOL were lowest before lung transplantation in patients with pulmonary complications after HSCT. Two years after lung transplantation, the dyspnea scores and performance status improved. However, recipients who were unemployed before lung transplant were likely to remain unemployed and continued to show poor HRQOL. The study showed poor recovery of HRQOL and the likelihood of failure to reintegrate into society within 2 years after lung transplantation. Hence, it is necessary to consider long-term follow-up, multidisciplinary treatment, rehabilitation, and physical training to improve social reintegration and HRQOL in patients undergoing LTx after HSCT [3].

# Patients with Primary Immunodeficiency

Patients with primary immunodeficiency, such as common variable deficiency, present a unique challenge for transplantation. Bone marrow transplantation can be curative with healthy bone marrow-derived immunity. However, patients with primary immunodeficiency often develop pulmonary complications secondary to recurrent infections, making them ineligible for even reduced intensity conditioning because of risk of mortality. On the other hand, these patients may develop end-stage bronchiectasis but are ineligible for LTx because of concerns of recurrent infections in the allograft.

In 2015, Szabolcs and colleagues reported the first successful combined sequential lung and bone marrow transplantation from an unrelated cadaveric donor in a 16-year-old girl with T-cell lymphopenia with long-term graft survival. After identification of an appropriate donor, bone marrow harvesting and cryopreservation were performed. The recipient underwent standard bilateral sequential LTx followed by standard immunosuppression. Three months after LTx, reduced intensity conditioning followed by cryopreserved, T-cell-depleted cadaveric bone marrow transplant was performed. Subsequently, the patient was noted to have 100% donor chimerism in whole blood and was completely weaned off all immunosuppression 3 years after transplant [34]. This report provided proof of concept to the hypothesis that persistent engraftment of the hematopoietic stem cells from an immunocompetent donor would result in donor-derived cellular immunity and may enable lifelong immune tolerance to the lung allograft. A clinical trial to evaluate the safety and efficacy of performing bilateral orthotopic lung transplantation followed by cadaveric HSCT from the same donor for patients with primary immunodeficiency disease and end-stage lung disease is currently underway [35].

## Conclusion

Lung transplantation for end-stage lung disease complicating HSCT remains a rare indication. Individuals being evaluated for LTx after HSCT are considered to be high-risk candidates due to the need for additional immunosuppression, presumed abnormal baseline immunology, risk for infection, nutritional deficiencies, extra pulmonary GVHD, and risk of recurrence of malignancy. The reported post-transplant outcomes in LTRs after HSCT are comparable to other LTx recipients, albeit the risk for infectious complications remains higher. Further research is required to determine the appropriate timing of referral and listing, post-transplant outcomes, and immunosuppressive and antimicrobial strategies, as well as supportive care in this patient population to assist HSCT and LTx programs to optimize resource utilization and outcomes.

## References


1. Styczyński J, Tridello G, Koster L, et al. Death after hematopoietic stem cell transplantation: changes over calendar year time, infections and associated factors. Bone Marrow Transplant. 2020;55(1):126–36. https://doi.org/10.1038/s41409-019-0624-z.
2. Chen-Yoshikawa TF, Sugimoto S, Shiraishi T, et al. Prognostic factors in lung transplantation after hematopoietic stem cell transplantation. Transplantation. 2018;102(1):154–61.
3. Hamada R, Oshima Y, Sato S, et al. Changes in the health-related quality of life and social reintegration status after lung transplantation following hematopoietic stem cell transplantation. Support Care Cancer. 2022;30(2):1831–9.
4. Hamada R, Oshima Y, Sato S, et al. Physical function after lung transplantation for late-onset non-infectious pulmonary complications after allogeneic hematopoietic stem cell transplantation. Support Care Center. 2021;29(9):5447–54.
5. Noguchi M, Chen-Yoshikawa TF, Arai Y, et al. Expanded indications for lung transplantation after hematopoietic stem cell transplantation. J Thorac Cardiovasc Surg. 2020;163(4):1549–1557.e4.
6. Greer M, Berastegui C, Jaksch P, et al. Lung transplantation after allogeneic stem cell transplantation: a pan-European experience. Eur Respir J. 2018;51(2):1701330. Published 2018 Feb 14. https://doi.org/10.1183/13993003.01330-2017.
7. Yusen RD, Edwards LB, Dipchand AI, et al. The registry of the International Society for Heart and Lung Transplantation: thirty-third adult lung and heart-lung transplant report-2016; focus theme: primary diagnostic indications for transplant. J Heart Lung Transplant. 2016;35(10):1170–84. https://doi.org/10.1016/j.healun.2016.09.001.
8. Calhoun JH, Levine S, Anzueto A, et al. Lung transplantation in a patient with a prior bone marrow transplant. Chest. 1992;102:948.
9. Said SA, Okamoto T, Sakanoue I, et al. Lung transplant for patient with idiopathic pneumonia syndrome.

Ann Thorac Surg. 2020;110(2):e87–9. https://doi.org/10.1016/j.athoracsur.2019.12.044.
10. Ueda S, Chen-Yoshikawa TF, Hijiya K, Date H. Lung transplantation after haematopoietic stem cell transplantation for Wiskott-Aldrich syndrome. Eur J Cardiothorac Surg. 2018;53(6):1286–7. https://doi.org/10.1093/ejcts/ezx461.
11. Weill D, Benden C, Corris PA, et al. A consensus document for the selection of lung transplant candidates: 2014—an update from the Pulmonary Transplantation Council of the International Society for Heart and Lung Transplantation. J Heart Lung Transplant. 2015;34(1):1–15.
12. Leard LE, Holm AM, Valapour M, et al. Consensus document for the selection of lung transplant candidates: an update from the International Society for Heart and Lung Transplantation. J Heart Lung Transplant. 2021;40(11):1349–79.
13. Gadre S, Turowski J, Budev M. Overview of lung transplantation, heart-lung transplantation, liver-lung transplantation, and combined hematopoietic stem cell transplantation and lung transplantation. Clin Chest Med. 2017;38(4):623–40.
14. Soubani AO, Kingah P, Alshabani K, Muma G, Haq A. Lung transplantation following hematopoietic stem cell transplantation: report of two cases and systematic review of literature. Clin Transpl. 2014;28(7):776–82. https://doi.org/10.1111/ctr.12378.
15. Holm AM, Riise GC, Hansson L, et al. Lung transplantation for bronchiolitis obliterans syndrome after Allo-SCT. Bone Marrow Transplant. 2013;48(5):703–7. https://doi.org/10.1038/bmt.2012.197.
16. Al-Adra DP, Hammel L, Roberts J, et al. Pre-existing melanoma and hematological malignancies, prognosis and timing to solid organ transplantation: a consensus expert opinion statement. Am J Transplant. 2021;21:475–83.
17. Greer M, Berastegui C, Jaksch P, et al. Lung transplantation after allogeneic stem cell transplantation: a pan-European experience. Eur Respir J. 2018;51(2):1701330.
18. Cheng GS, Edelman JD, Madtes DK, et al. Outcomes of lung transplantation after allogeneic hematopoietic stem cell transplantation. Biol Blood Marrow Transplant. 2014;20(8):1169–75.
19. Porteous MK, Lee JC. Primary graft dysfunction after lung transplantation. Clin Chest Med. 2017;38(4):641–54. https://doi.org/10.1016/j.ccm.2017.07.005.
20. Christie JD, Bellamy S, Ware LB, et al. Construct validity of the definition of primary graft dysfunction after lung transplantation. J Heart Lung Transplant. 2010;29(11):1231–9. https://doi.org/10.1016/j.healun.2010.05.013.
21. Kreisel D, Krupnick AS, Puri V, et al. Short- and long-term outcomes of 1000 adult lung transplant recipients at a single center. J Thorac Cardiovasc Surg. 2011;141(1):215–22. https://doi.org/10.1016/j.jtcvs.2010.09.009.
22. Kliman DS, Kotecha SR, Abelson DC, Snell GI, Glanville AR, Ma DDF. Favorable outcome of lung transplantation for severe pulmonary graft versus host disease: an Australian multicenter case series. Transplantation. 2019;103(12):2602–7. https://doi.org/10.1097/TP.0000000000002693.
23. Chen F, Yamane M, Inoue M, et al. Less maintenance immunosuppression in lung transplantation following hematopoietic stem cell transplantation from the same living donor. Am J Transplant. 2011;11(7):1509–16. https://doi.org/10.1111/j.1600-6143.2011.03591.x.
24. Sugimoto S, Miyoshi K, Kurosaki T, et al. Favorable survival in lung transplant recipients on preoperative low-dose, as compared to high-dose corticosteroids, after hematopoietic stem cell transplantation. Int J Hematol. 2018;107(6):696–702. https://doi.org/10.1007/s12185-018-2417-3.
25. Koenecke C, Hertenstein B, Schetelig J, et al. Solid organ transplantation after allogeneic hematopoietic stem cell transplantation: a retrospective, multicenter study of the EBMT. Am J Transplant. 2010;10(8):1897–906. https://doi.org/10.1111/j.1600-6143.2010.03187.x.
26. Brockmann JG, Broering DC, Raza SM, et al. Solid organ transplantation following allogeneic haematopoietic cell transplantation: experience from a referral organ transplantation center and systematic review of literature. Bone Marrow Transplant. 2019;54(2):190–203. https://doi.org/10.1038/s41409-018-0255-9.
27. Mesaki K, Sugimoto S, Otani S, et al. Pneumatosis intestinalis after lung transplantation for pulmonary graft-versus-host disease. J Thorac Dis. 2018;10(1):E42–5. https://doi.org/10.21037/jtd.2017.11.121.
28. Subramani MV, Pandit S, Gadre SK. Acute rejection and post lung transplant surveillance. Indian J Thorac Cardiovasc Surg. 2022;38(Suppl 2):271–9. https://doi.org/10.1007/s12055-021-01320-z.
29. Stewart S, Fishbein MC, Snell GI, et al. Revision of the 1996 working formulation for the standardization of nomenclature in the diagnosis of lung rejection. J Heart Lung Transplant. 2007;26(12):1229–42. https://doi.org/10.1016/j.healun.2007.10.017.
30. Levine DJ, Glanville AR, Aboyoun C, et al. Antibody-mediated rejection of the lung: a consensus report of the International Society for Heart and Lung Transplantation. J Heart Lung Transplant. 2016;35(4):397–406. https://doi.org/10.1016/j.healun.2016.01.1223.
31. Verleden GM, Glanville AR, Lease ED, et al. Chronic lung allograft dysfunction: definition, diagnostic criteria, and approaches to treatment—a consensus report from the pulmonary council of the ISHLT. J Heart Lung Transplant. 2019;38(5):493–503. https://doi.org/10.1016/j.healun.2019.03.009.
32. Holm AM, Riise GC, Brinch L, et al. Lung transplantation for bronchiolitis obliterans after allogeneic hematopoietic stem cell transplantation: unresolved questions. Transplantation. 2013;96(4):e21–2. https://doi.org/10.1097/TP.0b013e31829df2c0.
33. Riddell P, Vasudevan-Nampoothiri R, Ma J, Singer LG, Lipton JH, Juvet SC. Lung transplantation for late-onset non-infectious chronic pulmonary compli-

cations of allogeneic hematopoietic stem cell transplant. Respir Res. 2021;22(1):101. Published 2021 Apr 7. https://doi.org/10.1186/s12931-021-01699-8.
34. Szabolcs P, Buckley RH, Davis RD, et al. Tolerance and immunity after sequential lung and bone marrow transplantation from an unrelated cadaveric donor. J Allergy Clin Immunol. 2015;135(2):567–70. https://doi.org/10.1016/j.jaci.2014.07.058.
35. Sequential Cadaveric Lung and Bone Marrow Transplant for Immune Deficiency Diseases. ClinicalTrials.gov identifier: NCT01852370 https://clinicaltrials.gov/ct2/show/NCT01852370. Accessed 5 Jul 2022.

# 24 Outcomes in Critically Ill Allogeneic Hematopoietic Stem Cell Transplantation Recipients

Antoine Lafarge and Elie Azoulay

## Introduction

Allogeneic hematopoietic stem cell transplantation (Allo-HSCT) is a well-established therapeutic option for many malignancies such as acute myeloid and lymphoblastic leukemia, myelodysplastic syndromes, myeloproliferative neoplasms, and some nonmalignant life-threatening diseases. It is estimated that about 18,000 patients receive Allo-HSCT every year in Europe, the corresponding figure being 10,000 in the USA [1, 2].

## Intensive Care Unit Admission

Despite notable changes in the practice of Allo-HSCT in the past 30 years, including older age at Allo-HSCT and use of alternative stem cell sources, the proportion of Allo-HSCT recipients requiring intensive care unit (ICU) admission remains stable over time, a finding probably relevant to the greater use of reduced-intensity conditioning [3]. Similarly, Allo-HSCT recipients still display increased short and long-term mortality rates, mainly due to the relapse of primary disease and the high burden of nonrecurrence-related morbidity.

The likelihood of ICU admission varies from center to center, with published series reporting a wide range of admission rates from 5 to 57% [4, 5] (Table 24.1).

A. Lafarge · E. Azoulay (✉)
Critical Care Department, Saint Louis Hospital, Assistance Publique Hôpitaux de Paris (APHP), Paris Cité University, Paris, France
e-mail: elie.azoulay@aphp.fr



A. O. Soubani (ed.), *Pulmonary and Critical Care Considerations of Hematopoietic Stem Cell Transplantation*, https://doi.org/10.1007/978-3-031-28797-8_24

**Table 24.1** Key findings from five studies focusing on critically ill Allo-HSCT recipients

| Authors | Study period | ICU admission rate | Time from Allo-HSCT to ICU admission | ICU mortality | 1-year survival |
|---|---|---|---|---|---|
| Pichereau et al. (2020) [13] | 2005–2014 | 191/1212 (16%) | 145 days (29–446) | 35/191 (18%) | 75/191 (39%) |
| Lueck et al. (2018) [6] | 2000–2013 | 330/942 (35%) | 77 days (16–300) | 178/330 (54%) | 114/300 (38%) |
| Pène et al. (2006) [8] | 1997–2003 | | >30 days in 139/209 (66%) | 101/209 (48%) | 44/209 (21%) |
| Lengliné et al. (2015) [3] | 1997–2011 | 497/2286 (22%) | 73 days (14–239) | 194/497 (39%) | – |
| Benz et al. (2014) [4] | 1998–2007 | 33/250 (13%) | 72 days (7–870) | 21 (64%) | 9/33 (28%) |

## Risk Factors for ICU Admission

The risk for ICU admission is independently associated with acute graft-versus-host disease (aGVHD) grade II–IV and HLA mismatches, a finding probably due to the use of immunosuppressive therapies. In contrast, the stem cell source, donor relation, age of the patient, gender, ABO mismatch, as well as conditioning and TBI are not reported as risk factors for ICU admission [5].

## Timing of Intensive Care Unit Admission

Time between Allo-HSCT and ICU admission greatly differs according to series, but the majority of ICU admissions occur within 3 months after Allo-HSCT, during or immediately after the engraftment period [5]. However, Allo-HSCT recipients carry a substantial burden of late-onset morbidity, such as onco-hematological malignancies and cardiovascular diseases that may require ICU admission many years after Allo-HSCT. Accordingly, the delay between HSCT and ICU transfer is related to the reason for ICU admission [6].

## Indications of Intensive Care Unit Admission

Acute respiratory failure (ARF) represents the main reason for ICU admission. Causes of ARF are not always clearly reported but are dominated by pulmonary infections, acute cardiac failure, and intra-alveolar hemorrhage [6–9].

Other common reasons for ICU transfer are septic shock, neurological failure (including posterior reversible encephalopathy syndrome, drug toxicity, metabolic disorders, infectious causes, and cerebral hemorrhages), and acute kidney injury (sepsis, shock, and specific causes such as engraftment syndrome, veno-occlusive disease or thrombotic microangiopathy).

Documented infection rates vary from 50 to 70% [7, 8], involving mostly bacteria, way ahead of invasive fungal infections (mostly aspergillosis) and virus (mostly cytomegalovirus reactivation) [8].

## Autologous and Allogeneic HSCT Induce Different Patterns of Organ Dysfunction

Unlike Allo-HSCT, autologous HSCT (Auto-HSCT) has no therapeutic effect per se but can overcome the prolonged cytopenia induced by the therapeutic use of high-dose chemotherapies. Hence, the pattern of organ dysfunction is clearly different between critically ill Allo-HSCT and Auto-HSCT recipients. Less than 10% of Auto-HSCT recipients require ICU admission, mostly for chemotherapy-related toxicity and febrile neutropenia or sepsis [10, 11]. Studies including a mixture of both HSCT types should be interpreted carefully. Most of the literature specific to critically ill autologous HSCT patients show a favorable outcome that is not much different from other patients with hematological malignancies.

In this chapter, we sought to put forward five important tips for the management of critically ill Allo-HSCT recipients, encompassing prognosis evaluation and therapeutic strategy, as well as short- and long-term outcomes.

## The Number of Organ Dysfunction Is the Major Determinant of Mortality

The number of organ dysfunctions remains the main prognostic factor in critically ill Allo-HSCT recipients [3, 12, 13]. The number of organ dysfunctions is associated with both early (ICU and hospital mortality) [6, 12] and long-term mortality rates [3, 6, 13].

When Allo-HSCT patients are admitted to the ICU with only one or no organ failure, diagnostic and therapeutic procedures are associated with a better diagnostic yield or therapeutic response [11, 14]. However, ICU reality is more complex as it is mainly the combination of organ dysfunctions that require ICU admission [6], knowing that attempt to resuscitate multiple organ failure in the HSCT population is mostly associated with increased mortality [3, 11].

Acute respiratory failure (ARF) represents the main reason for critically ill Allo-HSCT recipients. Interestingly, ARF etiologies depend on the time since Allo-HSCT, the conditioning regimen, and the presence of GVHD. In addition, whether patients receive an antifungal or anti-pneumocystis prophylaxis is important. Overall, pulmonary infections, acute cardiac failure, and intra-alveolar hemorrhage are among the main ARF etiologies [5, 6, 8, 9].

Septic shock, neurological failure (including posterior reversible encephalopathy syndrome, drug toxicity, metabolic disorders, infectious causes, and cerebral hemorrhages), and acute kidney injury (sepsis, shock, and specific causes such as engraftment syndrome and veno-occlusive disease thrombotic microangiopathy) may also lead to ICU transfer.

## The Assessment of Acute GVHD (aGVHD) Trajectory Might Help to Identify Allo-HSCT Patients Who Could Benefit from Critical Care

Despite significant advances in the management of aGVHD, it still remains the leading Allo-HSCT complication and requires intense and aggressive immunosuppressive strategies [13]. Several studies published over the last decade emphasize on the grim survival associated with aGVHD. Mortality rates reach 70% in critically ill Allo-HSCT recipients with aGVHD requiring life-sustaining therapies, especially mechanical ventilation [3, 13]. The negative impact of aGVHD may be due to aGVHD-related organ involvement, incremental immunosuppression, opportunistic infections, and nutritional status degradation [13]. Thus, until recently, ICU admission of Allo-HSCT recipients with active and uncontrolled aGVHD was discouraged.

However, these reports always analyzed aGVHD as a binary variable, neglecting its dynamic assessment. Considering the aGVHD trajectory for the first time, Pichereau et al. considered different categories of patients, depending on whether they had a controlled, improving, or newly diagnosed (and untreated) aGVHD, as opposed to a refractory aGVHD. Their findings were that Allo-HSCT recipients without refractory aGVHD had nonsignificantly different day-90 survival. There was, however, a significantly increased mortality when aGVHD was refractory to immunosuppressive drugs.

While aGVHD remains a major determinant of mortality in critically ill Allo-HSCT recipients, these findings suggest that Allo-HSCT recipients in whom GVHD is not uncontrolled could benefit from ICU admission. The goals of care for these patients need, however, to be reassessed individually based on the patient's preferences and values, associated comorbid conditions, and frailty indexes.

## Early ICU Admission of Allo-HSCT Recipients Is Associated with Better Outcomes

Interestingly, Orvain et al. showed that Allo-HSCT recipients admitted earlier on to the ICU as soon as they show signs of organ injury fared better. Allo-HSCT recipients who were admitted later on following the first organ injury (>1 day) or with more organ injuries (>2 organ injuries) had a worse outcome. The development of a score combining these covariates (the number of organ injuries/day) further improved the prediction of in-hospital survival after ICU admission. Allo-HSCT recipients with higher organ injuries/day had significantly higher in-hospital mortality rate even after adjustment for refractory acute GVHD and the sequential organ failure assessment (SOFA) [12].

The benefit of an early ICU admission policy of onco-hematological patients has already been demonstrated but not specifically in Allo-HSCT recipients [6, 15, 16]. In a subgroup analysis, Bokhari et al. reported improved 6-month survival in HSCT recipients who were admitted earlier to the intensive care unit [17].

Multicenter studies are warranted to validate the injuries/day score and confirm the implementation of an early ICU admission policy in Allo-HSCT recipients. The benefit of such a strategy could rely on the early introduction of close monitoring, intensive diagnosis strategy, and optimized organ support on less injured patients.

## Need for Precision and Personalized Critical Care Management of Allo-HSCT Recipients

The dynamic assessment of aGVHD illustrates the evolution of critical care toward precision and personalized medicine. ICU admission should no longer be considered as a binary decision, and individuals' goals of critical care management must be defined as early as possible for each individual case.

When aGVHD is in remission, Allo-HSCT recipients should receive the same full code of ICU management as patients without aGVHD. In patients with active but controlled aGVHD, a time-limited trial of ICU management is in order. Unless aGVHD becomes uncontrolled or the underlying malignancy relapses, we recommend at least 14 days of full code management before reassessing the goals of care. However, in critically ill Allo-HSCT recipients with uncontrolled aGVHD despite high-dose steroids and additional immunosuppressors, ICU management is likely to be non-beneficial, and the goals of care should be shifted from curative to palliative [11, 13].

Beyond life-sustaining therapies in most severe Allo-HSCT recipients, ICU admission might be considered for less invasive strategies such as cardiac or pulmonary evaluation, diagnostic procedures, or close monitoring [6, 11].

Within a close relationship between hematologists and intensivists, the early assessment of the goals of critical care for every Allo-HSCT recipient should help align therapeutic objectives with patient expectations [11, 18].

## Long-Term Survival of Allo-HSCT Recipients Is Encouraging and No Longer Affected by a Former ICU Stay

As for other patients with hematological malignancies [14], both short- and long-term survival of critically ill HSCT patients have improved significantly in recent years [3, 6, 9]. ICU, hospital, and 1-year survival rates increased over time and now reach 60%, 43%, and 32%, respectively [6]. ICU admission policies and HSCT procedures may vary over time, but improved outcomes also involve most severe patients requiring life-sustaining therapies such as mechanical ventilation or vasoactive drugs, arguing for specific advances in critical care management [3, 6].

While the ICU admission remains clearly associated with poor outcomes in Allo-HSCT recipients, long-term survival is now comparable between ICU survivors and patients never admitted to the ICU [6].

These findings highlight the improvements in critical care management in recent years and emphasize the potential benefit of ICU admission that should be considered as a bridge to cure for critically ill Allo-HSCT recipients [11].

## Conclusion

As observed for other critically ill patients, ICU outcomes of Allo-HSCT recipients have dramatically improved over the last decades, including most severe patients requiring vasopressors and mechanical ventilation [3, 6]. This finding may rely on changes in HSCT procedures and immunosuppressive strategies, better triage, earlier ICU admission, and improved general critical care management.

About a third of Allo-HSCT recipients will require critical care management [6]. ICU admission remains clearly associated with shortened survival, but long-term outcomes of ICU survivors are not different anymore from patients that had never been in the ICU. Encouraging 5-year survival rates around 50% [6] is probably the strongest argument to maintain the doors of ICU widely opened to critically ill Allo-HSCT recipients without uncontrolled aGVHD.

The time for precision and personalized critical care management of Allo-HSCT recipients has come. Allo-HSCT recipients must be considered for intensive care, in terms of full code or 2-week ICU trial, as soon as they develop organ injury. The goals of care should be defined at ICU admission for every Allo-HSCT recipient, requiring a close collaboration between intensivists and hematologists in order to assess primary disease status, number of organ failures, aGVHD trajectory, and patient expectations. Hematologists and intensivists will for sure need to adapt their strategy with the growing use of genetically modified auto chimeric antigen receptor (CAR) T-cell therapy that will certainly modify the Allo-HSCT landscape (Fig. 24.1).

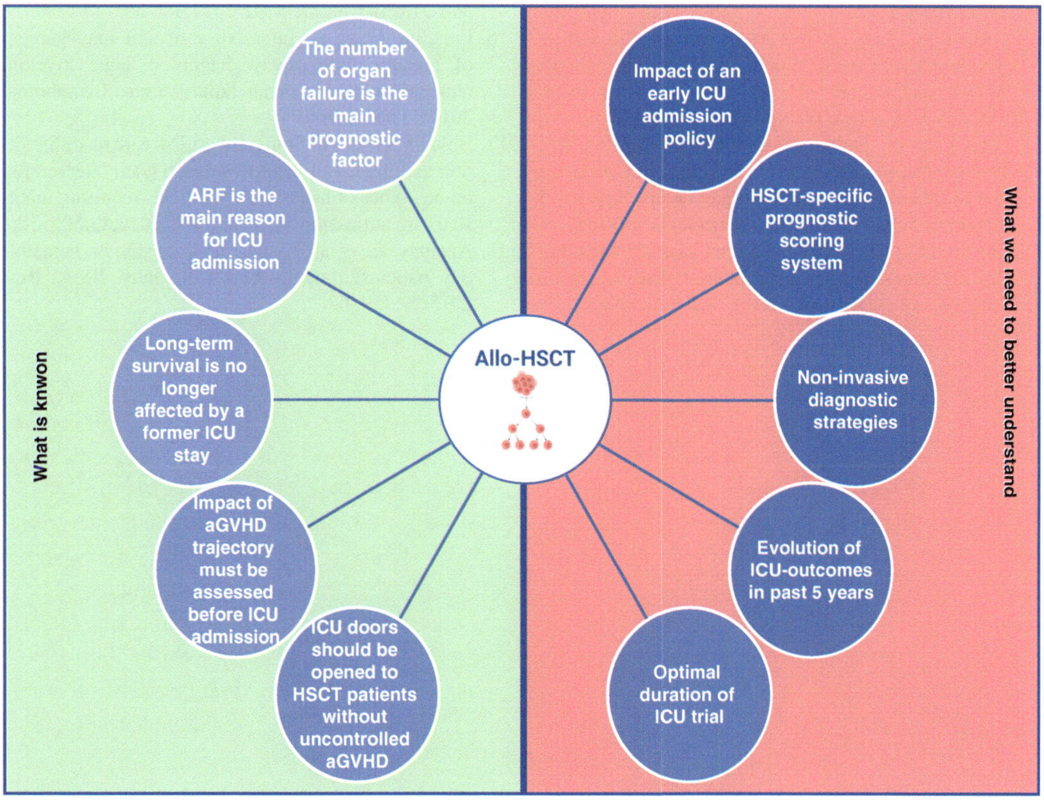


**Fig. 24.1** Outcomes in critically ill allogeneic hematopoietic stem cell transplantation recipients. *Allo-HSCT* allogeneic hematopoietic stem cell transplantation, *ARF* acute respiratory failure, *ICU* intensive care unit, *aGVHD* acute graft-versus-host disease

## References

1. Bhatia S, et al. Trends in late mortality and life expectancy after allogeneic blood or marrow transplantation over 4 decades: a blood or marrow transplant survivor study report. JAMA Oncol. 2021;7:1626–34.
2. D'Souza A, et al. Current use of and trends in hematopoietic cell transplantation in the United States. Biol Blood Marrow Transplant. 2020;26:e177–82.
3. Lengliné E, et al. Changes in intensive care for allogeneic hematopoietic stem cell transplant recipients. Bone Marrow Transplant. 2015;50:840–5.
4. Benz R, Schanz U, Maggiorini M, Seebach JD, Stussi G. Risk factors for ICU admission and ICU survival after allogeneic hematopoietic SCT. Bone Marrow Transplant. 2014;49:62–5.
5. Saillard C, et al. Critically ill allogeneic HSCT patients in the intensive care unit: a systematic review and meta-analysis of prognostic factors of mortality. Bone Marrow Transplant. 2018;53:1233–41.
6. Lueck C, et al. Improved short- and long-term outcome of allogeneic stem cell recipients admitted to the intensive care unit: a retrospective longitudinal analysis of 942 patients. Intensive Care Med. 2018;44:1483–92.
7. Saillard C, Blaise D, Mokart D. Critically ill allogeneic hematopoietic stem cell transplantation patients in the intensive care unit: reappraisal of actual prognosis. Bone Marrow Transplant. 2016;51:1050–61.
8. Pène F, et al. Outcome of critically ill allogeneic hematopoietic stem-cell transplantation recipients: a reappraisal of indications for organ failure supports. J Clin Oncol Off J Am Soc Clin Oncol. 2006;24:643–9.
9. Orvain C, et al. Different impact of the number of organ failures and graft-versus-host disease on the outcome of allogeneic stem cell transplantation recipients requiring intensive care. Transplantation. 2017;101:437–44.
10. Kerhuel L, Amorim S, Azoulay E, Thiéblemont C, Canet E. Clinical features of life-threatening complications following autologous stem cell transplantation in patients with lymphoma. Leuk Lymphoma. 2015;56:3090–5.
11. Lengliné E, Mirouse A, Azoulay E. Top ten tips for the management of critically ill hematopoietic stem cell transplantation recipients. Intensive Care Med. 2019;45:384–7.
12. Orvain C, et al. Allogeneic stem cell transplantation recipients requiring intensive care: time is of the essence. Ann Hematol. 2018;97:1601–9.
13. Pichereau C, et al. Trajectories of acute graft-versus-host disease and mortality in critically ill allogeneic-hematopoietic stem cell recipients: the Allo-GRRR-OH score. Bone Marrow Transplant. 2020;55:1966–74.
14. Azoulay E, et al. Outcomes of critically ill patients with hematologic malignancies: prospective Multicenter data from France and Belgium—a Groupe de Recherche Respiratoire en Réanimation Onco-Hématologique study. J Clin Oncol. 2013;31:2810–8.
15. Song J-U, et al. Early intervention on the outcomes in critically ill cancer patients admitted to intensive care units. Intensive Care Med. 2012;38:1505–13.
16. Lengliné E, et al. Intensive care unit management of patients with newly diagnosed acute myeloid leukemia with no organ failure. Leuk Lymphoma. 2012;53:1352–9.
17. Bokhari SWI, et al. Impact of critical care reconfiguration and track-and-trigger outreach team intervention on outcomes of haematology patients requiring intensive care admission. Ann Hematol. 2010;89:505–12.
18. Azoulay E, et al. Managing critically ill hematology patients: time to think differently. Blood Rev. 2015;29:359–67.

# Respiratory Support of the Critically Ill Hematopoietic Stem Cell Transplant Patient

25

Laveena Munshi and Dekel Stavi

## Introduction

Owing to advancements in oncology and critical care, the outcomes of acute respiratory failure (ARF) among cancer patients have improved significantly over the last three decades [1–4]. However, patients with cancer have a higher mortality rate than non-cancer cohorts (50–60% vs. 30–40%) in the setting of mechanical ventilation [2, 3, 5]. In more recent years, intensive care unit (ICU) mortality has continued to decrease steadily for most subtypes of cancer; however, in recent years, mortality across patients receiving hematopoietic stem cell transplant (HSCT) (specifically allogeneic) has plateaued [4].

Compared to other hematological malignant (HM) conditions and most other cancers, the HSCT population experiences a higher frequency of ARF necessitating ICU admission [6–8]. Approximately 25% of HSCT patients require an ICU admission within 1 year of procedure [1, 9]. The predominant cause of critical illness remains ARF. ICU mortality in this population in the setting of ARF ranges from 50% to 70%. Higher mortality rates are often related to the presence of invasive fungal infections or indeterminant ARF [10–16]. This high mortality rate is in contrast to 32% ARF mortality in the general population requiring ventilation [17] and 56% in an immunocompromised population requiring ventilation [18]. It remains unclear whether the higher mortality is predominantly due to (1) patient factors (e.g., greater propensity for frailty), (2) disease factors (e.g., higher severity of illness/more challenging organisms), (3) physician factors (e.g., preconceived perception of poor prognosis driving end-of-life conversations), (4) difference in mechanical ventilation practices (e.g., use of noninvasive devices), or (5) pathophysiologic differences in ARF.

This chapter will focus on respiratory support for the HSCT population in the setting of ARF. It is important to highlight that determining the cause of ARF through a safe and precise approach is possibly one of the most important principles in managing these patients as delays in diagnosis or indeterminant ARF carries a high mortality rate for this population [19–21].

L. Munshi (✉)
Interdepartmental Division of Critical Care Medicine, Mount Sinai Hospital, Sinai Health System, University of Toronto, Toronto, ON, Canada
e-mail: Laveena.Munshi@sinaihealth.ca

D. Stavi
Critical Care Medicine, Tel Aviv Sourasky Medical Center, Tel Aviv University, Tel Aviv, Israel
e-mail: dekelst@tlvmc.gov.il



A. O. Soubani (ed.), *Pulmonary and Critical Care Considerations of Hematopoietic Stem Cell Transplantation*, https://doi.org/10.1007/978-3-031-28797-8_25

## Features of Pulmonary Complications Following HSCT

There are distinct immunologic states that occur post-HSCT that render patients susceptible to specific etiologies of ARF following transplant (see Chap. 3). The differential for causes of ARF is vast with infectious and noninfectious causes occasionally occurring simultaneously. Knowing the timeline following transplant, prophylactic therapy received, type of immunosuppression, and duration of immunosuppression is imperative to inform investigative workup and approach to empiric therapy in the setting of severe illness. An early (0–100 days post-HSCT) and late (roughly beyond 100 days) timeline can be used to approach the etiology. Early can be categorized as pre-engraftment (first 30 days), peri-engraftment (within 7 days of engraftment), and early post-engraftment (30–100 days) [15, 22]. In a recent cohort study that assessed post-HSCT ARF in the first year, 65% were identified as severe, and 69% occurred in the first 100 days following the transplant. Occasionally, ARF can progress to the more severe form known as acute respiratory distress syndrome (ARDS). ARDS, as a syndrome, is intended to identify a process that results in diffuse alveolar damage. Neutrophil activation is a core process in ARDS; however, despite neutropenia, ARDS is known to occur in the HSCT population. More research is needed to inform whether the process of ARDS is similar in the general population compared to the HSCT cohort. This is imperative to informing support ventilatory care and best ICU practices for this population.

## Noninvasive and Invasive Respiratory Support

The goal of respiratory support is to improve patient's oxygenation, decrease respiratory work of breathing, and reverse any ventilation impairment. Respiratory support measures could be roughly divided into two categories: noninvasive respiratory support and invasive mechanical ventilation. Noninvasive devices may include high-flow nasal cannula (HFNC), continuous positive airway pressure (CPAP), and noninvasive mechanical ventilation (NIV).

The decision between noninvasive ventilation and upfront invasive mechanical ventilation (IMV) involves balancing the risks associated with coupling a patient to a ventilator and ventilator-associated lung injury against the risk of prolonged exposure to potentially injurious spontaneous breathing under a noninvasive strategy. Deciding between noninvasive and invasive may also be governed by the need for more invasive procedures that can be more safely executed under invasive mechanical ventilatory settings.

## Noninvasive Respiratory Support

HFNC uses a heated and humidified gas, providing a wide range of $FiO_2$ (0.21–1) and maximum flow up to 60–80 L/min. The high flows help minimize dilution of ambient air to ensure that the intended oxygen is delivered to the alveoli. An additional benefit is the creation of a low positive end expiratory pressure (PEEP), mucociliary clearance given the humidification, $CO_2$ washout from the upper airways, ease of use, and patient comfort [23]. CPAP and NIV use positive pressure ventilation through a tight-fitting face mask (oronasal or total face) or a helmet (plastic hood that is secured on the neck). Modes that are mainly used are continuous positive airway pressure (CPAP only), or pressure support (PS) ventilation in addition to CPAP, often termed bilevel positive airway pressure (BiPAP).

Historically, invasive mechanical ventilation in immunocompromised patients was associated with high mortality and was considered an unfavorable approach that should be avoided [24–27]. Given that historic trials demonstrated reduced need for intubation and mortality with an upfront approach of noninvasive ventilation, guideline recommendations suggested the use of noninvasive devices for this population. In a secondary analysis of a large epidemiologic study of ARDS, upfront NIV was used at a higher frequency in immunocompromised patients compared to non-immunocompromised patients [18]. However, subsequent evidence reflecting contemporary IMV and critical care practices have not shown the same benefit of NIV in this population.

### Non-immunocompromised Patient Population

Outside of the immunocompromised population, there has been a surge of evidence evaluating the comparative effectiveness of different noninvasive respiratory devices. A series of systematic reviews and meta-analyses have demonstrated that HFNC and NIV decrease the risks of intubation compared to standard oxygen therapies. In a comparative evaluation of HFNC, face mask NIV, and standard oxygen therapies, HFNC decreased the need for intubation in more severely hypoxemic patients and decreased 90-day mortality compared to face mask NIV and standard oxygen therapy [23]. Patients under NIV with a high tidal volume 1 h after initiation of NIV or more severely hypoxemic patients ($PaO_2/FiO_2 < 200$ mmHg) were more likely to be intubated. Patients with high tidal volumes on NIV had a higher mortality rate compared to the other modes. These findings, in general, raised enthusiasm for the use of HFNC and concern surrounding the use of NIV.

### Immunocompromised Patient Population

The EFRAIM study assessed 1611 immunocompromised patients with ARF and the initial approach of respiratory support [19]. The study evaluated the association between initial oxygen modality and need for IMV and in-hospital all-cause mortality. Among these patients, 54.9% were HM, 6.7% were post-auto-HSCT, and 9.7% were post-allo-HSCT. Factors that were associated with IMV included age, day-1 severity of illness, day-1 $PaO_2/FiO_2$, and ARF etiology (*Pneumocystis jirovecii* pneumonia, invasive pulmonary aspergillosis, and undetermined etiology). Factors that were associated with increased in-hospital mortality were age, indirect admission to the ICU, day-1 severity of illness, $PaO_2/FiO_2 < 100$, and indeterminate ARF etiology. Initial oxygen strategy was not associated with mortality [19].

Utility of face mask NIV and HFNC has been specifically evaluated across the general immunocompromised patient population. In a multicenter randomized controlled study (INVICTUS trial), the outcome of early face mask NIV vs. standard oxygen therapy in 374 critically ill immunocompromised patients with ARF did not reduce 28-day mortality, nor did it show any significant benefit for other secondary outcomes (need for intubation, severity of illness at day 3 of ICU admission, ICU-acquired infections, duration of mechanical ventilation, and ICU length of stay) [28].

Contemporary studies have further demonstrated that the frequency of face mask NIV failure is not uncommon, particularly across higher severities of illness as well as in patients with hematologic malignancies [28]. Furthermore, face mask NIV failure is associated with poor outcomes [19, 29]. In the large epidemiologic study of ARDS (LUNG SAFE study), upfront NIV was used in 15% of cases. NIV use was not restricted to primarily mild ARDS and was seen across all severities of ARDS: 22.2% of mild, 42.3% of moderate, and 47.1% of patients with severe ARDS. Increasing ARDS severity was associated with an increased incidence of NIV failure. Hospital mortality in patients with NIV success and failure was 16.1% and 45.4%, respectively. In a propensity score-matched analysis, ICU mortality was higher in patients who received upfront NIV compared to invasively ventilated patients with a $PaO_2/FiO_2$ lower than 150 mmHg [30]. A secondary analysis of this study focused on immunocompromised patients demonstrated that NIV was used more frequently as first-line respiratory support compared to the immunocompetent population [18]. While there may be a role for NIV in less-severe ARF, its routine role as first-line therapy for immunocompromised (and non-immunocompromised) patients has been called into question.

HFNC as compared to standard oxygen therapy was evaluated in a trial across 778 immunocompromised patients with ARF (the HIGH trial) [31]. Forty-five percent (348/778) of patients had an underlying hematologic malignancy with 48 auto-HSCT and 61 allo-HSCT. In this population, HFNC was not found to significantly decrease intubation or 28-day mortality [31]. Finally, a more recent trial by Coudroy et al. comparing face mask NIV to HFNC across 300 immunocompromised patients with ARF did not show any differences in 28-day mortality between HFNC and NIV alternating with HFNC.

## Placing Research into Context for the HSCT Patient Population

The current state of the literature does not definitively recommend one noninvasive oxygen strategy over another across immunocompromised patients. It is likely that there is not a one-size-fits-all approach to noninvasive respiratory support across patients (HSCT, immunocompromised nor immunocompetent). Different respiratory phenotypes likely exist and need to be tailored to individual patients. Currently, these phenotypes have not been defined, but future research should be dedicated to evaluating these. It may also be discovered that the clusters of phenotypes transverse the historic "immunocompromised vs. non-immunocompromised" categorization and even "hematologic oncology vs. solid tumor." Evidence to date has demonstrated certain risk factors more likely to be associated with noninvasive respiratory failure (particularly centered around face mask NIV but not specific to the HSCT or immunocompromised population).

Higher severity of ARF (i.e., $PaO_2/FiO_2 < 150$–200 mmHg), number of organs failed, and large tidal volumes 1 h after initiation have been found to be associated with face mask NIV failure and higher risk of death. The HACOR score is a composite score that considers heart rate, pH, level of consciousness, severity of hypoxemia, and respiratory rate, and when measured 1 h after NIV treatment, it may predict the need for intubation [32].

For HFNC, the ROX index ($SaO_2/FiO_2$/respiratory rate (RR)) was a tool validated to predict HFNC failure leading to IMV across patients with pneumonia [33]. As delayed intubation by using HFNC may be associated with higher mortality [34], it is of interest to develop a decision-making supporting tool to predict high risk of HFNC failure. The ROX index ($SpO_2/FiO_2/RR$) found that a score over 4.88 within 2–12 h of starting HFNC is associated with a lower risk of intubation (area under the curve [AUC] of the receiver operating characteristic [ROC] curve in the validation cohort was 0.703 [0.616–0.790] at 6 h and 0.752 [0.664–0.840] at 12 h) [33, 35]. The ROX index performance was also evaluated in immunocompromised patients and found a score of 4.88 still highly associated with HFNC failure and need for intubation but with poorer accuracy and predictability (AUC = 0.623) [36].

Spontaneous breathing may have beneficial physiological effects; however, an emerging area of interest surrounds the potential harm associated with spontaneous breathing. Large swings in intrathoracic pressure with vigorous breathing may also be injurious to the lungs. This concept has been labeled patient self-inflicted lung injury and is becoming increasingly recognized as a potential contributor to noninvasive respiratory support failure and/or mortality [37]. Ultimately, patients with an ARF trajectory that is about to peak/plateau and recover are likely the ones who would most benefit from noninvasive respiratory support compared to those who are still on their trajectory of worsening. Accurately identifying this cohort has not yet been accomplished; however, patients with more protracted ARF may be less likely to benefit from an upfront noninvasive device. Additional considerations specific to the HSCT population surround the need for invasive investigations to identify the cause of ARF for treatment to be tailored. In cases of diagnostic uncertainty, noninvasive techniques may lead to delays in diagnostic measures [19]. If bronchoscopy or computed tomography (CT) scans are necessary for the diagnostic workup and cannot safely be performed under noninvasive respiratory support due to hypoxemia risk, transitioning to IMV may be necessary to both support the patient and facilitate these investigations.

## Future Role of Noninvasive Respiratory Support

In addition to accurately identifying sub-phenotypes, matching noninvasive devices to these phenotypes, predicting trajectory of ARF, and better describing how to measure patient self-inflicted lung injury, new noninvasive devices are currently under evaluation with promising preliminary data. One of the greatest challenges with face mask NIV is patient tolerance. Helmet is a unique interface that can couple a patient noninvasively to NIV or CPAP using a transparent plastic hood. An exploratory trial evaluating helmet NIV compared to face mask NIV demonstrated improved mortality with the helmet interface [38]. The authors theorized that the mortality benefit might have been attributable to more effective PEEP application and tolerability with helmet compared to face mask. A network meta-analysis evaluated 25 trials comparing four different oxygen modalities (HFNC, face mask NIV/CPAP, helmet NIV/CPAP, or standard oxygen therapy). Helmet NIV (and face mask NIV) reduced intubation and mortality compared to the other modalities; however, this mortality benefit was no longer true with face mask NIV across patients with more severe ARF (studies with $PaO_2/FiO_2 < 200$ mmHg) [39]. The HENIVOT study was a multicenter randomized clinical trial that randomized 109 patients with COVID-19 and moderate to severe ARF to helmet ventilation for at least 48 h eventually followed by high-flow nasal oxygen ($n = 54$) or high-flow oxygen alone ($n = 55$). The median days free of respiratory support within 28 days were not significantly different between groups (primary outcome). The helmet group had significantly lower rate of endotracheal intubations and higher rate of days free of invasive mechanical ventilation within 28 days [40]. The option of helmet ventilation may offer some advantages in immunocompromised patients, but evidence is still lacking. Currently, there are a series of ongoing trials evaluating helmet compared to other modalities, and its role in immunocompromised, cancer, and HSCT patients has yet to be reported.

## Palliative Use of Noninvasive Respiratory Support

Noninvasive devices also serve the purpose of buying time for decision-making about escalating to IMV. Furthermore, an important aspect of HFNC specifically is its potential role in palliative care as it provides comfort and ease of use [41, 42].

## Invasive Mechanical Ventilation

Despite being a unique population, with distinct causes and mechanisms of severe respiratory failure pathophysiology, general ARDS categorization, prognostication, and management are currently generalized to the HSCT population [43]. However, as we better understand respiratory phenotypes, mechanisms of ARF across neutropenic/non-neutropenic patients, and their impact on respiratory physiology, our management may become more precisely tailored to the unique features of the specific patient. This is particularly important for patients with HSCT given the very heterogeneous causes of ARF that can develop post-transplant.

In a secondary analysis of the EFRAIM study evaluating the cohort that fulfilled criteria for ARDS, 52% were HM patients, 7% and 10% allo-HSCT and auto-HSCT [44]. ARDS of undetermined etiology, need for vasopressors, and need for renal replacement therapy were independently associated with hospital mortality. Higher plateau pressures (Pplat), higher driving pressures ($\Delta$Prs), and lower compliance (Crs) were associated with higher mortality. Interestingly, ARDS severity according to the Berlin definition, neutropenia on admission, and the type of underlying disease were not associated with mortality. These findings highlight the importance of striving for a sound diagnosis and the importance of implementing lung protective ventilation strategy in all critical care patients including in immunocompromised patients [44]. Interestingly, the lack of association between ARDS severities and outcome highlights the need for tailored evaluation of ARDS categorization in this cohort. More specifically, an observational study of HSCT patients with ARF reported contemporary outcomes in the setting of IMV [12]. Seventy patients from two centers, who needed IMV within 90 days of HSCT, were evaluated. ICU mortality was 63%, and 90-day mortality was 73%. Mortality was higher in patients who required a longer duration of MV with 76% mortality for those requiring MV over 14 days and 91% mortality for those requiring MV for more than 21 days. Most of the patients were intubated within 30 days of the HSCT, emphasizing the vulnerability of these patients in the pre- and peri-engraftment phases. Allo-HSCT (OR = 11.3), higher illness severity, and longer interval between HSCT and MV were found to be independently associated with higher all-cause mortality at 90 days. This study reflects persistent poor outcomes seen in the setting of IMV despite contemporary ICU practices across HSCT recipients and in particular across allo-HSCT patients.

Above all, a question that remains surrounds whether higher mortality in patients treated with IMV has a causal relation or is merely a consequence of a higher burden of disease and multiorgan involvement [16]. Once decision has been made to intubate and to proceed with IMV, the principles of "lung protective ventilation" should be followed to minimize the risk of ventilator-induced lung injury (VILI) [45–49] along with the emphasis on meticulous care and efforts to prevent additional complications that would act as a "second hit" such as preventing fluid overload and restriction of blood products, decreasing the risk of aspirations, adequate empiric antimicrobial treatment with de-escalation when appropriate, daily assessment of ventilation weaning, and early mobilization [49].

Given the conflicting body of evidence described above, when approaching an HSCT with ARF, considerations should include: patient severity, comfort and safety, the need for prompt diagnostic measures and associated safety, the different options of noninvasive support and their efficiency as well as the local experience, optimal timing for intubation, and implications on other aspects of care such as chemotherapy, nutrition, etc.

## Severe ARDS Adjunctive Measures and Extracorporeal Life Support (ECLS)

Currently, the approach to severe ARDS management in patients with HSCT is extrapolated from management used in the general population, with some exceptions. In the LUNG SAFE study of patients with ARDS, the frequency of the use of adjunctive measures such as neuromuscular blockade, recruitment maneuvers, prone positioning, inhaled vasodilators, high-frequency oscillatory ventilation, and extracorporeal life support was described. The secondary analysis focused on immunocompromised patients demonstrated that the adjuncts were used at the same frequency in the non-immunocompromised cohort with the exception of increased use of neuromuscular blockade. All adjuvants lack specific high-quality trial data evaluating their use across immunocompromised and specifically HSCT patients.

The one adjuvant measure that has been evaluated in this cohort is the use of extracorporeal life support (ECLS). ECLS is associated with significant health-care resource implications. Given this, most ECLS programs aim to restrict it to patients who would derive the greatest benefit. Historically, ECLS was discouraged in some programs across immunocompromised patients given their higher ARF mortality; however, with advancements in ARF outcomes and ECLS programs, its use has been expanded to select immunocompromised cohorts.

Several cohorts reported that 19–31% of ARDS patients treated with ECLS were immunocompromised [50–53]. A retrospective study that evaluated outcomes of 203 adult immunocompromised patients that were supported with ECLS for moderate to severe ARDS showed that 42% of the patients were weaned from ECLS. The overall survival rate was 30%. However, across all subtypes of immunocompromised patients, those with HM had the worse outcomes; 6-month survival varied between different immunocompromised groups with a 24% 6-month survival in the HM population. ECLS-related bleeding and nosocomial infections were frequent. A recent diagnosis of immunocompromised state, higher platelet counts, lower $CO_2$, and driving pressure were associated with better prognosis [54]. These findings have decreased enthusiasm for the application of ECLS across HM patients in general and specifically in the HSCT cohort. The more prolonged immunocompromised state, low platelet counts, and high frequency of indeterminate ARDS make this cohort less favorable candidates for ECLS. A recent cohort study of 297 patients with cancer who underwent veno-venous extra-

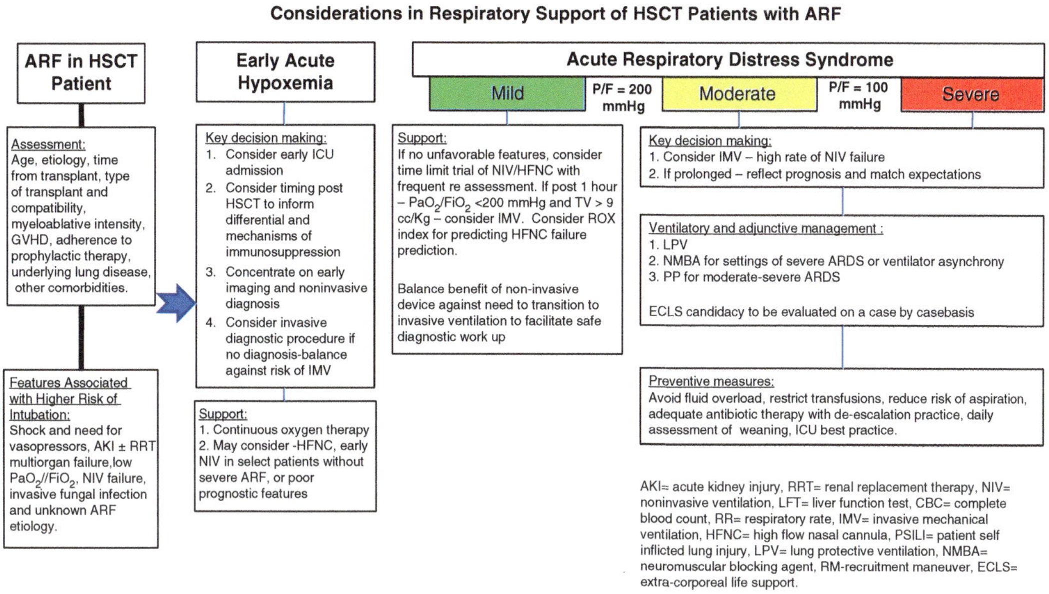


**Fig. 25.1** Considerations in respiratory support of HSCT patients with ARF

corporeal membrane oxygenation (ECMO) for ARF demonstrated a 27% 60-day overall survival. In a propensity score-matched analysis to patients who did not receive ECMO, there was no significant survival advance for treatment with ECMO [55].

For the HSCT population, Wohlfarth et al. studied ECLS use after allogeneic HSCT in 37 patients and found only 19% survival rate. However, ECLS survival was higher across patients who were cannulated more than 240 days post-transplant [56]. In a recent meta-analysis of ECMO use in patients with HSCT, survival rates were similarly low (13% in hospital mortality) [57]. Overall, data are still limited, and the approach to consideration should be taken on a case-by-case basis by an ECMO expert. Tools of prognostications, such as the RESP score (for hospital survival) and the PRESERVE score (for 6-month survival), have been created by analyzing an international ECLS registry or using a program-based cohort, respectively [52, 58]. Both recognized immunocompromised as a bad prognostic factor. However, the RESP score was validated in 2012 in which only 5% of the patients were diagnosed as immunocompromised and HSCT patients are not reported, and the PRESERVE score was validated in 2013, reporting 31% of patients who were immunocompromised and 9% with HM [51]. The low survival rates, the high rate of complications, and the high burden of ECLS raise numerous ethical questions about their use in this cohort, and more research is needed to inform optimal patient selection for severe ARF. Considerations for management are outlined in Fig. 25.1.

## Conclusion

Despite significant advances both in oncology and critical practice, post-HSCT patients are at high risk of developing ARF. While outcomes have improved, severe ARF is still associated with high mortality rates. Meticulous understanding of the pathophysiology, the risk factors, and cause is essential to tailoring effective therapy—ideally before the need for IMV. Further research of this unique population in critical care is needed to further our understanding of the mechanisms and causes of ARF. This is essential to develop studies targeted at evaluating optimal approaches to respiratory support (invasive and noninvasive) in this population.

## References


1. Ferreyro BL, Law AD, Munshi L. Acute respiratory distress syndrome following hematopoietic stem cell transplantation: one more piece in the puzzle. Ann Am Thorac Soc. 2021;18(6):950–2. https://doi.org/10.1513/AnnalsATS.202103-273ED.
2. Darmon M, Bourmaud A, Georges Q, et al. Changes in critically ill cancer patients' short-term outcome over the last decades: results of systematic review with meta-analysis on individual data. Intensive Care Med. 2019;45(7):977–87. https://doi.org/10.1007/s00134-019-05653-7.
3. Azoulay E, Pène F, Darmon M, et al. Managing critically ill hematology patients: time to think differently. Blood Rev. 2015;29(6):359–67. https://doi.org/10.1016/j.blre.2015.04.002.
4. Mokart D, Pastores SM, Darmon M. Has survival increased in cancer patients admitted to the ICU? Yes. Intensive Care Med. 2014;40(10):1570–2. https://doi.org/10.1007/s00134-014-3433-2.
5. Niederwieser D, Baldomero H, Szer J, et al. Hematopoietic stem cell transplantation activity worldwide in 2012 and a SWOT analysis of the worldwide network for blood and marrow transplantation group including the global survey. Bone Marrow Transplant. 2016;51(6):778–85. https://doi.org/10.1038/bmt.2016.18.
6. Afessa B, Abdulai RM, Kremers WK, Hogan WJ, Litzow MR, Peters SG. Risk factors and outcome of pulmonary complications after autologous hematopoietic stem cell transplant. Chest. 2012;141(2):442–50. https://doi.org/10.1378/chest.10-2889.
7. Bergeron A, Chevret S, de Latour RP, et al. Noninfectious lung complications after allogeneic haematopoietic stem cell transplantation. Eur Respir J. 2018;51(5):1702617. https://doi.org/10.1183/13993003.02617-2017.
8. Ho VT, Weller E, Lee SJ, Alyea EP, Antin JH, Soiffer RJ. Prognostic factors for early severe pulmonary complications after hematopoietic stem cell transplantation. Biol Blood Marrow Transplant. 2001;7(4):223–30. https://doi.org/10.1053/bbmt.2001.v7.pm11349809.
9. Herasevich S, Frank RD, Bo H, et al. Pretransplant risk factors can predict development of acute respiratory distress syndrome after hematopoietic stem cell transplantation. Ann Am Thorac Soc. 2021;18(6):1004–12. https://doi.org/10.1513/AnnalsATS.202004-336OC.
10. Saillard C, Darmon M, Bisbal M, et al. Critically ill allogenic HSCT patients in the intensive care unit: a systematic review and meta-analysis of prognostic factors of mortality. Bone Marrow Transplant. 2018;53(10):1233–41. https://doi.org/10.1038/s41409-018-0181-x.
11. Mokart D, van Craenenbroeck T, Lambert J, et al. Prognosis of acute respiratory distress syndrome in neutropenic cancer patients. Eur Respir J. 2012;40(1):169–76. https://doi.org/10.1183/09031936.00150611.
12. Hamidi M, Gossack-Keenan KL, Ferreyro BL, Angriman F, Rochwerg B, Mehta S. Outcomes of hematopoietic cell transplant recipients requiring invasive mechanical ventilation: a two-centre retrospective cohort study. Can J Anesth. 2019;66(12):1450–7. https://doi.org/10.1007/s12630-019-01439-z.
13. Chi AK, Soubani AO, White AC, Miller KB. An update on pulmonary complications of hematopoietic stem cell transplantation. Chest. 2013;144(6):1913–22. https://doi.org/10.1378/chest.12-1708.
14. Yadav H, Nolan ME, Bohman JK, et al. Epidemiology of acute respiratory distress syndrome following hematopoietic stem cell transplantation*. Crit Care Med. 2016;44(6):1082–90. https://journals.lww.com/ccmjournal/Fulltext/2016/06000/Epidemiology_of_Acute_Respiratory_Distress.9.aspx.
15. Wieruszewski PM, Herasevich S, Gajic O, Yadav H. Respiratory failure in the hematopoietic stem cell transplant recipient. World J Crit Care Med. 2018;7(5):62–72. https://doi.org/10.5492/wjccm.v7.i5.62.
16. Azoulay E, Mokart D, Kouatchet A, Demoule A, Lemiale V. Acute respiratory failure in immunocompromised adults. Lancet Respir Med. 2019;7(2):173–86. https://doi.org/10.1016/S2213-2600(18)30345-X.
17. Laffey JG, Bellani G, Pham T, et al. Potentially modifiable factors contributing to outcome from acute respiratory distress syndrome: the LUNG SAFE study. Intensive Care Med. 2016;42(12):1865–76. https://doi.org/10.1007/s00134-016-4571-5.
18. Cortegiani A, Madotto F, Gregoretti C, Bellani G, Laffey JG, Pham T. Immunocompromised patients with acute respiratory distress syndrome: secondary analysis of the LUNG SAFE database. Crit Care. 2018;22:157.
19. Azoulay E, Pickkers P, Soares M, et al. Acute hypoxemic respiratory failure in immunocompromised patients: the Efraim multinational prospective cohort study. Intensive Care Med. 2017;43(12):1808–19. https://doi.org/10.1007/s00134-017-4947-1.
20. Azoulay E, Mokart D, Rabbat A, et al. Diagnostic bronchoscopy in hematology and oncology patients with acute respiratory failure: prospective multicenter data*. Crit Care Med. 2008;36(1):100–7. https://journals.lww.com/ccmjournal/Fulltext/2008/01000/Diagnostic_bronchoscopy_in_hematology_and_oncology.14.aspx.
21. Azoulay É, Thiéry G, Chevret S, et al. The prognosis of acute respiratory failure in critically ill cancer patients. Medicine. 2004;83(6):360–70. https://doi.org/10.1097/01.md.0000145370.63676.fb.
22. Astashchanka A, Ryan J, Lin E, et al. Pulmonary complications in hematopoietic stem cell transplant recipients—a clinician primer. J Clin Med. 2021;10(15):3227. https://doi.org/10.3390/jcm10153227.

23. Frat JP, Thille AW, Mercat A, et al. High-flow oxygen through nasal cannula in acute hypoxemic respiratory failure. N Engl J Med. 2015;372(23):2185–96. https://doi.org/10.1056/nejmoa1503326.
24. Guideline. Guidelines for intensive care unit admission, discharge, and triage. Crit Care Med. 1999;27(3):633. https://journals.lww.com/ccmjournal/Fulltext/1999/03000/Guidelines_for_intensive_care_unit_admission.48.aspx.
25. Gruson D, Vargas F, Hilbert G, et al. Predictive factors of intensive care unit admission in patients with haematological malignancies and pneumonia. Intensive Care Med. 2004;30(5):965–71. https://doi.org/10.1007/s00134-004-2237-1.
26. Hilbert G, Gruson D, Vargas F, et al. Noninvasive ventilation in immunosuppressed patients with pulmonary infiltrates, fever, and acute respiratory failure. N Engl J Med. 2001;344(7):481–7. https://doi.org/10.1056/NEJM200102153440703.
27. Paz HL, Crilley P, Weinar M, Brodsky I. Outcome of patients requiring medical ICU admission following bone marrow transplantation. Chest. 1993;104(2):527–31. https://doi.org/10.1378/chest.104.2.527.
28. Lemiale V, Mokart D, Resche-Rigon M, et al. Effect of noninvasive ventilation vs oxygen therapy on mortality among immunocompromised patients with acute respiratory failure: a randomized clinical trial. JAMA. 2015;314(16):1711–9. https://doi.org/10.1001/jama.2015.12402.
29. Adda M, Coquet I, Darmon M, Thiery G, Schlemmer B, Azoulay É. Predictors of noninvasive ventilation failure in patients with hematologic malignancy and acute respiratory failure*. Crit Care Med. 2008;36(10):2766. https://journals.lww.com/ccmjournal/Fulltext/2008/10000/Predictors_of_noninvasive_ventilation_failure_in.9.aspx.
30. Bellani G, Laffey JG, Pham T, et al. Noninvasive ventilation of patients with acute respiratory distress syndrome: insights from the LUNG SAFE study. Am J Respir Crit Care Med. 2017;195(1):67–77. https://doi.org/10.1164/rccm.201606-1306OC.
31. Azoulay E, Lemiale V, Mokart D, et al. Effect of high-flow nasal oxygen vs standard oxygen on 28-day mortality in immunocompromised patients with acute respiratory failure: the HIGH randomized clinical trial. JAMA. 2018;320(20):2099–107. https://doi.org/10.1001/jama.2018.14282.
32. Magdy DM, Metwally A. The utility of HACOR score in predicting failure of high-flow nasal oxygen in acute hypoxemic respiratory failure. Adv Respir Med. 2021;89(1):23–9. https://doi.org/10.5603/ARM.a2021.0031.
33. Roca O, Messika J, Caralt B, et al. Predicting success of high-flow nasal cannula in pneumonia patients with hypoxemic respiratory failure: the utility of the ROX index. J Crit Care. 2016;35:200–5. https://doi.org/10.1016/j.jcrc.2016.05.022.
34. Kang BJ, Koh Y, Lim CM, et al. Failure of high-flow nasal cannula therapy may delay intubation and increase mortality. Intensive Care Med. 2015;41(4):623–32. https://doi.org/10.1007/s00134-015-3693-5.
35. Roca O, Caralt B, Messika J, et al. An index combining respiratory rate and oxygenation to predict outcome of nasal high-flow therapy. Am J Respir Crit Care Med. 2019;199(11):1368–76. https://doi.org/10.1164/rccm.201803-0589OC.
36. Lemiale V, Dumas G, Demoule A, et al. Performance of the ROX index to predict intubation in immunocompromised patients receiving high-flow nasal cannula for acute respiratory failure. Ann Intensive Care. 2021;11(1):17. https://doi.org/10.1186/s13613-021-00801-z.
37. Carteaux G, Parfait M, Combet M, Haudebourg AF, Tuffet S, Dessap AM. Patient self-inflicted lung injury: a practical review. J Clin Med. 2021;10(12):1–13. https://doi.org/10.3390/jcm10122738.
38. Patel BK, Wolfe KS, Pohlman AS, Hall JB, Kress JP. Effect of noninvasive ventilation delivered by helmet vs face mask on the rate of endotracheal intubation in patients with acute respiratory distress syndrome a randomized clinical trial. JAMA. 2016;315(22):2435–41. https://doi.org/10.1001/jama.2016.6338.
39. Ferreyro BL, Angriman F, Munshi L, et al. Association of noninvasive oxygenation strategies with all-cause mortality in adults with acute hypoxemic respiratory failure: a systematic review and meta-analysis. JAMA. 2020;324(1):57–67. https://doi.org/10.1001/jama.2020.9524.
40. Grieco DL, Menga LS, Cesarano M, et al. Effect of helmet noninvasive ventilation vs high-flow nasal oxygen on days free of respiratory support in patients with COVID-19 and moderate to severe hypoxemic respiratory failure: the HENIVOT randomized clinical trial. JAMA. 2021;325(17):1731–43. https://doi.org/10.1001/jama.2021.4682.
41. Hui D, Morgado M, Chisholm G, et al. High-flow oxygen and bilevel positive airway pressure for persistent dyspnea in patients with advanced cancer: a phase II randomized trial. J Pain Symptom Manag. 2013;46(4):463–73. https://doi.org/10.1016/j.jpainsymman.2012.10.284.
42. Epstein AS, Hartridge-Lambert SK, Ramaker JS, Voigt LP, Portlock CS. Humidified high-flow nasal oxygen utilization in patients with cancer at Memorial Sloan-Kettering Cancer Center. J Palliat Med. 2011;14(7):835–9. https://doi.org/10.1089/jpm.2011.0005.
43. Ranieri VM, Rubenfeld GD, Thompson BT, et al. Acute respiratory distress syndrome: the Berlin definition. JAMA. 2012;307(23):2526–33. https://doi.org/10.1001/jama.2012.5669.
44. Demoule A, Antonelli M, Schellongowski P, et al. Respiratory mechanics and outcomes in immunocompromised patients with ARDS: a secondary analysis of the EFRAIM study. Chest. 2020;158(5):1947–57. https://doi.org/10.1016/j.chest.2020.05.602.

45. Acute Respiratory Distress Syndrome Network. Ventilation with lower tidal volumes as compared with traditional tidal volumes for acute lung injury and the acute respiratory distress syndrome. N Engl J Med. 2000;342(18):1301–8. https://doi.org/10.1056/NEJM200005043421801.
46. Amato MBP, Meade MO, Slutsky AS, et al. Driving pressure and survival in the acute respiratory distress syndrome. N Engl J Med. 2015;372(8):747–55. https://doi.org/10.1056/nejmsa1410639.
47. National Heart, Lung, and Blood Institute Acute Respiratory Distress Syndrome (ARDS) Clinical Trials Network. Comparison of two fluid-management strategies in acute lung injury. N Engl J Med. 2006;354(24):2564–75. https://doi.org/10.1056/NEJMoa062200.
48. Fan E, del Sorbo L, Goligher EC, et al. An official American Thoracic Society/European Society of Intensive Care Medicine/Society of Critical Care Medicine clinical practice guideline: mechanical ventilation in adult patients with acute respiratory distress syndrome. Am J Respir Crit Care Med. 2017;195(9):1253–63. https://doi.org/10.1164/rccm.201703-0548ST.
49. Yadav H, Thompson BT, Gajic O. Is acute respiratory distress syndrome a preventable disease? Am J Respir Crit Care Med. 2017;195(6):725–36. https://doi.org/10.1164/rccm.201609-1767CI.
50. ANZICS Investigators. Extracorporeal membrane oxygenation for 2009 influenza a(H1N1) acute respiratory distress syndrome. JAMA. 2009;302(17):1888–95. https://doi.org/10.1001/jama.2009.1535.
51. Schmidt M, Zogheib E, Rozé H, et al. The PRESERVE mortality risk score and analysis of long-term outcomes after extracorporeal membrane oxygenation for severe acute respiratory distress syndrome. Intensive Care Med. 2013;39(10):1704–13. https://doi.org/10.1007/s00134-013-3037-2.
52. Schmidt M, Bailey M, Sheldrake J, et al. Predicting survival after extracorporeal membrane oxygenation for severe acute respiratory failure: the respiratory extracorporeal membrane oxygenation survival prediction (RESP) score. Am J Respir Crit Care Med. 2014;189(11):1374–82. https://doi.org/10.1164/rccm.201311-2023OC.
53. Combes A, Hajage D, Capellier G, et al. Extracorporeal membrane oxygenation for severe acute respiratory distress syndrome. N Engl J Med. 2018;378(21):1965–75. https://doi.org/10.1056/NEJMoa1800385.
54. Schmidt M, Schellongowski P, Patroniti N, et al. Six-month outcome of immunocompromised patients with severe acute respiratory distress syndrome rescued by extracorporeal membrane oxygenation an international multicenter retrospective study. Am J Respir Crit Care Med. 2018;197(10):1297–307. https://doi.org/10.1164/rccm.201708-1761OC.
55. Kochanek M, Kochanek J, Boll B, et al. Veno-venous extracorporeal membrane oxygenation (vv-ECMO) for severe respiratory failure in adult cancer patients: a retrospective multicenter analysis. Intensive Care Med. 2020;48:332–42.
56. Wohlfarth P, Beutel G, Lebiedz P, et al. Characteristics and outcome of patients after allogeneic hematopoietic stem cell transplantation treated with extracorporeal membrane oxygenation for acute respiratory distress syndrome*. Crit Care Med. 2017;45(5):e500.
57. Sim JJL, Mitra S, Ling RR, et al. Extracorporeal membrane oxygenation in patients with hematologic malignancies: a systematic review and meta-analysis. Ann Hematol. 2022;101:1395–406.
58. Schmidt M, Combes A, Shekar K. ECMO for immunosuppressed patients with acute respiratory distress syndrome: drawing a line in the sand. Intensive Care Med. 2019;45(8):1140–2. https://doi.org/10.1007/s00134-019-05632-y.

# Cardiovascular Considerations in Patients Undergoing Hematopoietic Stem Cell Transplantation

26

Alexi Vasbinder and Salim S. Hayek

The number of hematopoietic stem cell transplantations (HSCT) continues to steadily increase as indications for HSCT have broadened. Advances in management have led to improvement in the safety and efficacy of HSCT, expanding its use to older adults, often with multiple comorbidities and who are at higher risk of cardiovascular disease.

Despite the significant improvement in survival afforded by HSCT, the therapy is associated with significant acute and long-term complications, resulting in a high burden of morbidity and mortality. Patients undergoing HSCT are subject to challenges to nearly all organs due to the toxicity of conditioning regimens and ensuing hyperinflammatory responses, often leading to hemodynamic instability and exacerbation of underlying comorbidities. Cardiovascular complications such as cardiomyopathy, arrhythmias, acute thrombosis, pulmonary hypertension, and pericardial effusions are among the potential adverse events occurring during HSCT [1]. Long-term cardiovascular complications of HSCT such as heart failure and atherosclerotic disease are increasingly recognized as the number of survivors grows. The incidence of cardiac complications is related to a variety of factors such as age at transplant, comorbid conditions, prior cardiotoxic cancer treatments, type of HSCT, and the specific conditioning regimen.

Elderly patients and those with preexisting cardiovascular disease, who represent a growing proportion of HSCTs performed annually in the United States, are at a greater risk of developing cardiac complications [2]. These concerns have led to cardiovascular evaluations becoming a core component of the pre-transplant assessment. Until recently, cardiac complications have largely been managed by restricting the eligible HSCT population by age and excluding those with impaired cardiac function. However, this approach has become less justifiable as contemporary HSCT protocols aim at minimizing toxicities and improving outcomes.

An understanding of the incidence, risk factors, and mechanisms of cardiovascular complications can assist clinicians in appropriate risk stratification and guide management strategies to improve HSCT outcomes. This chapter aims to summarize available data on the incidence of acute and long-term cardiotoxicities and potential mechanisms of cardiac complications and provide guidance surrounding the cardiovascular management of patients throughout the transplant process from the pre-transplant assessment to survivorship.

A. Vasbinder · S. S. Hayek (✉)
Department of Internal Medicine, Division of Cardiology, University of Michigan, Ann Arbor, MI, USA
e-mail: avasbind@med.umich.edu; shayek@med.umich.edu



A. O. Soubani (ed.), *Pulmonary and Critical Care Considerations of Hematopoietic Stem Cell Transplantation*, https://doi.org/10.1007/978-3-031-28797-8_26

## Incidence and Risk Factors of Acute and Long-Term Cardiac Complications

Cardiac complications can occur acutely during inpatient hospitalization and years after HSCT. The incidence of cardiac complications varies widely depending on the study. Estimating the incidence of complications is challenging given the varying diagnostic criteria for cardiotoxicity, surveillance techniques, and heterogeneous populations across studies. The initial report of HSCT-related cardiotoxicity was published in 1976, which described post-mortem cardiac histopathologic findings in 29 patients with leukemia, aplastic anemia, or metastatic cancer undergoing allogeneic HSCT [3]. Infiltration of immune cells and extensive myocardial necrosis, fibrin deposits, and extravasation of red blood cells were noted in some patients. In this early era of HSCT, cardiovascular complications including heart failure, pericarditis, and arrhythmias were reported in 43% of recipients and were attributed to the toxicity of high-intensity conditioning regimens and total body irradiation [4]. The landscape of HSCT has rapidly evolved to improve safety; however, contemporary data on the trends in the incidence of cardiac complications are limited. Based on available data, the incidence of cardiovascular complications is related to factors such as age, comorbid medical conditions, prior cardiotoxicity chemotherapy or radiation, the type of HSCT (autologous versus allogeneic), and the specific conditioning or maintenance regimen (Table 26.1).

**Table 26.1** Incidence of and risk factors of acute and chronic cardiovascular complications following HSCT

| | Incidence | Risk factors |
|---|---|---|
| *Acute* | | |
| Arrhythmias | 2–10% | Age<br>Anthracycline use<br>Lower ejection fraction at baseline<br>History of arrhythmias<br>Baseline renal dysfunction |
| Acute heart failure | 0.4–2.2% | Age<br>History of cardiovascular disease<br>Anthracycline use<br>Lower ejection fraction at baseline<br>High-dose cyclophosphamide |
| Pericarditis/myocarditis | <1–2% | Chest radiation<br>Immune-checkpoint inhibitors |
| Pericardial effusion | <1–3% | High-dose cyclophosphamide<br>Graft-vs.-host disease<br>Infection |
| *Chronic* | | |
| Vascular diseases<br>Stroke<br>Myocardial infarction<br>Ischemic heart disease<br>Hypertension | 4–47% | Age<br>Anthracycline use<br>Chest radiation<br>Hypertension<br>Diabetes<br>Smoking<br>Physical inactivity<br>Dyslipidemia<br>Obesity<br>Allogeneic HSCT |
| Heart failure | 2–9.1% | Age<br>Sex<br>Anthracycline use<br>Chest radiation<br>Hypertension<br>Diabetes<br>Smoking<br>History of ischemic heart disease<br>High-dose cyclophosphamide |

## Incidence of Acute Complications

Overall, severe cardiac complications during HSCT such as myocardial infarctions, large pericardial effusions, and cardiac tamponade are rare, occurring in fewer than 1% of patients [5]. Heart failure was a dreaded complication of older conditioning regimens with high doses of cyclophosphamide, reportedly occurring in upwards of 28% of HSCT recipients [5, 6]. Studies of HSCT patients who received contemporary conditioning regimens estimate the incidence of heart failure ranges from 0.4% to 2.2% [5, 7–9]. Arrhythmias are the most frequent acute cardiac complication during HSCT, with an estimated incidence of 2–10% in adult recipients [7, 10–12]. Of these, atrial fibrillation, atrial flutter, and other supraventricular tachycardias are the most common, with lethal arrhythmias such as ventricular tachycardias occurring rarely [10, 12]. A large, retrospective study of 2821 recipients who underwent HSCT between 1977 and 1997 identified 26 recipients (0.9%) who experienced major or lethal cardiotoxicity in the first 100 days post-HSCT defined as death from cardiovascular cause, congestive heart failure requiring inotropic support, cardiac tamponade, or significant electrocardiographic abnormalities [13]. The development of arrhythmias post-transplant has been associated with poor in-hospital outcomes and greater 1-year mortality [11, 14].

## Incidence of Long-Term Complications

HSCT survivors remain at an elevated risk of cardiovascular complications for 10 to 20 years following transplantation compared to the general population. Long-term complications have been extensively documented and appear to be more common than acute cardiotoxicity. In an observational study of 1244 patients who underwent autologous HSCT, the incidence of congestive heart failure was 4.8% at 5 years and 9.1% at 15 years post-HSCT [15]. In addition to heart failure, long-term HSCT survivors experience a greater incidence of ischemic heart disease, stroke, vascular disease, rhythm disorders, hypertension, hyperlipidemia, and diabetes mellitus compared to the general population [16, 17]. Estimates of these complications vary greatly due to population risk profile differences; however, it is suggested the 10-year cumulative incidence ranges from 18% to 47% [16].

## Risk Factors for Cardiovascular Complications

### Patient Factors

Pre-transplant risk factors can be categorized as non-modifiable or modifiable. Non-modifiable risk factors include age at transplantation and sex. Age is a well-known risk factor for cardiovascular events in the general population. Unsurprisingly, older age at transplantation has been associated with nearly all cardiovascular complications occurring after HSCT, including arrhythmias and the long-term development of heart failure [12, 18, 19]. The risk of long-term heart failure increases with age, where recipients older than 55 years have four times greater risk compared to recipients younger than 39 years [18]. This is likely explained by the structural and functional changes that occur in aging hearts as well as the larger burden of cardiovascular risk factors associated with aging, such as diabetes, hypertension, and obesity [12, 18, 20]. This has important implications for the management of HSCT recipients as the number of HSCT in older adults continues to increase, with 26% of allogeneic recipients and 36% of autologous recipients older than 65 years of age as of 2019 [21]. Women may be at a twofold greater risk of developing heart failure compared to men independently of age, cardiovascular risk factors, underlying diagnosis, and treatment regimen [18]. Similar associations have been reported for the risk of other cancer treatment-induced cardiotoxicities, such as anthracycline-induced cardiotoxicity [22]. Although the underlying mechanism is unclear, differences in body composition and adipose tissue distribution have been proposed as potential explanations [23].

Preexisting cardiomyopathy, most often defined by reduced left ventricular ejection fraction, has been associated with an increased risk of acute and long-term heart failure after HSCT as well as atrial arrhythmias in early studies [14, 24, 25]. Often, patients with reduced ejection fraction are excluded from receiving HSCT; however, more recent data do not support the widespread exclusion of these patients. Multiple studies have reported similar mortality and cardiovascular event rates in patients with a reduced pre-HSCT ejection fraction compared to control groups with an ejection fraction of ≥50% [26, 27].

Comorbidities prior to and after HSCT have frequently been cited as important risk factors for the development of both acute and long-term cardiovascular complications. Recipients of HSCT typically have a higher prevalence of hypertension, renal disease, dyslipidemia, and diabetes compared to the general population [16, 17, 28, 29]. This is in part due to cancer and cardiovascular disease having shared risk factors, in addition to the impact of long-term immunosuppressive therapy, exposure to total body irradiation, and the development of growth hormone deficiency or hypothyroidism related to HSCT. Elevated body mass index, a history of smoking, and physical inactivity have also been identified as risk factors for acute and long-term cardiovascular complications of HSCT such as heart failure and stroke [15, 18, 30, 31].

### Disease-Related Factors

Cardiac involvement of the primary disease treated by HSCT, for example, systemic sclerosis and amyloidosis, can increase the risk of cardiovascular morbidity and mortality after HSCT [32]. Systemic sclerosis is a rare, life-threatening, autoimmune disease characterized by skin and visceral fibrosis as a result of increased collagen deposition [33, 34]. Mortality associated with this condition is high with a 5-year survival rate as low as 70%, with most deaths attributed to cardiac causes [35, 36]. Sclerosis can occur in multiple organs, including the lungs, kidneys, and heart, resulting in altered renal function, pulmonary hypertension, and respiratory failure typically as a result of cardiac failure [37]. Recent clinical trials have demonstrated the benefit of autologous HSCT in improving organ function, quality of life, and long-term survival in individuals with systemic sclerosis; however, the presence of extensive cardiac involvement remains a strong predictor of mortality [38–40]. Primary amyloidosis results from the abnormal production of immunoglobulin light chains by plasma cells and their deposition in multiple organs, including the heart [41]. Cardiac amyloidosis typically presents as restrictive cardiomyopathy often associated with serious arrhythmias [42]. Individuals with cardiac amyloidosis are particularly sensitive to shifts in fluid volume and require close monitoring of volume status during HSCT [42].

### Prior Cancer Therapy

Anthracyclines are a component of the treatment regimen for a variety of hematologic and non-hematologic malignancies. Anthracyclines directly target the cardiomyocytes by inhibiting topoisomerase II leading to mitochondrial dysfunction, the production of reactive oxygen species, and DNA double-strand breaks, resulting in cardiomyopathy and a progressive decline in systolic function [43]. Many recipients of HSCT will have received anthracyclines prior to HSCT or as part of their conditioning regimen. Anthracycline exposure prior to HSCT has been linked to an increased risk of heart failure and cardiovascular death in a dose-dependent manner [13, 14, 18]. Particularly, cumulative doses greater than 250 mg/m$^2$ have been identified as an important risk factor [18].

A number of newer therapies, including monoclonal antibodies [44, 45], proteasome inhibitors [46, 47], immunomodulatory agents [48, 49], and tyrosine kinase inhibitors [50–52], have been associated with unique cardiovascular adverse effects (Table 26.2). These therapies are used in the treatment of hematologic malignan-

**Table 26.2** Cardiovascular complications of therapeutics that may be used during HSCT

| Therapeutics | Complication |
|---|---|
| *Calcineurin inhibitors* | |
| Tacrolimus<br>Cyclosporine | Hypertension |
| *Alkylating agents* | |
| Busulfan | Cardiac tamponade, heart failure, pericardial effusion |
| Cyclophosphamide | Myocarditis, pericarditis, atrial fibrillation, pericardial effusion, heart failure |
| Melphalan | Heart failure, pericarditis |
| Carmustine | Myocardial ischemia |
| *Anthracyclines* | |
| Doxorubicin | Cardiomyopathy, heart failure |
| *Antimetabolite* | |
| Cytarabine | Dysrhythmia, congestive heart failure, pericarditis |
| *Radiation* | Coronary artery disease, cardiomyopathy |
| *Tyrosine kinase inhibitors* | |
| Ibrutinib | Atrial fibrillation, hypertension, cardiomyopathy, heart failure, QT prolongation, premature ventricular contractions, non-sustained ventricular tachycardia, ventricular fibrillation |
| Idelalisib<br>Duvelisib | Atrial fibrillation, peripheral edema |
| Copanlisib | Hypertension |
| Ivosidenib<br>Enasidenib | QT prolongation |
| Ruxolitinib | Hypertension |
| Fedratinib | Heart failure, peripheral edema |
| Imatinib<br>Sorafenib | Heart failure |
| Dasatinib | Heart failure, QT prolongation, pleural effusion, pericardial effusion |
| Nilotinib | QT prolongation, myocardial infarction, peripheral arterial disease |
| Bosutinib | Peripheral arterial disease, acute coronary syndrome, hypertension, peripheral edema, heart failure, atrial fibrillation, QT prolongation, pericardial effusion |
| Ponatinib | Heart failure, atrial fibrillation, myocardial infarction, hypertension, peripheral arterial disease, stroke, venous thromboembolism |
| Gilteritinib | Peripheral edema, QT prolongation |
| Midostaurin | Hypertension, pericardial effusion, pulmonary hypertension |
| *Proteasome inhibitors* | |
| Bortezomib | Heart failure, myocardial infarction, atrial fibrillation, atrio-ventricular block, premature atrial or ventricular complexes, sinus bradycardia, sinus tachycardia, ventricular tachycardia |
| Carfilzomib | Heart failure, pulmonary edema, hypertension |
| *Immunomodulators* | |
| Thalidomide<br>Lenalidomide | Sinus bradycardia, atrial fibrillation, ventricular tachycardia, atrial and venous thromboembolisms |
| Pomalidomide | Atrial fibrillation |
| *Monoclonal antibodies* | |
| Rituximab | Hypertension, hypotension, atrial fibrillation |
| Nivolumab<br>Pembrolizumab | Myocarditis, pericardial disease, cardiomyopathy, ventricular tachycardia |

cies, HSCT conditioning, and post-HSCT maintenance. Cardiovascular events associated with these therapies are often rare, resulting in sparse data.

## Mechanisms of Cardiovascular Complications

The pathogenesis of cardiovascular disease after HSCT is multifactorial and is the result of multiple cardiovascular insults throughout the HSCT process. Direct endothelial injury can occur because of the conditioning regimen—which often includes a combination of high-dose chemotherapy and total body irradiation—and the hyper-inflammatory nature of the HSCT process itself and its consequences such as graft-vs.-host disease (GVHD) and engraftment syndrome. However, these effects are more likely to lead to complications in recipients who present with a high burden of cardiovascular risk factors [53].

High-dose alkylating agents, frequently given as part of conditioning regimens, are cytotoxic and lead to cardiac injury through inflammatory and oxidative stress pathways. Of the alkylating agents, cyclophosphamide is the most commonly included and is well established as a major contributor of cardiotoxicity [54]. A number of cardiovascular complications have been documented with cyclophosphamide use including heart failure, atrial arrhythmias, pericardial effusion, and myocarditis [55]. Cardiotoxicities from busulfan, carmustine, and melphalan are rarer but may present as dysrhythmia, pericarditis, heart failure, and myocardial ischemia and often occur in combination with cyclophosphamide [56–59]. The exact cardiotoxic mechanisms of alkylating agents are not fully understood but involve a combination of inflammation, oxidative stress, alterations in calcium homeostasis, and programmed cell death [60]. The increased production of reactive oxygen species by alkylating agents reduces nitric oxide availability, resulting in endothelial cell dysfunction [61]. Alkylating agents increase the permeability of the mitochondrial membrane to calcium, leading to calcium overload and impairing mitochondrial production of adenosine triphosphate, further exacerbating reactive oxygen species production [62]. Alkylating agents also cause direct injury to endothelial cells leading to the extravasation of toxic metabolites that can damage the myocardium, resulting in edema, interstitial hemorrhage, and the formation of micro-thrombosis [60]. Alkylating agents activate p53, a protein that plays an important role in apoptosis, leading to programmed cell death within the myocardium [63].

Chronic inflammation and oxidative stress due to endothelial injury are key to the development of long-term atherosclerosis and coronary artery disease after HSCT [31, 53, 64]. Radiation therapy causes direct cellular injury leading to an upregulation of pro-inflammatory markers and oxidative stress-mediated chronic inflammation [65, 66]. Chronic oxidative stress and a hyper-inflammatory state lead to endothelial cell proliferation, impaired remodeling, vascular thickening, fibrosis, and thrombi formation in arteries, which can progress to premature atherosclerosis and coronary artery disease [67].

Endothelial injury and atherogenesis are also a consequence of GVHD. GVHD is a common complication of allogeneic HSCT that results from immune recognition of host cells leading to cytokine production and direct attack by donor T cells on host tissues [68]. This inflammatory state promotes vascular injury and plaque instability leading to accelerated atherosclerosis and predisposing recipients to arterial complications [53, 64, 69]. Allogeneic-HSCT recipients are at a threefold higher risk of stroke, coronary artery disease, and peripheral artery disease compared to autologous transplantation recipients [70]. Additionally, the treatment of GVHD, which includes the use of immunosuppressants, such as corticosteroids and calcineurin inhibitors, has been implicated with the exacerbation of cardiovascular risk factors such as dyslipidemia, hypertension, and insulin resistance [71]. Indeed, recipients of allogeneic HSCT have a higher prevalence of cardiovascular risk factors such as hypertension, diabetes, and dyslipidemia post-HSCT [16]. Newer therapies used to treat GVHD, including ibrutinib, also carry the risk of new-onset atrial fibrillation and hypertension [72].

Post-conditioning, infusion of the hematopoietic stem cells, and engraftment itself can impact hemodynamics. Dimethyl sulfoxide, a standard cryoprotective agent used to preserve hematopoietic stem cells, has been linked to cardiac events, including hypertension and bradycardia, which are generally manageable [73]. Contributors to the effect of dimethyl sulfoxide include its dose, cell lysis products, red blood cell content, total nuclear cell content, acute volume expansion, and the age of the recipient [73]. Engraftment syndrome is an early complication of HSCT characterized by the release of pro-inflammatory cytokines, resulting in activated leukocytes, endothelial injury, and vascular leak [74]. This hyper-inflammatory state can exacerbate preexisting cardiovascular conditions, notably heart failure with preserved ejection fraction, arrhythmias, and stress-induced cardiomyopathy [74].

Reduced-intensity conditioning was developed as an alternative for patients who are less likely to tolerate conventional myeloablative conditioning [75]. Reduced-intensity conditioning has been associated with a lower risk of cardiotoxicity compared to conventional conditioning; however, early and late cardiac events still occur [14, 75, 76]. Additional data are needed to better delineate the incidence of cardiovascular complications associated with reduced-intensity conditioning.

## Role of the Cardio-oncology Team

Given the concern for cardiovascular complications related to HSCT, a thorough cardiovascular evaluation has become a core component of the pre-transplant assessment. The role of the cardiovascular specialist is to advise on the risks of cardiovascular complications related to HSCT, optimize the cardiovascular status of patients, and provide guidance as to the inpatient management of preexisting cardiovascular comorbidities and potential complications.

## The Pre-HSCT Cardiovascular Assessment

Currently, there are no published guidelines on pre-HSCT cardiovascular screening or assessment. Recommendations are mostly expert opinion based and are largely derived from data around chemotherapy-induced cardiotoxicity. The protocols for pre-HSCT assessment, however, vary widely, with most centers establishing their own institutional guidelines for determining HSCT eligibility and referring for a cardiovascular evaluation. There are no absolute cardiovascular contraindications to HSCT in the stable outpatient. However, high-risk cardiovascular conditions with poor cardiac reserve such as advanced heart failure, untreated severe valvular heart disease, and severe triple vessel or left main obstructive coronary artery disease are associated with poor outcomes regardless of HSCT and preclude candidacy unless a pre-HSCT intervention is possible. Thus, the most important step in the pre-transplant assessment is to rule out the presence of high-risk cardiovascular disease through a detailed history and physical exam, along with indicated testing.

The focus on the pre-HSCT cardiovascular assessment is on the concept of "cardiovascular reserve," or the ability of the heart to withstand stressors imparted by the HSCT process, including the cardiotoxicity of conditioning regimens, rapid volume shifts, and increased oxygen demand due to the anemia and the systemic inflammatory response. Quantifying cardiovascular reserve relies on a detailed assessment of symptoms attributable to cardiovascular disease, functional status, risk factors, signs of increased intracardiac pressures on exam, and lastly cardiovascular structure and function.

## History and Physical Exam

The history component should include a detailed review of traditional and nontraditional cardiovascular risk factors including prior anthracycline, radiation therapy, and other cancer therapeutics administered. An assessment of exercise tolerance is crucial, as the absence of symptoms of heart failure in patients with poor exercise capacity is much less meaningful. Poor cardiopulmonary fitness is common in patients with multimorbidity, especially those with cancer, who experience rapid muscle wasting and adverse effects related to their treatment. The lack of improvement after a 2-week daily exercise regimen suggests pathology beyond frailty that warrants investigation. The physical exam can help determine the contribution of cardiovascular disease to the decrease in function through assessment of signs of heart failure [77]. Notably, the presence of jugular venous distention should prompt additional workup given its high positive predictive value for heart failure, while a confirmed low jugular venous pulse is reassuring.

## Risk Models

Identifying HSCT recipients at risk of cardiovascular complications is challenging due to the variability of recipient characteristics and large number of influencing factors. As a result, several risk prediction models have been developed to help identify candidates at high risk of late cardiovascular complications. Most models were developed based on data from large-scale, prospective cohort studies of childhood cancer survivors and HSCT recipients [78, 79]. One model created to predict heart failure prior to the age of 40 was formed based on sex, age at cancer diagnosis, chest radiotherapy, and anthracycline dose [78]. Scores were used to create low-, moderate-, and high-risk groups with corresponding incidences of heart failure of 0.5% in the low-risk group and 11.7% in the high-risk group. A second model was developed to predict ischemic heart disease prior to the age of 50 [79]. This model included sex, chemotherapy, and radiotherapy. In an analogous manner, low-, medium-, and high-risk cohorts were formed with cumulative incidences of ischemic heart disease of <5% in the low-risk groups compared with 20% for high-risk groups.

A recent risk model for developing long-term heart failure and coronary artery disease derived from adult HSCT survivors included age, anthracycline dose, chest radiation, hypertension, diabetes, and smoking history [80]. Risk scores were collapsed to form low-, intermediate-, and high-risk groups, corresponding to 10-year cumulative incidences of cardiovascular disease of 3.7%, 9.9%, and 26.2%, respectively. Overall, these risk models exhibited modest discrimination ability and are not routinely incorporated in the pre-HSCT assessment. Additionally, these models were developed in cohorts where patients received HSCT between 1970 and 2004. Thus, further validation of these models is needed to account for changes in conditioning regimens, the use of reduced-intensity conditioning, and introduction of novel therapeutics.

## Cardiac Structure and Function

Assessment of cardiac function is performed routinely pre-HSCT given many candidates are at higher risk of cardiomyopathy by virtue of their prior exposure to cardiotoxic therapies. Most institutional guidelines exclude patients with an ejection fraction ≤35% from HSCT candidacy. The data surrounding that exclusion criterion is limited, and it is likely that a subset of patients with preexisting cardiomyopathy would fare well through HSCT [27, 81, 82]. Echocardiography is preferred as the initial test as it allows for examination of various parameters beyond left ventricular function including chamber sizes, valvular regurgitation or stenosis, and estimation of intracardiac pressures (diastolic function). Multiple-gated acquisition (MUGA) scan can be useful when echocardiographic images are poor despite contrast but provides more limited data (chamber sizes and biventricular ejection fraction). Cardiac magnetic resonance imaging is not typically necessary in a pre-HSCT evaluation unless performed for other indications.

## Assessing for Ischemia

Review of previously performed computed tomography (CT) imaging studies can provide valuable information with regard to the presence of coronary and aortic calcifications. Signs of atherosclerotic disease should prompt initiation of statin therapy in the absence of contraindications. Consider further evaluation for high-risk ischemia in HSCT candidates with a high pretest probability of coronary artery disease and poor exercise tolerance, with or without angina. Coronary CT angiography and myocardial perfusion imaging are both useful modalities to evaluate for high-risk ischemic heart disease. Coronary angiography and revascularization should be limited in patients with high-risk coronary artery disease and those with angina refractory to medical therapy to avoid delaying HSCT.

## Pre-HSCT Management of Cardiovascular Comorbidities

Every effort at optimizing the cardiovascular status of patients should be made prior to HSCT. This includes treating reversible disease and ensuring patients with cardiomyopathy are euvolemic, on a stable diuretic regimen, with optimal blood pressure control, and on guideline-directed medical therapy at maximally tolerated doses. While this process is likely to require multiple clinic visits, we recommend expediting testing and optimization of medical therapy to maximize the potential to recover cardiac function and avoid delaying HSCT. Patients who have adequate cardiopulmonary reserve, defined as not experiencing cardiovascular symptoms that are lifestyle limiting, and that are on an optimal medication regimen should be able to undergo HSCT safely regardless of whether their cardiac function, as measured by left ventricualr ejection fraction (LVEF), has recovered. Lack of recovery of cardiac function alone should not preclude candidacy for HSCT. Excluding patients from HSCT for cardiovascular reasons should be limited to the rare patient with severe, non-treatable disease and poor cardiopulmonary reserve with a life expectancy of <1 year. Lastly, providing guidance to the hematology/oncology teams as to the management of the likely exacerbation of comorbid cardiovascular conditions such as heart failure and atrial fibrillation during transplant is essential.

## Special Considerations for Inpatient Management of Cardiovascular Complications

Recommendations on the cardiovascular management of patients undergoing HSCT focus on the early identification of cardiovascular complications in patients at risk. Large volumes of intravenous fluids are administered during HSCT; thus, patients with or at risk of heart failure should have their weights monitored daily, with administration of diuretics for changes in weight of 2–3 lbs in 24 h to avoid hypervolemia. Volume shifts and systemic inflammation related to engraftment or infections can trigger supraventricular arrhythmias, most commonly atrial fibrillation. If the patient is asymptomatic and hemodynamically stable, avoiding aggressive rate control is recommended. A very common trigger and sustaining factor of atrial fibrillation is hypervolemia; thus, a diligent assessment for weight gain, jugular venous distention, and other signs of hypervolemia should always be performed at diagnosis and treated with diuretics prior to initiating rate control. Cardioversion should also be avoided unless in emergent situations given patients undergoing HSCT are often thrombocytopenic and cannot be anticoagulated. Special considerations must be given in these patients due to the frequent drug-drug interactions with concurrent cancer therapeutics related to alterations in the cytochrome P450 or P-glycoprotein metabolism [83, 84].

## Survivorship

HSCT survivors experience a higher burden of cardiovascular risk factors and long-term events including cardiomyopathy, ischemic heart disease, stroke, peripheral vascular disease, and rhythm disorders compared to the general population. Guidelines on screening and preventative measures for vascular complications in long-term HSCT survivors have been published by the American Society for Blood and Bone Marrow Transplantation [85, 86]. The optimization of cardiovascular risk factors and monitoring are cornerstones of the long-term cardiovascular management of HSCT survivors. There are no data to guide the optimal frequency of monitoring in HSCT survivors, with existing guidelines focusing on the cardiovascular monitoring of the broader adult cancer survivor population. A 3-month cardiovascular assessment post-HSCT in patients with preexisting cardiovascular disease is typical in many institutions, with earlier evaluations in patients who experienced complications during HSCT. Patients are then seen every 1–3 years, with factors such as cardiovascular comorbidity burden and active conditions dictating the frequency of monitoring [87]. Every visit should represent an opportunity to address risk factors such as smoking, hypertension, hyperlipidemia, and diabetes mellitus. HSCT survivors on immunosuppressive therapies associated with hyperlipidemia should undergo measurement of lipid profiles every 3–6 months until therapy is terminated [87, 88]. Similarly, HSCT survivors are at higher risk of developing diabetes mellitus, which should be screened yearly. Survivorship clinics have been devised in many institutions with a focus on risk factor screening and optimizing through both pharmacologic therapy and lifestyle modification.

Given the overall higher risk of this patient population, a low threshold to evaluate for cardiovascular origins of symptoms should be maintained [89]. Routine imaging during or after HSCT is not typically recommended for low-risk, asymptomatic individuals. Individuals who are considered high risk for developing cardiovascular complications may benefit from routine imaging surveillance during treatment with echocardiography being the preferred method [89]. There are no guidelines recommending specific time intervals for imaging surveillance; thus, this should be determined in collaboration with cardiology based on clinical judgment and patient characteristics. Additionally, it is recommended that asymptomatic, high-risk individuals receive an echocardiogram 1 year after completion of HSCT; however, more frequent assessments may be warranted if clinically appropriate [87, 89].

## Conclusion

Hematopoietic stem cell transplantation is increasingly used for the management of many malignancies. Older patients with multimorbidity, including cardiovascular disease, are more commonly being considered candidates for HSCT. Short- and long-term cardiovascular complications of HSCT are diverse, with complex pathophysiology and interaction with preexisting disease. While data guiding the pre-HSCT and post-HSCT cardiovascular assessment of patients are lacking, specialists in cardio-oncology can play a crucial role in minimizing the impact of preexisting cardiovascular disease on transplant outcomes and address cardiovascular complications both during HSCT and in survivorship.

## References


1. Rotz SJ, Ryan TD, Hayek SS. Cardiovascular disease and its management in children and adults undergoing hematopoietic stem cell transplantation. J Thromb Thrombolysis. 2021;51(4):854–69.
2. D'Souza A, Lee S, Zhu X, Pasquini M. Current use and trends in hematopoietic cell transplantation in the United States. Biol Blood Marrow Transplant. 2017;23(9):1417–21.
3. Buja LM, Ferrans VJ, Graw RG Jr. Cardiac pathologic findings in patients treated with bone marrow transplantation. Hum Pathol. 1976;7(1):17–45.
4. Cazin B, Gorin NC, Laporte J, Gallet B, Douay L, Lopez M, et al. Cardiac complications after bone marrow transplantation. A report on a series of 63 consecutive transplantations. Cancer. 1986;57(10):2061–9.
5. Murdych T, Weisdorf DJ. Serious cardiac complications during bone marrow transplantation at the University of Minnesota, 1977–1997. Bone Marrow Transplant. 2001;28(3):283–7.
6. Goldberg MA, Antin JH, Guinan EC, Rappeport JM. Cyclophosphamide cardiotoxicity: an analysis of dosing as a risk factor. Blood. 1986;68(5):1114–8.
7. Alblooshi R, Kanfar S, Lord B, Atenafu EG, Michelis FV, Pasic I, et al. Clinical prevalence and outcome of cardiovascular events in the first 100 days postallogeneic hematopoietic stem cell transplant. Eur J Haematol. 2021;106(1):32–9.
8. Gul Z, Bashir Q, Cremer M, Yusuf SW, Gunaydin H, Arora S, et al. Short-term cardiac toxicity of autologous hematopoietic stem cell transplant for multiple myeloma. Leuk Lymphoma. 2015;56(2):533–5.
9. Mo X-D, Xu L-P, Liu D-H, Zhang X-H, Chen H, Chen Y-H, et al. Heart failure after allogeneic hema-

topoietic stem cell transplantation. Int J Cardiol. 2013;167(6):2502–6.

10. Chiengthong K, Lertjitbanjong P, Thongprayoon C, Bathini T, Sharma K, Prasitlumkum N, et al. Arrhythmias in hematopoietic stem cell transplantation: a systematic review and meta-analysis. Eur J Haematol. 2019;103(6):564–72.
11. Tonorezos ES, Stillwell EE, Calloway JJ, Glew T, Wessler JD, Rebolledo BJ, et al. Arrhythmias in the setting of hematopoietic cell transplants. Bone Marrow Transplant. 2015;50(9):1212–6.
12. Singla A, Hogan WJ, Ansell SM, Buadi FK, Dingli D, Dispenzieri A, et al. Incidence of supraventricular arrhythmias during autologous peripheral blood stem cell transplantation. Biol Blood Marrow Transplant. 2013;19(8):1233–7.
13. Sakata-Yanagimoto M, Kanda Y, Nakagawa M, Asano-Mori Y, Kandabashi K, Izutsu K, et al. Predictors for severe cardiac complications after hematopoietic stem cell transplantation. Bone Marrow Transplant. 2004;33(10):1043–7.
14. Peres E, Levine JE, Khaled YA, Ibrahim RB, Braun TM, Krijanovski OI, et al. Cardiac complications in patients undergoing a reduced-intensity conditioning hematopoietic stem cell transplantation. Bone Marrow Transplant. 2010;45(1):149–52.
15. Armenian SH, Sun C-L, Francisco L, Steinberger J, Kurian S, Wong FL, et al. Late congestive heart failure after hematopoietic cell transplantation. J Clin Oncol. 2008;26(34):5537.
16. Armenian SH, Sun C-L, Vase T, Ness KK, Blum E, Francisco L, et al. Cardiovascular risk factors in hematopoietic cell transplantation survivors: role in development of subsequent cardiovascular disease. Blood. 2012;120(23):4505–12.
17. Chow EJ, Mueller BA, Baker KS, Cushing-Haugen KL, Flowers MED, Martin PJ, et al. Cardiovascular hospitalizations and mortality among recipients of hematopoietic stem cell transplantation. Ann Intern Med. 2011;155(1):21–32.
18. Armenian SH, Sun C-L, Shannon T, Mills G, Francisco L, Venkataraman K, et al. Incidence and predictors of congestive heart failure after autologous hematopoietic cell transplantation. Blood. 2011;118(23):6023–9.
19. Steuter JA, Villanueva MLH, Loberiza FR, Armitage JO, Bociek RG, Ganti AK, et al. Factors affecting the development of atrial fibrillation and atrial flutter (AF/AFL) following autologous hematopoietic SCT (auto-HSCT). Bone Marrow Transplant. 2013;48(7):963–5.
20. Rodgers JL, Jones J, Bolleddu SI, Vanthenapalli S, Rodgers LE, Shah K, et al. Cardiovascular risks associated with gender and aging. J Cardiovasc Dev Dis. 2019;6(2):19.
21. D'Souza A, Fretham C, Lee SJ, Arora M, Brunner J, Chhabra S, et al. Current use of and trends in hematopoietic cell transplantation in the United States. Biol Blood Marrow Transplant. 2020;26(8):e177–e82.
22. Majhail NS, Ness KK, Burns LJ, Sun C-L, Carter A, Francisco L, et al. Late effects in survivors of Hodgkin and non-Hodgkin lymphoma treated with autologous hematopoietic cell transplantation: a report from the bone marrow transplant survivor study. Biol Blood Marrow Transplant. 2007;13(10):1153–9.
23. Lipshultz SE, Lipsitz SR, Mone SM, Goorin AM, Sallan SE, Sanders SP, et al. Female sex and higher drug dose as risk factors for late cardiotoxic effects of doxorubicin therapy for childhood cancer. N Engl J Med. 1995;332(26):1738–44.
24. Fujimaki K, Maruta A, Yoshida M, Sakai R, Tanabe J, Koharazawa H, et al. Severe cardiac toxicity in hematological stem cell transplantation: predictive value of reduced left ventricular ejection fraction. Bone Marrow Transplant. 2001;27(3):307–10.
25. Armenian SH, Chow EJ. Cardiovascular disease in survivors of hematopoietic cell transplantation. Cancer. 2014;120(4):469–79.
26. Qazilbash MH, Amjad AI, Qureshi S, Qureshi SR, Saliba RM, Khan ZU, et al. Outcome of allogeneic hematopoietic stem cell transplantation in patients with low left ventricular ejection fraction. Biol Blood Marrow Transplant. 2009;15(10):1265–70.
27. Tang WHW, Thomas S, Kalaycio M, Sobecks R, Andresen S, Jarvis J, et al. Clinical outcomes of patients with impaired left ventricular ejection fraction undergoing autologous bone marrow transplantation: can we safely transplant patients with impaired ejection fraction? Bone Marrow Transplant. 2004;34(7):603–7.
28. Baker KS, Ness KK, Steinberger J, Carter A, Francisco L, Burns LJ, et al. Diabetes, hypertension, and cardiovascular events in survivors of hematopoietic cell transplantation: a report from the bone marrow transplantation survivor study. Blood. 2007;109(4):1765–72.
29. Taskinen M, Saarinen-Pihkala UM, Hovi L, Lipsanen-Nyman M. Impaired glucose tolerance and dyslipidaemia as late effects after bone-marrow transplantation in childhood. Lancet. 2000;356(9234):993–7.
30. André T, Jakob P, Dorota W, Alicia R, Jean-Luc H, Tamas M, et al. Late cardiovascular events after allogeneic hematopoietic stem cell transplantation: a retrospective multicenter study of the late effects Working Party of the European Group for blood and marrow transplantation. Haematologica. 2008;93(8):1203–10.
31. Armenian SH, Sun C-L, Mills G, Teh JB, Francisco L, Durand J-B, et al. Predictors of late cardiovascular complications in survivors of hematopoietic cell transplantation. Biol Blood Marrow Transplant. 2010;16(8):1138–44.
32. D'Souza A, Dispenzieri A, Wirk B, Zhang M-J, Huang J, Gertz MA, et al. Improved outcomes after autologous hematopoietic cell transplantation for light chain amyloidosis: a Center for International Blood and Marrow Transplant Research Study. J Clin Oncol. 2015;33(32):3741–9.
33. Gabrielli A, Avvedimento EV, Krieg T. Scleroderma. N Engl J Med. 2009;360(19):1989–2003.
34. Hoogen F, Khanna D, Fransen J, Johnson SR, Baron M, Tyndall A, et al. 2013 classification crite-

ria for systemic sclerosis: an American College of Rheumatology/European League against rheumatism collaborative initiative. 2013.
35. Desai CS, Lee DC, Shah SJ. Systemic sclerosis and the heart: current diagnosis and management. Curr Opin Rheumatol. 2011;23(6):545.
36. Fransen J, Popa-Diaconu D, Hesselstrand R, Carreira P, Valentini G, Beretta L, et al. Clinical prediction of 5-year survival in systemic sclerosis: validation of a simple prognostic model in EUSTAR centres. Ann Rheum Dis. 2011;70(10):1788–92.
37. Tyndall AJ, Bannert B, Vonk M, Airò P, Cozzi F, Carreira PE, et al. Causes and risk factors for death in systemic sclerosis: a study from the EULAR scleroderma trials and research (EUSTAR) database. Ann Rheum Dis. 2010;69(10):1809–15.
38. Burt RK, Shah SJ, Dill K, Grant T, Gheorghiade M, Schroeder J, et al. Autologous non-myeloablative haemopoietic stem-cell transplantation compared with pulse cyclophosphamide once per month for systemic sclerosis (ASSIST): an open-label, randomised phase 2 trial. Lancet. 2011;378(9790):498–506.
39. van Laar JM, Farge D, Sont JK, Naraghi K, Marjanovic Z, Larghero J, et al. Autologous hematopoietic stem cell transplantation vs intravenous pulse cyclophosphamide in diffuse cutaneous systemic sclerosis: a randomized clinical trial. JAMA. 2014;311(24):2490–8.
40. Burt RK, Oliveira MC, Shah SJ, Moraes DA, Simoes B, Gheorghiade M, et al. Cardiac involvement and treatment-related mortality after non-myeloablative haemopoietic stem-cell transplantation with unselected autologous peripheral blood for patients with systemic sclerosis: a retrospective analysis. Lancet. 2013;381(9872):1116–24.
41. Hassan W, Al-Sergani H, Mourad W, Tabbaa R. Amyloid heart disease. New frontiers and insights in pathophysiology, diagnosis, and management. Tex Heart Inst J. 2005;32(2):178–84.
42. Falk RH, Alexander KM, Liao R, Dorbala S. AL (light-chain) cardiac amyloidosis: a review of diagnosis and therapy. J Am Coll Cardiol. 2016;68(12):1323–41.
43. Cardinale D, Iacopo F, Cipolla CM. Cardiotoxicity of anthracyclines. Front Cardiovasc Med. 2020;7:26.
44. Giudice V, Vecchione C, Selleri C. Cardiotoxicity of novel targeted hematological therapies. Life (Basel). 2020;10(12):344.
45. Corrigendum to: cardiovascular toxicities associated with immune checkpoint inhibitors. Cardiovasc Res. 2019;115(5):868.
46. Nowis D, Maczewski M, Mackiewicz U, Kujawa M, Ratajska A, Wieckowski MR, et al. Cardiotoxicity of the anticancer therapeutic agent bortezomib. Am J Pathol. 2010;176(6):2658–68.
47. Xiao Y, Yin J, Wei J, Shang Z. Incidence and risk of cardiotoxicity associated with bortezomib in the treatment of cancer: a systematic review and meta-analysis. PLoS One. 2014;9(1):e87671.
48. Quach H, Ritchie D, Stewart AK, Neeson P, Harrison S, Smyth MJ, et al. Mechanism of action of immunomodulatory drugs (IMiDS) in multiple myeloma. Leukemia. 2010;24(1):22–32.
49. Fahdi IE, Gaddam V, Saucedo JF, Kishan CV, Vyas K, Deneke MG, et al. Bradycardia during therapy for multiple myeloma with thalidomide. Am J Cardiol. 2004;93(8):1052–5.
50. McMullen JR, Boey EJH, Ooi JYY, Seymour JF, Keating MJ, Tam CS. Ibrutinib increases the risk of atrial fibrillation, potentially through inhibition of cardiac PI3K-Akt signaling. Blood. 2014;124(25):3829–30.
51. Ganatra S, Sharma A, Shah S, Chaudhry GM, Martin DT, Neilan TG, et al. Ibrutinib-associated atrial fibrillation. JACC Clin Electrophysiol. 2018;4(12):1491–500.
52. Pineda-Gayoso R, Alomar M, Lee DH, Fradley MG. Cardiovascular toxicities of Bruton's tyrosine kinase inhibitors. Curr Treat Options in Oncol. 2020;21(8):67.
53. Scott JM, Armenian S, Giralt S, Moslehi J, Wang T, Jones LW. Cardiovascular disease following hematopoietic stem cell transplantation: pathogenesis, detection, and the cardioprotective role of aerobic training. Crit Rev Oncol Hematol. 2016;98:222–34.
54. Braverman AC, Antin JH, Plappert MT, Cook EF, Lee RT. Cyclophosphamide cardiotoxicity in bone marrow transplantation: a prospective evaluation of new dosing regimens. J Clin Oncol. 1991;9(7):1215–23.
55. Goldberg MA, Antin JH, Guinan EC, Rappeport JM. Cyclophosphamide cardiotoxicity: an analysis of dosing as a risk factor, vol. 68; 1986. p. 1114.
56. Vaickus L, Letendre L. Pericarditis induced by high-dose cytarabine therapy. Arch Intern Med. 1984;144(9):1868–9.
57. Kanj SS, Sharara AI, Shpall EJ, Jones RB, Peters WP. Myocardial ischemia associated with high-dose carmustine infusion. Cancer. 1991;68(9):1910–2.
58. Olivieri A, Corvatta L, Montanari M, Brunori M, Offidani M, Ferretti GF, et al. Paroxysmal atrial fibrillation after high-dose melphalan in five patients autotransplanted with blood progenitor cells. Bone Marrow Transplant. 1998;21(10):1049–53.
59. Van Besien K, Devine S, Wickrema A, Jessop E, Amin K, Yassine M, et al. Regimen-related toxicity after fludarabine–melphalan conditioning: a prospective study of 31 patients with hematologic malignancies. Bone Marrow Transplant. 2003;32(5):471–6.
60. Ayza MA, Zewdie KA, Tesfaye BA, Wondafrash DZ, Berhe AH. The role of antioxidants in ameliorating cyclophosphamide-induced cardiotoxicity. Oxidative Med Cell Longev. 2020;2020:4965171.
61. Dhesi S, Chu MP, Blevins G, Paterson I, Larratt L, Oudit GY, et al. Cyclophosphamide-induced cardiomyopathy: a case report, review, and recommendations for management. J Investig Med High Impact Case Rep. 2013;1(1):2324709613480346.
62. Al-Nasser IA. In vivo prevention of cyclophosphamide-induced Ca2+ dependent damage of rat heart and liver mitochondria by cyclospo-

rin a. Comp Biochem Physiol A Mol Integr Physiol. 1998;121(3):209–14.
63. Asiri YA. Probucol attenuates cyclophosphamide-induced oxidative apoptosis, p53 and Bax signal expression in rat cardiac tissues. Oxidative Med Cell Longev. 2010;3(5):308–16.
64. Rovó A, Tichelli A. Cardiovascular complications in long-term survivors after allogeneic hematopoietic stem cell transplantation. Semin Hematol. 2012;49(1):25–34.
65. Han X, Zhou Y, Liu W. Precision cardio-oncology: understanding the cardiotoxicity of cancer therapy. NPJ Precis Oncol. 2017;1(1):31.
66. Taunk NK, Haffty BG, Kostis JB, Goyal S. Radiation-induced heart disease: pathologic abnormalities and putative mechanisms. Front Oncol. 2015;5:39.
67. Cuomo JR, Sharma GK, Conger PD, Weintraub NL. Novel concepts in radiation-induced cardiovascular disease. World J Cardiol. 2016;8(9):504–19.
68. Ghimire S, Weber D, Mavin E, Wang XN, Dickinson AM, Holler E. Pathophysiology of GvHD and other HSCT-related major complications. Front Immunol. 2017;8:79.
69. Tichelli A, Gratwohl A. Vascular endothelium as 'novel' target of graft-versus-host disease. Best Pract Res Clin Haematol. 2008;21(2):139–48.
70. Tichelli A, Bucher C, Rovó A, Stussi G, Stern M, Paulussen M, et al. Premature cardiovascular disease after allogeneic hematopoietic stem-cell transplantation. Blood. 2007;110(9):3463–71.
71. Miller LW. Cardiovascular toxicities of immunosuppressive agents. Am J Transplant. 2002;2(9):807–18.
72. Bachier C, Eiznhamer D, Milgroom A, Lenco M, Patel N, Skaar JR. Costs and adverse events associated with ibrutinib or ruxolitinib in chronic graft-versus-host disease. Blood. 2020;136:14–5.
73. Konuma T, Ooi J, Takahashi S, Tomonari A, Tsukada N, Kobayashi T, et al. Cardiovascular toxicity of cryopreserved cord blood cell infusion. Bone Marrow Transplant. 2008;41(10):861–5.
74. Spitzer TR. Engraftment syndrome: double-edged sword of hematopoietic cell transplants. Bone Marrow Transplant. 2015;50(4):469–75.
75. Sengsayadeth S, Savani BN, Blaise D, Malard F, Nagler A, Mohty M. Reduced intensity conditioning allogeneic hematopoietic cell transplantation for adult acute myeloid leukemia in complete remission—a review from the acute Leukemia working party of the EBMT. Haematologica. 2015;100(7):859–69.
76. Duléry R, Mohty R, Labopin M, Sestili S, Malard F, Brissot E, et al. Early cardiac toxicity associated with post-transplant cyclophosphamide in allogeneic stem cell transplantation. JACC CardioOncol. 2021;3(2):250–9.
77. Thibodeau JT, Drazner MH. The role of the clinical examination in patients with heart failure. JACC Heart Fail. 2018;6(7):543–51.
78. Chow EJ, Chen Y, Kremer LC, Breslow NE, Hudson MM, Armstrong GT, et al. Individual prediction of heart failure among childhood cancer survivors. J Clin Oncol. 2015;33(5):394.
79. Chow EJ, Chen Y, Hudson MM, Feijen EAM, Kremer LC, Border WL, et al. Prediction of ischemic heart disease and stroke in survivors of childhood cancer. J Clin Oncol. 2018;36(1):44.
80. Armenian SH, Yang D, Teh JB, Atencio LC, Gonzales A, Wong FL, et al. Prediction of cardiovascular disease among hematopoietic cell transplantation survivors. Blood Adv. 2018;2(14):1756–64.
81. Hertenstein B, Stefanic M, Schmeiser T, Scholz M, Göller V, Clausen M, et al. Cardiac toxicity of bone marrow transplantation: predictive value of cardiologic evaluation before transplant. J Clin Oncol. 1994;12(5):998–1004.
82. Lehmann S, Isberg B, Ljungman P, Paul C. Cardiac systolic function before and after hematopoietic stem cell transplantation. Bone Marrow Transplant. 2000;26(2):187–92.
83. van Leeuwen RWF, Jansman FGA, van den Bemt PMLA, de Man F, Piran F, Vincenten I, et al. Drug–drug interactions in patients treated for cancer: a prospective study on clinical interventions. Ann Oncol. 2015;26(5):992–7.
84. Fradley MG, Beckie TM, Brown SA, Cheng RK, Dent SF, Nohria A, et al. Recognition, prevention, and management of arrhythmias and autonomic disorders in cardio-oncology: a scientific statement from the American Heart Association. Circulation. 2021;144(3):e41–55.
85. Coghlan JG, Handler CE, Kottaridis PD. Cardiac assessment of patients for haematopoietic stem cell transplantation. Best Pract Res Clin Haematol. 2007;20(2):247–63.
86. Rizzo JD, Wingard JR, Tichelli A, Lee SJ, Van Lint MT, Burns LJ, et al. Recommended screening and preventive practices for long-term survivors after hematopoietic cell transplantation: joint recommendations of the European Group for Blood and Marrow Transplantation, the Center for International Blood and Marrow Transplant Research, and the American Society of Blood and Marrow Transplantation. Biol Blood Marrow Transplant. 2006;12(2):138–51.
87. Majhail NS, Rizzo JD, Lee SJ, Aljurf M, Atsuta Y, Bonfim C, et al. Recommended screening and preventive practices for long-term survivors after hematopoietic cell transplantation. Rev Bras Hematol Hemoter. 2012;34(2):109–33.
88. DeFilipp Z, Duarte RF, Snowden JA, Majhail NS, Greenfield DM, Miranda JL, et al. Metabolic syndrome and cardiovascular disease after hematopoietic cell transplantation: screening and preventive practice recommendations from the CIBMTR and EBMT. Biol Blood Marrow Transplant. 2016;22(8):1493–503.
89. Armenian SH, Lacchetti C, Barac A, Carver J, Constine LS, Denduluri N, et al. Prevention and monitoring of cardiac dysfunction in survivors of adult cancers: American Society of Clinical Oncology clinical practice guideline. J Clin Oncol. 2017;35(8):893–911.

# 27 Renal Considerations in Critically Ill Hematopoietic Stem Cell Transplant Patients

Abinet Aklilu and Amanda DeMauro Renaghan

## Introduction

In this chapter, we review renal complications of hematopoietic stem cell transplantation (HSCT). We discuss the epidemiology of acute kidney injury (AKI) following HSCT, potentially modifiable pre- and post-transplant risk factors, etiologies, pathophysiology, diagnosis, prevention, and treatment. AKI post-HSCT commonly refers to the first 100 days post-transplant. However, we recognize patients may present to the intensive care unit (ICU) at different times post-transplant.

## Epidemiology of AKI in HSCT

AKI is a common complication of HSCT. Incidence of 20–92% has been reported in the first 100 days post-transplant; this wide range is attributed to evolving definitions of AKI, differences in severity of illness in the populations assessed, and progress in peri-transplant care [1–3]. Incidence also varies by donor type and conditioning regimen (autologous, 12–50%; non-myeloablative allogeneic, 29–54%; myeloablative allogeneic, 19–66%) [1, 2]. Overall, non-myeloablative HSCT has been associated with lower incidence and less severe AKI compared with myeloablative allogeneic HSCT, which uses more intensive conditioning [2–5]. However, the data are not robust, and in a more recent study using the Kidney Disease: Improving Global Outcomes (KDIGO) definition of AKI, a higher incidence was observed in those who underwent non-myeloablative conditioning [6]. This may be due to the underlying characteristics of non-myeloablative transplant recipients, including older age, baseline chronic kidney disease (CKD), and prior failed high-dose HSCT, which are known risk factors for AKI in this popu-

A. Aklilu
Section of Nephrology, Yale University School of Medicine, New Haven, CT, USA

A. D. Renaghan (✉)
Division of Nephrology, University of Virginia Health System, Charlottesville, VA, USA
e-mail: ajd9y@virginia.edu


A. O. Soubani (ed.), *Pulmonary and Critical Care Considerations of Hematopoietic Stem Cell Transplantation*, https://doi.org/10.1007/978-3-031-28797-8_27

lation [6]. Autologous transplantation appears to have the lowest risk of AKI, likely related to the absence of graft-versus-host disease (GVHD), lack of calcineurin inhibitor (CNI) exposure, and more rapid engraftment [7–9].

Severe AKI requiring kidney replacement therapy (KRT) has been reported in 12–24% of patients in older studies and carries poorer prognosis [4]. A more recent study of 616 allogeneic HSCT recipients using KDIGO AKI criteria revealed a 64% incidence of AKI by day 100, with only 3% of patients requiring KRT and only 24% of patients surviving to discharge when dialysis was required [6]. Incidence of AKI in HSCT recipients admitted to the ICU is consistently high, on average around 60–65% [7, 10]. KRT requirement is higher in critically ill HSCT recipients (50–72%) and is associated with high mortality, especially when co-occurring with other organ dysfunction [7, 10].

## Outcomes of Post-HSCT AKI

AKI is an independent risk factor for in-hospital mortality [11, 12]. In both adult and pediatric HSCT populations, all stages of AKI in the first 100 days post-transplant are associated with reduced 1-year overall survival [5, 13, 14]. Mortality is highest in those requiring dialysis (83–88% versus 47% with stage I AKI and 17% without AKI) [4, 10, 13]. Severe AKI is also associated with indicators of critical illness such as sepsis, liver dysfunction, and ventilator requirement [13].

AKI is a risk factor for CKD, which is itself a risk factor for premature mortality [15]. In one recent meta-analysis, renal recovery occurred in 58% of AKI survivors and only 10% of those requiring dialysis [16]. Average CKD incidence (varying definitions) by 6–12 months post-transplant has been reported in 20%, up to 66%, and 12–20% of myeloablative, non-myeloablative, and autologous HSCT recipients, respectively [5, 17–19]. In another study of non-myeloablative HSCT patients, prevalence of CKD (defined as glomerular filtration rate (GFR) <60 mL/min/1.73 m$^2$) at 12 months was lower at 7% but increased to 14% at 24 months and 22% at 48 months [20]. Total body irradiation (TBI), previous HSCT, chronic CNI use, and chronic GVHD are independent predictors of CKD after non-myeloablative transplant [20, 21]. Female sex and pre-transplant CKD increase the risk of CKD after myeloablative HSCT [22].

## Predictors of AKI

Risk of AKI after HSCT varies by patient characteristics, including baseline renal reserve, conditioning and donor type, post-transplant complications and associated exposures, and timing of AKI diagnosis. The hematopoietic cell transplantation-specific comorbidity index (HCT-CI), a marker of pre-transplant comorbidity and an established prognostic factor for overall survival and non-relapse mortality, is the most important predictor of severe AKI [6, 23, 24]. Particularly in critically ill patients, older age, Sequential Organ Failure Assessment (SOFA) score, history of hypertension, and nephrotoxin exposure are independent predictors of AKI [7]. In a cohort of 207 patients who underwent allogeneic HSCT, the presence of infection (37%) and acute GVHD (20.7%) were the strongest predictors of AKI, while exposure to CNIs, antimicrobials, engraftment syndrome (ES), transplant-associated thrombotic microangiopathy (TA-TMA), and Cytomegalovirus (CMV) reactivation contributed to a lower degree [23].

## Pathogenesis of AKI in Critically Ill Patients After HSCT

AKI after HSCT is often multifactorial. Here, we highlight several important etiologies of post-transplant AKI, including several entities unique to this population (Table 27.1). AKI is most frequently observed approximately 2 weeks after myeloablative allogeneic HSCT and 26–60 days after non-myeloablative HSCT; however, the timing is highly variable [9]. A timeline of causes of AKI following HSCT is provided in Fig. 27.1.

**Table 27.1** Etiologies of renal injury in critically ill HSCT recipients

| Etiology of kidney injury | Time of peak incidence | Diagnosis | Risk factors | Prevention and management |
|---|---|---|---|---|
| Marrow infusion syndrome [44, 45] | 24–48 h post-transplant | GFR drop in the setting of fever, hypotension and GI symptoms, hematuria, and urine sediment with granular casts | Exposure to the cryoprotectant DMSO | Alkalinization of urine<br>Forced diuresis with mannitol |
| Engraftment syndrome [30, 31] | 7–9 days post-transplant; about 4 days after engraftment | GFR drop in the setting of fever, non-cardiogenic pulmonary edema, and erythematous rash | Baseline proteinuria, AL amyloidosis, POEMS | Supportive care<br>Steroids<br>Monitor for infection |
| Sinusoidal obstruction syndrome [27, 61, 74, 96, 100, 120] | 12 days post-transplant (often <21 days but may present >21 days) | ≥5% weight gain, bilirubin >2 mg/dL, hepatomegaly, ascites | Older age, allogeneic HSCT, unrelated donor, underlying liver dysfunction, high-dose conditioning, pre-transplant ADC | Prophylaxis with ursodiol and defibrotide in high-risk patients<br>Management similar to HRS + defibrotide |
| GVHD [33, 34, 74, 75, 79] | aGVHD <100 days post-transplant<br>cGVHD >100 days post-transplant | Proteinuria and GFR decline in the setting of other GVHD features (skin rash, GI and other system involvement) | High-intensity conditioning regimen, TBI, cGVHD common in non-myeloablative HSCT | Prevention (MTX, T-cell depletion)<br>Supportive care infection prevention<br>Optimize immunosuppression, optimize nutrition |
| TA-TMA [103, 111–114] | Variable | Hemolytic anemia, thrombocytopenia, GFR decline, hypertension, proteinuria | GVHD, TBI, underlying endothelial dysfunction, CNI exposure | Possible withdrawal of CNI<br>Consideration of rituximab or eculizumab (selected patients) |
| Viral nephritis (BK, adenovirus) [46, 48, 51, 118, 119] | Peak immunosuppression | GFR decline, viremia, viruria | High-intensity conditioning | Reduction of immunosuppression (BK virus)<br>Infectious disease consult for consideration of antiviral therapy |
| Acute GN [29, 34, 42] | ~6 months post-transplant | Nephrotic syndrome with nephrotic-range proteinuria, hypoalbuminemia, edema | GVHD, cancer recurrence | Nephrology consult and urgent kidney biopsy to preserve renal function<br>Multidisciplinary management of immunosuppression |

*ADC* antibody-drug conjugate, *aHUS* atypical hemolytic uremic syndrome, *AKI* acute kidney injury, *CNI* calcineurin inhibitor, *DAH* diffuse alveolar hemorrhage, *DMSO* dimethyl sulfoxide, *GFR* glomerular filtration rate, *GI* gastrointestinal, *GVHD* graft-versus-host disease, *GN* glomerulonephritis, *HRS* hepatorenal syndrome, *HSCT* hematopoietic stem cell transplant, *MTX* methotrexate, *POEMS* polyneuropathy, organomegaly, endocrinopathy, monoclonal gammopathy, and skin abnormalities, *TBI* total body irradiation, *TA-TMA* transplant-associated thrombotic microangiopathy, *RBCs* red blood cells

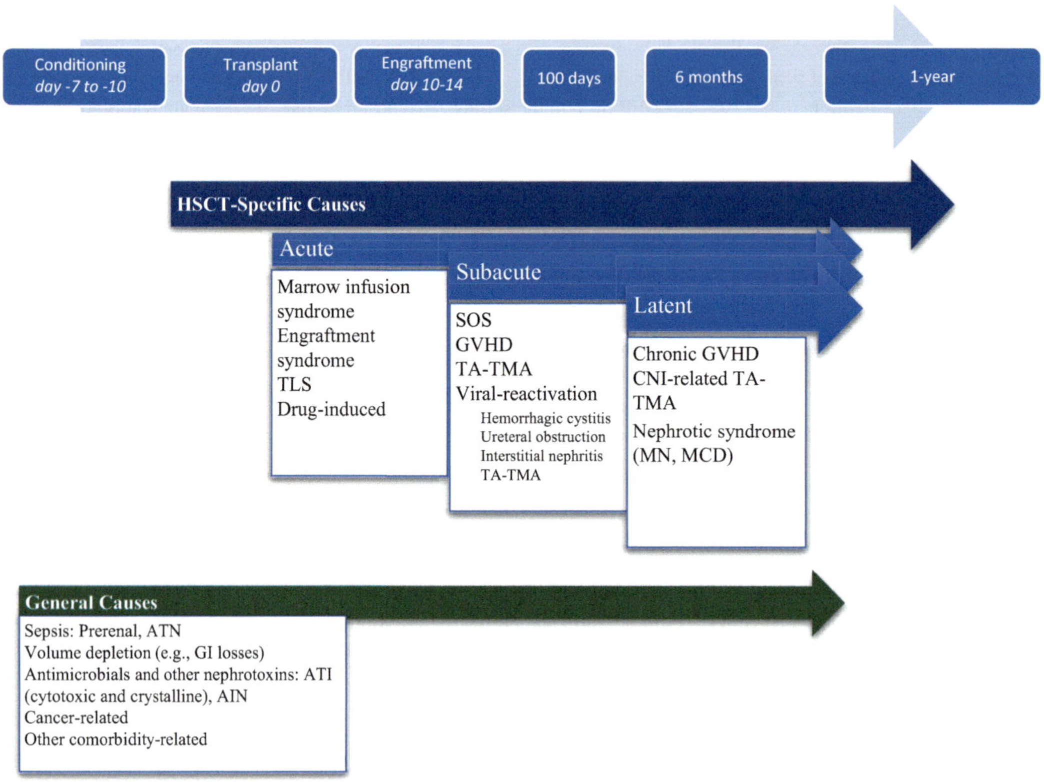


**Fig. 27.1** Timeline of etiologies of AKI in critically ill HSCT recipients. *AKI* acute kidney injury, *AIN* acute interstitial nephritis, *ATI* acute tubular injury, *ATN* acute tubular necrosis, *CNI* calcineurin inhibitors, *GVHD* graft-versus-host disease, *MCD* minimal change disease, *MN* membranous nephropathy, *SOS* sinusoidal obstruction syndrome, *TA-TMA* transplant-associated thrombotic microangiopathy, *TLS* tumor lysis syndrome

## Prerenal and Cytokine Release Syndromes

### Sepsis

Sepsis and circulatory shock are the most common causes of AKI in critically ill HSCT recipients [7, 10]. Exposure to nephrotoxic antimicrobials also contributes, as detailed below.

### Hepatic Sinusoidal Obstruction Syndrome (SOS)

Previously known as veno-occlusive disease (VOD), SOS classically occurs within the first 21 days after HSCT, though delayed-onset cases (44.5 days) have been described [25, 26]. SOS has been reported in up to 60% of HSCT recipients (estimated mean incidence, 13.7%) and is more likely to occur after allogeneic as compared with autologous transplant [25, 26]. Severe cases were previously associated with >80% mortality; however, both incidence and prognosis have improved with recent advances in prevention and treatment [25, 26].

*SOS* presents as a form of hepatorenal syndrome with edema, weight gain, jaundice, and right upper quadrant pain. Oliguria and rising creatinine follow. Urine sodium concentration is low (<10 mEq/L), and urinalysis and microscopy are typically bland, though granular casts may be seen with progression to acute tubular necrosis (ATN). SOS is caused by damage to hepatic sinusoidal endothelial cells in zone 3 of the liver around the central veins, with resultant subendothelial deposition of fibrin and other blood products leading to sinusoidal obstruction and portal hypertension [25]. Risk factors include exposure to gemtuzumab ozogamicin and inotuzumab ozogamicin prior to transplantation, high-intensity conditioning regimens (particularly busulfan-thiothepa, busulfan-cyclophosphamide, fludarabine, and TBI based), and CNI use [27, 28]. In addition to cytokine release, glutathione depletion as a result of chemotherapeutic drug detoxification contributes to centrilobular hepatocellular necrosis and fibrosis [25, 26].

#### Engraftment Syndrome

ES occurs around the time of neutrophil engraftment and is seen most commonly after autologous transplantation [29, 30]. It is characterized by fever, non-cardiogenic pulmonary edema, and erythematous rash and may present with multi-organ involvement. >90% incidence of AKI has been reported, with >50% of patients having stage III AKI and 27% requiring dialysis [31]. Etiology is believed to be neutrophil degranulation and inflammatory cytokine release during engraftment [31]. Baseline proteinuria was the only significant predictor in one study [31].

### Complement- and Immune-Related AKI

#### Graft-Versus-Host Disease

GVHD is a major complication of allogeneic HSCT and can arise at any point after transplant. Acute GVHD occurs within 100 days post-transplant, with a median time of around 21 days, and is recognized in 20–68% of those admitted to the ICU [10, 32, 33]. Chronic GVHD occurs after 100 days post-transplant and is a major risk factor for post-HSCT CKD [34]. Whereas acute GVHD is a result of donor-derived cytotoxic T-cells and cytokine-related tissue aggression, chronic GVHD (cGVHD) arises from both autoimmune causes and immunosuppression [33, 35].

GVHD has been associated with various types of kidney injury, including prerenal AKI (by way of gastrointestinal losses in the setting of gut GVHD), TA-TMA, and post-transplant glomerulonephritis (GN). Additionally, direct kidney injury may present as interstitial inflammation and renal tubular injury as a result of cytokine release [33, 36]. Renal biopsy reveals evidence of renal tubular injury (ATN) and/or tubulitis and interstitial infiltration by lymphocytes and mononuclear cells (Fig. 27.2a, b) [36, 37].

#### Transplant-Associated Thrombotic Microangiopathy

TA-TMA is a multi-organ disease that often involves the kidneys. It typically presents 6–12 months after transplant but may occur earlier [29]. Incidence varies widely due to different diagnostic criteria. Patients present with evidence of microangiopathic hemolytic anemia, reduced GFR, proteinuria, and hypertension. Both endothelial injury and complement activation have been implicated, with decreased levels of vascular endothelial growth factor (VEGF) and activation of the alternative complement pathway contributing to pathogenesis [38, 39]. Risk factors include older age, unrelated donor type, high-dose busulfan conditioning, TBI (especially when performed without renal shielding), exposure to calcineurin and mTOR inhibitors, GVHD, and infections such as BK, CMV, and adenovirus [38, 39]. Biopsy reveals endothelial cell swelling, mesangiolysis, and fibrin thrombi in arterioles and glomeruli (Fig. 27.2c) [29, 40].

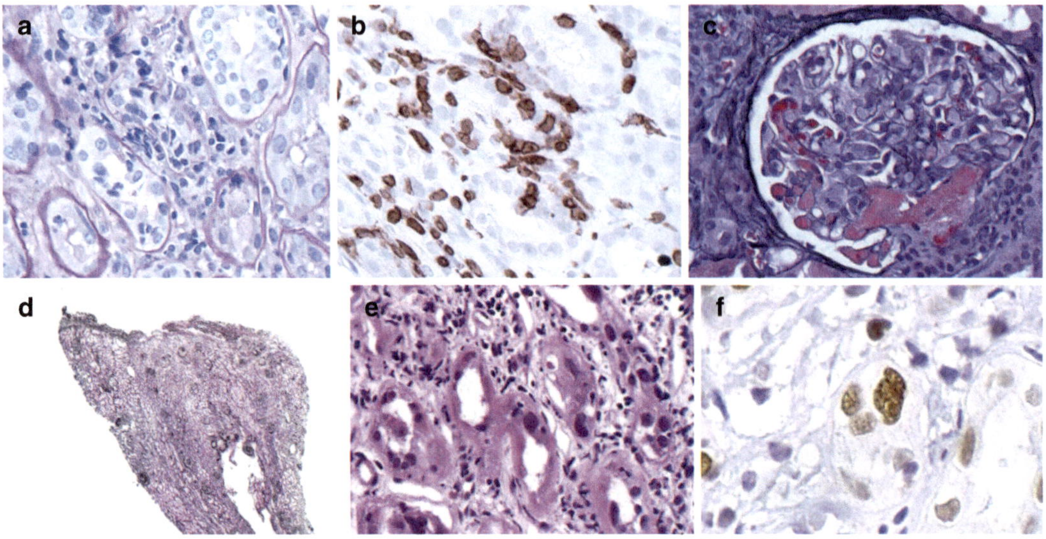

**Fig. 27.2** Renal manifestations of post-HSCT complications. Graft-versus-host disease—(**a**) Light microscopy demonstrating interstitial infiltration and tubulitis and tubular basement membrane damage (PAS stain, ×400 magnification). (**b**) Immunohistochemistry showing CD3+ lymphocytes in the interstitium. CNI nephrotoxicity—(**c**) TMA involving the glomerular tuft and vascular pole in the setting of CNI use (Jones silver stain). (**d**) Striped interstitial fibrosis in the setting of CNI use (Jones silver stain, low power). Polyoma (BK) virus-associated nephropathy (BKVAN)—(**e**) Viral inclusions in tubular epithelial cells along with interstitial infiltrate of plasma cells, lymphocytes, and occasional polymorphonuclear neutrophils (PAS, ×200 magnification). (**f**) Immunohistochemistry showing nuclear inclusions with antibody staining for simian kidney virus (SV40, ×400 magnification). (*Used with permission from Koratala et al., 2020* [37] *(A&B), Lusco et al., 2017* [40] *(C&D), Atlas of Renal Pathology, 2001* [47] *(E&F)*)

## Acute Glomerulonephritis

Although biopsy is underperformed in the HSCT population due to thrombocytopenia and coagulopathy, various glomerular lesions have been reported when performed for investigation of proteinuria. Membranous glomerulonephritis and minimal change disease are the most commonly described etiologies of post-transplant nephrotic syndrome (NS) [41]. While post-transplant NS appears to be strongly associated with the tapering of immunosuppression and presence of GVHD, it remains unclear if NS is caused by GVHD or other factors [41–43]. In some cases, GN may be related to recurrence of the original malignancy (e.g., amyloidosis, multiple myeloma).

## Transplant- or Tumor-Related AKI

### Marrow Infusion Syndrome

Exposure to toxic cell lysis products and cryoprotectants such as dimethyl sulfoxide (DMSO) used during the process of stem cell preservation may cause hemolysis on infusion and subsequently lead to heme precipitation in distal renal tubules, resulting in tubular obstruction (pigment nephropathy) [44]. Patients present with fever, hypotension, and gastrointestinal symptoms, typically within 24–48 h of transplant [45]. This complication is now infrequent, likely related to advances in cell preservation.

### Tumor Lysis Syndrome

Tumor lysis syndrome is a rare complication in HSCT, as most patients are in remission or have low tumor burden at the time of transplant. AKI results from tubular damage secondary to intratubular obstruction from uric acid or calcium phosphate crystals [5, 45].

## Viral Infections

BK virus and adenovirus infections are common in the heavily immunosuppressed HSCT population. BK virus reactivation in the urogenital system may manifest as interstitial nephritis (BK virus-associated nephropathy, BKVAN), hemorrhagic cystitis, or urinary obstruction. In patients with BKVAN, kidney biopsy specimens demonstrate a pleomorphic interstitial infiltrate, interstitial edema, tubulitis, and tubular injury; infected tubular epithelial cells may have enlarged nuclei with amorphous inclusions (Fig. 27.2e) [46, 47]. Infected epithelial cells stain positive for SV40 on immunohistochemistry (Fig. 27.2f) [46, 47]. BK hemorrhagic cystitis is most often seen in association with high BK viremia [48]. Large bladder clots may lead to obstruction and, in some cases, require surgical evacuation [49]. Obstruction may also result from ureteral stenosis, though this complication is more common among kidney transplant recipients [50]. Adenovirus may cause acute interstitial nephritis but more commonly causes hemorrhagic cystitis [51]. Both BK and adenovirus have been associated with endothelial injury leading to TA-TMA [38, 39, 49]. Particularly, high BK viremia (>10,000 copies/uL) has been associated with higher incidence of TA-TMA as compared with low BK viremia (70% versus 18%) [49]. Post-transplant BK viruria has also been associated with progressively worsening renal function and mortality [48].

## Nephrotoxins in HSCT

### Calcineurin Inhibitors

The CNIs tacrolimus and cyclosporine are used to prevent GVHD and frequently contribute to post-transplant AKI. These drugs cause afferent arteriolar vasoconstriction with resultant ischemic tubular injury, especially in predisposed patients (hypovolemic or on agents that alter renal hemodynamics) [5]. In cases of acute CNI nephrotoxicity, kidney biopsy demonstrates isometric vacuolization of the proximal tubular epithelium and vascular injury with loss of smooth muscles, myocyte cytoplasmic vacuolization, and dropout from necrosis or apoptosis [40]. Additionally, CNIs may produce endothelial injury through oxidative stress and activation of the alternative complement pathway, contributing to TA-TMA [5, 29].

### Antimicrobials

Antimicrobial agents may lead to various types of kidney injury peri-transplant. Aminoglycosides cause direct proximal tubular injury, whereas amphotericin causes cell membrane injury in the distal tubules, resulting in tubular damage and distal renal tubular acidosis [52]. Ciprofloxacin, acyclovir, and sulfamethoxazole can cause crystalline nephropathy, particularly at high doses and rapid infusions and especially in the setting of volume depletion [45, 52]. Vancomycin is a known cause of acute tubular injury and acute interstitial nephritis and has been associated with increased nephrotoxicity when administered concurrently with piperacillin-tazobactam [53, 54].

### Conditioning Regimen

Both myeloablative and less intensive conditioning regimens have been associated with AKI. High-dose busulfan-, fludarabine-, and TBI-based regimens have been linked to TA-TMA [38].

## Diagnosis

Evaluation of AKI after HSCT is similar to that for the general population, but with special attention to the timing of AKI in relation to transplant, type of transplant, and conditioning regimen [55]. Assessment includes a careful history and physical examination, urinalysis, urine microscopy, urine protein-to-creatinine ratio, and kidney ultrasound [45]. Additional workup for transplant-specific causes of AKI such as CNI toxicity (blood tacrolimus or cyclosporine concentrations), TA-TMA (complete blood count, platelet count, review of the peripheral blood smear for schistocytes, serum markers of hemolysis [lactate dehydrogenase, haptoglobin], serum complement testing [C3, C4, CH50, soluble C5b-9]), hepatic SOS (bilirubin levels, urine sodium, liver ultrasound), and blood BK and adenovirus viral loads should be considered in the appropriate clinical contexts [56–63]. Diagnostic criteria for specific entities, including hepatic SOS and TA-TMA, are detailed elsewhere [56–62].

## Biomarkers

Patients undergoing HSCT may have fluctuations in nutritional status, muscle mass, and weight that influence serum creatinine values and, subsequently, the creatinine-based GFR estimates used to select and dose medications before and after HSCT [63, 64]. Further, as serum creatinine concentration is a late marker of injury, diagnosis of AKI may be delayed in the post-transplant setting [65]. Because detection of subclinical kidney damage and early diagnosis and treatment of AKI are vital for improved patient outcomes, there has been significant recent interest in identifying new biomarkers. Several novel AKI biomarkers (e.g., serum cystatin C, urine neutrophil gelatinase-associated lipocalin [NGAL], urine liver-type fatty acid-binding protein, urinary elafin, and urine alpha macroglobulin) have been evaluated in the research setting but have not entered routine clinical use [66–71]. Increased serum concentrations of neutrophil extracellular traps (NETs) have been shown to predict TA-TMA; however, prospective studies in larger patient populations are necessary [72].

## Role of Kidney Biopsy

While there are no established guidelines addressing the role of kidney biopsy after HSCT, biopsy should be considered when there is AKI of unclear etiology despite the above workup, delayed kidney recovery refractory to initial modifications in therapy, or nephrotic-range proteinuria. Because many transplant patients are thrombocytopenic and/or coagulopathic, biopsy should be performed with appropriate transfusion support and a multidisciplinary approach to patient care [45].

## Management of Post-HSCT AKI

Strategies for the prevention and treatment of post-HSCT AKI are shown in Table 27.1.

## Monitoring and Prevention

Identification of preexisting kidney disease and selection of reduced-intensity conditioning regimens, where appropriate, may help reduce incidence of AKI after HSCT [63, 73]. Post-transplant, careful volume management is critical to AKI prevention, with regular monitoring of weight, blood pressure, intake, and output. Nephrotoxic medications and iodinated contrast agents should be used cautiously, and complications that predispose to AKI such as infections and gastrointestinal GVHD treated promptly [1, 45, 65].

Recent developments that may lower the risk of post-transplant AKI include the use of (1) CNI-free (e.g., cyclophosphamide-based) regimens for GVHD prophylaxis; (2) personalized drug-dosing protocols tailored to individual-patient drug levels; and (3) drug selection and dosing guided by gene polymorphisms involved in the metabolism of chemotherapeutic agents [45, 65, 74–79]. Animal studies are ongoing to investigate the potential nephroprotective role of drugs that impact the renin-angiotensin-aldosterone system after TBI or CNI exposure [80, 81].

## Treatment

### General Measures

In many cases, treatment of AKI after HSCT is supportive. Nephrotoxic medications should be stopped when possible, and medication doses adjusted for level of kidney function [45]. If CNI trough concentrations are elevated, dose reduction should be considered [55]. Care must be taken to prevent and mitigate fluid overload, which has been linked with increased mortality [82–85]. Swift diagnosis of HSCT-specific complications is critical for timely intervention; early nephrology consultation should be considered.

### Kidney Replacement Therapy Considerations

At present, no consensus guidelines exist regarding the best timing of dialysis initiation after post-HSCT AKI. Data supporting earlier (versus later) initiation of KRT in this context come primarily from the pediatric population, with a small recent study demonstrating good outcomes in children with hepatic SOS, AKI, and fluid overload treated with a standardized fluid balance protocol and early initiation of KRT [63, 86]. KRT initiation when there is evidence of pulmonary edema, worsening oxygenation, no response to diuretic dose escalation, and oliguria has been suggested [63].

No randomized controlled trials (RCTs) have compared intermittent hemodialysis (IHD) with continuous renal replacement therapy (CRRT) in the post-HSCT setting, and choice of KRT modality is usually based on hemodynamic stability and volume status [55]. There is some evidence that continuous therapies are associated with less increase in intracranial pressure than IHD, thus making CRRT potentially more appropriate in cases of SOS [55, 87, 88]. Additionally, daily obligate fluid intake after HSCT is often considerable, and fluid balance may be controlled most easily with a continuous modality [55].

## Disease-Specific Considerations

### Hepatic Sinusoidal Obstruction Syndrome

Strategies for the prevention of SOS combine two approaches: (1) reversal of SOS risk factors and (2) pharmacologic intervention [89, 90]. The use of heparin for SOS prophylaxis remains controversial, with two RCTs (one with unfractionated heparin and one with low-molecular-weight heparin) demonstrating a beneficial effect and a subsequent meta-analysis including the above RCTs showing no significant benefit [91–93]. Large RCTs are needed to properly evaluate its use. Data regarding the value of ursodeoxycholic acid for SOS prevention are inconclusive; however, administration of prophylactic ursodeoxycholic acid has been associated with less liver toxicity, less acute GVHD, and improved survival, supporting its use [94]. Defibrotide, an agent with anti-thrombotic, pro-fibrinolytic, and anti-ischemic properties, has shown efficacy in pediatric and high-risk adult allogeneic-HSCT recipients when used for SOS prophylaxis [95, 96]. Additionally, early treatment with defibrotide has shown improved survival in those with severe/very severe SOS as compared with supportive care alone [90, 97–100].

In patients with suspected or established SOS, exposure to hepatotoxic and nephrotoxic drugs should be minimized [101]. Management should aim at preserving intravascular volume and renal blood flow while addressing peripheral edema and ascites with judicious use of diuretics and therapeutic paracentesis [63, 101]. As above, if hemodialysis is indicated, CRRT may be preferred to handle high obligate daily fluid intake and prevent intracranial pressure increase [63, 86–88].

### Transplant-Associated Thrombotic Microangiopathy

Patients with suspected or confirmed TA-TMA should be supported with platelet and red blood cell transfusions and appropriate volume management [38]. Precipitating viral infections and acute GVHD should be sought and treated accordingly [38]. In patients receiving CNIs or mTOR inhibitors for GVHD prophylaxis, replacement with alternative agents (e.g., corticosteroids, mycophenolate mofetil, IL-2 inhibitors, anti-CD20 agents) may be considered, although more evidence is needed [38, 102, 103]. The role of therapeutic plasma exchange remains uncertain, with studies confounded by disease severity, heterogeneous outcome measurements, withdrawal of offending agents, and concomitant administration of other therapies [39, 58, 104–106].

Data regarding the use of immunomodulatory therapies for TA-TMA are limited, with most published experience coming from small observational studies and from the pediatric literature; use should be individualized and with expert guidance. Limited reports in pediatric and adult patients have demonstrated up to 80% response rates with the use of the anti-CD20 monoclonal antibody rituximab [107–110]. Additionally, the discovery of alternative complement pathway abnormalities in the pathophysiology of TA-TMA has led to the use of the C5 inhibitor eculizumab [111–114]. Data come primarily from the pediatric population, with a recent relatively large study of 64 children with high-risk TA-TMA demonstrating 66% 1-year post-HSCT survival after receiving eculizumab, compared with 16.7% in a previously reported untreated cohort [113]. Similar benefits have been reported in adult patients with TA-TMA treated with eculizumab, making this therapy a potential option in selected patients with evidence of complement dysregulation [111, 112, 114]. Defibrotide has been tried in the treatment of TA-TMA with some success [115, 116]. A recent pilot study of 25 high-risk pediatric patients demonstrated a reduced incidence of TA-TMA with administration of prophylactic defibrotide (4% as compared with an 18–40% incidence in a similar population) [117].

#### Viral Infections

Treatment of viral nephritis is often challenging and should be aimed at treating the underlying viral infection (e.g., reduction of immunosuppression for BK virus; cidofovir for adenovirus) [118, 119]. Patients with hemorrhagic cystitis and/or ureteral stenosis must be monitored for urinary obstruction.

## Conclusion

Post-HSCT outcomes have overall improved with progress in recognition of risk factors and specific management of HSCT complications, as well as advancements in critical care. However, AKI remains a common complication and a significant risk factor for early mortality. AKI can occur at any time after transplant in the critically ill patient with a history of HSCT and may present with different pathologies that require targeted interventions. It is essential to identify high-risk individuals and employ preventive measures where appropriate, diagnose AKI early, identify and withdraw offending agents, treat any underlying conditions, monitor renal function, and optimize volume status.

## References

1. Kanduri SR, et al. Incidence and mortality of acute kidney injury in patients undergoing hematopoietic stem cell transplantation: a systematic review and meta-analysis. Q J Med. 2020;113(9):621–32.
2. Krishnappa V, et al. Acute kidney injury in hematopoietic stem cell transplantation: a review. Int J Nephrol. 2016;2016:5163789.
3. Liu H, et al. A multicenter, retrospective study of acute kidney injury in adult patients with nonmyeloablative hematopoietic SCT. Bone Marrow Transplant. 2010;45(1):153–8.
4. Zager RA, et al. Acute renal failure following bone marrow transplantation: a retrospective study of 272 patients. Am J Kidney Dis. 1989;13(3):210–6.
5. Parikh CR, Coca SG. Acute renal failure in hematopoietic cell transplantation. Kidney Int. 2006;69(3):430–5.
6. Abramson M, et al. Acute kidney injury in the modern era of allogeneic hematopoietic stem cell transplantation. Clin J Am Soc Nephrol. 2021:CJN.19801220.
7. Darmon M, et al. Acute kidney injury in critically ill patients with haematological malignancies: results of a multicentre cohort study from the Groupe de Recherche en Réanimation Respiratoire en Onco-Hématologie. Nephrol Dialysis Transpl. 2015;30(12):2006–13.
8. Fadia A, et al. Incidence and outcome of acute renal failure complicating autologous stem cell transplantation for AL amyloidosis. Kidney Int. 2003;63(5):1868–73.
9. Merouani A, et al. Renal function in high dose chemotherapy and autologous hematopoietic cell support treatment for breast cancer. Kidney Int. 1996;50(3):1026–31.
10. Canet E, et al. Acute kidney injury in critically ill Allo-HSCT recipients. Bone Marrow Transplant. 2014;49(8):1121–2.
11. Wang HE, et al. Acute kidney injury and mortality in hospitalized patients. Am J Nephrol. 2012;35(4):349–55.
12. Chertow GM, et al. Acute kidney injury, mortality, length of stay, and costs in hospitalized patients. J Am Soc Nephrol. 2005;16(11):3365–70.
13. Parikh CR, et al. Renal dysfunction in allogeneic hematopoietic cell transplantation. Kidney Int. 2002;62(2):566–73.
14. Kizilbash SJ, et al. Acute kidney injury and the risk of mortality in children undergoing hematopoietic stem cell transplantation. Biol Blood Marrow Transplant. 2016;22(7):1264–70.
15. Tonelli M, et al. Chronic kidney disease and mortality risk: a systematic review. J Am Soc Nephrol. 2006;17(7):2034–47.
16. Kanduri SR, et al. Kidney recovery from acute kidney injury after hematopoietic stem cell transplant: a systematic review and meta-analysis. Cureus. 2021;13(1):e12418.

17. Wu Q, et al. Chronic kidney disease after autologous stem cell transplantation: analysis of a single center experience. Int Urol Nephrol. 2014;46(7):1403–10.
18. Hingorani S. Chronic kidney disease after liver, cardiac, lung, heart-lung, and hematopoietic stem cell transplant. Pediatr Nephrol. 2008;23(6):879–88.
19. Weiss AS, et al. Chronic kidney disease following non-myeloablative hematopoietic cell transplantation. Am J Transplant. 2006;6(1):89–94.
20. Kersting S, Verdonck LF. Chronic kidney disease after nonmyeloablative stem cell transplantation in adults. Biol Blood Marrow Transplant. 2008;14(4):403–8.
21. Abboud I, Peraldi MN, Hingorani S. Chronic kidney diseases in long-term survivors after allogeneic hematopoietic stem cell transplantation: monitoring and management guidelines. Semin Hematol. 2012;49(1):73–82.
22. Kersting S, et al. Chronic kidney disease after myeloablative allogeneic hematopoietic stem cell transplantation. Biol Blood Marrow Transplant. 2007;13(10):1169–75.
23. Kagoya Y, et al. Pretransplant predictors and posttransplant sequels of acute kidney injury after allogeneic stem cell transplantation. Biol Blood Marrow Transplant. 2011;17(3):394–400.
24. Sorror ML, et al. Comorbidity and disease status–based risk stratification of outcomes among patients with acute myeloid leukemia or myelodysplasia receiving allogeneic hematopoietic cell transplantation. J Clin Oncol. 2007;25(27):4246–54.
25. Coppell JA, et al. Hepatic veno-occlusive disease following stem cell transplantation: incidence, clinical course, and outcome. Biol Blood Marrow Transplant. 2010;16(2):157–68.
26. Ozkan HA, Ozkan SG. Hepatic veno-occlusive disease (sinusoidal obstruction syndrome) after hematopoietic stem cell transplantation in adult patients: diagnosis, incidence, prophylaxis, and treatment. Transfus Apher Sci. 2022;61:103372.
27. Corbacioglu S, Jabbour EJ, Mohty M. Risk factors for development of and progression of hepatic veno-occlusive disease/sinusoidal obstruction syndrome. Biol Blood Marrow Transplant. 2019;25(7):1271–80.
28. Hwang DY, et al. High pre-transplant serum ferritin and busulfan-thiotepa conditioning regimen as risk factors for hepatic sinusoidal obstructive syndrome after autologous stem cell transplantation in patients with malignant lymphoma. Leuk Lymphoma. 2016;57(1):51–7.
29. Singh N, et al. Kidney complications of hematopoietic stem cell transplantation. Am J Kidney Dis. 2013;61(5):809–21.
30. Cornell RF, Hari P, Drobyski WR. Engraftment syndrome after autologous stem cell transplantation: an update unifying the definition and management approach. Biol Blood Marrow Transplant. 2015;21(12):2061–8.
31. Irazabal MV, et al. Acute kidney injury during leukocyte engraftment after autologous stem cell transplantation in patients with light-chain amyloidosis. Am J Hematol. 2012;87(1):51–4.
32. Platon L, et al. A reappraisal of ICU and long-term outcome of allogeneic hematopoietic stem cell transplantation patients and reassessment of prognosis factors: results of a 5-year cohort study (2009–2013). Bone Marrow Transplant. 2016;51(2):256–61.
33. Pichereau C, et al. Trajectories of acute graft-versus-host disease and mortality in critically ill allogeneic-hematopoietic stem cell recipients: the Allo-GRRR-OH score. Bone Marrow Transplant. 2020;55(10):1966–74.
34. Fraile P, et al. Chronic graft-versus-host disease of the kidney in patients with allogenic hematopoietic stem cell transplant. Eur J Haematol. 2013;91(2):129–34.
35. Magenau J, Runaas L, Reddy P. Advances in understanding the pathogenesis of graft-versus-host disease. Br J Haematol. 2016;173(2):190–205.
36. Higo S, et al. Acute graft-versus-host disease of the kidney in allogeneic rat bone marrow transplantation. PloS One. 2014;9(12):e115399.
37. Koratala A, et al. Graft-versus-host disease of the kidney. Hematol Oncol Stem Cell Ther. 2020;13(3):178–9.
38. Wanchoo R, et al. Emerging concepts in hematopoietic stem cell transplantation–associated renal thrombotic microangiopathy and prospects for new treatments. Am J Kidney Dis. 2018;72(6):857–65.
39. Laskin BL, et al. Small vessels, big trouble in the kidneys and beyond: hematopoietic stem cell transplantation–associated thrombotic microangiopathy. Blood. 2011;118(6):1452–62.
40. Lusco MA, et al. AJKD atlas of renal pathology: calcineurin inhibitor nephrotoxicity. Am J Kidney Dis. 2017;69(5):e21–2.
41. Beyar-Katz O, et al. Adult nephrotic syndrome after hematopoietic stem cell transplantation: renal pathology is the best predictor of response to therapy. Biol Blood Marrow Transplant. 2016;22(6):975–81.
42. Niscola P, et al. The management of membranous glomerulopathy in allogeneic stem cells transplantation: updated literature. Cardiovasc Hematol Agents Med Chem. 2013;11(1):67–76.
43. Brukamp K, et al. Nephrotic syndrome after hematopoietic cell transplantation: do glomerular lesions represent renal graft-versus-host disease? Clin J Am Soc Nephrol. 2006;1(4):685–94.
44. Pulla B, Barri YM, Anaissie E. Acute renal failure following bone marrow transplantation. Ren Fail. 1998;20(3):421–35.
45. Renaghan AD, et al. Acute kidney injury and CKD associated with hematopoietic stem cell transplantation. Clin J Am Soc Nephrol. 2020;15(2):289–97.
46. Lusco MA, et al. AJKD atlas of renal pathology: polyomavirus nephropathy. Am J Kidney Dis. 2016;68(6):e37–8.
47. Fogo A. Polyoma virus infection. Am J Kidney Dis. 2001;37(1):E1–2.
48. Abudayyeh A, et al. Symptomatic BK virus infection is associated with kidney function decline

and poor overall survival in allogeneic hematopoietic stem cell recipients. Am J Transplant. 2016;16(5):1492–502.
49. Haines HL, et al. Blood, and not urine, BK viral load predicts renal outcome in children with hemorrhagic cystitis following hematopoietic stem cell transplantation. Biol Blood Marrow Transplant. 2011;17(10):1512–9.
50. Hwang YY, et al. BK virus-associated bilateral ureteric stenosis after haematopoietic SCT: viral kinetics and successful treatment. Bone Marrow Transplant. 2013;48(5):745–6.
51. Ito M, et al. Necrotizing tubulointerstitial nephritis associated with adenovirus infection. Hum Pathol. 1991;22(12):1225–31.
52. Downes KJ, et al. Mechanisms of antimicrobial-induced nephrotoxicity in children. J Antimicrob Chemother. 2020;75(1):1–13.
53. Filippone EJ, Kraft WK, Farber JL. The nephrotoxicity of vancomycin. Clin Pharmacol Ther. 2017;102(3):459–69.
54. Hammond DA, et al. Systematic review and meta-analysis of acute kidney injury associated with concomitant vancomycin and piperacillin/tazobactam. Clin Infect Dis. 2017;64(5):666–74.
55. Kennedy CMC. Kidney disease in liver, cardiac, lung, and hematopoietic stem cell transplantation in comprehensive clinical nephrology. Amsterdam: Elsevier; 2019. p. 1272–1281.e1.
56. Cho BS, et al. Validation of recently proposed consensus criteria for thrombotic microangiopathy after allogeneic hematopoietic stem-cell transplantation. Transplantation. 2010;90(8):918–26.
57. Jodele S, et al. Diagnostic and risk criteria for HSCT-associated thrombotic microangiopathy: a study in children and young adults. Blood. 2014;124(4):645–53.
58. Ho VT, et al. Blood and marrow transplant clinical trials network toxicity committee consensus summary: thrombotic microangiopathy after hematopoietic stem cell transplantation. Biol Blood Marrow Transplant. 2005;11(8):571–5.
59. Jones RJ, et al. Venoocclusive disease of the liver following bone marrow transplantation. Transplantation. 1987;44(6):778–83.
60. McDonald GB, et al. Venoocclusive disease of the liver after bone marrow transplantation: diagnosis, incidence, and predisposing factors. Hepatology. 1984;4(1):116–22.
61. Mohty M, et al. Revised diagnosis and severity criteria for sinusoidal obstruction syndrome/veno-occlusive disease in adult patients: a new classification from the European Society for Blood and Marrow Transplantation. Bone Marrow Transplant. 2016;51(7):906–12.
62. Ruutu T, et al. Diagnostic criteria for hematopoietic stem cell transplant-associated microangiopathy: results of a consensus process by an International Working Group. Haematologica. 2007;92(1):95–100.
63. Wanchoo R, et al. Acute kidney injury in hematopoietic stem cell transplantation. Curr Opin Crit Care. 2019;25(6):531–8.
64. Hingorani S, et al. Estimating GFR in adult patients with hematopoietic cell transplant: comparison of estimating equations with an iohexol reference standard. Clin J Am Soc Nephrol. 2015;10(4):601–10.
65. Jagus D, et al. Kidney dysfunction after hematopoietic cell transplantation-etiology, management, and perspectives. Hematol Oncol Stem Cell Ther. 2018;11(4):195–205.
66. Benoit SW, et al. A novel strategy for identifying early acute kidney injury in pediatric hematopoietic stem cell transplantation. Bone Marrow Transplant. 2019;54(9):1453–61.
67. Deger SM, et al. Early diagnostic markers for detection of acute kidney injury in allogeneic hematopoietic stem cell transplant recipients. Exp Clin Transplant. 2020;18(1):98–105.
68. Hingorani S, et al. Urinary elafin and kidney injury in hematopoietic cell transplant recipients. Clin J Am Soc Nephrol. 2015;10(1):12–20.
69. Morito T, et al. Early identification of acute kidney injury after hematopoietic stem cell transplantation by the measurement of urinary biomarkers. Nihon Jinzo Gakkai Shi. 2011;53(8):1150–8.
70. Shingai N, et al. Urinary liver-type fatty acid-binding protein linked with increased risk of acute kidney injury after allogeneic stem cell transplantation. Biol Blood Marrow Transplant. 2014;20(12):2010–4.
71. Taghizadeh-Ghehi M, et al. Urine neutrophil gelatinase associated lipocalin as an early marker of acute kidney injury in hematopoietic stem cell transplantation patients. Ren Fail. 2015;37(6):994–8.
72. Arai Y, et al. Serum neutrophil extracellular trap levels predict thrombotic microangiopathy after allogeneic stem cell transplantation. Biol Blood Marrow Transplant. 2013;19(12):1683–9.
73. Parikh CR, et al. Comparison of ARF after myeloablative and nonmyeloablative hematopoietic cell transplantation. Am J Kidney Dis. 2005;45(3):502–9.
74. Bejanyan N, et al. Sirolimus and mycophenolate mofetil as calcineurin inhibitor-free graft-versus-host disease prophylaxis for reduced-intensity conditioning umbilical cord blood transplantation. Biol Blood Marrow Transplant. 2016;22(11):2025–30.
75. Jacoby E, et al. Single-agent post-transplantation cyclophosphamide as graft-versus-host disease prophylaxis after human leukocyte antigen-matched related bone marrow transplantation for pediatric and young adult patients with hematologic malignancies. Biol Blood Marrow Transplant. 2016;22(1):112–8.
76. McCune J, et al. Personalized dosing of cyclophosphamide in the total body irradiation–cyclophosphamide conditioning regimen: a phase II trial in patients with hematologic malignancy. Clin Pharmacol Therapeut. 2009;85(6):615–22.
77. Punt AM, et al. Simultaneous quantification of busulfan, clofarabine and F-ARA-A using isotope labelled

standards and standard addition in plasma by LC-MS/MS for exposure monitoring in hematopoietic cell transplantation conditioning. J Chromatogr B Analyt Technol Biomed Life Sci. 2017;1055–1056:81–5.
78. Rocha V, et al. Association of drug metabolism gene polymorphisms with toxicities, graft-versus-host disease and survival after HLA-identical sibling hematopoietic stem cell transplantation for patients with leukemia. Leukemia. 2009;23(3):545–56.
79. Sanghavi K, et al. Personalized fludarabine dosing to reduce nonrelapse mortality in hematopoietic stem-cell transplant recipients receiving reduced intensity conditioning. Transl Res. 2016;175:103–115 e4.
80. Mortensen LA, Bistrup C, Thiesson HC. Does mineralocorticoid receptor antagonism prevent calcineurin inhibitor-induced nephrotoxicity? Front Med (Lausanne). 2017;4:210.
81. Moulder JE, Cohen EP, Fish BL. Captopril and losartan for mitigation of renal injury caused by single-dose total-body irradiation. Radiat Res. 2011;175(1):29–36.
82. Foland JA, et al. Fluid overload before continuous hemofiltration and survival in critically ill children: a retrospective analysis. Crit Care Med. 2004;32(8):1771–6.
83. Goldstein SL, et al. Pediatric patients with multi-organ dysfunction syndrome receiving continuous renal replacement therapy. Kidney Int. 2005;67(2):653–8.
84. Grams ME, et al. Fluid balance, diuretic use, and mortality in acute kidney injury. Clin J Am Soc Nephrol. 2011;6(5):966–73.
85. Sethi SK, et al. Unique considerations in renal replacement therapy in children: core curriculum 2014. Am J Kidney Dis. 2014;63(2):329–45.
86. Raina R, et al. The role of continuous renal replacement therapy in the management of acute kidney injury associated with sinusoidal obstruction syndrome following hematopoietic cell transplantation. Pediatr Transplant. 2018;22(2).
87. Arroyo VFJ. Hepatorenal syndrome, in comprehensive clinical nephrology. Amsterdam: Elsevier; 2019. p. 859–869.e1.
88. Gonwa TA, Wadei HM. The challenges of providing renal replacement therapy in decompensated liver cirrhosis. Blood Purif. 2012;33(1–3):144–8.
89. Cheuk DK, et al. Interventions for prophylaxis of hepatic veno-occlusive disease in people undergoing haematopoietic stem cell transplantation. Cochrane Database Syst Rev. 2015;5:CD009311.
90. Mohty M, et al. Sinusoidal obstruction syndrome/veno-occlusive disease: current situation and perspectives—a position statement from the European Society for Blood and Marrow Transplantation (EBMT). Bone Marrow Transplant. 2015;50(6):781–9.
91. Attal M, et al. Prevention of hepatic veno-occlusive disease after bone marrow transplantation by continuous infusion of low-dose heparin: a prospective, randomized trial. Blood. 1992;79(11):2834–40.
92. Imran H, et al. Use of prophylactic anticoagulation and the risk of hepatic veno-occlusive disease in patients undergoing hematopoietic stem cell transplantation: a systematic review and meta-analysis. Bone Marrow Transplant. 2006;37(7):677–86.
93. Or R, et al. Low molecular weight heparin for the prevention of veno-occlusive disease of the liver in bone marrow transplantation patients. Transplantation. 1996;61(7):1067–71.
94. Ruutu T, et al. Ursodeoxycholic acid for the prevention of hepatic complications in allogeneic stem cell transplantation. Blood. 2002;100(6):1977–83.
95. Corbacioglu S, et al. Defibrotide for prophylaxis of hepatic veno-occlusive disease in paediatric haemopoietic stem-cell transplantation: an open-label, phase 3, randomised controlled trial. Lancet. 2012;379(9823):1301–9.
96. Picod A, et al. Defibrotide for sinusoidal obstruction syndrome/veno-occlusive disease prophylaxis in high-risk adult patients: a single-center experience study. Biol Blood Marrow Transplant. 2018;24(7):1471–5.
97. Corbacioglu S, et al. Defibrotide in the treatment of children with veno-occlusive disease (VOD): a retrospective multicentre study demonstrates therapeutic efficacy upon early intervention. Bone Marrow Transplant. 2004;33(2):189–95.
98. Richardson P, et al. Publisher correction: systematic review of defibrotide studies in the treatment of veno-occlusive disease/sinusoidal obstruction syndrome (VOD/SOS). Bone Marrow Transplant. 2019;54(12):2117–9.
99. Richardson PG, et al. Phase 3 trial of defibrotide for the treatment of severe veno-occlusive disease and multi-organ failure. Blood. 2016;127(13):1656–65.
100. Richardson PG, et al. Earlier defibrotide initiation post-diagnosis of veno-occlusive disease/sinusoidal obstruction syndrome improves day +100 survival following haematopoietic stem cell transplantation. Br J Haematol. 2017;178(1):112–8.
101. Carreras E. How I manage sinusoidal obstruction syndrome after haematopoietic cell transplantation. Br J Haematol. 2015;168(4):481–91.
102. Cutler C, et al. Sirolimus and thrombotic microangiopathy after allogeneic hematopoietic stem cell transplantation. Biol Blood Marrow Transplant. 2005;11(7):551–7.
103. Rosenthal J. Hematopoietic cell transplantation-associated thrombotic microangiopathy: a review of pathophysiology, diagnosis, and treatment. J Blood Med. 2016;7:181–6.
104. George JN, et al. Thrombotic thrombocytopenic purpura-hemolytic uremic syndrome following allogeneic HPC transplantation: a diagnostic dilemma. Transfusion. 2004;44(2):294–304.
105. Jodele S, et al. Does early initiation of therapeutic plasma exchange improve outcome in pediatric stem cell transplant-associated thrombotic microangiopathy? Transfusion. 2013;53(3):661–7.

106. Sartain S, et al. Therapeutic plasma exchange does not improve renal function in hematopoietic stem cell transplantation-associated thrombotic microangiopathy: an institutional experience. Biol Blood Marrow Transplant. 2019;25(1):157–62.
107. Au WY, et al. Successful treatment of thrombotic microangiopathy after haematopoietic stem cell transplantation with rituximab. Br J Haematol. 2007;137(5):475–8.
108. Vasko R, et al. Plasmapheresis-refractory thrombotic microangiopathy in a hematopoietic stem cell transplant recipient. Ther Apher Dial. 2011;15(5):507–9.
109. Marr H, et al. Successful treatment of transplant-associated microangiopathy with rituximab. N Z Med J. 2009;122(1292):72–4.
110. Ostronoff M, et al. Life-threatening hemolytic-uremic syndrome treated with rituximab in an allogeneic bone marrow transplant recipient. Bone Marrow Transplant. 2007;39(10):649–51.
111. de Fontbrune FS, et al. Use of eculizumab in patients with allogeneic stem cell transplant-associated thrombotic microangiopathy: a study from the SFGM-TC. Transplantation. 2015;99(9):1953–9.
112. Dhakal P, et al. Eculizumab in transplant-associated thrombotic microangiopathy. Clin Appl Thromb Hemost. 2017;23(2):175–80.
113. Jodele S, et al. Complement blockade for TA-TMA: lessons learned from a large pediatric cohort treated with eculizumab. Blood. 2020;135(13):1049–57.
114. Rudoni J, et al. Eculizumab for transplant-associated thrombotic microangiopathy in adult allogeneic stem cell transplant recipients. Eur J Haematol. 2018;101(3):389–98.
115. Corti P, et al. Defibrotide as a promising treatment for thrombotic thrombocytopenic purpura in patients undergoing bone marrow transplantation. Bone Marrow Transplant. 2002;29(6):542–3.
116. Devadas SK, et al. Successful treatment of transplant associated thrombotic microangiopathy (TA-TMA) with low dose defibrotide. Indian J Hematol Blood Transfus. 2018;34(3):469–73.
117. Higham CS, et al. A pilot trial of prophylactic defibrotide to prevent serious thrombotic microangiopathy in high-risk pediatric patients. Pediatr Blood Cancer. 2022;69:e29641.
118. Lekakis LJ, et al. BK virus nephropathy after allogeneic stem cell transplantation: a case report and literature review. Am J Hematol. 2009;84(4):243–6.
119. Neofytos D, et al. Treatment of adenovirus disease in stem cell transplant recipients with cidofovir. Biol Blood Marrow Transplant. 2007;13(1):74–81.
120. Dalle JH, Giralt SA. Hepatic veno-occlusive disease after hematopoietic stem cell transplantation: risk factors and stratification, prophylaxis, and treatment. Biol Blood Marrow Transplant. 2016;22(3):400–9.

# 28 Gastrointestinal and Hepatic Considerations in Critically Ill Hematopoietic Stem Cell Transplantation Patient

Mohammed Almakadi, Ali Alahmari, and Amal Albeihany

## Introduction

Hematopoietic stem cell transplantation (HSCT) has made groundbreaking progress to become the foundation of therapy for many hematological conditions primarily, or upon disease recurrence since its inception in the 1970s. Scientists and clinicians have worked hand in hand to untangle so many knots in the biological success of stem cell transplantation to evolve from syngeneic to allogeneic sources of hematopoietic stem cells. The path from experimental trials of HSCT to becoming a standard of care therapy exceeding 1 million HSCT procedures worldwide [1] has been difficult as mortality in the early days following stem cell infusion was very high. In addition, the biology behind transplant-related problems was so complex [2]. Despite that, the huge collaborative efforts from all stakeholders made HSCT safely accessible for the treatment of many malignant and nonmalignant hematological conditions [3, 4]. In addition to using allogeneic HSCT to cure for a variety of conditions that cause a state of bone marrow failure, autologous source of HSCT has become the mainstay for securing rapid hematopoietic recovery following high-dose chemotherapy regimen for certain conditions like multiple myeloma. These high-dose chemotherapy protocols are meant to "wipe" residual disease cells in the body yet have a prolonged myeloablative effect on the bone marrow that can be recuperated hastily by means of autologous stem cell infusion [5].

Despite the curative potential of HSCT and the utmost effort to make the process less toxic, HSCT-associated morbidity and mortality are sometimes inevitable. Aside from patients' related factors and the underlying disease status, HSCT complications are largely related to the overall HSCT protocol. The preparative regimens for HSCT are largely dictated by the underlying disease biology and the availability of matched human leukocyte antigen (HLA) donor. However, the modifications in HSCT preparative regimens along with further enhancements in supportive therapies throughout the whole process that the current field has adopted to lessen HSCT-related complications resulted in significant reduction in these complications [6–8].

M. Almakadi (✉) · A. Albeihany
Oncology Center, King Faisal Specialist Hospital and Research Center, Madinah, Saudi Arabia
e-mail: malmakadi@kfshrc.edu.sa

A. Alahmari
Oncology Center, King Faisal Specialist Hospital and Research Center, Riyadh, Saudi Arabia



A. O. Soubani (ed.), *Pulmonary and Critical Care Considerations of Hematopoietic Stem Cell Transplantation*, https://doi.org/10.1007/978-3-031-28797-8_28

**Table 28.1** List of critical HSCT-related hepatobiliary and gastrointestinal tract complications

| |
|---|
| 1. Airway compromise due to severe mucositis |
| 2. Sepsis/septic shock |
| 3. Complicated neutropenic enterocolitis |
| 4. Bowel perforation |
| 5. Gastrointestinal bleeding |
| 6. Disseminated intravascular coagulation |
| 7. Secondary severe electrolyte derangements |
| 8. Hepatic failure |
| 9. Sinusoidal obstruction syndrome with multiorgan failure |

Patients undergoing HSCT are at potential risk for admission to the intensive care unit (ICU) as part of their maximized supportive care for critical HSCT-related adverse events, like organ failure and sepsis [9]. Following ICU admission, mortality rate of HSCT recipients can reach up to 70% with a reduction in 1-year overall survival by around 30% in comparison to HSCT recipients not requiring ICU care [10, 11] (Table 28.1). These worse outcomes of HSCT can vary between specialized centers in HSCT; however, this calls for further advancements in the collective efforts and treatments' guidelines shouldered by healthcare providers that should begin with prioritized and ongoing up-to-date education to spread the awareness about early recognition of HSCT complications, potential prevention measures, and effective accurate timely management according to the current body of evidence.

## Patient's Assessment

When HSCT is planned, HSCT recipients and their potential donors undergo thorough clinical, laboratory, and diagnostic assessments to be cleared for the HSCT process. This routinely includes screening for certain infections, which includes but not limited to human immunodeficiency virus (HIV), viral hepatitis, cytomegalovirus (CMV), and Epstein-Barr virus (EBV). Current modifications into preparative chemotherapy regimen prior to stem cell infusion have allowed many patients with liver dysfunction, who were historically deemed "unfit" for receiving HSCT, to be potential candidates for HSCT. Reduced-intensity conditioning (RIC) or non-myeloablative conditioning chemotherapy has resulted in less transplant-induced hepatic injury. However, allowing for more individualized patients with liver dysfunction and immune-mediated inflammatory conditions like inflammatory bowel disease (IBD) to challenge their ways through HSCT hurdles presented to the treating teams potentially unpredictable tenuous patients that require highest care and support with expected increased risk for decompensated liver function, gastrointestinal tract (GIT) complications, and increased morbidity and mortality. These can be lessened drastically by implementing rigorous hepatic and GIT assessments to ensure fitness for HSCT [12, 13].

## Allogeneic HSCT

First, we will begin discussing issues related to hepatobiliary (HB) or GIT complications in allogeneic HSCT recipients. The days counting begin from the day of stem cell infusion, which is referred to as Day 0. The overall assessment of critically ill allogeneic HSCT recipients with HB or GIT abnormalities should account for the occurrence of signs and/or symptoms of GIT or HB derangements in relation to the timeline of the allogeneic HSCT process (Table 28.2).

**Table 28.2** Time-specific allogeneic HSCT hepatobiliary and gastrointestinal tract complications

| Condition | Timeframe |
|---|---|
| Chemotherapy-induced toxicity | From initiation of conditioning chemotherapy until around Day 14 |
| Mucositis | Following initiation of conditioning chemotherapy until around Day 14 |
| Neutropenic enterocolitis | Following initiation of conditioning chemotherapy until around Day 14 |
| Sinusoidal obstruction syndrome | Within the first 21 days |
| Acute graft-versus-host disease | From around Day 14 until around Day 100 |
| Chronic graft-versus-host disease | From around Day 100 onward |

## Early HSCT Period (Up to Day 100)

HB and GIT abnormalities in critically ill patients that occur very early in the HSCT period are more likely to be related to the baseline health of the liver and GIT than due to the transplant process. It is crucial to assess whether the abnormality is a worsening of an underlying chronic process, recurrence of a recent illness, or a new insult. The host immune system is most vulnerable during this period while awaiting stem cells to engraft and repopulate the bone marrow. Thus, it is important to consider infectious etiologies early on when facing critically ill HSCT patients with complaints that can be manifestations of infections. The major complications to be aware of during the early HSCT period are as follows.

### Pain

One of the most foreseeable complications during the early phase of this period affecting more than 75% of HSCT recipients is mucositis. This occurs due to the breakdown of the mucosal lining of the GIT as a result of conditioning chemotherapy regimens [14]. Patients can suffer from oral pain and dysphagia that can significantly affect their hydration and food intake. Sterile mucositis may take 2–3 weeks to heal as neutrophil count recovers following conditioning chemotherapy. Furthermore, mucositis can occur due to CMV, herpes simplex virus (HSV), candidiasis, and bacterial infections. The incidence of the majority of these infections has become significantly lower following the implementation of routine anti-infective prophylaxis. Mucositis is an important complication to prevent and recognize because it can lead to upper airway edema that could impose airway threat requiring invasive intervention. Strategies to shorten the duration of mucositis and lessen the severity of symptoms include frequent mouth rinsing, use of ice chips, bicarbonate-based mouth rinses, topical anesthetics, and opioids. Generous parenteral hydration and nutrition should be initiated for patients with severe cases to avoid renal injury and hasten their recovery [15].

Commonly occurring systemic infections with secondary evidence of transaminitis, liver dysfunction, or hyperbilirubinemia should be investigated like critically ill patients who are not HSCT recipients. HSCT recipients who experience tender hepatomegaly should prompt workup for fungal infection including dedicated imaging and liver biopsy if feasible to rule out fungal abscesses for better sensitive selection of antifungal strategy [16]. Patients who are transfusion dependents due to certain underlying conditions are at risk for iron overload, which has been associated with increased risk for invasive mold infections [17].

Other causes of abdominal pain during this period include peptic ulcer disease, pancreatitis, or cholecystitis. These conditions can be very challenging to manage due to expected patients' low blood counts that can preclude surgical interventions [15]. Although it is rare, acute pancreatitis can occur secondary to commonly used medications in HSCT recipients like trimethoprim/sulfamethoxazole, cyclosporine, and corticosteroids. The management is mainly supportive and to hold or discontinue offending drugs [18]. Another important, yet rare cause of abdominal pain is intestinal pseudo-obstruction. It occurs due to increased inflammatory state from sepsis, or prolonged use of narcotics, or due to electrolyte disturbances. Treatment is mainly conservative by maximizing supportive therapy and addressing the potential underlying etiology [19]. Clinicians taking care of HSCT recipients in the ICU should always have a high index of suspicion toward early warning symptoms and signs so they can initiate appropriate management sooner to defer unnecessary early surgical interventions that can bring significant mortality and morbidity. Early successful and aggressive supportive management is associated with better outcomes [20].

### Diarrhea

Diarrhea usually affects the majority of HSCT patients due to toxicity of radiation or high-dose chemotherapy conditioning within the following first 2 weeks causing severe mucosal inflammation that can be debilitating due to fluid losses and electrolyte disturbances [21, 22]. Infectious causes of diarrhea constitute up to 15% of cases; however, diarrhea in HSCT patients should always trigger infectious causes workup to rule out *Clostridium difficile* infection [22]. Endoscopic evaluation with or without biopsy procedure might be necessary in some cases, but it can be limited by the degree of cytopenia secondary to bone marrow suppression.

### Neutropenic Enterocolitis

Neutropenic enterocolitis (NE) can be a life-threatening complication that occurs in patients with neutropenia. Cell-toxic radiation or chemotherapy compromises the mucosal integrity of the GIT in neutropenic patients becoming an "open door" for microbial translocation. Typhlitis refers to cecal inflammation in patients with neutropenia [23]. The microbial spectrum is variable including gram-negative bacilli (*Pseudomonas aeruginosa, Escherichia coli, Klebsiella* species), gram-positive cocci (enterococci, *Streptococcus viridans*), anaerobes (*Clostridium* species, *Bacteroides* species), and fungi (*Candida species*) [24].

The diagnosis necessitates clinical suspicion when neutropenic patients present with fever and abdominal pain that is commonly located in the right lower quadrant. Severe cases leading to bowel perforation can manifest with abdominal distension, gastrointestinal bleeding, peritonitis, and shock [24]. Computed tomography (CT) is the best diagnostic modality if NE is suspected that can show mucosal thickening, fat stranding, and pneumatosis in severe cases [25].

In general, patients with NE should receive expedited aggressive supportive therapy according to the severity of the condition and occurrence of complications. This includes bowel rest, intravenous (IV) hydration, nutritional support, blood product transfusion, and broad-spectrum antibiotics. Antifungals should be considered if fever persists longer than 72 h despite appropriate antibacterial coverage [26]. When appropriate, granulocyte colony-stimulating factor (G-CSF) should be considered in severe cases to accelerate neutrophil recovery [24].

### Acute Graft-Versus-Host Disease (GVHD)

GVHD is a common complication of HSCT that can affect multiple organs because of immunological attack of the donor's lymphoid cells against the "foreign" recipient's tissues. It is usually biphasic. The acute phase of GVHD typically manifests with GIT, skin, and liver involvements. Chronic GVHD will be discussed later in this chapter. GVHD can still occur despite current advances in prophylactic immunosuppressive therapy in up to 50% of allogeneic HSCT patients [27–29].

Acute GVHD of the GIT presents with nausea, vomiting, decreased oral intake, and commonly diarrhea [30]. Hepatic involvement can be suggested if patients develop worsening liver enzymes. The diagnosis requires tissue biopsy confirmation, and the severity of the symptoms needs to be graded to direct choice of therapy [31]. Treatment is mainly supportive care, and systemic and local corticosteroids are the principal first-line therapy [32]. Unfortunately, prognosis can be worse in severe cases and sometimes fatal in refractory cases [33].

### Jaundice

In preparation for HSCT, patients require conditioning chemotherapy that can cause transaminitis or impairment of liver function [16, 34]. In addition, this period is characterized by inevitable reactivation of donor's acquired or recipient's dormant infections due to immunosuppressive therapy. Severe cases of acute viral hepatitis typically happen due to reactivation of adenovirus, herpes simplex virus, varicella zoster virus, EBV, and hepatitis B virus [35]. Hepatitis C and CMV can rarely cause severe cases of hepatitis [12]. To prevent patients from acquiring most of these infections, early use of anti-infective prophylaxis is essential. In case of hepatitis B, longer duration of antiviral prophylaxis is recommended even after full immune reconstitution as fulminant hepatitis B cases can still occur with premature discontinuation of antiviral prophylaxis [36]. Resistant fungal infections should be suspected in patients on prophylactic antifungals, and the antifungal regimen should be adjusted. However, it is not unusual for some fungal infections to show a state of refractoriness to antifungal treatment that can begin to resolve after full recovery of healthy neutrophils production [37].

Hepatic sinusoidal obstruction syndrome (SOS) can be a serious complication during this period, and it is hallmarked by the co-occurrence of tender hepatomegaly, hyperbilirubinemia, and weight gain due to fluid retention [38]. Despite certain patient-related risk factors that can increase the likelihood of developing hepatic SOS, the adoption of RIC along with the limited usage of certain high-risk conditioning regimen like high-dose cyclophosphamide or total body irradiation has led to a drastic reduction in the incidence and severity of SOS [16, 39].

There should be a high index of suspicion for SOS in all allogeneic HSCT recipients who develop painful hepatomegaly, ascites, jaundice, refractory thrombocytopenia, and/or weight gain typically within 21 days from stem cell infusion. Other than transjugular liver biopsy, no certain tests can provisionally confirm this condition [35, 40]. After ruling out mimickers, the diagnosis of hepatic SOS is mainly clinically suggested that can be based on the revised European Society for Blood and Marrow Transplantation (EBMT) criteria. Accordingly, classical SOS diagnosis requires the presence of hyperbilirubinemia ≥2 mg/dL *and* two of the following: tender hepatomegaly, weight gain >5%, or ascites. Late-onset SOS (≥21 days after HSCT) diagnosis requires classical SOS criteria; or histopathological-proven SOS; or ultrasound or hemodynamic evidence of SOS *and* at least two of the following: hyperbilirubinemia ≥2 mg/dL, tender hepatomegaly, weight gain >5%, or ascites [41]. Other clinical criteria for diagnosing SOS include the modified Seattle criteria [42] and the Baltimore criteria [43].

The current backbone of therapy for SOS is prevention. Once clinically suspected, the revised EBMT grading system categorizes patients into mild, moderate, severe, and very severe [41]. Severe cases of SOS have a mortality rate reaching up to 80% majorly due to cardiopulmonary or renal failure rather than hepatic failure [44, 45]. In all cases, the main goal is to keep patients in euvolemic state using diuretics and fluid removal, and minimizing hepatotoxic medications. Patients should be weighed daily to assess their weight loss response. Ursodeoxycholic acid (UDCA) is very effective as primary prophylaxis against SOS by reducing hydrophobicity of bile acids and should be continued even if SOS develops [46]. Additionally in severe cases, defibrotide has shown some survival benefits in addition to aggressive supportive therapy [47].

## Late HSCT Period (Day 100+)

This period usually coincides with gradual tapering of immunosuppressive therapy following stem cells engraftment. Majority of HSCT-related complications during this late period and onward are either a continuum or recurrence of an earlier event. The most important complications are as follows.

### Chronic GVHD

Chronic GVHD involves chronic inflammation and fibrosis leading sometimes to permanent damage of the affected organs. It is hallmarked by inflammation akin to what happens in acute GVHD, but it persists longer due to imbalanced regulatory immune responses against chronic inflammation. This is coupled with an aberrant tissue repair mechanism leading to tissue fibrosis and scarring [48].

If the GIT is affected by chronic GVHD, patients will have narrowing and strictures that can cause luminal obstruction. Progression of early lesions can be slowed medically; however, advanced strictures may require repetitive interventional or surgical corrections [15]. Chronic GVHD of the liver can present as hepatitis that can be managed by increasing immunosuppression therapy with or without addition of corticosteroids [49].

### Iron Overload

Patients with hematological malignancies on chemotherapy usually receive multiple packed red blood cell transfusions to supplement their physiological recovery while the bone marrow is recovering from myelosuppression. The inevitable consequence of these multiple transfusions is hemosiderosis that should be addressed once patients become transfusion independent before it leads to organ damage. In the majority of cases, patients will undergo therapeutic phlebotomies. In a few cases when patients cannot tolerate therapeutic phlebotomy sessions, they are managed with iron chelators [50].

## Autologous HSCT

Majority of the complications following autologous HSCT are related to the conditioning chemotherapy regimen. Autologous HSCT recipients commonly sustain GIT injury, especially mucositis. They are also at risk for developing HB chemotherapy-induced cytotoxic injury that can be serious, requiring removal of any additionally hepatotoxic medication and maximizing supportive care [51]. In addition, all autologous HSCT patients will become neutropenic, which can increase the risk for infections, especially serious bacterial infections [52]. They are also at risk for typhlitis or NE. If NE occurs, it should be managed aggressively as described previously.

## References


1. Gratwohl A, et al. One million haemopoietic stem-cell transplants: a retrospective observational study. Lancet Haematol. 2015;2(3):e91–100.
2. Singh AK, McGuirk JP. Allogeneic stem cell transplantation: a historical and scientific overview. Cancer Res. 2016;76(22):6445–51.
3. Burt RK, et al. Clinical applications of blood-derived and marrow-derived stem cells for nonmalignant diseases. JAMA. 2008;299(8):925–36.
4. Gratwohl A, et al. Hematopoietic stem cell transplantation: a global perspective. JAMA. 2010;303(16):1617–24.
5. Barlogie B, et al. High-dose melphalan with autologous bone marrow transplantation for multiple myeloma. Blood. 1986;67(5):1298–301.
6. McSweeney PA, et al. Hematopoietic cell transplantation in older patients with hematologic malignancies: replacing high-dose cytotoxic therapy with graft-versus-tumor effects. Blood. 2001;97(11):3390–400.
7. Alyea EP, et al. Impact of conditioning regimen intensity on outcome of allogeneic hematopoietic cell transplantation for advanced acute myelogenous leukemia and myelodysplastic syndrome. Biol Blood Marrow Transplant. 2006;12(10):1047–55.
8. Luger SM, et al. Similar outcomes using myeloablative vs reduced-intensity allogeneic transplant preparative regimens for AML or MDS. Bone Marrow Transplant. 2012;47(2):203–11.
9. Benz R, et al. Risk factors for ICU admission and ICU survival after allogeneic hematopoietic SCT. Bone marrow transplantation. 2014;49(1):62–5.
10. Hahn T, et al. Significant improvement in survival after allogeneic hematopoietic cell transplantation during a period of significantly increased use, older recipient age, and use of unrelated donors. J Clin Oncol. 2013;31(19):2437–49.
11. Bayraktar UD, Nates JL. Intensive care outcomes in adult hematopoietic stem cell transplantation patients. World J Clin Oncol. 2016;7(1):98–105.
12. Strasser SI, et al. Hepatitis C virus infection and bone marrow transplantation: a cohort study with 10-year follow-up. Hepatology. 1999;29(6):1893–9.
13. Mehta K, et al. In-patient outcomes of hematopoietic stem cell transplantation in patients with immune mediated inflammatory diseases: a nationwide study. Sci Rep. 2018;8(1):6825.
14. Vera-Llonch M, et al. Oral mucositis and outcomes of allogeneic hematopoietic stem-cell transplantation in patients with hematologic malignancies. Support Care Cancer. 2007;15(5):491–6.
15. Tuncer HH, et al. Gastrointestinal and hepatic complications of hematopoietic stem cell transplantation. World J Gastroenterol. 2012;18(16):1851–60.
16. McDonald GB. Hepatobiliary complications of hematopoietic cell transplantation, 40 years on. Hepatology. 2010;51(4):1450–60.
17. Kontoyiannis DP, et al. Increased bone marrow iron stores is an independent risk factor for invasive aspergillosis in patients with high-risk hematologic malignancies and recipients of allogeneic hematopoietic stem cell transplantation. Cancer. 2007;110(6):1303–6.
18. Shore T, et al. Pancreatitis post-bone marrow transplantation. Bone Marrow Transplant. 1996;17(6):1181–4.
19. Yahng SA, et al. Acute colonic pseudo-obstruction following allogeneic stem cell transplantation successfully treated by neostigmine. Blood Res. 2013;48(2):145–8.
20. Tarantino G, et al. Gastrointestinal complications after allogeneic hematopoietic stem cell transplant: a multidisciplinary approach with early endoscopic evaluation. Clin Hematol Int. 2021;3(4):161–8.
21. Goldberg J, et al. Gastrointestinal toxicity from the preparative regimen is associated with an increased risk of graft-versus-host disease. Biol Blood Marrow Transplant. 2005;11(2):101–7.
22. Robak K, et al. Diarrhea after allogeneic stem cell transplantation: beyond graft-versus-host disease. Eur J Gastroenterol Hepatol. 2017;29(5):495–502.
23. Rolston KV, Bodey GP, Safdar A. Polymicrobial infection in patients with cancer: an underappreciated and underreported entity. Clin Infect Dis. 2007;45(2):228–33.
24. Nesher L, Rolston KV. Neutropenic enterocolitis, a growing concern in the era of widespread use of aggressive chemotherapy. Clin Infect Dis. 2013;56(5):711–7.
25. Kirkpatrick ID, Greenberg HM. Gastrointestinal complications in the neutropenic patient: characterization

and differentiation with abdominal CT. Radiology. 2003;226(3):668–74.
26. Mullassery D, et al. Diagnosis, incidence, and outcomes of suspected typhlitis in oncology patients--experience in a tertiary pediatric surgical center in the United Kingdom. J Pediatr Surg. 2009;44(2):381–5.
27. Filipovich AH, et al. National Institutes of Health consensus development project on criteria for clinical trials in chronic graft-versus-host disease: I. diagnosis and staging working group report. Biol Blood Marrow Transplant. 2005;11(12):945–56.
28. Jagasia M, et al. Risk factors for acute GVHD and survival after hematopoietic cell transplantation. Blood. 2012;119(1):296–307.
29. Lee SE, et al. Risk and prognostic factors for acute GVHD based on NIH consensus criteria. Bone Marrow Transplant. 2013;48(4):587–92.
30. Weisdorf DJ, et al. Acute upper gastrointestinal graft-versus-host disease: clinical significance and response to immunosuppressive therapy. Blood. 1990;76(3):624–9.
31. Rowlings PA, et al. IBMTR severity index for grading acute graft-versus-host disease: retrospective comparison with Glucksberg grade. Br J Haematol. 1997;97(4):855–64.
32. Martin PJ, et al. First- and second-line systemic treatment of acute graft-versus-host disease: recommendations of the American Society of Blood and Marrow Transplantation. Biol Blood Marrow Transplant. 2012;18(8):1150–63.
33. Leisenring WM, et al. An acute graft-versus-host disease activity index to predict survival after hematopoietic cell transplantation with myeloablative conditioning regimens. Blood. 2006;108(2):749–55.
34. Bodge MN, et al. Preparative regimen dosing for hematopoietic stem cell transplantation in patients with chronic hepatic impairment: analysis of the literature and recommendations. Biol Blood Marrow Transplant. 2014;20(5):622–9.
35. Sakai M, et al. Severe hepatocellular injury after hematopoietic cell transplant: incidence, etiology and outcome. Bone Marrow Transplant. 2009;44(7):441–7.
36. Wu Y, Huang H, Luo Y. Management of hepatitis B virus in allogeneic hematopoietic stem cell transplantation. Front Immunol. 2020;11:610500.
37. Marotta G, et al. Complete resolution of hepatic aspergillosis after non-myeloablative hematopoietic stem cell transplantation in a patient with acute myeloid leukemia. Hematology. 2005;10(5):383–6.
38. Chitturi S, Farrell GC. Etiopathogenesis of nonalcoholic steatohepatitis. Semin Liver Dis. 2001;21(1):27–41.
39. Donelli MG, et al. Pharmacokinetics of anticancer agents in patients with impaired liver function. Eur J Cancer. 1998;34(1):33–46.
40. Carreras E, et al. Transjugular liver biopsy in BMT. Bone Marrow Transplant. 1993;11(1):21–6.
41. Mohty M, et al. Revised diagnosis and severity criteria for sinusoidal obstruction syndrome/veno-occlusive disease in adult patients: a new classification from the European Society for Blood and Marrow Transplantation. Bone Marrow Transplant. 2016;51(7):906–12.
42. McDonald GB, et al. Venoocclusive disease of the liver after bone marrow transplantation: diagnosis, incidence, and predisposing factors. Hepatology. 1984;4(1):116–22.
43. Jones RJ, et al. Venoocclusive disease of the liver following bone marrow transplantation. Transplantation. 1987;44(6):778–83.
44. Coppell JA, et al. Hepatic veno-occlusive disease following stem cell transplantation: incidence, clinical course, and outcome. Biol Blood Marrow Transplant. 2010;16(2):157–68.
45. Carreras E. How I manage sinusoidal obstruction syndrome after haematopoietic cell transplantation. Br J Haematol. 2015;168(4):481–91.
46. Cheuk DK, et al. Interventions for prophylaxis of hepatic veno-occlusive disease in people undergoing haematopoietic stem cell transplantation. Cochrane Database Syst Rev. 2015;5:CD009311.
47. Richardson PG, et al. Phase 3 trial of defibrotide for the treatment of severe veno-occlusive disease and multi-organ failure. Blood. 2016;127(13):1656–65.
48. Cooke KR, et al. The biology of chronic graft-versus-host disease: a task force report from the National Institutes of Health consensus development project on criteria for clinical trials in chronic graft-versus-host disease. Biol Blood Marrow Transplant. 2017;23(2):211–34.
49. Akpek G, et al. Hepatitic variant of graft-versus-host disease after donor lymphocyte infusion. Blood. 2002;100(12):3903–7.
50. Koreth J, Antin JH. Iron overload in hematologic malignancies and outcome of allogeneic hematopoietic stem cell transplantation. Haematologica. 2010;95(3):364–6.
51. Lambertenghi Deliliers G, Annaloro C, Lambertenghi Deliliers D. Complications of autologous hematopoietic stem cell transplantation. Haematologia (Budap). 2000;30(4):253–62.
52. Mossad SB, et al. Early infectious complications in autologous bone marrow transplantation: a review of 219 patients. Bone Marrow Transplant. 1996;18(2):265–71.

# 29 Neurologic Considerations in Critically Ill Hematopoietic Stem Cell Transplantation Patients

Kiddy Levente Ume and Rajat Dhar

## Introduction

Hematopoietic stem cell transplantation (HSCT) as a treatment for hematological malignancies and genetic disorders has been on the rise in recent years [1]. The use of reduced-intensity conditioning (RIC) regimens and improvements in supportive care have allowed the expansion of HSCT to patient populations that were considered ineligible in the past (e.g., elderly patients with advanced disease and more comorbidities); however, such patients are more prone to post-transplantation complications [2]. Neurological complications are a significant cause of both early and delayed morbidity and contribute to transplant-related mortality (TRM) [3]. A landmark study of 302 consecutive HSCT patients from the early twenty-first century found that complications affecting the central nervous system (CNS) occurred in 18% at 100 days and 23% at 1 year (Fig. 29.1) [4]. Survival was worse in those with CNS complications. The most common complications observed were drug neurotoxicities, especially posterior reversible encephalopathy syndrome (PRES), other metabolic encephalopathies, and CNS infections. Similar rates of complications and their negative prognostic implications have since been corroborated in several further studies [5, 6], with some demonstrating that most complications occur early after transplantation [3, 7]. However, other complications can occur months to years after HSCT, so careful screening and vigilant surveillance remain critical. The tension between more careful drug dosing, prophylaxis, and monitoring, balanced against more vulnerable patients undergoing HSCT, means that the incidence of complications has not changed significantly, remaining around 20% in many contemporary studies [3, 6, 8]. The most common presentations included seizures and altered mental status (encephalopathy). However, these are nonspecific and may be preceded by more subtle symptoms and signs, such as headache, tremor, or visual disturbances, making accurate and specific diagnoses challenging early on. The heterogeneity in presentation and ascertainment also explains why estimates of incidence vary greatly; a study including minor complications found a total incidence of 56% [9]. Table 29.1 provides a

K. L. Ume · R. Dhar (✉)
Department of Neurology (Division of Neurocritical Care), Washington University in St. Louis School of Medicine, St. Louis, MO, USA
e-mail: ume@wustl.edu; dharr@wustl.edu



A. O. Soubani (ed.), *Pulmonary and Critical Care Considerations of Hematopoietic Stem Cell Transplantation*, https://doi.org/10.1007/978-3-031-28797-8_29

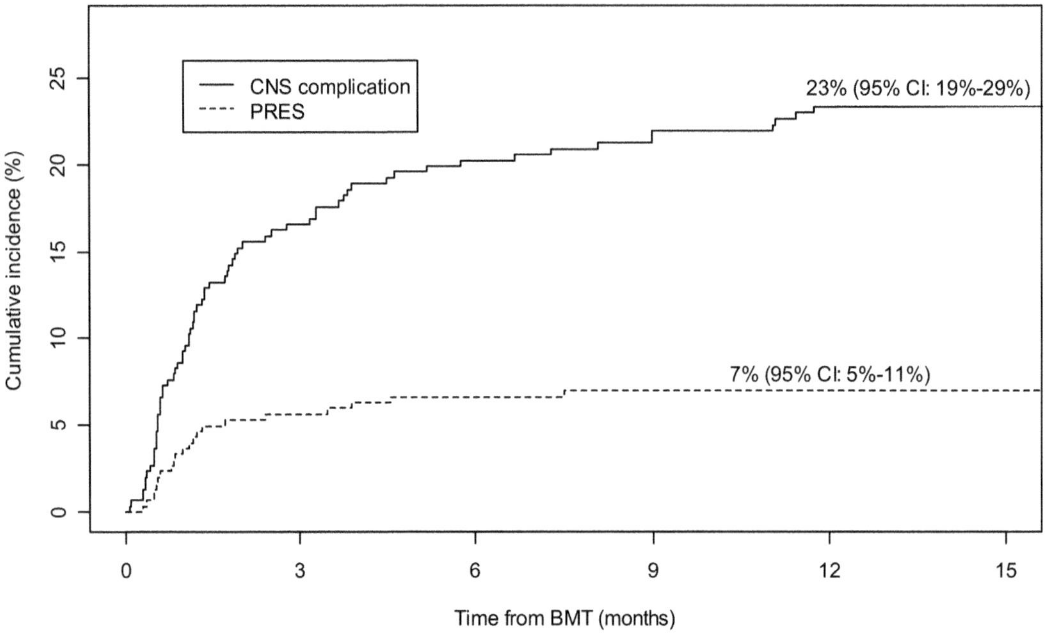


**Fig. 29.1** The cumulative incidences of all CNS complications and of PRES after HSCT [With permission from Siegal D, et al. Central nervous system complications after allogeneic hematopoietic stem cell transplantation: incidence, manifestations, and clinical significance. Biol Blood Marrow Transplant. 2007;13(11):1369–79]

**Table 29.1** Major diagnostic considerations for common neurologic presentations after HSCT, divided by those occurring early versus late after transplant

| Presenting syndrome | Early (<60 days after HSCT) | Late (≥60 days after HSCT) |
|---|---|---|
| Seizures | • PRES<br>• Other drug toxicity<br>• Subdural hematoma | • Drug toxicity<br>– Cytotoxic agents<br>– Antibiotics<br>• CNS infections |
| Delirium/ encephalopathy | • Metabolic: uremia or hepatic failure, SIRS, sepsis<br>• PRES<br>• Meningitis | • Metabolic<br>• Viral or fungal encephalitis<br>• PML<br>• IRIS (rare) |
| Focal deficits | • Subdural hematoma<br>• Acute ischemic or hemorrhagic stroke | • Brain abscess: fungal or bacterial<br>• GVHD<br>– Vasculitis<br>– CNS demyelinating disease |
| Generalized weakness | • Deconditioning<br>• Critical illness myopathy or neuropathy<br>• Immune-mediated polyneuropathy (GBS) | • Immune-mediated polyneuropathy (GBS)<br>• Drug toxicity<br>– Steroid myopathy<br>– Tacrolimus-induced polymyositis or plexitis<br>• GVHD<br>– Myasthenia gravis<br>– Myositis |

*PRES* posterior reversible encephalopathy syndrome, *PML* progressive multifocal leukoencephalopathy, *SIRS* systemic inflammatory response syndrome, *IRIS* immune reconstitution inflammatory syndrome, *GBS* Guillain-Barré syndrome, *GVHD* graft-versus-host disease

high-level overview, highlighting major differential diagnoses to be considered for common neurological presentations in the early or delayed periods after HSCT. The remainder of this chapter provides greater details into specific complications and their evaluation and management, with a focus on those likely to occur in the critical care setting.

## Drug-Related Neurotoxicity

Transplant patients are exposed to numerous potentially neurotoxic medications as part of their management. Neurological complications can result from immunosuppressants, cytotoxic agents, monoclonal antibodies, antibiotics, or a combination of these. Drug–drug interactions may play a pivotal role when several drugs with potentially different neurotoxicities are administered simultaneously [10].

### Calcineurin Inhibitors

Calcineurin inhibitors (CNIs), such as cyclosporine and tacrolimus, are immunosuppressants frequently used for prophylaxis of graft-versus-host disease (GVHD) and carry a high risk of drug-related neurotoxicity [11]. They work by binding to proteins called immunophilins to form a complex that inhibits calcineurin. This results in inhibition of calcium-dependent signaling pathways that release interleukin-2 and activate T cells [12]. The exact mechanism of their neurotoxicity remains unclear, but previous studies point to neuronal apoptosis mainly involving oligodendrocytes [13], leading to a disruption of the blood–brain barrier [14] and resulting in the development of vasogenic edema [15]. Dysregulation of neuronal excitability through calcineurin inhibition may also contribute [16]. Although levels of CNIs may be elevated or toxicity may follow drug loading, drug levels are often normal in those with symptoms. Additional factors that may play a role in toxicity include high blood pressure, hypomagnesemia, renal dysfunction, and umbilical cord blood transplant [6].

CNI toxicity may present with a myriad of symptoms often beginning with relatively minor complaints (e.g. headache, paresthesias, tremor – seen in up to half of treated patients), with early neuropsychiatric (e.g., insomnia, anxiety, agitation) and visual disturbances. These symptoms may occur in isolation (if detected early and treatment is modified) or progress to the development of overt delirium with hallucinations and delusions that may culminate in seizures and persistent encephalopathy. Seizures are a particularly common presentation of CNI toxicity. Postictal focal deficits, aphasia, and cortical blindness have also been described [10]. A peculiar state of akinetic mutism has been reported with tacrolimus [17, 18].

The radiographic hallmark of CNI neurotoxicity is PRES, an entity consisting of a magnetic resonance imaging (MRI) pattern of multifocal or confluent areas of T2 and FLAIR-signal hyperintensity (i.e., vasogenic edema) most often in the white matter of occipital lobes, but occasionally involving other sites, such as the cerebellum, brainstem, or basal ganglia [19] (Fig. 29.2). It is one of the most common neurological complications after HSCT: a prospective series found PRES in 7% of HSCT recipients by 1 year, with most cases being diagnosed within the first 30–100 days [4] (Fig. 29.1). Critically, PRES is rapidly reversible if recognized promptly and the inciting agent is stopped. Blood pressure control and correction of hypomagnesemia should also be considered. Anticonvulsant agents, commonly non-enzyme inducers such as levetiracetam, should be provided to those with seizures but can be discontinued after a few weeks once PRES resolves. If PRES is not recognized and it progresses, hemorrhage and permanent neurological deficits can develop [18].

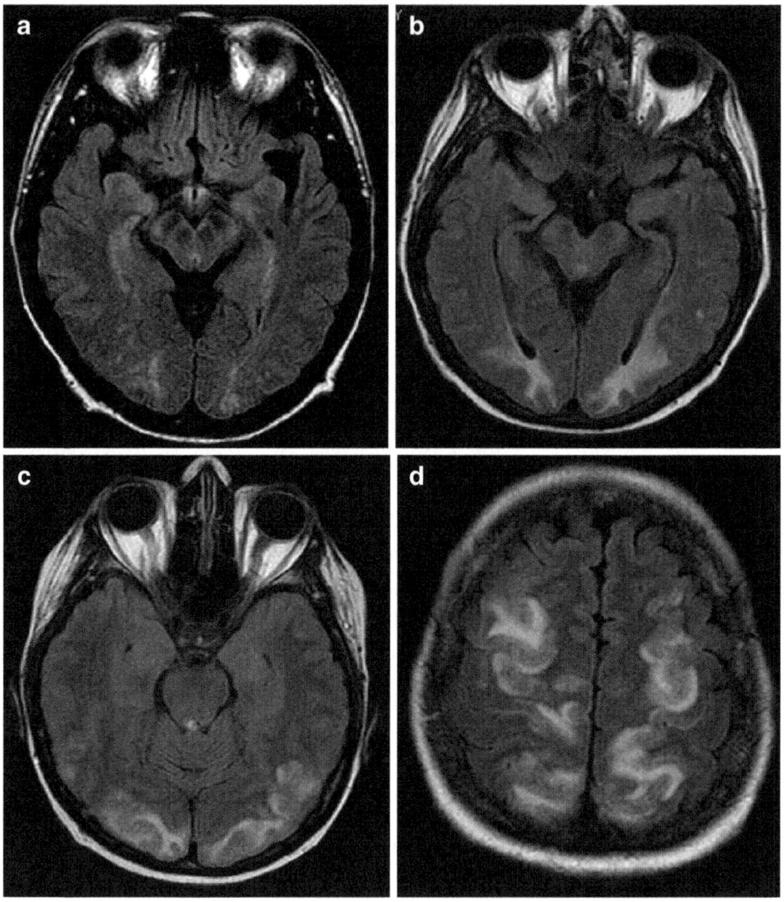


**Fig. 29.2** Axial FLAIR images of the brain demonstrating mild (**a**), moderate (**b**), and severe (**c** and **d**) forms of PRES [With permission from Siegal D, et al. Central nervous system complications after allogeneic hematopoietic stem cell transplantation: incidence, manifestations, and clinical significance. Biol Blood Marrow Transplant. 2007;13(11):1369–79]

## Cytotoxic Agents

Busulfan, a total-body-irradiation-sparing agent used in HSCT, is known for causing direct neurotoxicity and decreasing the seizure threshold in a dose-dependent fashion. It crosses the blood–brain barrier and can accumulate in the cerebrospinal fluid [10]. Seizures can occur in up to 10% of patients [20]. This risk can be lowered by up to eightfold by using prophylactic antiseizure medications [21]. Existing data support the use of benzodiazepines, most notably clonazepam and lorazepam, to prevent busulfan-induced seizures [22]. In addition, second-generation antiepileptic drugs, such as levetiracetam, can be added, but phenytoin should be avoided due to possible toxicities and its ability to induce busulfan metabolism [22]. Fludarabine, another cytotoxic agent, has been linked to PRES as well as another white matter syndrome termed acute toxic leukoencephalopathy (ATL). This involves the deep and periventricular white matter more symmetrically and is more likely to have diffusion-weighted changes on MRI. PRES and ATL combined were seen in 2.4% of fludarabine exposures in one series [23]. PRES was more likely to present with seizures and hypertension, while ATL was more likely to present with cognitive disturbances and focal neurological deficits. Survival was worse in those with either toxicity, but neurological deficits were more persistent and more deaths were directly attributable to ATL. Ifosfamide, an isomer of cyclophosphamide, has been associated with encephalopathy, delirium, seizures, and cerebellar dysfunction, especially in the setting of low albumin [24]. Methylene blue [25] and vitamin B1 (thiamine) [26] have been proposed as beneficial in treating

**Table 29.2** Drugs associated with neurological symptoms and syndromes

| Neurological symptom/ syndrome | Drug |
|---|---|
| PRES | CNI (e.g., cyclosporine, tacrolimus)<br>Fludarabine, etoposide<br>Steroids<br>Acyclovir<br>Monoclonal antibodies |
| Acute toxic leukoencephalopathy | Fludarabine<br>Methotrexate<br>Cranial irradiation |
| Other nonspecific severe encephalopathy | Fludarabine, ifosfamide, carmustine<br>Cefepime, acyclovir<br>Amphotericin B (w/wo parkinsonism) |
| Seizures | Busulfan, cytarabine<br>β-Lactam antibiotics<br>Drugs that cause PRES and ATL |
| Lymphocytic meningitis | Cytarabine, thiotepa<br>ATG, OKT3 |
| PML | Alemtuzumab, rituximab |
| Cerebellar toxicity | Cytarabine, ifosfamide<br>Metronidazole |
| Neuropathy | Carmustine, etoposide<br>Metronidazole |
| Hallucinations | Voriconazole |

*PRES* posterior reversible encephalopathy syndrome, *CNI* calcineurin inhibitor, *ATL* acute toxic leukoencephalopathy, *ATG* antithymocyte globulin, *PML* progressive multifocal leukoencephalopathy

ifosfamide-associated neurotoxicity. A summary of the spectrum of neurological symptoms and syndromes associated with both cytotoxic agents and other drug classes encountered after HSCT is provided in Table 29.2.

## Monoclonal Antibodies

Alemtuzumab, an anti-CD52 monoclonal antibody, and rituximab, a chimeric anti-CD20 monoclonal antibody, have both been associated with an elevated risk of progressive multifocal leukoencephalopathy (PML). This is a subacute demyelinating disease caused by JC virus infection/reactivation (discussed in detail in the section on Infectious Complications). Symptoms include cognitive decline, aphasia, and ataxia [10]. Other monoclonal antibodies have recently been applied for reducing tumor burden or promoting long-term disease control (tyrosine kinase inhibitors or, more recently, blinatumomab) and have been implicated in the development of PRES and other toxic encephalopathies causing confusion or aphasia [27, 28].

## Antimicrobials

Acyclovir, which is used for herpes simplex virus (HSV)/varicella-zoster virus (VZV) prophylaxis and treatment, may cause neurologic complications especially in those with renal impairment [10, 29]. Approximately 90% of the drug is renally excreted, so its half-life and serum levels are markedly elevated in renal disease [30]. 9-Carboxymethoxymethylguanine (CMMG) is an acyclovir metabolite, present in serum and cerebral spinal fluid. Significantly higher serum CMMG levels have been demonstrated in patients with neuropsychiatric disturbances [31]. The most common presentation is encephalopathy, but symptoms ranging from tremor to seizures and coma have been described. PRES can also occur with acyclovir [32]. One of the commonly used antifungals, voriconazole, can induce visual hallucinations that are reversible after discontinuation [33]. Amphotericin B therapy has been rarely associated with development of reversible encephalopathy and parkinsonism [34]. β-lactam antibiotics may cause seizures if given in high doses relative to renal function and/or body weight [35]. Cefepime, a fourth-generation cephalosporin commonly prescribed in intensive care units, is frequently associated with encephalopathy but can also cause myoclonus, seizures, and coma. Its neurotoxic effects are more pronounced during concomitant renal insufficiency [36]. There are several reports on the neurotoxic effects of carbapenems especially on their potential to lower seizure thresholds [37]. Other antibiotics with potential neurotoxic effects include linezolid, which may predispose patients to serotonin syndrome and can rarely cause encephalopathy and peripheral neuropathy [38, 39], and metronidazole, which can induce cerebellar dysfunction [40], sensorimotor peripheral neuropathy, optic neuropathy, and autonomic dysfunction [41].

## Metabolic Encephalopathy

A variety of metabolic disturbances commonly seen in the ICU can cause alterations in the level and content of consciousness (i.e., delirium). These are subsumed under the broad term, metabolic encephalopathies, including those due to uremia, hepatic dysfunction, electrolyte disturbances, and sepsis/multi-organ failure. The hallmarks of metabolic encephalopathy are its lack of lateralizing neurological deficits and fluctuating course. The brainstem reflexes (e.g., pupillary light reflexes) and eye movements are generally preserved, as opposed to what may be seen in structural brain damage [10]. However, most of those with delirium and/or coma after HSCT require brain imaging to exclude an occult structural lesion. Electroencephalography (EEG) may also be helpful to rule out subclinical seizures, in cases of fluctuating or unexplained encephalopathy or coma. Myoclonus, rapid arrhythmic muscle jerking, can be seen in conjunction with metabolic disturbances and, especially when multifocal, is much more likely metabolic than due to structural or epileptiform etiologies. In some cases, negative myoclonus (i.e., asterixis) can be detected. Delirium has been reported in as many as 73% of HSCT cases early after transplant [42]. In HSCT patients, uremic encephalopathy can be associated with CNI nephrotoxicity and/or thrombotic microangiopathy/hemolytic-uremic syndrome [10]. Hepatic encephalopathy can be of toxic, infectious, or autoimmune etiology or in some cases result from veno-occlusive disease. In lieu of clear uremic or hepatic etiology, metabolic encephalopathy can occur from critical illness, systemic inflammatory response syndrome (SIRS), or sepsis and is often exacerbated by concurrent sedation and hospital delirium. Treatment of the underlying cause of delirium is the key to its reversal. Similarly, prognosis depends on the reversibility of the underlying disorder.

## Wernicke's Encephalopathy

Wernicke's encephalopathy (WE) is an acute neuropsychiatric syndrome precipitated by thiamine deficiency. It is classically characterized by the triad of confusion (or coma), ataxia, and ophthalmoplegia, though not all features have to be present. WE may be confirmed by pathognomonic features on MRI: symmetric signal abnormalities in the medial thalami, mammillary bodies, tectal plate, periaqueductal area, and around the third ventricle. Frank WE has been reported rarely after HSCT but may be under-diagnosed. This is especially important because it is reversible and permanent morbidity preventable by early replacement of thiamine. Risk factors for nutritional deficiency should be sought, including anorexia, vomiting, stomatitis, GVHD, and use of Total Parenteral Nutrition lacking thiamine. Thiamine may also be metabolized more rapidly in states of stress, and conversion to its biologically active form may be inhibited by CNIs and chemotherapeutic agents [43]. Concerns over occult thiamine deficiency contributing to the high incidence of delirium after HSCT led to the recent completion of a pilot randomized study of aggressive thiamine repletion in HSCT patients at a single center. Although delirium was not prevented by treatment, notably half of those in the placebo group developed thiamine deficiency by day 8 [43]. Risk factors for delirium included development of infections and receipt of corticosteroids (as well as polypharmacy with opioids and benzodiazepines).

## Cerebrovascular Disease

Even disorders of the cerebral blood vessels may not present with focal neurological deficits (i.e., as a typical stroke) in those with HSCT but instead, given their frequent multifocal nature, present with nonspecific encephalopathy, weakness, and/or seizures. Brain imaging is critical to evaluate for structural brain lesions in most cases. HSCT patients are more susceptible to both ischemic and hemorrhagic cerebrovascular complications. Hemorrhagic complications are frequently related to coagulopathy, especially thrombocytopenia [44]. Hypertension, low fibrinogen level, and acute GVHD may all contribute to the development of hemorrhages [45]. Subdural hematomas (SDH) (Fig. 29.3) are the most frequent intracranial hemorrhagic complication in HSCT, occurring in 2–3% of patients [46]. Treatment usually centers on conservative measures, such as platelet transfusion and correction of coagulopathy. Neurosurgical intervention (craniotomy/craniectomy and/or subdural drain placement) is reserved for subdural hematomas with neurological deterioration and increasing mass effect. Primary intraparenchymal hemorrhage is less common than SDH and is typically non-operable and often fatal [17]. These may also relate to hypertension and coagulopathy but may signal an underlying mass lesion or CNS infection.

Acute ischemic strokes are less common but may be associated with a hypercoagulable state, cerebral vasculitis, or with thromboembolism from atrial fibrillation. HSCT patients may also develop ischemic strokes from infection-related cerebrovascular events, so cultures and other testing for infections are important in the evaluation of stroke [47]. Transplant patients that have significant vascular risk factors (diabetes, hypertension, hyperlipidemia) may develop strokes related to atherothrombosis. Antiplatelets or antithrombotic agents are frequently contraindicated (due to concurrent thrombocytopenia, or, in some cases, septic embolism). Global or watershed ischemic injury from hypotension, hypoxemia, or cardiac arrest can occur in critically ill transplant patients. Chronic GVHD can manifest in CNS vasculitis and ischemic or hemorrhagic infarcts (discussed further under the "Immune-Mediated Complications" section). HSCT patients also have an 8–20% risk for venous thromboembolism due to the underlying malignancy, their chemotherapy regimens, the immobility during hospitalization, transplant-associated thrombotic microangiopathy (TA-TMA), and the use of central venous catheters [48]. Rare cases of cerebral venous sinus thromboses (CVST) have been described, mainly manifesting in multifocal intraparenchymal hemorrhages [49]. The treatment of venous thromboembolism can be challenging, as the options are limited in thrombocytopenic patients and require extensive risk-benefit assessments. Finally, TA-TMA is a multisystem disorder associated with widespread complement activation and endothelial injury, manifesting as hemolytic anemia and renal dysfunction [50]. It can also cause neurological symptoms such as headache, confusion, or seizures in one-third, though frank ischemic stroke seems rare [51]. In addition, it may result in intracerebral hemorrhage or PRES from uncontrolled acute hypertension [52]. Eculizumab, a terminal complement inhibitor, has recently shown promise in the management of TA-TMA [53].

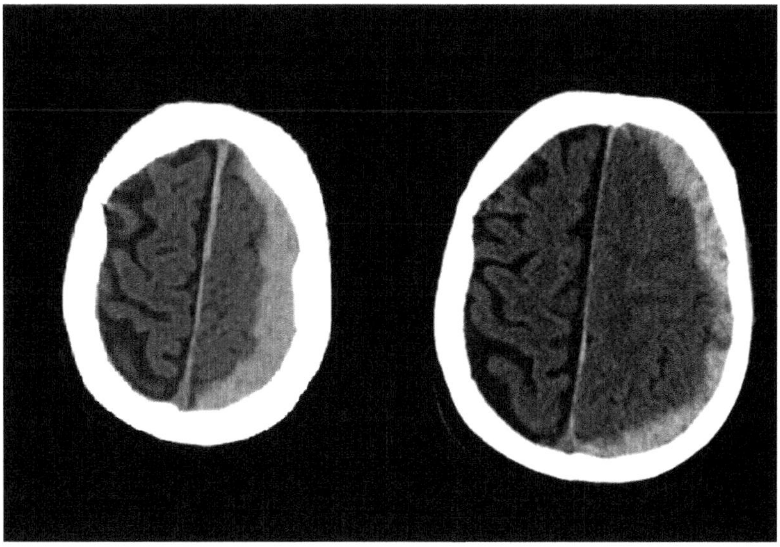

**Fig. 29.3** Axial CT image of acute left-sided subdural hematoma

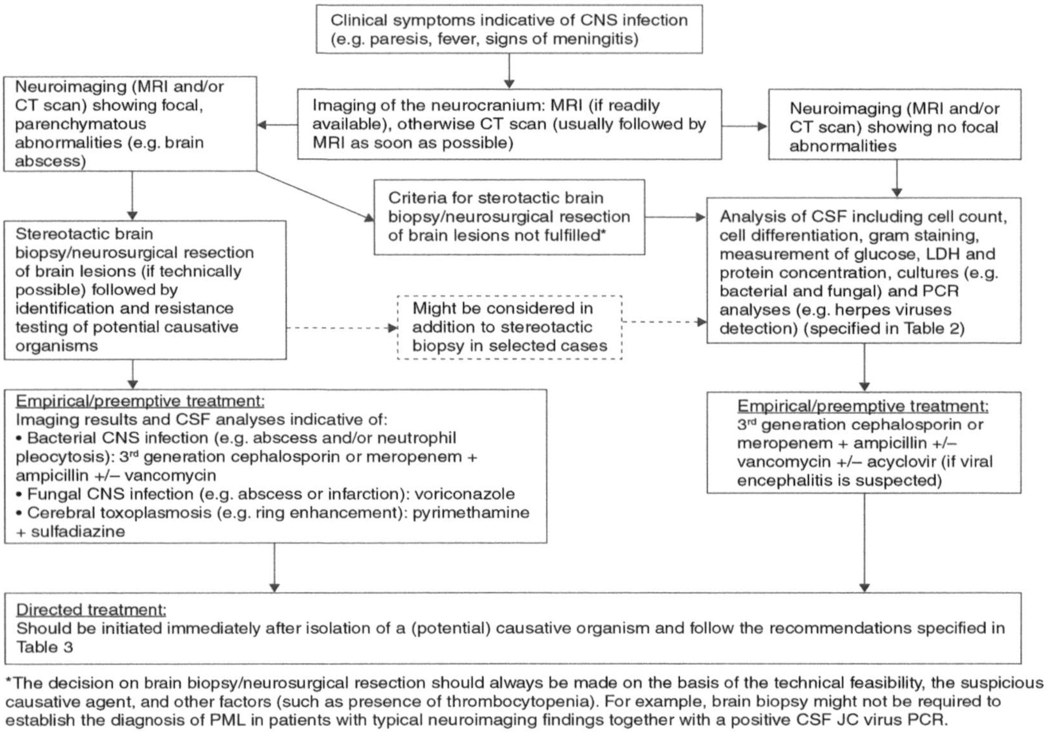


**Fig. 29.4** Diagnostic and therapeutic approach to patients with concern for CNS infection [With permission from M. Schmidt-Hieber, et al. CNS infections in patients with hematological disorders (including allogeneic stem-cell transplantation)—Guidelines of the Infectious Diseases Working Party (AGIHO) of the German Society of Hematology and Medical Oncology (DGHO), Annals of Oncology, Volume 27, Issue 7, 2016, pages 1207–1225, ISSN 0923–7534, https://doi.org/10.1093/annonc/mdw155]

## Infectious Complications

Allogeneic HSCT recipients are at a relatively high risk for opportunistic CNS infections, with an incidence ranging from 4% to 15% [54, 55]. Risk factors include severe GVHD and the use of high doses of immunosuppressive drugs [56]. The most common CNS infections are related to fungi and toxoplasmosis, but bacterial and viral infections also occur [57]. CNS infections may present with diffuse meningoencephalitis or with solitary or more often multiple mass lesions. Timing may be helpful: in the early period with severe neutropenia, bacterial meningitis and complications of sepsis are most likely; then while cellular immunity is suppressed, fungal and viral infections are more common. Neurologic symptoms include seizures, encephalopathy, new focal neurologic signs, and cranial nerve deficits; the classic signs such as headache and neck stiffness may be attenuated or absent [10]. MRI (ideally with contrast) and cerebrospinal fluid (CSF) analysis are the mainstay of the workup. In some cases, a tissue sample may be required to establish the diagnosis (e.g., stereotactic brain biopsy or resection of a brain mass lesion). The 2016 AGIHO and DGHO guidelines for the diagnostic algorithm and management approach of CNS infections in HSCT patients are summarized in Fig. 29.4 [58].

### Fungal Infections

Aspergillosis is the most common fungal infection with an incidence of 4–10% [59]. CNS involvement is usually disseminated lung involvement or from cranial sinuses and is seen in up to half of those with invasive aspergillosis [60]. The clinical presentation is nonspecific and may include fever and encephalopathy with or without focal signs or meningeal irritation [10]. However, signs and symptoms may progress rapidly [61]. CSF is nonspecific and aspergillus is rarely cultured. Serum or bronchoalveolar aspergillus galactomannan testing is the gold standard for diagnosis [62]. Neuroimaging can be helpful: computed tomography (CT) may show low-density lesions, while MRI may reveal more lesions that exhibit weak or absent contrast enhancement [63]. Given the frequent vascular involvement, septic infarcts and mycotic aneurysms can occur; microhemorrhages may be seen on gradient-echo or susceptibility-weighted MRI [64]. Treatment consists of either amphotericin B or voriconazole, the latter may be favored for its better CNS penetration [65]. Given the poor prognosis, combination therapy may be worth trying; addition of caspofungin to voriconazole may have a synergistic effect [66]. Despite treatment, CNS aspergillosis in HSCT patients has a dismal prognosis and is almost invariably fatal.

The incidence of CNS candidiasis has decreased with the widespread use of prophylactic fluconazole [62]. Although *Candida albicans* is the most common species (identified in 30–40%), other non-albicans *Candida* species are now frequently reported [67]. Presentation is commonly with nonspecific encephalopathy, headache, fever, and less commonly seizures. Diagnosis can be difficult. CSF analysis may show pleocytosis with elevated protein and low glucose levels, but these changes can be absent in immunosuppressed patients [67]. CSF culture may be positive for *Candida* species, but repeat testing may be useful in ruling out contamination. Measuring CSF mannan (a *Candida* antigen) is a promising technique for distinguishing CNS candidiasis from contamination [67]. Indwelling CNS devices should be removed as soon as candidiasis is suspected. Liposomal amphotericin B is the treatment of choice, with voriconazole as an alternative for treatment refractory cases [62].

*Cryptococcus* infection is rarely reported in HSCT patients [10]. Presentation is often rapid, with fever, confusion, headache, and diplopia [67]. CT scans may be normal or reveal meningeal enhancement, single or multiple nodules (cryptococcomas), cerebral edema, or hydrocephalus. MRI scans are more sensitive, showing multiple enhancing nodules within the brain parenchyma, meninges, basal ganglia, and midbrain [68]. Antigen detection using polymerase chain reaction (PCR) of body fluids has high sensitivity and specificity, though *Cryptococcus neoformans* can also be identified with India ink staining of the CSF [67]. Cases with elevated opening pressure should undergo serial large volume lumbar punctures or insertion of a temporary lumbar drain [68]. Liposomal amphotericin B and flucytosine are the mainstay of treatment followed by fluconazole until immune reconstitution [68].

Histoplasmosis is extremely rare even in hyperendemic areas [69]. Signs and symptoms of *Histoplasma capsulatum* infection include fever, chills, myalgias, dry cough, and chest discomfort. The disease may become disseminated, and if untreated, it is usually fatal with a reported mortality rate of 67% in HSCT recipients [70]. Itraconazole and amphotericin are the first-line therapies [71]. Mucormycosis can also affect HSCT patients, causing rapidly invasive nasal, oral, or sinus infections. Surgical debridement and combination therapy with lipid formulations of amphotericin and echinocandins are standard treatment. Despite treatment, mucormycosis is often fatal.

## Toxoplasmosis

*Toxoplasma gondii* is the most common protozoal infection in transplant recipients and an important cause of brain abscesses in this population [54]. Toxoplasmosis can occur in 1–8% of HSCT patients, depending on the seroprevalence in the given population [72]. It often presents within the first 100 days with altered mental status, variable fever, and focal neurological deficits [73]. Risk factors include *T. gondii* seropositivity, unrelated donor graft, receiving T-cell-depleted transplants, prior graft-versus-host disease (GVHD), or inability to take trimethoprim-sulfamethoxazole (TMP/SMX) prophylaxis [74]. Toxoplasmosis causes multiple brain abscesses, typically in the basal ganglia or at the gray-white junction, associated with ring enhancement on CT and MRI [75]. These do not typically exhibit diffusion-weighted imaging (DWI) restriction on MRI, unlike typical bacterial abscesses. Obstructive hydrocephalus can also occur. CSF *Toxoplasma* PCR is the mainstay of diagnosis, although histological diagnosis can be made by stereotactic brain biopsy if required [10]. Trimethoprim-sulfamethoxazole (TMP/SMX) with clindamycin or pyrimethamine is the current treatment of choice. Early diagnosis improves treatment response, but mortality remains at approximately 50% [76].

## Viral Infections

Human herpesvirus 6 (HHV-6) is the most common causative agent of viral CNS infection in HSCT patients, but several other viruses can be implicated, some with overlapping presentations and other with distinct features [57]. The pattern of presentation, diagnostic evaluation, and management of various common viral CNS infections is compared in Table 29.3. HHV-6 infection is the major cause of post-transplant acute limbic encephalitis (PALE) and most commonly occurs in the weeks to months after HSCT [57, 77]. Alterations in behavior/personality, short-term memory impairment, and seizures are common presentations [78]. Cytomegalovirus (CMV) or VZV infections may present with predominant ventriculitis, myelitis (spinal cord involvement), or even radiculomyelitis, the latter two both pre-

**Table 29.3** Comparison of the manifestations, patterns, and treatments for viral infections that may involve the CNS after HSCT

| VIRUS | HSV | HHV-6 | CMV | VZV | EBV |
|---|---|---|---|---|---|
| Relative frequency | Reactivation common but rare in CNS | Most common | Rare | Rare (more with GVHD) | Somewhat rare |
| Timing | Subacute to delayed | Subacute | Subacute to delayed | Subacute to delayed | Delayed |
| Pattern of presentation | | | | | |
| Meningoencephalitis | + | + | ± | + (seizures) | – |
| Limbic involvement | ++ | ++ | – | – | – |
| Ventricular | – | – | ++ | – | – |
| Myelitis | – | ± | ++ | ++ | ± |
| Other features | Orofacial or genital reactivation | SIADH | Retinitis | Dermatomal zoster<br>Cranial nerve palsies, hearing loss | PTLD |
| Diagnosis | | | | | |
| CSF | Pleocytosis<br>PCR useful | Mild pleocytosis<br>PCR useful | PCR useful | PCR useful | Flow cytometry and PCR |
| MRI | Mesial temporal | Mesial temporal | Periventricular | Basal ganglia, thalami, periventricular, frequently exhibit reduced DWI signal | Subcortical ± ring-enhancing |
| Treatment | Acyclovir | Ganciclovir or foscarnet | Ganciclovir or foscarnet | Acyclovir | Reduction of immunosuppression, rituximab, adoptive T-cell therapy |

*DWI* diffusion-weighted imaging, *PTLD* post-transplant lymphoproliferative disorder, *SIADH* syndrome of inappropriate antidiuretic hormone

senting with weakness in the legs and bladder dysfunction [79]. CSF analysis often reveals lymphocytic pleocytosis and elevated protein, with PCR testing identifying the specific causative virus. Despite treatment, mortality can be high for many viral infections (as high as 90%) [80]; long-term disability is common [81, 82].

## Progressive Multifocal Leukoencephalopathy

JC virus reactivation can also occur in immunocompromised hosts and manifest in progressive multifocal leukoencephalopathy (PML). PML remains less commonly seen than in HIV/AIDS with an estimated incidence of 1.24 per 1000 post-transplantation years [83]. Symptoms (e.g., cognitive decline, aphasia, motor deficits) develop gradually over weeks to months and occur in a delayed fashion (on average 17 months) after transplant. MRI typically reveals asymmetric multifocal white matter lesions that are non-enhancing. The gold standard for diagnosis is brain biopsy, but positive PCR for JC virus in CSF can now confirm PML without need for biopsy. Sensitivity of PCR is high but can be negative in some cases [84]. The disease usually progresses relentlessly. While there is no specific therapy for PML, reducing immunosuppression is often attempted. Mortality is extremely high (approx. 80%) with a median survival of 6 months. Survivors are usually left with significant neurological deficits.

## Bacterial Infections

HSCT patients have an increased risk of developing bacterial infections due to underlying neutropenia, mucosal barrier disruption, immunosuppressive treatment, and/or GVHD. Patients can develop invasive pneumococcal disease or other systemic infections that can be associated with bacterial meningitis. Fever and encephalopathy are the two most common presenting symptoms. Classical meningeal signs can be absent in the setting of an impaired inflammatory response [10]. The most common organisms include *Streptococcus pneumoniae*, *Neisseria meningitidis*, *Listeria monocytogenes*, *Staphylococcus aureus*, *Haemophilus influenzae*, and *Enterococcus* species [85]. *Listeria* can cause a rhombencephalitis, with involvement of the brainstem and cranial nerves. In HSCT patients, vaccination against encapsulated bacteria (*S. pneumoniae*, *Neisseria meningitidis*, *H. influenzae*) is mandatory [86]. The incidence of *Listeria* meningitis has significantly declined with TMP/SMX prophylaxis. The mainstay of diagnosing bacterial meningitis is a lumbar puncture with CSF showing marked pleocytosis, markedly elevated protein, and decreased glucose (below 40% of serum glucose). CSF changes in HSCT patients are often less pronounced, with nucleated counts usually staying below 1000/mL [85]. Early empiric broad-spectrum antibiotics are crucial.

Brain abscesses typically present with fever, headache, altered mental status, and rapidly progressive neurological deficits. More than 90% of brain abscesses in transplant recipients are fungal or parasitic (toxoplasmosis), discussed above. Bacterial abscesses are usually polymicrobial, with streptococci, Enterobacteriaceae, and anaerobic bacteria dominating [87]. *Pseudomonas* can also occur. Abscesses from opportunistic organisms such as *Listeria*, *Nocardia*, and *Actinomyces* present a greater challenge in management and portend a poorer prognosis [88]. Lumbar puncture can be considered in instances where there is limited mass effect, but its diagnostic yield is variable. CSF pleocytosis may be modest or absent, and CSF cultures are commonly negative. Brain imaging is critical to diagnosis, revealing hypoattenuation on CT with potential contrast enhancement and T2 hyperintensity on MRI with avid homogeneous diffusion restriction and characteristic ring enhancement [89]. Management consists of broad-spectrum antibiotics with consideration for surgical aspiration or excision if location is accessible. Patients failing to improve after initial medical management may require drainage. Despite treatment, outcome is poor with a high mortality [87].

## Immune-Mediated Complications

### Acute Immune-Mediated Polyneuropathy (Guillain-Barré Syndrome)

Guillain-Barré syndrome (GBS) is an autoimmune condition that occurs in up to 1% of transplant recipients, typically within the first 3 months after HSCT [90]. It is characterized by symmetrical ascending motor weakness progressing over days to a few weeks with sensory loss and areflexia. Bulbar dysfunction is common, and one quarter progress to respiratory failure requiring mechanical ventilation. GBS is due to an aberrant autoimmune response targeting peripheral nerves and their roots [91]. In addition to typical clinical features, cerebrospinal fluid (CSF) analysis revealing cytoalbuminologic dissociation (combination of a normal cell count and increased protein level) is diagnostic. However, a normal CSF protein level, especially in the first week after onset, does not exclude GBS. Early initiation of intravenous immunoglobulins (IVIG) or plasma exchange (PLEX) is of proven benefit and crucial, especially in patients with rapidly progressive weakness. Patients often require close monitoring (including respiratory vital capacity) and may benefit from intensive care admission for aggressive supportive care [91]. HSCT patients treated with alemtuzumab for RIC may have a higher incidence of polyneuropathy and/or myelitis that can mimic GBS and can be triggered by viral reactivation [92].

### Neurological Manifestations of Chronic Graft-Versus-Host Disease

Neurological manifestations of chronic GVHD are rare, occurring months to years after HSCT, and can affect both the peripheral and the central nervous system. Myositis occurs in 2–3% and is characterized by moderate-severe proximal muscle weakness [93]. Its hallmark features are myalgia and a markedly elevated serum creatine kinase (CK) [94]. Myositis associated with chronic GVHD does not affect the overall prognosis and treatment response [95]. Prompt treatment with steroids often results in full recovery, but there is a lack of consensus guidelines dictating therapy [96]. Polymyositis (as well as brachial plexitis [97]) can also be associated with tacrolimus therapy [98]. The presence of myalgia, elevated serum CK, and the inflammatory features on needle electromyography (EMG) can help distinguish GVHD-associated polymyositis from steroid-induced myopathy, which may also present with proximal muscle weakness. Muscle biopsy can further establish the diagnosis.

Myasthenia gravis (MG) is a rare manifestation of chronic GVHD (below 1%), typically seen several months to years after HSCT [99]. Occasionally, it may occur without other symptoms of chronic GVHD [93]. Symptoms include fatigable muscle weakness, ptosis, dysphagia, dysarthria, diplopia, and facial, limb, and/or axial muscle weakness. Patients at high risk for developing MG after allogeneic HSCT have been shown to express specific human leukocyte antigens (HLAs), particularly HLA-Cw1, HLA-Cw7, and HLA-DR2 [100]. GVHD-associated MG is characterized by the invariable presence of serum anti-acetylcholine receptor antibodies and absence of thymoma [100]. However, it is important to note that up to 40% of HSCT recipients have positive anti-acetylcholine receptor antibodies without disease, so its diagnostic value for MG is questionable without proper clinical correlation [101]. Electrophysiological testing can be diagnostic for this neuromuscular junction disorder, revealing a progressive decrease in the muscle action potential with repetitive nerve stimulation [10]. Treatment consists of cholinesterase inhibitors, steroids, and immunosuppression. Severe exacerbations with respiratory weakness may require intensive care admission and mechanical ventilation. Such acute myasthenic crisis may respond to IVIG or PLEX.

Chronic GVHD can have CNS manifestations, including small- or medium-vessel vasculitis, immune-mediated encephalitis, or a demyelinating (multiple sclerosis-like) disease pattern [10]. However, these are very rare, generally require the presence of GVHD manifestations in other organs, and should only be diagnosed after exclusion of other neurological complications such as CNS infections. Small-vessel vasculitis is often characterized by multifocal nonspecific symptoms with a progressive relapsing course [93]. In contrast, medium-vessel vasculitis often presents with focal neurological signs such as hemiparesis or aphasia. Inflammatory markers may be normal, explained by sustained immunosuppressive therapy [102]. To establish the diagnosis of inflammatory vasculopathy, vascular imaging (CT angiography, magnetic resonance angiography, conventional angiography) may reveal the typical beading appearance (i.e., multifocal segmental narrowing of cerebral arteries). Although brain biopsy is required to confirm the diagnosis, it is rarely performed, and its sensitivity can be low based on sampling. Treatment of cerebral vasculitis consists of corticosteroids, usually in combination with cyclophosphamide, for 3 to 6 months until the induction of remission [10]. Demyelination related to GVHD in the CNS may affect the optic nerves, the spinal cord, or the cerebral white matter [103, 104]. Typically, such demyelination takes a relapsing–remitting course similar to multiple sclerosis [93]. Diagnosis is based upon brain MRI (white matter lesions, some of which enhance with gadolinium due to active disease) and CSF analysis (pleocytosis, IgG elevation, and oligoclonal bands). The distinction between the demyelinating complications of chronic GVHD from de novo demyelinating diseases is not possible based on clinical, laboratory, or imaging findings [93]. Thus, the diagnosis can only be established in the presence of other manifestations of chronic GVHD. Other pathologies causing white matter lesions should also be considered (e.g., PRES, PML, viral encephalitis). Treatment of CNS demyelinating disease consists of pulse-dosed corticosteroids for 3–5 days followed by immunosuppressive therapy (e.g., rituximab).

## Immune Reconstitution Inflammatory Syndrome (IRIS)

IRIS is an increasingly recognized entity seen in the context of the restoration of the immune system after immunosuppression and treatment of opportunistic infection [105]. IRIS occurs when the immune response becomes dysregulated and exaggerated as a shift occurs from an immunosuppressed to pro-inflammatory state. This has primarily been described with antiretroviral treatment of HIV patients but is increasingly recognized in immunocompromised transplant recipients who develop and are treated for an infection [106]. Neurologic signs of IRIS may include clinical or radiologic evidence of inflammation (e.g., contrast enhancement of leptomeninges, CSF pleocytosis but negative cultures). It can otherwise mimic recurrent infection, and so repeat cultures and close evaluation for residual infection are mandatory [52]. Treatment consists of supportive care, but prednisone 1–2 mg/kg or equivalent for 1–2 weeks can be considered in severe cases [107].

## Cytokine Release Syndrome

Haploidentical hematopoietic cell transplantation (haplo-HCT) offers a crucial alternative to traditional HLA-matched HSCT for patients with active disease in need of expedient HCT [108]. Cytokine release syndrome (CRS) is a potentially life-threatening complication usually observed after haplo-HCT or adoptive T-cell therapies [109]. The syndrome is characterized by systemic inflammation – fevers, vascular leak, hypotension, and respiratory and renal insufficiency—in the context of elevated inflammatory markers and cytokine levels, such as IL-6, IL-2, IFN-$\gamma$, and tumor necrosis factor [109]. Neurotoxicity can occur with symptoms including encephalopathy, cranial nerve palsies, ataxia, aphasia, and hemiparesis. Anti-IL-6 receptor therapies such as tocilizumab can be used to disrupt the toxic effects associated with CRS [109].

## Neuro-diagnostics

Neuroimaging should be obtained for almost all acute neurologic symptoms in transplant recipients, even if associated with clear metabolic precipitant; this is especially true for focal deficits or seizures with focal semiology. Computed tomography (CT) of the head is a reasonable and rapidly available first-line investigation that will reveal major lesions such as intracranial hemorrhages, brain abscesses, or cerebral edema but will often miss acute ischemia and other subtle or evolving lesions. MRI is much more sensitive to ischemia and smaller lesions and should be performed in the presence of persistent focal deficits or unexplained mental status changes. Contrast administration is preferable as this will enhance the detection of infectious and inflammatory disorders but should be avoided in the presence of renal insufficiency (for both iodinated CT and gadolinium-based MR contrast). Notably, inflammatory/infectious lesions may not enhance as avidly in transplant recipients as in normal patients.

EEG evaluation should be performed to rule out non-convulsive seizures in those with unexplained encephalopathy after imaging and systemic studies have been unrevealing, or if subtle signs of seizure are seen (e.g., nystagmus, eye deviation, twitching). Urgent EEG should be obtained in any patient with convulsive seizures who has not awoken or is not returning at least toward baseline mentation within a few hours. Prolonged EEG monitoring may be preferable in patients with persistent coma or fluctuations to optimize detection of intermittent seizures. Even in the absence of seizures, EEG can reveal epileptiform discharges or periodic patterns that may presage a risk of imminent seizures (warranting prolonged monitoring) or could highlight focal or hemispheric slowing that suggests an underlying structural brain lesion. Nerve conduction studies and electromyography (EMG) may be useful for unexplained or unclear neuromuscular symptoms or deficits. It can differentiate diffuse weakness due to demyelinating disorders like Guillain-Barré syndrome (GBS) from critical illness polyneuropathy, which has an axonal pattern. CSF testing should be performed in any cases with suspected CNS infections, or for cases of suspected GBS.

## References

1. Passweg JR, Baldomero H, Bader P, Bonini C, Cesaro S, Dreger P, et al. Hematopoietic SCT in Europe 2013: recent trends in the use of alternative donors showing more haploidentical donors but fewer cord blood transplants. Bone Marrow Transplant. 2015;50(4):476–82. https://doi.org/10.1038/bmt.2014.312.
2. Hahn T, McCarthy PL Jr, Hassebroek A, Bredeson C, Gajewski JL, Hale GA, et al. Significant improvement in survival after allogeneic hematopoietic cell transplantation during a period of significantly increased use, older recipient age, and use of unrelated donors. J Clin Oncol. 2013;31(19):2437–49. https://doi.org/10.1200/JCO.2012.46.6193.
3. Dowling MR, Li S, Dey BR, McAfee SL, Hock HR, Spitzer TR, et al. Neurologic complications after allogeneic hematopoietic stem cell transplantation: risk factors and impact. Bone Marrow Transplant. 2018;53(2):199–206. https://doi.org/10.1038/bmt.2017.239.
4. Siegal D, Keller A, Xu W, Bhuta S, Kim DH, Kuruvilla J, et al. Central nervous system complications after allogeneic hematopoietic stem cell transplantation: incidence, manifestations, and clinical significance. Biol Blood Marrow Transplant. 2007;13(11):1369–79. https://doi.org/10.1016/j.bbmt.2007.07.013.
5. Bhatt VR, Balasetti V, Jasem JA, Giri S, Armitage JO, Loberiza FR Jr, et al. Central nervous system complications and outcomes after allogeneic hematopoietic stem cell transplantation. Clin Lymphoma Myeloma Leuk. 2015;15(10):606–11. https://doi.org/10.1016/j.clml.2015.06.004.
6. Balaguer-Rosello A, Bataller L, Pinana JL, Montoro J, Lorenzo I, Villalba A, et al. Noninfectious neurologic complications after allogeneic hematopoietic stem cell transplantation. Biol Blood Marrow Transplant. 2019;25(9):1818–24. https://doi.org/10.1016/j.bbmt.2019.05.024.
7. Barba P, Pinana JL, Valcarcel D, Querol L, Martino R, Sureda A, et al. Early and late neurological complications after reduced-intensity conditioning allogeneic stem cell transplantation. Biol Blood Marrow Transplant. 2009;15(11):1439–46. https://doi.org/10.1016/j.bbmt.2009.07.013.
8. Colombo AA, Marchioni E, Diamanti L, Di Matteo AM, Baldanti F, Furione M, et al. Neurological complications involving the central nervous system after allogeneic hematopoietic stem cell transplantation during a period of evolution in transplant modalities: a cohort analysis. Transplantation. 2017;101(3):616–23. https://doi.org/10.1097/TP.0000000000001257.
9. Antonini G, Ceschin V, Morino S, Fiorelli M, Gragnani F, Mengarelli A, et al. Early neurologic complications following allogeneic bone marrow transplant for leukemia: a prospective study. Neurology. 1998;50(5):1441–5.
10. Maffini E, Festuccia M, Brunello L, Boccadoro M, Giaccone L, Bruno B. Neurologic complications after allogeneic hematopoietic stem cell transplantation. Biol Blood Marrow Transplant. 2017;23(3):388–97. https://doi.org/10.1016/j.bbmt.2016.12.632.
11. Masetti R, Cordelli DM, Zama D, Vendemini F, Biagi C, Franzoni E, et al. PRES in children under-

going hematopoietic stem cell or solid organ transplantation. Pediatrics. 2015;135(5):890–901. https://doi.org/10.1542/peds.2014-2325.
12. Ho S, Clipstone N, Timmermann L, Northrop J, Graef I, Fiorentino D, et al. The mechanism of action of cyclosporin a and FK506. Clin Immunol Immunopathol. 1996;80(3 Pt 2):S40–5.
13. McDonald JW, Goldberg MP, Gwag BJ, Chi SI, Choi DW. Cyclosporine induces neuronal apoptosis and selective oligodendrocyte death in cortical cultures. Ann Neurol. 1996;40(5):750–8. https://doi.org/10.1002/ana.410400511.
14. Dawson TM. Immunosuppressants, immunophilins, and the nervous system. Ann Neurol. 1996;40(4):559–60. https://doi.org/10.1002/ana.410400403.
15. Lavigne CM, Shrier DA, Ketkar M, Powers JM. Tacrolimus leukoencephalopathy: a neuropathologic confirmation. Neurology. 2004;63(6):1132–3. https://doi.org/10.1212/01.wnl.0000138568.60774.e4.
16. Gijtenbeek JM, van den Bent MJ, Vecht CJ. Cyclosporine neurotoxicity: a review. J Neurol. 1999;246(5):339–46.
17. Najima Y, Ohashi K, Miyazawa M, Nakano M, Kobayashi T, Yamashita T, et al. Intracranial hemorrhage following allogeneic hematopoietic stem cell transplantation. Am J Hematol. 2009;84(5):298–301. https://doi.org/10.1002/ajh.21382.
18. Dhar R. Neurologic complications of transplantation. Neurocrit Care. 2018;28(1):4–11. https://doi.org/10.1007/s12028-017-0387-6.
19. Bartynski WS. Posterior reversible encephalopathy syndrome, part 1: fundamental imaging and clinical features. AJNR Am J Neuroradiol. 2008;29(6):1036–42. https://doi.org/10.3174/ajnr.A0928.
20. De La Camara R, Tomas JF, Figuera A, Berberana M, Fernandez-Ranada JM. High dose busulfan and seizures. Bone Marrow Transplant. 1991;7(5):363–4.
21. Caselli D, Rosati A, Faraci M, Podda M, Ripaldi M, Longoni D, et al. Risk of seizures in children receiving busulphan-containing regimens for stem cell transplantation. Biol Blood Marrow Transplant. 2014;20(2):282–5. https://doi.org/10.1016/j.bbmt.2013.10.028.
22. Eberly AL, Anderson GD, Bubalo JS, McCune JS. Optimal prevention of seizures induced by high-dose busulfan. Pharmacotherapy. 2008;28(12):1502–10. https://doi.org/10.1592/phco.28.12.1502.
23. Beitinjaneh A, McKinney AM, Cao Q, Weisdorf DJ. Toxic leukoencephalopathy following fludarabine-associated hematopoietic cell transplantation. Biol Blood Marrow Transplant. 2011;17(3):300–8. https://doi.org/10.1016/j.bbmt.2010.04.003.
24. Gonzalez-Angulo AM, Orzano JA, Davila E. Ifosfamide-induced encephalopathy. South Med J. 2002;95(10):1215–7.
25. Raj AB, Bertolone SJ, Jaffe N. Methylene blue reversal of ifosfamide-related encephalopathy. J Pediatr Hematol Oncol. 2004;26(2):116. https://doi.org/10.1097/00043426-200402000-00010.
26. Lombardi G, Zustovich F, Nicoletto MO, Donach M, Pastorelli D. Important role of thiamine in preventing ifosfamide-induced encephalopathy. J Oncol Pharm Pract. 2010;16(2):135–6. https://doi.org/10.1177/1078155209342134.
27. Przybylyski A, Esper P. Early recognition and management of posterior reversible encephalopathy syndrome: a newly recognized complication in patients receiving tyrosine kinase inhibitors. Clin J Oncol Nurs. 2016;20(3):305–8. https://doi.org/10.1188/16.CJON.305-308.
28. Filippidou M, Avgerinou G, Katsibardi K, Gavra M, Pons R, Kattamis A. Delayed-onset severe neurotoxicity related to blinatumomab in an adolescent patient with refractory acute lymphoblastic leukemia. Pediatr Blood Cancer. 2021;68(7):e29040. https://doi.org/10.1002/pbc.29040.
29. Wade JC, Meyers JD. Neurologic symptoms associated with parenteral acyclovir treatment after marrow transplantation. Ann Intern Med. 1983;98(6):921–5. https://doi.org/10.7326/0003-4819-98-6-921.
30. Haefeli WE, Schoenenberger RA, Weiss P, Ritz RF. Acyclovir-induced neurotoxicity: concentration-side effect relationship in acyclovir overdose. Am J Med. 1993;94(2):212–5. https://doi.org/10.1016/0002-9343(93)90186-s.
31. Hellden A, Odar-Cederlof I, Diener P, Barkholt L, Medin C, Svensson JO, et al. High serum concentrations of the acyclovir main metabolite 9-carboxymethoxymethylguanine in renal failure patients with acyclovir-related neuropsychiatric side effects: an observational study. Nephrol Dial Transplant. 2003;18(6):1135–41. https://doi.org/10.1093/ndt/gfg119.
32. Mahad DJ, Hellden A, Jarvis J, Mitra D, Gholkar A, Chinnery PF. Aciclovir induced posterior leucoencephalopathy. J Neurol Neurosurg Psychiatry. 2005;76(9):1308–9. https://doi.org/10.1136/jnnp.2004.059824.
33. Zonios DI, Gea-Banacloche J, Childs R, Bennett JE. Hallucinations during voriconazole therapy. Clin Infect Dis. 2008;47(1):e7–e10. https://doi.org/10.1086/588844.
34. Kulkantrakorn K, Selhorst JB, Petruska PJ. Cytosine arabinoside and amphotericin B-induced parkinsonism. Ann Neurol. 1996;39(3):413–4. https://doi.org/10.1002/ana.410390326.
35. Schliamser SE, Cars O, Norrby SR. Neurotoxicity of beta-lactam antibiotics: predisposing factors and pathogenesis. J Antimicrob Chemother. 1991;27(4):405–25. https://doi.org/10.1093/jac/27.4.405.
36. Fugate JE, Kalimullah EA, Hocker SE, Clark SL, Wijdicks EF, Rabinstein AA. Cefepime neurotoxicity in the intensive care unit: a cause of severe, underappreciated encephalopathy. Crit Care. 2013;17(6):R264. https://doi.org/10.1186/cc13094.

37. Norrby SR. Neurotoxicity of carbapenem antibiotics: consequences for their use in bacterial meningitis. J Antimicrob Chemother. 2000;45(1):5–7. https://doi.org/10.1093/jac/45.1.5.
38. Ferry T, Ponceau B, Simon M, Issartel B, Petiot P, Boibieux A, et al. Possibly linezolid-induced peripheral and central neurotoxicity: report of four cases. Infection. 2005;33(3):151–4. https://doi.org/10.1007/s15010-005-4057-9.
39. Fletcher J, Aykroyd LE, Feucht EC, Curtis JM. Early onset probable linezolid-induced encephalopathy. J Neurol. 2010;257(3):433–5. https://doi.org/10.1007/s00415-009-5340-y.
40. Hari A, Srikanth BA, Lakshmi GS. Metronidazole induced cerebellar ataxia. Indian J Pharm. 2013;45(3):295–7. https://doi.org/10.4103/0253-7613.111903.
41. Hobson-Webb LD, Roach ES, Donofrio PD. Metronidazole: newly recognized cause of autonomic neuropathy. J Child Neurol. 2006;21(5):429–31. https://doi.org/10.1177/08830738060210051201.
42. Fann JR, Roth-Roemer S, Burington BE, Katon WJ, Syrjala KL. Delirium in patients undergoing hematopoietic stem cell transplantation. Cancer. 2002;95(9):1971–81. https://doi.org/10.1002/cncr.10889.
43. Nakamura ZM, Deal AM, Park EM, Quillen LJ, Chien SA, Stanton KE, et al. A randomized double-blind placebo-controlled trial of intravenous thiamine for prevention of delirium following allogeneic hematopoietic stem cell transplantation. J Psychosom Res. 2021;146:110503. https://doi.org/10.1016/j.jpsychores.2021.110503.
44. Labrador J, Lopez-Anglada L, Perez-Lopez E, Lozano FS, Lopez-Corral L, Sanchez-Guijo FM, et al. Analysis of incidence, risk factors and clinical outcome of thromboembolic and bleeding events in 431 allogeneic hematopoietic stem cell transplantation recipients. Haematologica. 2013;98(3):437–43. https://doi.org/10.3324/haematol.2012.069559.
45. Zhang XH, Wang QM, Chen H, Chen YH, Han W, Wang FR, et al. Clinical characteristics and risk factors of intracranial hemorrhage in patients following allogeneic hematopoietic stem cell transplantation. Ann Hematol. 2016;95(10):1637–43. https://doi.org/10.1007/s00277-016-2767-y.
46. Colosimo M, McCarthy N, Jayasinghe R, Morton J, Taylor K, Durrant S. Diagnosis and management of subdural haematoma complicating bone marrow transplantation. Bone Marrow Transplant. 2000;25(5):549–52. https://doi.org/10.1038/sj.bmt.1702166.
47. Coplin WM, Cochran MS, Levine SR, Crawford SW. Stroke after bone marrow transplantation: frequency, aetiology and outcome. Brain. 2001;124(Pt 5):1043–51. https://doi.org/10.1093/brain/124.5.1043.
48. Kansu E. Thrombosis in stem cell transplantation. Hematology. 2012;17(Suppl 1):S159–62. https://doi.org/10.1179/102453312X13336169156735.
49. Harvey CJ, Peniket AJ, Miszkiel K, Patterson K, Goldstone AH, Mackinnon S, et al. MR angiographic diagnosis of cerebral venous sinus thrombosis following allogeneic bone marrow transplantation. Bone Marrow Transplant. 2000;25(7):791–5. https://doi.org/10.1038/sj.bmt.1702238.
50. Khosla J, Yeh AC, Spitzer TR, Dey BR. Hematopoietic stem cell transplant-associated thrombotic microangiopathy: current paradigm and novel therapies. Bone Marrow Transplant. 2018;53(2):129–37. https://doi.org/10.1038/bmt.2017.207.
51. Uderzo C, Bonanomi S, Busca A, Renoldi M, Ferrari P, Iacobelli M, et al. Risk factors and severe outcome in thrombotic microangiopathy after allogeneic hematopoietic stem cell transplantation. Transplantation. 2006;82(5):638–44. https://doi.org/10.1097/01.tp.0000230373.82376.46.
52. Bonardi M, Turpini E, Sanfilippo G, Mina T, Tolva A, Zappoli TF. Brain imaging findings and neurologic complications after allogenic hematopoietic stem cell transplantation in children. Radiographics. 2018;38(4):1223–38. https://doi.org/10.1148/rg.2018170139.
53. Zhang R, Zhou M, Qi J, Miao W, Zhang Z, Wu D, et al. Efficacy and safety of eculizumab in the treatment of transplant-associated thrombotic microangiopathy: a systematic review and meta-analysis. Front Immunol. 2020;11:564647. https://doi.org/10.3389/fimmu.2020.564647.
54. Maschke M, Dietrich U, Prumbaum M, Kastrup O, Turowski B, Schaefer UW, et al. Opportunistic CNS infection after bone marrow transplantation. Bone Marrow Transplant. 1999;23(11):1167–76. https://doi.org/10.1038/sj.bmt.1701782.
55. de Medeiros BC, de Medeiros CR, Werner B, Neto JZ, Loddo G, Pasquini R, et al. Central nervous system infections following bone marrow transplantation: an autopsy report of 27 cases. J Hematother Stem Cell Res. 2000;9(4):535–40. https://doi.org/10.1089/152581600419215.
56. Hanajiri R, Kobayashi T, Yoshioka K, Watanabe D, Watakabe K, Murata Y, et al. Central nervous system infection following allogeneic hematopoietic stem cell transplantation. Hematol Oncol Stem Cell Ther. 2017;10(1):22–8. https://doi.org/10.1016/j.hemonc.2016.08.008.
57. Schmidt-Hieber M, Schwender J, Heinz WJ, Zabelina T, Kuhl JS, Mousset S, et al. Viral encephalitis after allogeneic stem cell transplantation: a rare complication with distinct characteristics of different causative agents. Haematologica. 2011;96(1):142–9. https://doi.org/10.3324/haematol.2010.029876.
58. Schmidt-Hieber M, Silling G, Schalk E, Heinz W, Panse J, Penack O, et al. CNS infections in patients with hematological disorders (including allogeneic stem-cell transplantation)-guidelines of the infectious diseases working party (AGIHO) of the German Society of Hematology and Medical Oncology (DGHO). Ann Oncol. 2016;27(7):1207–25. https://doi.org/10.1093/annonc/mdw155.

59. Jantunen E, Volin L, Salonen O, Piilonen A, Parkkali T, Anttila VJ, et al. Central nervous system aspergillosis in allogeneic stem cell transplant recipients. Bone Marrow Transplant. 2003;31(3):191–6. https://doi.org/10.1038/sj.bmt.1703812.
60. Jantunen E, Ruutu P, Niskanen L, Volin L, Parkkali T, Koukila-Kahkola P, et al. Incidence and risk factors for invasive fungal infections in allogeneic BMT recipients. Bone Marrow Transplant. 1997;19(8):801–8. https://doi.org/10.1038/sj.bmt.1700737.
61. Ruhnke M, Kofla G, Otto K, Schwartz S. CNS aspergillosis: recognition, diagnosis and management. CNS Drugs. 2007;21(8):659–76. https://doi.org/10.2165/00023210-200721080-00004.
62. Rahi MS, Jindal V, Pednekar P, Parekh J, Gunasekaran K, Sharma S, et al. Fungal infections in hematopoietic stem-cell transplant patients: a review of epidemiology, diagnosis, and management. Ther Adv Infect Dis. 2021;8:20499361211039050. https://doi.org/10.1177/20499361211039050.
63. Server A, Bargallo N, Floisand Y, Sponheim J, Graus F, Hald JK. Imaging spectrum of central nervous system complications of hematopoietic stem cell and solid organ transplantation. Neuroradiology. 2017;59(2):105–26. https://doi.org/10.1007/s00234-017-1804-4.
64. Guermazi A, Gluckman E, Tabti B, Miaux Y. Invasive central nervous system aspergillosis in bone marrow transplantation recipients: an overview. Eur Radiol. 2003;13(2):377–88. https://doi.org/10.1007/s00330-002-1480-5.
65. Herbrecht R, Denning DW, Patterson TF, Bennett JE, Greene RE, Oestmann JW, et al. Voriconazole versus amphotericin B for primary therapy of invasive aspergillosis. N Engl J Med. 2002;347(6):408–15. https://doi.org/10.1056/NEJMoa020191.
66. Perea S, Gonzalez G, Fothergill AW, Kirkpatrick WR, Rinaldi MG, Patterson TF. In vitro interaction of caspofungin acetate with voriconazole against clinical isolates of aspergillus spp. Antimicrob Agents Chemother. 2002;46(9):3039–41. https://doi.org/10.1128/AAC.46.9.3039-3041.2002.
67. Mattiuzzi G, Giles FJ. Management of intracranial fungal infections in patients with haematological malignancies. Br J Haematol. 2005;131(3):287–300. https://doi.org/10.1111/j.1365-2141.2005.05749.x.
68. Bicanic T, Harrison TS. Cryptococcal meningitis. Br Med Bull. 2004;72:99–118. https://doi.org/10.1093/bmb/ldh043.
69. Vail GM, Young RS, Wheat LJ, Filo RS, Cornetta K, Goldman M. Incidence of histoplasmosis following allogeneic bone marrow transplant or solid organ transplant in a hyperendemic area. Transpl Infect Dis. 2002;4(3):148–51. https://doi.org/10.1034/j.1399-3062.2002.01016.x.
70. Agrawal V, Brinda BJ, Farag SS. Histoplasma capsulatum infection in an allogeneic hematopoietic stem cell transplant patient receiving voriconazole prophylaxis. Case Rep Hematol. 2020;2020:8124137. https://doi.org/10.1155/2020/8124137.
71. Wheat LJ, Freifeld AG, Kleiman MB, Baddley JW, McKinsey DS, Loyd JE, et al. Clinical practice guidelines for the management of patients with histoplasmosis: 2007 update by the infectious diseases Society of America. Clin Infect Dis. 2007;45(7):807–25. https://doi.org/10.1086/521259.
72. Martino R, Maertens J, Bretagne S, Rovira M, Deconinck E, Ullmann AJ, et al. Toxoplasmosis after hematopoietic stem cell transplantation. Clin Infect Dis. 2000;31(5):1188–95. https://doi.org/10.1086/317471.
73. Prestes DP, Mendes C, Batista MV, Ramos JF, Junior JS, Okay TS, et al. A case-series of toxoplasmosis in hematopoietic stem cell transplantation: still a concern for endemic countries. Bone Marrow Transplant. 2018;53(10):1336–9. https://doi.org/10.1038/s41409-018-0179-4.
74. Fricker-Hidalgo H, Bulabois CE, Brenier-Pinchart MP, Hamidfar R, Garban F, Brion JP, et al. Diagnosis of toxoplasmosis after allogeneic stem cell transplantation: results of DNA detection and serological techniques. Clin Infect Dis. 2009;48(2):e9–e15. https://doi.org/10.1086/595709.
75. Busemann C, Ribback S, Zimmermann K, Sailer V, Kiefer T, Schmidt CA, et al. Toxoplasmosis after allogeneic stem cell transplantation—a single centre experience. Ann Hematol. 2012;91(7):1081–9. https://doi.org/10.1007/s00277-012-1406-5.
76. Kitahara M, Hiroshima Y, Norose K, Hikosaka K, Kazumoto H, Uematsu N, et al. Clinical characteristics and incidence of toxoplasmosis after autologous hematopoietic stem cell transplantation: a retrospective study and literature review. Transpl Infect Dis. 2021;23(6):e13726. https://doi.org/10.1111/tid.13726.
77. Ogata M, Fukuda T, Teshima T. Human herpesvirus-6 encephalitis after allogeneic hematopoietic cell transplantation: what we do and do not know. Bone Marrow Transplant. 2015;50(8):1030–6. https://doi.org/10.1038/bmt.2015.76.
78. Ogata M, Satou T, Kadota J, Saito N, Yoshida T, Okumura H, et al. Human herpesvirus 6 (HHV-6) reactivation and HHV-6 encephalitis after allogeneic hematopoietic cell transplantation: a multicenter, prospective study. Clin Infect Dis. 2013;57(5):671–81. https://doi.org/10.1093/cid/cit358.
79. Steer CB, Szer J, Sasadeusz J, Matthews JP, Beresford JA, Grigg A. Varicella-zoster infection after allogeneic bone marrow transplantation: incidence, risk factors and prevention with low-dose aciclovir and ganciclovir. Bone Marrow Transplant. 2000;25(6):657–64. https://doi.org/10.1038/sj.bmt.1702190.
80. Reddy SM, Winston DJ, Territo MC, Schiller GJ. CMV central nervous system disease in stem-cell transplant recipients: an increasing complication of drug-resistant CMV infection and protracted immunodeficiency. Bone Marrow Transplant.

2010;45(6):979–84. https://doi.org/10.1038/bmt.2010.35.
81. Tyler KL. Herpes simplex virus infections of the central nervous system: encephalitis and meningitis, including Mollaret's. Herpes. 2004;11(Suppl 2):57A–64A.
82. Styczynski J, Reusser P, Einsele H, de la Camara R, Cordonnier C, Ward KN, et al. Management of HSV, VZV and EBV infections in patients with hematological malignancies and after SCT: guidelines from the second European conference on infections in leukemia. Bone Marrow Transplant. 2009;43(10):757–70. https://doi.org/10.1038/bmt.2008.386.
83. Mateen FJ, Muralidharan R, Carone M, van de Beek D, Harrison DM, Aksamit AJ, et al. Progressive multifocal leukoencephalopathy in transplant recipients. Ann Neurol. 2011;70(2):305–22. https://doi.org/10.1002/ana.22408.
84. Sheikh SI, Stemmer-Rachamimov A, Attar EC. Autopsy diagnosis of progressive multifocal leukoencephalopathy with JC virus-negative CSF after cord blood stem-cell transplantation. J Clin Oncol. 2009;27(23):e46–7. https://doi.org/10.1200/JCO.2009.22.4451.
85. van Veen KE, Brouwer MC, van der Ende A, van de Beek D. Bacterial meningitis in hematopoietic stem cell transplant recipients: a population-based prospective study. Bone Marrow Transplant. 2016;51(11):1490–5. https://doi.org/10.1038/bmt.2016.181.
86. Johnston BL, Conly JM. Immunization for bone marrow transplant recipients. Can J Infect Dis. 2002;13(6):353–7.
87. Hagensee ME, Bauwens JE, Kjos B, Bowden RA. Brain abscess following marrow transplantation: experience at the Fred Hutchinson Cancer Research Center, 1984-1992. Clin Infect Dis. 1994;19(3):402–8. https://doi.org/10.1093/clinids/19.3.402.
88. Patel K, Clifford DB. Bacterial brain abscess. Neurohospitalist. 2014;4(4):196–204. https://doi.org/10.1177/1941874414540684.
89. Faehndrich J, Weidauer S, Pilatus U, Oszvald A, Zanella FE, Hattingen E. Neuroradiological viewpoint on the diagnostics of space-occupying brain lesions. Clin Neuroradiol. 2011;21(3):123–39. https://doi.org/10.1007/s00062-011-0073-6.
90. Bulsara KR, Baron PW, Tuttle-Newhall JE, Clavien PA, Morgenlander J. Guillain-Barre syndrome in organ and bone marrow transplant patients. Transplantation. 2001;71(8):1169–72. https://doi.org/10.1097/00007890-200104270-00026.
91. Willison HJ, Jacobs BC, van Doorn PA. Guillain-barre syndrome. Lancet. 2016;388(10045):717–27. https://doi.org/10.1016/S0140-6736(16)00339-1.
92. Avivi I, Chakrabarti S, Kottaridis P, Kyriaku C, Dogan A, Milligan DW, et al. Neurological complications following alemtuzumab-based reduced-intensity allogeneic transplantation. Bone Marrow Transplant. 2004;34(2):137–42. https://doi.org/10.1038/sj.bmt.1704538.
93. Grauer O, Wolff D, Bertz H, Greinix H, Kuhl JS, Lawitschka A, et al. Neurological manifestations of chronic graft-versus-host disease after allogeneic haematopoietic stem cell transplantation: report from the consensus conference on clinical practice in chronic graft-versus-host disease. Brain. 2010;133(10):2852–65. https://doi.org/10.1093/brain/awq245.
94. Stephenson AL, Mackenzie IR, Levy RD, Road J. Myositis associated graft-versus-host-disease presenting as respiratory muscle weakness. Thorax. 2001;56(1):82–4. https://doi.org/10.1136/thorax.56.1.82.
95. Parker P, Chao NJ, Ben-Ezra J, Slatkin N, Openshaw H, Niland JC, et al. Polymyositis as a manifestation of chronic graft-versus-host disease. Medicine (Baltimore). 1996;75(5):279–85. https://doi.org/10.1097/00005792-199609000-00004.
96. Limaye S, Limaye V. Clinical characteristics of myositis associated with graft-versus-host disease. Curr Rheumatol Rep. 2021;23(5):30. https://doi.org/10.1007/s11926-021-00996-x.
97. Al Masri O, Fathallah W, Quader S. Recovery of tacrolimus-associated brachial neuritis after conversion to everolimus in a pediatric renal transplant recipient--case report and review of the literature. Pediatr Transplant. 2008;12(8):914–7. https://doi.org/10.1111/j.1399-3046.2008.00961.x.
98. Vattemi G, Marini M, Di Chio M, Colpani M, Guglielmi V, Tomelleri G. Polymyositis in solid organ transplant recipients receiving tacrolimus. J Neurol Sci. 2014;345(1–2):239–43. https://doi.org/10.1016/j.jns.2014.07.036.
99. Tse S, Saunders EF, Silverman E, Vajsar J, Becker L, Meaney B. Myasthenia gravis and polymyositis as manifestations of chronic graft-versus-host-disease. Bone Marrow Transplant. 1999;23(4):397–9. https://doi.org/10.1038/sj.bmt.1701575.
100. Mackey JR, Desai S, Larratt L, Cwik V, Nabholtz JM. Myasthenia gravis in association with allogeneic bone marrow transplantation: clinical observations, therapeutic implications and review of literature. Bone Marrow Transplant. 1997;19(9):939–42. https://doi.org/10.1038/sj.bmt.1700759.
101. Lefvert AK, Bjorkholm M. Antibodies against the acetylcholine receptor in hematologic disorders: implications for the development of myasthenia gravis after bone marrow grafting. N Engl J Med. 1987;317(3):170. https://doi.org/10.1056/NEJM198707163170315.
102. Sostak P, Saam T, Hacker M, Schankin C, Wagner J, Kolb HJ, et al. Large vessel vasculitis: manifestation of graft-versus-host disease? J Neurol. 2009;256(11):1947–9. https://doi.org/10.1007/s00415-009-5272-6.
103. Sakai M, Ohashi K, Ohta K, Yamashita T, Akiyama H, Kisida S, et al. Immune-mediated myelopathy following allogeneic stem cell transplantation. Int J Hematol. 2006;84(3):272–5. https://doi.org/10.1532/IJH97.06060.

104. Solaro C, Murialdo A, Giunti D, Mancardi G, Uccelli A. Central and peripheral nervous system complications following allogeneic bone marrow transplantation. Eur J Neurol. 2001;8(1):77–80. https://doi.org/10.1046/j.1468-1331.2001.00160.x.
105. Airas L, Paivarinta M, Roytta M, Karhu J, Kauppila M, Itala-Remes M, et al. Central nervous system immune reconstitution inflammatory syndrome (IRIS) after hematopoietic SCT. Bone Marrow Transplant. 2010;45(3):593–6. https://doi.org/10.1038/bmt.2009.186.
106. Sun HY, Singh N. Opportunistic infection-associated immune reconstitution syndrome in transplant recipients. Clin Infect Dis. 2011;53(2):168–76. https://doi.org/10.1093/cid/cir276.
107. Murthy AR, Marulappa R, Hegde U, Kappadi D, Ambikathanaya UK, Nair P. Treatment guidelines and prognosis of immune reconstitution inflammatory syndrome patients: a review. J Int Oral Health. 2015;7(4):92–5.
108. Abboud R, Keller J, Slade M, DiPersio JF, Westervelt P, Rettig MP, et al. Severe cytokine-release syndrome after T cell-replete peripheral blood haploidentical donor transplantation is associated with poor survival and anti-IL-6 therapy is safe and well tolerated. Biol Blood Marrow Transplant. 2016;22(10):1851–60. https://doi.org/10.1016/j.bbmt.2016.06.010.
109. Lee DW, Gardner R, Porter DL, Louis CU, Ahmed N, Jensen M, et al. Current concepts in the diagnosis and management of cytokine release syndrome. Blood. 2014;124(2):188–95. https://doi.org/10.1182/blood-2014-05-552729.

# 30 Hematological Considerations in Critically Ill Hematopoietic Stem Cell Transplantation Patients

Abhinav Deol

## Introduction

Hematopoietic stem cell transplant (HSCT) is an essential tool in the management of various hematological malignancies. The source of stem cells in HSCT patients can be autologous or allogeneic. Allogeneic stem cell sources can be from a fully matched sibling donor, matched unrelated donor, mismatched unrelated donor, or haplo-identical donor [1]. In addition, cord blood stem cells can be used as a source of allogeneic stem cells; however, the use of cord blood transplant especially for adult patients is rapidly declining due to the advances in preventing graft-versus-host disease (GVHD) in haplo-identical stem cell transplant by using post-transplant cyclophosphamide [2]. Patients undergoing HSCT received a preparative regimen consisting of chemotherapy and/or radiation followed by infusion of stem cells after which it takes about 2 weeks for count recovery. In the setting of allogeneic (allo) HSCT, patients also receive appropriate GVHD prophylaxis based on the source of stem cells [1]. During the course of HSCT, patients may need management in the intensive care unit at various time points due to inherent complications that may develop during the HSCT journey. This chapter will address some of the common hematological problems seen in critically ill HSCT patients.

## Laboratory Analysis and Venous Access

Critically ill HSCT patients should have a daily CBC with a differential. Type and screen should be available in the blood bank to be able to have blood products available in a timely manner for these patients. In absence of active bleeding, coagulation profile should be monitored twice a week. If there is any suspicion of hemolysis, bilirubin, lactate dehydrogenase, haptoglobin, reticulocyte count, isohemagglutinin levels, and Coombs test should be monitored. Peripheral blood smear evaluation can provide additional information if thrombotic microangiopathy is suspected.

Most patients who have recently undergone HSCT will have a central venous catheter (CVC). In the absence of infection, all efforts should be made to maintain central venous access in these critically ill HSCT patients as these patients especially during the early peri-transplant period will require blood transfusions and intravenous antibiotics due to marrow aplasia from the preparative regimen.

A. Deol (✉)
Department of Oncology, Wayne State University/Karmanos Cancer Institute, Detroit, MI, USA
e-mail: deola@karmanos.org



A. O. Soubani (ed.), *Pulmonary and Critical Care Considerations of Hematopoietic Stem Cell Transplantation*, https://doi.org/10.1007/978-3-031-28797-8_30

## Transfusion Support

During the HSCT process, patients need transfusion support during the period between preparative regimen and engraftment of blood counts. Blood products that may need to be transfused are platelets and packed red blood cells. Patients who develop bleeding diathesis may need fresh frozen plasma or cryoprecipitate infusions in certain situations. Usually, blood product transfusion requirement resolves with engraftment, which normally is seen about 2–3 weeks after infusion of the stem cells. However, in the setting of delayed or failed engraftment and ABO incompatibility, transfusion support may be needed for a longer period. As a rule, blood products transfused to these immunocompromised patients should be irradiated and leukoreduced [3]. The irradiation prevents development of transfusion-associated graft-versus-host disease, and leukoreduction has been shown to reduce the risk of Cytomegalovirus (CMV) transmission, febrile non-hemolytic transfusion reactions, and alloimmunization. Irradiation of blood products with minimum 2500 cGy eliminates T-lymphocyte growth [4]. Pre-storage leukocyte reduction is standard in many countries with national blood banking programs.

## Packed Red Blood Cell Transfusion

The reason for low hemoglobin in critically ill HSCT patients can be multifactorial. The underlying reason for low hemoglobin should be understood to provide appropriate management. The common reasons for low hemoglobin are due to marrow aplasia/hypoplasia due to preparative regimen, viral infections (like parvovirus, cytomegalovirus, Epstein-Barr virus), medications, hemolysis, and/or active bleeding (due to damage to mucosal surfaces from preparative regime, infections like CMV, graft-versus-host disease, or coagulopathy). In addition to treatment of the underlying cause or waiting for the marrow function, it is critical for these patients to receive transfusion support during this period. Multiple studies have shown that in the absence of active bleeding, maintaining hemoglobin >7 provides similar outcomes compared to higher thresholds [5]. In critically ill patients who have comorbid conditions like cardiovascular disease, a higher threshold for packed red blood cell (PRBC) support may be needed. PRBC transfusion support is relatively simple in patients undergoing autologous HSCT. These patients receive ABO-compatible PRBC transfusions to maintain hemoglobin levels at aforementioned levels. However, patients who undergo HSCT from an allogeneic source may have differences in blood group between the donor and the recipient. The ABO incompatibility in allogeneic HSCT can be minor (when the donor has isohemagglutinins directed against the recipient RBC antigens), major (when the recipient plasma contains isohemagglutinins directed at donor RBC antigens), or bidirectional. ABO type O blood can be safely transfused in patients who have minor, major, or bidirectional ABO incompatibility between the donor and the recipient during the peri-transplant period. Table 30.1 shows compatible blood products that can be used in patients who undergo ABO-incompatible HSCT. Usually by about 2

**Table 30.1** Blood transfusion support in ABO-incompatible HSCT

| ABO incompatibility | RBC transfusion | Platelet/plasma transfusion |
|---|---|---|
| *Major mismatch* Example: donor blood group B to recipient blood group 0 | Transfuse group O red cells till anti-B titer is undetectable and recipient types as blood group B | Donor type platelet/plasma (group B) |
| *Minor mismatch* Example: donor blood group O to recipient blood group A | Transfuse group O red cells | Platelet and plasma that lack anti-A isohemagglutinin |
| *Bidirectional mismatch* Example: donor blood group A to recipient blood group B | Transfuse group 0 red cells | AB group plasma and platelet products |

months post-transplant, the isohemagglutinin titers become undetectable; however, this may take a longer time in patients who receive reduced-intensity conditioning regimens [6, 7].

## Platelet Transfusion

Platelet transfusion support is required in some critically ill HSCT patients. This is usually during the peri-transplant period when their marrow function is suppressed due to the underlying disease or the preparative regimen. In addition, some patients may need prolonged platelet transfusion support if they have persistent severe thrombocytopenia due to delayed engraftment, infections, GVHD, etc. Platelet products, which are used for infusion, can be from pooled donor or single-donor apheresis products. Platelet transfusions are associated with the highest number of infusion reactions [8], and appropriate use of platelet products is needed in these critically ill patients. Table 30.1 shows compatible blood products for patients who have undergone ABO-incompatible allo-HSCT.

There are randomized studies that looked at patients with acute myeloid leukemia undergoing induction/consolidation chemo or patients with other hematological malignancies undergoing autologous HSCT where patients were prophylactically transfused platelets when their platelet count dropped below 10,000/μL vs. platelet transfusion only when there was evidence of bleeding [9, 10]. These studies showed no significant difference in rates of significant bleeding in the two groups. However, these studies did not include critically ill HSCT patients or patients who underwent allogeneic HSCT. In the absence of bleeding, the majority of the groups recommend prophylactic platelet transfusions to keep platelet count >10,000/μL in critically ill HSCT patients. There is a dearth of data in this setting to know if a lower threshold will lead to similar outcomes in these patients. Guidelines about platelet thresholds in patients who have bleeding are not based on randomized studies, but most transplant physicians recommend keeping platelets around 30,000–50,000/μL to stop and prevent bleeding in these scenarios. Prophylactic platelet transfusions prior to procedures are another gray area in general without many randomized well-designed studies. The Society of Interventional Radiology in 2019 recommended platelet transfusion for platelet count $<20 \times 10^9$/L in patients undergoing procedures with low bleeding risk and platelet transfusion for count $<50 \times 10^9$/L in patients undergoing procedures with high bleeding risk [11]. However, these recommendations are not based on randomized studies and are expert panel recommendations.

## Platelet Refractoriness

The American Society of Clinical Oncology clinical practice guidelines updated in 2018 based on informal consensus recommended platelet counts should be performed within 1 h after transfusion when refractoriness is suspected [12]. In order to consider a diagnosis of platelet refractoriness, patients should have infusion of fresh ABO-compatible platelets on two separate occasions that lead to poor increment. In this situation, determination of alloantibodies should be obtained. Patients who are confirmed to have alloimmunization should receive platelet transfusions from histocompatible donors matched for HLA-A and HLA-B antigens. Most blood banks work with blood suppliers like the Red Cross, who have access to lists of such donors. Histocompatible platelet units can often be identified using a platelet cross-matching technique especially for patients whose HLA type cannot be determined or who have uncommon HLA types for whom suitable donors cannot be identified. This technique may also be used for patients who do not respond to HLA-matched platelets [13].

## Fresh Frozen Plasma and Cryoprecipitate

Fresh frozen plasma infusion is indicated when the critically ill HSCT patients develop coagulopathy due to deficiency of various coagulation factors [14]. This can be seen in severe liver dysfunction, which can be seen in HSCT patients because of organ damage due to preparative regimen, sinusoidal obstructive syndrome, or development of severe graft-versus-host disease. Cryoprecipitate may be utilized in these patients in the setting of hypofibirinogenemia [15].

## Granulocyte Colony-Stimulating Factors

Granulocyte colony-stimulating factors (G-CSF) shorten the duration of severe neutropenia after marrow suppressive chemotherapy. G-CSF use post-transplant shortens the duration of neutropenia and duration of hospitalization [16]. ASCO guidelines recommend the use of G-CSF post-auto-HSCT for the previously stated reasons [17]. However, there have been concerns regarding the use of G-CSF post-allo-HSCT, which in some studies was shown to increase risk of development of GVHD [16]. A meta-analysis of randomized controlled trials published in 2006 found that G-CSF use after allo-HSCT reduced the risk of documented infections and did not have a statistically significant effect on grade 2 to 4 acute GVHD or treatment-related mortality [18]. Based on these data, the ASCO guidelines do not have a strong recommendation against or in favor of using G-CSF in the post-allo-HSCT setting [17]. In some patients, G-CSF may need to be used after the peri-transplant period when the marrow function is suppressed due to infections or GVHD.

## Delayed Engraftment/Graft Failure

The Center for International Blood and Marrow Transplant Research (CIBMTR) defines neutrophil engraftment as first of 3 days when absolute neutrophil count is >500/mm$^3$ for three consecutive days and platelet engraftment as first of 7 days without transfusion support where the platelet count is >20,000/mm$^3$. Graft failure is defined as non-engraftment of neutrophils by day 28 post-HSCT. If there are concerns for delayed/non-engraftment, an extensive infectious workup is usually done to rule out infectious etiologies, and a bone marrow biopsy evaluation including chimerism studies is needed to confirm the diagnosis. Management includes stopping immunosuppression for delayed engraftment and use of eltrombopag [19] to enhance marrow recovery, and in some select situations, a second HSCT may be warranted.

## Hemolytic Anemia and Pure Red Cell Aplasia

Common causes of hemolysis in HSCT patients include drugs, infections, ABO incompatibility, or thrombotic microangiopathy. In this section, the focus will be on management of drug-induced hemolytic anemia and pure red cell aplasia. During the transplant process and recovery, patients are on multiple drugs during various phases of the transplant process like chemotherapeutic agents, immunosuppressive agents, and antibiotics. Incidence of hemolytic anemia has been estimated to be around 1.5 to 4.5% [20, 21]. Risk factors, which may increase the risk of development of hemolytic anemia, are use of unrelated donor and development of chronic GVHD [22]. If blood transfusions are indicated, cross matching may be unable to identify compatible RBC units, as the autoantibodies are directed against highly prevalent antigens. In this situation, close coordination with the blood bank team may be needed to get appropriate units released as delay in transfusion during severe hemolysis may be life threatening. Once diagnosis is confirmed in laboratory studies and is not improved with stopping drugs, which may be implicated, corticosteroids are started, usually at a dose of 1 mg/kg. In patients who do not respond to steroids, other immunosuppressive agents like rituximab may be needed [21]. Recent reports suggest a role for the anti-CD38 monoclonal antibody daratumumab (FDA approved for Light chain amyloidosis and multiple myeloma) in refractory hemolytic anemia and pure red cell aplasia [23, 24].

## Transplant-Associated Thrombotic Microangiopathy

Transplant-associated thrombotic microangiopathy (TA-TMA) develops in patients post-HSCT due to endothelial damage and complement activation [25]. The inciting event leading to the development of TA-TMA can be immune dysregulation and/or tissue damage due to preparative chemotherapy, total body irradiation, or GVHD. The incidence of this diagnosis post-HSCT has not been well documented, and this entity may be underdiagnosed in HSCT patients due to overlap with various other complications seen in this patient population. Various groups have reported incidence of TA-TMA to be between 1% and 40% using different diagnostic criteria [26, 27]. The mortality rate of TA-TMA has been reported to be 40–84% in various reports [26, 27]. Patients usually present with renal dysfunction in the presence of anemia and thrombocytopenia; often these patients rapidly develop multi-organ failure. Risk factors associated with development of TA-TMA have been identified as older age, female gender, HLA-mismatched/unrelated donors, use of busulfan/total body irradiation during preparative regimen, and drugs like calcineurin inhibitors (CNI) that are used to prevent GVHD post-allo-HSCT [28]. Various groups have proposed different criteria for the diagnosis of TA-TMA. Recently, the European Society for Blood and Marrow Transplantation (EBMT), American Society of Transplantation and Cellular Therapy (ASTCT)/Center for International Blood and Marrow Transplant Research (CIBMTR), and Asia-Pacific Blood and Marrow Transplantation (APBMT) group have released a consensus statement for harmonizing definitions for diagnostic criteria of TA-TMA. They proposed that either patients have biopsy-proven evidence of TMA or using modified Jodele criteria as shown in Table 30.2 where TA-TMA is diagnosed when ≥4/7 following features occur twice within 14 days. In addition, ADAMTS13 activity should be measured to exclude the diagnosis of acquired thrombotic thrombocytopenic purpura. A genetic mutation can be identified in about two-thirds of the patients with this diagnosis, which is similar to those seen in atypical hemolytic uremic syndrome.

**Table 30.2** Modified Jodele criteria for the diagnosis of transplant-associated thrombotic microangiopathy

| *Clinical/lab findings* | *Definitions* | |
|---|---|---|
| Anemia | Defined as failure to achieve transfusion independence despite neutrophil engraftment, hemoglobin decline by ≥1 g/dL, or new onset transfusion dependence | ≥4/7 criteria occurring more than two times in 14 days |
| Thrombocytopenia | Defined as failure to achieve platelet engraftment, higher than expected transfusion needs, refractory to platelet transfusions, or ≥50% reduction in baseline platelet count after full platelet engraftment | |
| Lactate dehydrogenase | Elevated | |
| Schistocytes | Present on peripheral smear | |
| Hypertension | ≥140/90 in those ≥18 years old, or ≥99th percentile in those <18 years old | |
| sC5b-9 | Elevated | |
| Proteinuria | >1 mg/mg random urine protein/creatinine ratio | |

Response to plasma exchange is underwhelming in patients with TA-TMA, and this modality should not be used for patients with this diagnosis [29, 30]. Patients diagnosed with TA-TMA should be taken off CNI [29]. Some patients will have improvement after stopping CNI. Eculizumab is an antibody that inhibits the activation of complement system by blocking the cleavage of C5 into C5a and C5b, which has been shown to reverse end-organ damage and restore hematologic parameters of patients diagnosed with TA-TMA in various case reports and case series [31–34]. Given the poor prognosis of patients diagnosed with TA-TMA who do not respond to CNI withdrawal, the use of eculizumab should be considered in critically ill HSCT patients diagnosed with TA-TMA [35].

## Secondary Hemophagocytic Lymphohistiocytosis/Macrophage Activation Syndrome

Secondary hemophagocytic lymphohistiocytosis (sHLH) is also sometimes referred to as macrophage activation syndrome (MAS), wherein a hyper-inflammatory state develops in patients due to underlying infection, malignancy, or immune dysregulated state [36]. sHLH/MAS has been reported mainly after allo-HSCT, but there are rare reports of this entity being diagnosed after autologous HSCT. There are reports that suggest the incidence of sHLH/MAS to be around 3–4% with mortality of patients diagnosed with this condition to be around 60–80% [37]. A recent survey from the European Society for Blood and Marrow Transplantation (EBMT) estimated the incidence of sHLH/MAS to be around 1% and 0.15% after allo-HSCT and autologous HSCT, respectively [38]. Diagnosis can be challenging especially as these patients can be critically ill due to few different reasons. Unfortunately, there are no validated algorithms for diagnosing HLH in the post-HSCT setting. In this setting, algorithms used in non-HSCT patients such as HLH-2004 criteria [36] or H score [39] as shown in Table 30.3 have been used to diagnose patients with post-HSCT sHLH/MAS. Significantly elevated ferritin, viral infections like Epstein-Barr virus or cytomegalovirus, and unexplained cytopenias are findings that may raise initial suspicion for sHLH/MAS. Other markers like soluble IL-2 levels, fibrinogen, and triglyceride levels should be checked in this setting. As this condition can be rapidly fatal, if there is clinical suspicion with some of the initial laboratory studies suggestive of sHLH/MAS, treatment should start emergently as this condition can be rapidly fatal. However, there is no clear consensus on the treatment of sHLH/MAS in the post-HSCT setting, but general principles of management of this condition [36], which include treating the inciting event and immune suppression, are utilized in HSCT patients. Immune-suppressive approaches including corticosteroids, immunoglobulin infusions, chemotherapeutic agents like etoposide, cytokine blocking agents like tocilizumab (IL-6 receptor blocking antibody) [40], anakinra (IL-1 receptor antagonist) [41], and more recently ruxolitinib (JAK1/2 inhibitor) [42] have been utilized. In addition to treatment with immunosuppressive agents, it is imperative for these patients to get appropriate supportive care including transfusion support and antibiotics.

**Table 30.3** H score for the diagnosis of secondary hemophagocytic lymphohistiocytosis (sHLH)

| Clinical/laboratory parameter | Qualifier | Score |
|---|---|---|
| Underlying immune-suppressive condition | No | 0 |
| | Yes | 18 |
| Temperature (C) | <38.4 | 0 |
| | 38.4–39.4 | 33 |
| | >39.4 | 49 |
| Number of cytopenias[a] | 1 lineage | 0 |
| | 2 lineages | 24 |
| | 3 lineages | 34 |
| Ferritin (ng/mL) | <2000 | 0 |
| | 2000–6000 | 35 |
| | >6000 | 50 |
| Triglycerides (mmols/L) | <1.5 | 0 |
| | 1.5–4 | 44 |
| | >4 | 64 |
| Fibrinogen (g/L) | >2.5 | 0 |
| | ≤2.5 | 30 |
| ALT/SGOT (IU/L) | <30 | 0 |
| | ≥30 | 19 |
| Hemophagocytosis on bone marrow biopsy | No | 0 |
| | Yes | 35 |

(Patients with a score of ≥250 have >99% probability of having sHLH)

[a]Hemoglobin ≤9.2 g/dL, platelet count ≤110,000/mm$^3$, and leukocyte count ≤5000/mm$^3$

## Conclusion

Critically ill HSCT patients need close cooperation between various teams to ensure an optimal outcome for these patients. Prompt identification of underlying etiology and appropriate management can be life saving for these patients who have the potential to be cured of their underlying malignancy after recovery from the HSCT procedure. The recovery for some patients can be prolonged, but they should be provided with the supportive care as needed to manage them through some expected HSCT complications as majority of the patients have relatively good performance status and organ function prior to them becoming critically ill especially during the peri-transplant period.

## References

1. Copelan EA. Hematopoietic stem-cell transplantation. N Engl J Med. 2006;354(17):1813–26.
2. Fuchs EJ, O'Donnell PV, Eapen M, Logan B, Antin JH, Dawson P, Devine S, Horowitz MM, Horwitz ME, Karanes C, Leifer E, Magenau JM, McGuirk JP, Morris LE, Rezvani AR, Jones RJ, Brunstein CG, Blood and Marrow Transplant Clinical Trials Network. Double unrelated umbilical cord blood vs. HLA-haploidentical bone marrow transplantation: the BMT CTN 1101 trial. Blood. 2021;137(3):420–8.
3. The Trial to Reduce Alloimmunization to Platelets Study Group. Leukocyte reduction and ultraviolet B irradiation of platelets to prevent alloimmunization and refractoriness to platelet transfusions. N Engl J Med. 1997;337:1861–70.
4. Moroff G, Leitman SF, Luban NL. Principles of blood irradiation, dose validation, and quality control. Transfusion. 1997;37:1084–92.
5. Tay J, Allan DS, Chatelein E, et al. Transfusion of red cells in hematopoietic stem cell transplantation (TRIST study): a randomized controlled trial evaluating 2 red cell transfusion thresholds. Blood. 2016;128:1032.
6. Mielcarek M, Leisenring W, Torok-Storb B, Storb R. Graft-versus-host disease and donor-directed hemagglutinin titers after ABO-mismatched related and unrelated marrow allografts: evidence for a graft-versus-plasma cell effect. Blood. 2000;96(3):1150–6.
7. Remberger M, Watz E, Ringdén O, Mattsson J, Shanwell A, Wikman A. Major ABO blood group mismatch increases the risk for graft failure after unrelated donor hematopoietic stem cell transplantation. Biol Blood Marrow Transplant. 2007;13(6):675–82.
8. Narayan S, Poles D, Serious Hazards or Transfusion (SHOT) Steering Group, et al. The 2021 annual SHOT report, 2022.
9. Wandt H, Schaefer-Eckart K, Wendelin K, et al. Therapeutic platelet transfusion versus routine prophylactic transfusion in patients with haematological malignancies: an open-label, multicentre, randomized study. Lancet. 2012;380:1309–16.
10. Crighton GL, Estcourt LJ, Wood EM, Trivella M, Doree C, Stanworth S. A therapeutic-only versus prophylactic platelet transfusion strategy for preventing bleeding in patients with haematological disorders after myelosuppressive chemotherapy or stem cell transplantation. Cochrane Database Syst Rev. 2015;2015(9):CD010981.
11. Patel IJ, Rahim S, Davidson JC, Hanks SE, Tam AL, Walker TG, Wilkins LR, Sarode R, Weinberg I. Society of interventional radiology consensus guidelines for the periprocedural management of thrombotic and bleeding risk in patients undergoing percutaneous image-guided interventions-part ii: recommendations: endorsed by the Canadian association for interventional radiology and the cardiovascular and interventional radiological society of Europe. J Vasc Interv Radiol. 2019;30(8):1168–84.
12. Schiffer CA, Bohlke K, Delaney M, Hume H, Magdalinski AJ, McCullough JJ, Omel JL, Rainey JM, Rebulla P, Rowley SD, Troner MB, Anderson KC. Platelet transfusion for patients with cancer: American society of clinical oncology clinical practice guideline update. J Clin Oncol. 2018;36(3):283–99.
13. Vassallo RR, Fung M, Rebulla P, et al. Utility of cross-matched platelet transfusions in patients with hypoproliferative thrombocytopenia: a systematic review. Transfusion. 2014;54:1180–91.
14. Consensus Conference. Fresh-frozen plasma. Indications and risks. JAMA. 1985;253(4):551–3.
15. Franchini M, Lippi G. Fibrinogen replacement therapy: a critical review of the literature. Blood Transfus. 2012;10(1):23–7.
16. Singh V, Jang H, Kim S, Ayash L, Alavi A, Ratanatharathorn V, Uberti JP, Deol A. G-CSF use post peripheral blood stem cell transplant is associated with faster neutrophil engraftment, shorter hospital stay and increased incidence of chronic GVHD. Leuk Lymphoma. 2021;62(2):446–53.
17. Smith TJ, Bohlke K, Lyman GH, Carson KR, Crawford J, Cross SJ, Goldberg JM, Khatcheressian JL, Leighl NB, Perkins CL, Somlo G, Wade JL, Wozniak AJ, Armitage JO, American Society of Clinical Oncology. Recommendations for the use of WBC growth factors: American society of clinical oncology clinical practice guideline update. J Clin Oncol. 2015;33(28):3199–212.
18. Dekker A, Bulley S, Beyene J, Dupuis LL, Doyle JJ, Sung L. Meta-analysis of randomized controlled trials of prophylactic granulocyte colony-stimulating factor and granulocyte-macrophage colony-stimulating factor after autologous and allogeneic stem cell transplantation. J Clin Oncol. 2006;24(33):5207–15.

19. Marotta S, Marano L, Ricci P, Cacace F, Frieri C, Simeone L, Trastulli F, Vitiello S, Cardano F, Pane F, Risitano AM. Eltrombopag for post-transplant cytopenias due to poor graft function. Bone Marrow Transplant. 2019;54(8):1346–53.
20. Wang M, Wang W, Abeywardane A, Adikarama M, McLornan D, Raj K, de Lavallade H, Devereux S, Mufti GJ, Pagliuca A, Potter VT, Mijovic A. Autoimmune hemolytic anemia after allogeneic hematopoietic stem cell transplantation: analysis of 533 adult patients who underwent transplantation at King's college hospital. Biol Blood Marrow Transplant. 2015;21(1):60–6.
21. González-Vicent M, Sanz J, Fuster JL, Cid J, de Heredia CD, Morillo D, Fernández JM, Pascual A, Badell I, Serrano D, Fox L, de la Serna J, Benito A, Couselo JM, Molina B, Díaz MÁ, Sanz MÁ. Autoimmune hemolytic anemia (AIHA) following allogeneic hematopoietic stem cell transplantation (HSCT): a retrospective analysis and a proposal of treatment on behalf of the Grupo Español De Trasplante de Medula Osea en Niños (GETMON) and the Grupo Español de Trasplante Hematopoyetico (GETH). Transfus Med Rev. 2018;S0887-7963(17):30164–5.
22. Sanz J, Arriaga F, Montesinos P, Ortí G, Lorenzo I, Cantero S, Puig N, Moscardó F, de la Rubia J, Sanz G, Sanz MA. Autoimmune hemolytic anemia following allogeneic hematopoietic stem cell transplantation in adult patients. Bone Marrow Transplant. 2007;39(9):555–61.
23. Chapuy CI, Kaufman RM, Alyea EP, Connors JM. Daratumumab for delayed red-cell engraftment after allogeneic transplantation. N Engl J Med. 2018;379(19):1846–50.
24. Rautenberg C, Kaivers J, Germing U, Haas R, Ackerstaff S, Hoffmann T, Kobbe G, Schroeder T. Daratumumab for treatment of pure red cell aplasia after allogeneic stem cell transplantation. Bone Marrow Transplant. 2020;55(6):1191–3.
25. Young JA, Pallas CR, Knovich MA. Transplant-associated thrombotic microangiopathy: theoretical considerations and a practical approach to an unrefined diagnosis. Bone Marrow Transplant. 2021;56(8):1805–17.
26. Gavriilaki E, Sakellari I, Batsis I, Mallouri D, Bousiou Z, Vardi A, Yannaki E, Constantinou V, Tsompanakou A, Vadikoliou C, Kaloyannidis P, Bamihas G, Anagnostopoulos A. Transplant-associated thrombotic microangiopathy: incidence, prognostic factors, morbidity, and mortality in allogeneic hematopoietic cell transplantation. Clin Transplant. 2018;32(9):e13371.
27. Epperla N, Li A, Logan B, Fretham C, Chhabra S, Aljurf M, Chee L, Copelan E, Freytes CO, Hematti P, Lazarus HM, Litzow M, Nishihori T, Olsson RF, Prestidge T, Saber W, Wirk B, Yared JA, Loren A, Pasquini M. Incidence, risk factors for and outcomes of transplant-associated thrombotic microangiopathy. Br J Haematol. 2020;189(6):1171–81.
28. Jodele S, Davies SM, Lane A, Khoury J, Dandoy C, Goebel J, Myers K, Grimley M, Bleesing J, El-Bietar J, Wallace G, Chima RS, Paff Z, Laskin BL. Diagnostic and risk criteria for HSCT-associated thrombotic microangiopathy: a study in children and young adults. Blood. 2014;124(4):645–53.
29. Ho VT, Cutler C, Carter S, Martin P, Adams R, Horowitz M, et al. Blood and marrow transplant clinical trials network toxicity committee consensus summary: thrombotic microangiopathy after hematopoietic stem cell transplantation. Biol Blood Marrow Transplant. 2005;11:571–5.
30. Epperla N, Li A, Logan B, Fretham C, Chhabra S, Aljurf M, et al. Incidence, risk factors for and outcomes of transplant-associated thrombotic microangiopathy. Br J Haematol. 2020;189:1171–81.
31. Okano M, Sakata N, Ueda S, Takemura T. Recovery from life-threatening transplantation-associated thrombotic microangiopathy using eculizumab in a patient with very severe aplastic anemia. Bone Marrow Transplant. 2014;49(8):1116–8.
32. Chapin J, Shore T, Forsberg P, Desman G, Van Besien K, Laurence J, et al. Hematopoietic transplant-associated thrombotic microangiopathy: case report and review of diagnosis and treatments. Clin Adv Hematol Oncol. 2014;12(9):565–73.
33. Bohl SR, Kuchenbauer F, von Harsdorf S, Kloevekorn N, Schonsteiner SS, Rouhi A, et al. Thrombotic microangiopathy after allogeneic stem cell transplantation: a comparison of eculizumab therapy and conventional therapy. Biol Blood Marrow Transplant. 2017;23(12):2172–7.
34. Rudoni J, Jan A, Hosing C, Aung F, Yeh J. Eculizumab for transplant-associated thrombotic microangiopathy in adult allogeneic stem cell transplant recipients. Eur J Haematol. 2018;101(3):389–98.Zhang R, Zhou M, Qi J, Miao W, Zhang Z, Wu D, Han Y. Efficacy and safety of eculizumab in the treatment of transplant-associated thrombotic microangiopathy: a systematic review and meta-analysis. Front Immunol. 2021;11:564647.
35. La Rosée P, Horne AC, Hines M, von Bahr T, Greenwood RM, Berliner N, Birndt S, Gil-Herrera J, Girschikofsky M, Jordan MB, Kumar A, van Laar JAM, Lachmann G, Nichols KE, Ramanan AV, Wang Y, Wang Z, Janka G, Henter J-I. Recommendations for the management of hemophagocytic lymphohistiocytosis in adults. Blood. 2019;133(23):2465–77.
36. Sandler RD, Carter S, Kaur H, Francis S, Tattersall RS, Snowden JA. Haemophagocytic lymphohistiocytosis (HLH) following allogeneic haematopoietic stem cell transplantation (HSCT)-time to reappraise with modern diagnostic and treatment strategies? Bone Marrow Transplant. 2020;55(2):307–16. https://doi.org/10.1038/s41409-019-0637-7.
37. Sandler RD, Tattersall RS, Schoemans H, Greco R, Badoglio M, Labopin M, Alexander T, Kirgizov K, Rovira M, Saif M, Saccardi R, Delgado J, Peric Z, Koenecke C, Penack O, Basak G, Snowden

JA. Diagnosis and management of secondary HLH/MAS following HSCT and CAR-T cell therapy in adults; a review of the literature and a survey of practice within EBMT centres on behalf of the Autoimmune Diseases Working Party (ADWP) and Transplant Complications Working Party (TCWP). Front Immunol. 2020;11:524.
38. Fardet L, Galicier L, Lambotte O, Marzac C, Aumont C, Chahwan D, Coppo P, Hejblum G. Development and validation of the HScore, a score for the diagnosis of reactive hemophagocytic syndrome. Arthritis Rheumatol. 2014;66(9):2613–20.
39. Dufranc E, Del Bello A, Belliere J, Kamar N, Faguer S, TAIDI (Toulouse Acquired Immune Deficiency and Infection) Study Group. IL6-R blocking with tocilizumab in critically ill patients with hemophagocytic syndrome. Crit Care. 2020;24(1):166.
40. Bami S, Vagrecha A, Soberman D, Badawi M, Cannone D, Lipton JM, Cron RQ, Levy CF. The use of anakinra in the treatment of secondary hemophagocytic lymphohistiocytosis. Pediatr Blood Cancer. 2020;67(11):e28581.
41. Goldsmith SR, Rehman SSU, Shirai CL, Vij K, DiPersio JF. Resolution of secondary hemophagocytic lymphohistiocytosis after treatment with the JAK1/2 inhibitor ruxolitinib. Blood Adv. 2019;3(23):4131–5.

# Pulmonary and Critical Care Considerations in Pediatric Hematopoietic Stem Cell Transplantation Patient

31

Yiouli Ktena and Kenneth R. Cooke

## Introduction

Hematopoietic stem cell transplantation (HSCT) is curative for an ever-increasing number of children with malignant and non-malignant conditions. Approximately 2500 pediatric procedures are performed annually in the USA [1, 2]. Although HSCT is undertaken with curative intent, relapse of underlying malignancies and post-HSCT complications limit successful outcomes. In aggregate, pulmonary dysfunction, transplant-related thrombotic microangiopathy (TA-TMA), and veno-occlusive disease are major contributors to the development of multiorgan dysfunction syndrome [3] and intensive care admissions [4, 5] in pediatric and young adult HSCT recipients. The significance of respiratory failure in this setting was further underscored by a NIH workshop convened in 2018 specifically to identify clinical challenges and scientific knowledge gaps regarding pulmonary dysfunction after pediatric HSCT [6]. This chapter will explore the state of the science and remaining challenges related to these transplant-related complications and associated critical care considerations in pediatric HSCT recipients.

## Pulmonary Dysfunction Following Pediatric HSCT

### Overview

Lung dysfunction occurs frequently following HSCT in the immediate post-transplant period and in the months and years that follow and significantly contributes to transplant-related morbidity and mortality [7–12]. Pulmonary toxicity requiring mechanical ventilation after HSCT occurs in 10–39% of pediatric, adolescent, and young adult (AYA) patients and often results in death, underscoring its severity and impact on outcomes [4, 7, 13–15]. Importantly, allogeneic HSCT has been increasingly used to treat non-malignant disorders (sickle cell disease, immune deficiencies, and metabolic disorders) wherein pulmonary disease pre-exists/co-exists, increasing the likelihood of post-transplant lung dysfunction. Additionally, conditioning regimens, immunosuppression, opportunistic infections, and graft-versus-host reactions may contribute to lung toxicity pre- and post-HSCT. In one report, 40% of long-term survivors of allogeneic HSCT for pediatric hematologic malignancies had abnormal pulmonary function tests (PFT) pre-transplant, and nearly two-thirds developed

Y. Ktena · K. R. Cooke (✉)
Department of Oncology, Pediatric Blood and Marrow Transplantation Program, The Sidney Kimmel Comprehensive Cancer Center, The Johns Hopkins University School of Medicine, Baltimore, MD, USA
e-mail: kcooke5@jhmi.edu



A. O. Soubani (ed.), *Pulmonary and Critical Care Considerations of Hematopoietic Stem Cell Transplantation*, https://doi.org/10.1007/978-3-031-28797-8_31

abnormal PFTs following HSCT [16]. Unfortunately, current retrospective/registry data lack the granularity, accuracy, and completeness to identify pre-transplant pulmonary phenotypes that may predict, or associate with lung dysfunction post-transplant. Similarly, there are few prospective studies in children describing pulmonary risk before HSCT or longitudinal studies characterizing pulmonary toxicity afterwards. In addition, clinical definitions for conditions unique to adult HSCT patients such as bronchiolitis obliterans syndrome (BOS) may be less applicable in children, undoubtedly contributing to reported variations in the incidence and outcomes of these conditions. Prompt and accurate diagnosis of lung dysfunction in the pediatric population is also impacted by the lack of effective, reliable, monitoring of lung function in young and/or critically ill children [17–19] and the low sensitivity and specificity of imaging techniques [20]. Developing longitudinal, prospective cohorts of pediatric HSCT recipients using PFTs, prognostic biomarkers, and enhanced diagnostic and imaging techniques could improve outcomes [12].

## Clinical Phenotypes

Pulmonary diagnoses following HSCT can be considered infectious or non-infectious [8, 21]. Infectious lung injury remains problematic, particularly in patients with acute or chronic graft-versus-host disease (GVHD). Historically, one-half of all pulmonary complications after HSCT were secondary to infection, but the current use of broad-spectrum, antimicrobial agents has tipped the balance toward non-infectious causes [22]. Non-infectious lung injury can be acute or chronic depending on the time of onset after HSCT, nature of the immune response (inflammatory vs. fibrotic), and tempo of disease progression [22, 23].

The clinical spectrum of acute, non-infectious lung dysfunction includes idiopathic pneumonia syndrome (IPS), diffuse alveolar hemorrhage (DAH), transfusion-related acute lung injury (TRALI), and pulmonary thrombotic microangiopathy (TMA) [8]. These disorders develop in the context of cytotoxicity of anti-neoplastic therapies, infusion of blood products, inflammation engendered during HSCT, or combinations thereof [8, 22]. IPS is defined as widespread alveolar injury following HSCT occurring in the absence of active infection, cardiogenic dysfunction, or iatrogenic fluid overload [8, 21]. The diagnostic criteria include clinical signs and symptoms of pneumonia, non-lobar radiographic infiltrates, abnormal pulmonary function, and absence of infection as determined by bronchoalveolar lavage (BAL) or lung biopsy preferably including multiplex PCR-based assays [24]. The updated definition of IPS classifies non-infectious lung disease by anatomical site [8]. IPS typically presents within the first 120 days of HSCT [8, 21]. Historically, the incidence of IPS following myeloablative conditioning ranged from 3% to 15% in adults and children [8, 11, 21, 25–28]. The implementation of reduced-intensity conditioning regimens coupled with enhanced contemporary, molecular diagnostic techniques has reduced the incidence of IPS [12, 24, 29, 30].

A subset of patients with IPS may develop DAH, characterized by progressive shortness of breath, cough, and hypoxemia with or without fever [31]. Classically, the diagnosis of DAH is based on progressively bloodier aliquots of BAL fluid, but frank hemoptysis is rare. Challenges associated with timely BAL in children highlight the importance of a clinical diagnosis. DAH has been reported in 5–12% of adult HSCT recipients [22] and generally occurs within the first 2 to 3 months after transplant [22, 31]. A disproportionately higher incidence of DAH post-HSCT is reported in children with mucopolysaccharidosis [32]. DAH can occur with or without infection; both forms are associated with poor outcomes following conventional therapy, including high-dose steroids [33]. Pulmonary TMA is another complication in pediatric and adult HSCT recipients that is associated with high mortality. TMA in the lungs presents as pulmonary hypertension, often leading to acute hypoxia, cardiopulmonary compromise, and death [34–36]. TRALI is one of the leading causes of mortality following infusions of plasma containing blood products. Initially reported in as many as 1:5000 units transfused, estimates of 1:64,000 transfusions in more recent reports suggest that the occurrence is far less frequent [37–39]. Symptoms present acutely, with the onset of dyspnea and respiratory distress being typically 6–8 h following blood product transfusion. Chest radiographs reveal diffuse pulmonary infiltrates reflecting edema from increased pulmonary vascular permeability. Treatment is generally supportive. Discontinuation of the blood product, corticosteroid administration, forced diuresis, and respiratory support results in recovery within 3 to 4 days in the majority of patients.

Sub-acute/chronic (occurring or persisting 0.5 to 2 years after HSCT), non-infectious, pulmonary complications contribute to significant morbidity after allo-HSCT. Pediatric studies are few and small, highlighting a need for further studies particularly in the context of a developing lung. HSCT recipients can develop obstructive lung disease (OLD) or restrictive lung disease (RLD), resulting from fibrotic remodeling, either primarily around the small airways/bronchioles or within gas exchange regions (e.g., interstitial fibrosis), respectively [23, 40, 41]. RLD can develop in association with previous chest wall/thoracic surgery and/or radiation therapy and in patients who develop acute lung injury (e.g., IPS) and acute GVHD. In the sub-acute setting, RLD may occur with cryptogenic organizing pneumonia (COP) /bronchiolitis obliterans organizing pneumonia (BOOP) [42] or in the context of chronic, fibrotic, interstitial lung disease [22]. BOS after HSCT is often reflective of pulmonary GVHD. BOS is associated with OLD with air trapping demonstrated by chest radiographs, computerized tomography (CT) imaging, and spirometry (reduced $FEV_1$/FVC ratio). BOS is a clinical diagnosis based on a scoring system designed for adult lung transplant patients, predicated upon a decline in $FEV_1$ and/or $FEF_{25-75\%}$. A modified version of the NIH criteria for the diagnosis of BOS in HSCT patients was developed for adults but has yet to be validated in children [43]. A rapid decline in $FEV_1$ has been demonstrated during the 6 months prior to the diagnosis of chronic GVHD/BOS in two adult cohorts [44], and a 10% decline in $FEV_1$ from baseline increases the risk of developing BOS [45]. Once BOS is diagnosed, reversing changes from fibrosis is challenging particularly when patients have already become symptomatic. Hence, early detection of pulmonary dysfunction is believed to be critical to initiate pre-emptive therapies in pediatric HCT recipients [46–48]. Frequent PFTs should be obtained post-transplant, particularly in those with baseline abnormalities and/or significant non-pulmonary GVHD. Two pediatric cohorts demonstrated that PFTs are more sensitive than clinical exam for the early detection and diagnosis of BOS; those investigators recommend monitoring PFTs longitudinally beyond 12 months post-HSCT in at-risk patients [49, 50]. Home-based, hand-held spirometry correlates with traditional laboratory spirometry in adults following lung transplantation [51] and HSCT [44, 52] and warrants similar evaluation in children.

## Risk Factors

Numerous patient-specific factors influence the risk of developing pulmonary complications after HSCT. Indications for transplant, especially in non-malignant conditions, may include disorders with baseline airway/parenchymal abnormalities or predisposition to pre-transplant pulmonary complications. A thorough medical history may reveal factors affecting pre-transplant lung function. Previous cancer therapy, underlying genetic variants, particular phyla within the individual microbiome, pre-transplant conditioning, and early post-transplant inflammation can all contribute to lung abnormalities and influence the likelihood of long-term complications. For example, 10–15% of children pre-transplant demonstrate abnormal forced and static lung volumes, and over 50% demonstrate decreased diffusing capacity, placing them at risk of immediate pulmonary complications and abnormal lung function and mortality post-transplant [53–55]. Furthermore, a higher pre-transplant lung function score based on the estimation of expiratory flow ($FEV_1$) and diffusion (DLCO) is associated with increased risk of respiratory failure and death post-transplant. Pre-existing impaired lung function and total body irradiation (TBI)-based regimens correlated with the lowest survival in a retrospective study of adults [56]. Similarly, pulmonary disease and lower pre-transplant forced vital capacity z-scores along with abnormalities in chest CT scans have been associated with poor recovery of lung function [57] and a higher risk of immune-mediated lung injury [58] post HSCT, respectively. The development of a risk score based on pre-transplant pulmonary function and imaging, stem cell source, donor type, HLA match, conditioning regimen intensity and composition, fecal microbiota diversity, Day +7 GVHD biomarkers, and presence of comorbidities including prior infections and pre-existing renal and cardiac impairment may help stratify patients at risk for pulmonary complications after HSCT.

## Diagnostic Challenges Unique to Pediatric HSCT Patients

The treatment of lung dysfunction after HSCT requires attention to pulmonary and non-pulmonary causes. Respiratory distress may progress rapidly once identified; hence, a timely work-up including assessment of pulmonary and cardiac function, imaging, and procurement of samples to rule out infection is critical for optimizing outcomes. Initial chest imaging may identify the presence of lobar, multilobar, or diffuse pulmonary infiltrates. Echocardiography may reveal pulmonary hypertension or left heart dysfunction. While such findings impact the decision-making process, they are non-diagnostic. Challenges with effective and reliable monitoring of lung function in young and/or critically ill children [59] including imaging techniques that only offer low sensitivity and specificity [20, 59–62] represent major obstacles to the prompt and accurate diagnosis of lung injury. While successful spirometry is reported in patients as young as 3 years [63] and acceptability of testing can be as high as 87% in 5-year-old patients [64], consistent measurements of $FEV_1$ in young children present significant challenges as well. $FEV_{0.5}$ (0.5 s), a measurement found to be more reproducible in pre-school children with cystic fibrosis [65] than $FEV_1$, could be evaluated as an early physiological biomarker of BOS. Forced oscillometry testing (FOT) is a feasible, yet to be validated, technique in preschoolers, which detects changes in pulmonary resistance and compliance [66]. In addition, the lung clearance index (LCI), measured using the multiple breath washout technique (MBW), has demonstrated greater sensitivity than standard PFTs in detecting airway changes in adults post-HSCT [61, 67]. Novel parameters of respiratory function assessed by quantitative CT (e.g., parametric response mapping (PRM)) [68] and specific-gas mapping [69] also need to be tested prospectively in childhood. Hyperpolarized $^{129}Xe$ MRI, feasible in children unable to perform reliable spirometry, can differentiate cystic fibrosis patients with early lung obstruction from age-matched controls [70]. The development and validation of novel criteria to predict risk, follow the trajectory of lung function, and diagnose BOS in pediatric HSCT populations are needed [71].

In the absence of obvious, non-pulmonary causes of lung dysfunction, bronchoscopy with BAL should be considered to distinguish infectious from non-infectious etiologies and to initiate appropriate management. However, this remains an area of active debate [72]. Complication rates from bronchoscopy procedures in adults were less than 2% in three large series [73–75], and similar findings need to be replicated in children. The diagnostic yield from BAL fluid ranges from 31% to 67% depending on the timing post-HSCT of respiratory distress, the time elapsed between the onset of symptoms and BAL, and the start of antimicrobial therapy [74–77]. BAL within 4 days of the appearance of pulmonary infiltrates increases the overall diagnostic yield [76]. The therapeutic and diagnostic impact of lung biopsy in children with pulmonary dysfunction after HSCT has been recently reported [78]. The diagnostic utility of serum and lung biomarkers in lung injury among HSCT recipients with IPS [79, 80] is described in a consensus statement [8].

## Mechanisms of Lung Injury Following HSCT

The mechanisms contributing to non-infectious pulmonary complications following HSCT are complex. The pathophysiology of IPS has been explored in various lines of laboratory investigation [8, 22] and translational research efforts [79, 81, 82]. Data from established, pre-clinical models support a shift in perspective away from simply viewing the lung as an indirect target of collateral damage from systemic inflammation and toward a scenario wherein the lung is specifically vulnerable to two pathways of immune-mediated injury, which include the recruitment of donor-derived, cytotoxic effector cells and inflammatory cytokine release [8, 22]. These distinct but interrelated pathways involve (1) components of the adaptive and innate immune responses, (2) synergistic interactions between lymphoid [83, 84] and myeloid cells, and (3) release of soluble inflammatory chemokines [85–88] and cytokines including TNF-α [25, 89–92], INF-γ [93, 94], and IL-6 [95]. Furthermore, they orchestrate the sequential recruitment of donor-derived immune cells (T-lymphocytes, macrophages, monocytes, and neutrophils) to the lung and ultimately contribute to tissue damage and dysfunction [8]. Laboratory insights have been translated back to the clinic for pediatric patients with IPS in the form of novel strategies to mitigate the lethal effects of this complication [80, 81, 96]. Importantly, proteomic studies from three human clinical studies revealed striking similarities among mechanisms contributing to IPS in humans and mice, underscored a role for the acute-phase response (TNF-α/IL-6) signaling pathway, and illuminated a possible role for pulmonary vascular endothelial injury in the development of lung dysfunction. Endothelial cell (EC) damage has been implicated as a direct contributor to the development of several complications following allogeneic HSCT, including DAH and TMA [97–99]. EC activation and injury are also observed after clinical and experimental IPS [80, 83, 90, 100] and likely contribute other late effects after HSCT for pediatric and AYA patients [101]. Moreover, the proteomic studies uncovered biomarkers predictive of IPS development and response to therapy [82] and identified several novel pathways ripe for further exploration [81, 82, 95]. Importantly, other investigators studying clinical serum and BAL samples have been corroborated and extended these observations by identifying biomarker panels that associate with IPS [79, 102] and predict respiratory failure [103].

As noted above, chronic pulmonary dysfunction following allogeneic HSCT can manifest as either OLD or RLD [22, 23, 40, 42]. The pathophysiology of lung fibrosis after HSCT is complex and incompletely understood, highlighting significant knowledge gaps with respect to the biology of and approach to therapy for this spectrum of disorders [40, 104, 105]. These limitations stem from the (1) lack of consistent approaches to monitor for respiratory compromise and accurately diagnose the cause of lung dysfunction; (2) absence of correlative data obtained from afflicted HSCT recipients, and, until recently, (3) paucity of suitable preclinical animal models for either form of chronic lung disease [40, 106]. Fibrosis refers to the excessive deposition of extracellular matrix, primarily cross-linked fibrillar collagens, by persistently or abnormally activated fibroblasts. Resultant scarring usually causes architectural distortion and physiological dysfunction of tissues and organs [40, 107, 108]. When developing in the context of pulmonary GVHD, fibrosis is thought to involve a persistent or recurrent antigenic stimulus, which elicits chronic inflammation [22, 23, 40]. In this context, a *tri-phasic model* recently proposed for the development of chronic GVHD [40] can be applied to the development of chronic pulmonary dysfunction after HSCT [23, 40]. This model involves acute inflammation, which may be subclinical (Phase I) [8], dysregulated immunity (Phase II), along with dysfunctional repair, and propagation of chronic inflammation resulting in the deposition of collagen and fibrosis (Phase III) (Fig. 31.1). When this occurs in and around bronchial structures, obliteration of small airways and significant, "fixed" OLD ensues. By contrast, fibroblast proliferation and intra-septal collagen deposition may ultimately result in interstitial fibrosis, volume loss, and impaired gas exchange, characteristic of severe RLD [40]. Recently, murine systems have revealed that dysregulation of other factors including aberrant B-cell immunity with associated auto-/allo-antibody production [109–113], disruption of the balance of M1/

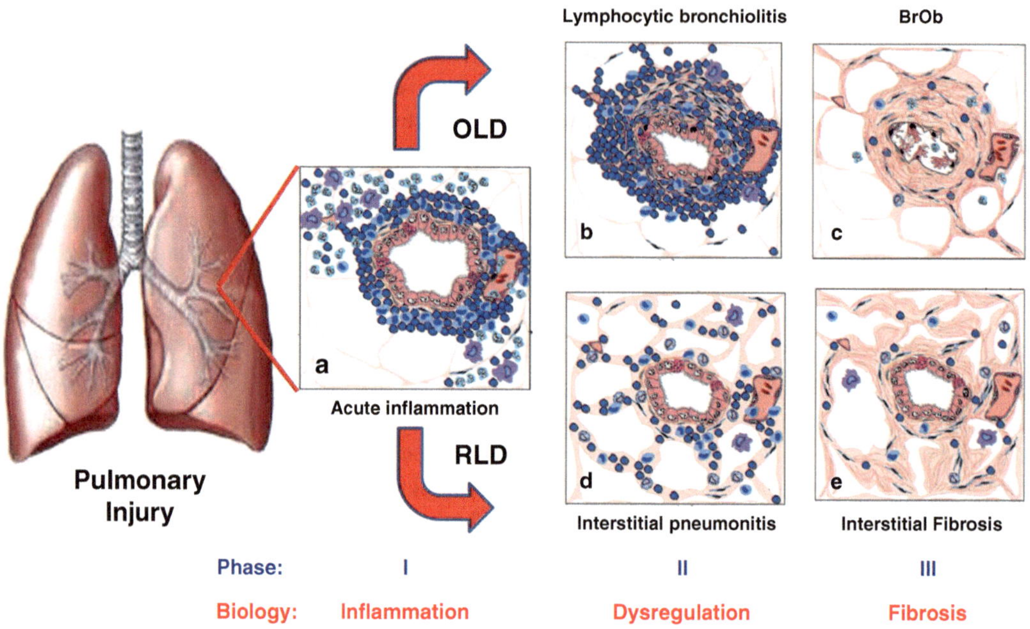


**Fig. 31.1** Tri-phasic model of non-infectious lung injury after allogeneic HSCT. A tri-phasic model of chronic GVHD is proposed for the development of lung dysfunction after allogeneic HSCT. In Phase I, acute lung injury occurs as a consequence of an allogeneic immune response and results in the influx of donor immune cells into an inflamed pulmonary parenchyma (**a**). Persistence of an inflammatory signal in the setting of dysregulated immunity promotes the transition from acute to chronic injury in Phase II (**b** and **d**). If the inciting injurious event predominantly involves bronchiolar epithelial cells, Phase II is associated with the development of chronic bronchiolitis (**b**). In the context of aberrant repair, chronic inflammation proceeds to Phase III. Lung fibroblasts increase dramatically in number and contribute to the enhanced deposition of collagen and granulation tissue in and around bronchial structures, ultimately resulting in complete obliteration of small airways and fixed obstructive lung disease (OLD) characteristic of bronchiolitis obliterans (BrOb) (**c**). If, by contrast, the principal target of chronic inflammation is the alveolar epithelium, leukocyte recruitment and matrix deposition during Phase II contribute to interstitial pneumonitis (**d**). Fibroblast proliferation and intra-septal collagen deposition during Phase III ultimately results in interstitial thickening, septal fibrosis, significant volume reduction, and development of severe restrictive lung disease (RLD) and interstitial fibrosis (**e**)

M2 macrophage function [114], and release of pro-inflammatory cytokines including TNF-α [115, 116] may all be operative during the development of pulmonary fibrosis [40].

The role of the microbiome in the development of lung toxicity after HSCT has been the focus of recent investigation. Inflammation and injury may result from disturbances in microbe-host interaction balance [117]. For example, the γ-proteobacterial domination of fecal microbiota pre-transplant predicted pulmonary complications and mortality in a cohort of adults receiving allogeneic HSCT [118]. Studies demonstrating that genetic variations in bactericidal/permeability-increasing protein and NOD2/CARD15 influence the risk of developing airflow decline after allogeneic HSCT [119, 120] underscore the possible effects of the microbiome and function of the intestinal barrier on the development of BOS. Hence, interventions to preserve the respiratory and gut-lung microbiome axis pre- and post-transplant may decrease pulmonary risk. Moreover, the impact of the lung microbiome and prior infections as triggers of dysregulated immunity and repair contributing to fibrotic lung injury that may appear "non-infectious" in etiology at later time points is a topic of active investigation [121–124]. Newer methods including metagenomic sequencing, gene-expression profiling, and proteomics could help clarify these relationships and their effects on disease severity and lung function in the long term [125].

## Treatment of Pulmonary Complications in Pediatric HSCT Patients

Conducting clinical trials in relatively small, heterogeneous, pediatric populations with acute or chronic pulmonary complications following HSCT is challenging [126]. For example, three pediatric reports [27, 28, 127] confirmed that IPS remains a serious complication following HSCT with high mortality (50–80%) and poor (18–30%) response to treatment. The use of high-dose steroids to pediatric HSCT recipients with non-infectious, acute lung injury has produced mixed results. The Pediatric Acute Lung Injury Consensus Conference (PALICC) recommends future studies be completed to identify specific populations that might benefit from glucocorticoid therapy [128]. To this end, early-phase prospective studies [80, 96] and two retrospective reports [129, 130] suggested that treatment of IPS with corticosteroids and etanercept, a soluble TNF-α binding protein, may improve survival. A subsequent multicenter, open-label, Phase II, pediatric study found that the administration of corticosteroids combined with etanercept was safe and resulted in response rates of 71% with Day +28- and 1-year survival rates of 89% and 63%, respectively [81]. Of note, this trial had uniform eligibility (excluding age), dosing schedules, and assessments with a parallel Phase III IPS study in adults [131]. However, the 1-year overall survival for adults was extremely poor (<25%) in both arms. Importantly, the pediatric trial ended early as an efficacy stopping rule was met, whereas the adult trial was terminated early for poor accrual; only 34 out of a targeted 120 patients were randomized, which undoubtedly impacted the interpretation of results [131]. Despite these advances in pediatric patients with IPS [81], not all patients responded to TNF-α neutralization. Hence, the utility of cytokine analysis and additional targetable protein biomarkers such as Ang-2 [97, 132] in further optimizing the recognition and treatment of IPS requires additional study. For example, a retrospective trial revealed that elevated levels of suppression of tumorigenicity/stimulation-2 (ST2), a biomarker implicated in acute lung injury and GVHD, when combined with elevated levels of IL-6 and sTNFR1 were most predictive in diagnosing IPS even before clinical signs and symptoms were present [79]. These findings were recently extended by Rowen and colleagues who showed that a biomarker panel including ST2, IL-6, and sTNFR1 could, as early as day 7 after HSCT, predict respiratory failure and associated mortality in a cohort of predominantly pediatric HSCT recipients [103]. Hence, pre-emptive, combinatorial, anti-cytokine strategies for patients at a high risk for IPS and respiratory failure may have merit.

DAH is associated with mortality as high as 85% in adult and pediatric HSCT patients [8, 22, 31]. Studies report minimal benefit with high-dose steroids with or without aminocaproic acid (Amicar™) therapy; a recent, single-center, retrospective review of 119 adults with DAH treated with varying doses of steroids revealed Day +100 and overall mortality rates of 85% and 95%, respectively. Two-thirds of cases were non-infectious in origin and could be classified as IPS [133]. Anecdotal reports of inhaled recombinant Factor VIIa therapy suggest benefit, and this approach appears well tolerated despite a risk of endotracheal tube occlusion from sudden clot formation [134, 135]. Future considerations should include combining non-infectious DAH and IPS together for inclusion in multi-center studies of targetable inflammatory cytokines and other novel therapies for pediatric patients. An approach to HSCT patients with acute pulmonary dysfunction is proposed in Fig. 31.2.

Standard treatments for non-infectious forms of OLD and RLD remain suboptimal; no agent or combination of agents has been particularly effective. However, a number of new therapeutic strategies have been employed for BOS [136]. The administration of etanercept and combination therapy with "FAM" (fluticasone, azithromycin, and montelukast) have shown promise in improving [137] and potentially stabilizing [138] lung function, respectively. Both studies were early-phase, open-label trials, and therefore, results need to be interpreted in the context of the known natural history of BOS, which can include stabilization of disease with time [45, 139]. A very small, randomized study showed no effect

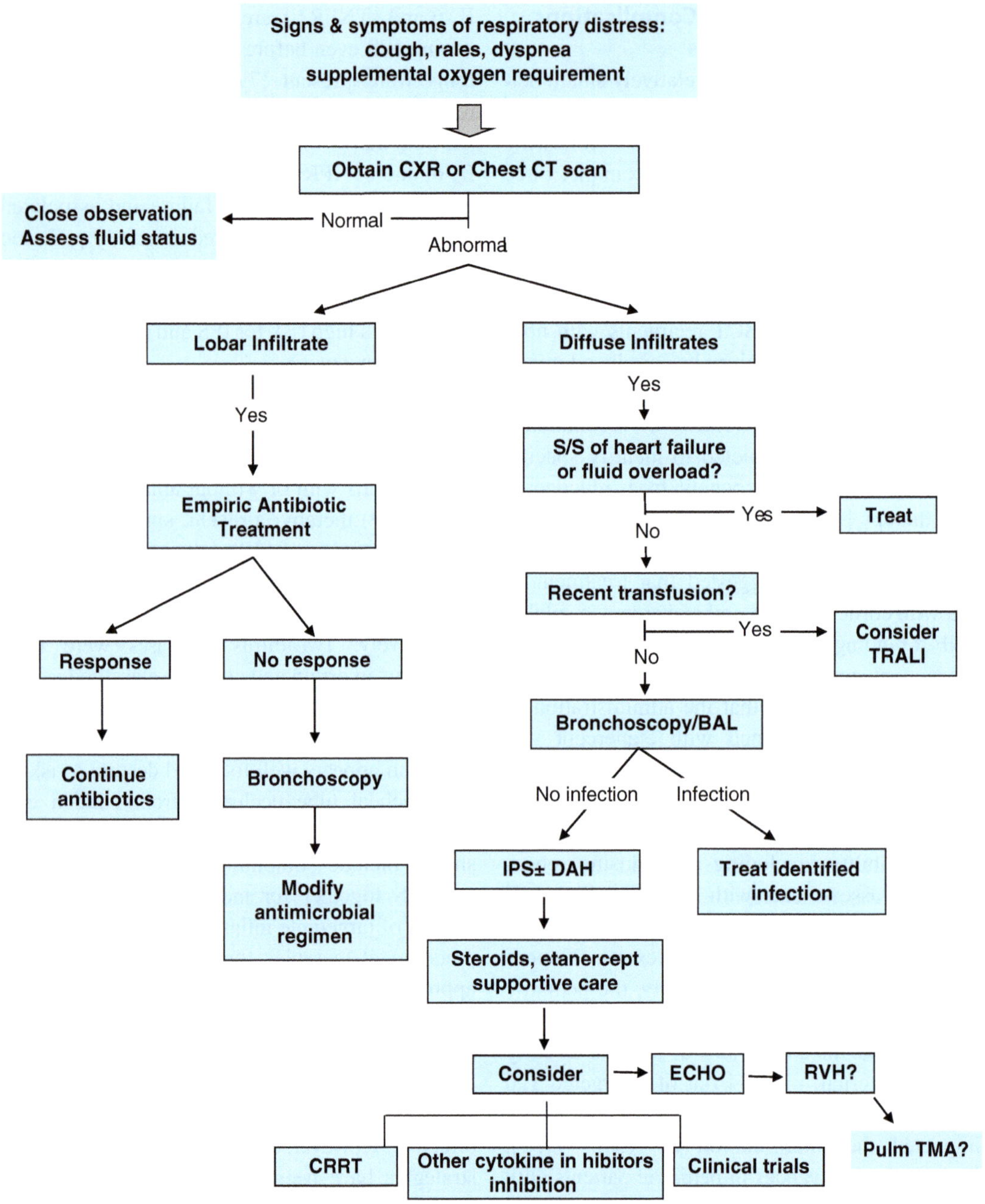


**Fig. 31.2** Approach to patients with acute pulmonary dysfunction. The comprehensive approach to HSCT patients with acute pulmonary dysfunction is complex. It requires the completion of a thorough history (including recent blood products) and physical exam and the timely determination of the severity of respiratory impairment. An initial assessment of the need for supplemental oxygen support, overall fluid balance, renal function, and cardiac output should be followed by radiographic imagining. Results of the initial work-up will guide subsequent decision-making toward the initiation of empiric antimicrobial therapy versus consultation with medical and surgical specialists and consideration of bronchoscopy/broncho-alveolar lavage to rule out infectious causes of lung inflammation. When pulmonary dysfunction is determined to be non-infectious in origin and immunosuppressive therapy is considered, enrollment on open clinical trials is desirable whenever possible. *CXR* chest X-ray, *CT* computerized tomography, *BAL* broncho-alveolar lavage, *IPS* idiopathic pneumonia syndrome, *DAH* diffuse alveolar hemorrhage, *TRALI* transfusion-related acute lung injury, *CRRT* continuous renal replacement therapy, *RVH* right ventricular hypertrophy, *Pulm-TMA* pulmonary thrombotic microangiopathy

of FAM over placebo for severe BOS [140, 141]. Interestingly, long-term administration of azithromycin, a component of FAM, as prophylaxis against pulmonary injury was recently found to increase the risk of malignant relapse [142], and this may be secondary to significant immune modulatory effects of the drug [143]. The impact of FAM on relapse or the development of secondary malignancy when used to treat patients with chronic GVHD and BOS remains to be fully elucidated [144–146]. By contrast, treatment with formoterol and budesonide may improve FEV1 in patients with moderately severe BOS when detected early [147].

Laboratory insights currently being translated into clinical medicine regarding the role of B-cells [111, 148] and JAK pathways [149] may pave the way for novel strategies to treat chronic pulmonary dysfunction in children and adults as agents, including ibrutinib and ruxolitinib, are now approved for the treatment of steroid-resistant chronic GVHD in individuals as young as 12 years. It remains unclear whether established pulmonary fibrosis following HSCT in childhood is reversible. Accordingly, the antifibrotic drug nintedanib, FDA-approved for idiopathic pulmonary fibrosis, is currently being tested in children with fibrosis from multiple causes. Normalization of lung function after initial impairment improves survival to rates comparable to long-term HSCT survivors with normal baseline PFTs [150], highlighting the importance of pulmonary surveillance and early intervention.

## Transplant-Associated Microangiopathy (TA-TMA)

Transplant-associated thrombotic microangiopathy (TA-TMA) describes multisystem complications occurring after HSCT that are characterized by microangiopathic changes [34]. The diagnosis of TA-TMA is based on clinical criteria and the relatively acute onset of anemia and thrombocytopenia with evidence of RBC fragmentation in the peripheral blood smear [34, 35, 151, 152]. Concomitant acute renal dysfunction, often associated with proteinuria and hypertension, occurs in the majority of patients. Neurologic, pulmonary [36] and gastrointestinal symptoms can also be observed. In this context, TA-TMA is now believed to be a multi-visceral disorder [34]. The onset of TA-TMA usually occurs within the first 100 days after HSCT but has also been recognized months after the procedure. Given the close association of TA-TMA with calcineurin inhibitors, GVHD, and infections, the syndrome is reported less frequently after autologous HSCT (approximately 2.6%) compared with the allogeneic setting where the incidence is in the 10–15% range and even higher in some recent pediatric reports [35, 153].

Damage to the vascular endothelium is central to the pathogenesis of TA-TMA, which may represent a common thread underlying several other post-transplant complications [97–99]. Approximately 12–18% of patients with TA-TMA will have severe disease affecting their overall survival. Proteinuria and elevated soluble membrane attack complex levels at TA-TMA diagnosis are poor prognostic markers that warrant prompt consideration for clinical interventions [35]. Unfortunately, there is currently no standard treatment for TA-TMA. There is consensus, however, that rapid withdrawal of potentially offending drugs such as calcineurin inhibitors or sirolimus should be the primary intervention. Aggressive management of concurrent GVHD and infections is also crucial because these are common causes of mortality in patients with TA-TMA and can be triggers of EC injury. Plasma exchange (PE) has demonstrated limited efficacy and has not been endorsed as a standard treatment; early implementation in pediatric patients may rescue some patients with renal failure, but outcomes remain poor [154]. Recent reports have revealed that activation and dysregulation of the alternative pathway of complement may contribute to endothelial damage incurred during TA-TMA [155]. Indeed, the role of complement activation and associated genetic susceptibility to the development of TMA was demonstrated in a prospective study in pediatric HSCT recipients [155]. To this end, early intervention with the terminal complement blocking agent eculizumab has been effective in treating some, but not all, patients with TMA [156–158]. The effectiveness of eculizumab appears to depend on precise personalized drug dosing regimens [159]. Other interventions suggested for TMA have included agents that stabilize vascular endothelial integrity and function [160].

## Veno-Occlusive Disease/Sinusoidal Obstruction Syndrome (VOD/SOS)

Veno-occlusive disease/sinusoidal obstruction syndrome (VOD/SOS) is another endothelial injury complication associated with high-dose chemotherapy and HSCT and often includes multiorgan dysfunction. VOD/SOS results from direct injury to sinusoidal endothelium, hepatocytes, and the central venules in zone 3 of the liver acinus that ultimately progresses to veno-occlusion and sinusoidal obstruction [161–165]. The diagnosis of VOD/SOS is based on the classical triad of weight gain, painful hepatomegaly, and jaundice as initially characterized by the transplant programs at Johns Hopkins and the Fred Hutchinson Cancer Research Center. The diagnostic criteria were recently updated and expanded to include platelet refractory thrombocytopenia, which is often seen in pediatric patients, and reversal of portal venous flow on Doppler ultrasound of the liver [165]. As with TA-TMA, making the diagnosis of VOD/SOS can be challenging because the signs and symptoms of this condition often overlap those of other transplant-related complications [165]. The incidence of VOD/SOS depends upon several factors, including type of transplant (allogeneic > autologous), patient age (pediatric > adult), conditioning regimen intensity (myeloablative > reduced intensity), pre-existing risk factors, and criteria used to make the clinical diagnosis. The incidence of VOD/SOS reported in the contemporary literature ranges from 10 to 20% after allogeneic HSCT using myeloablative conditioning (and has high as 60% in a subset of pediatric patients) to 0 to 10% following reduced-intensity allogeneic HSCT and as low as 5% following autologous HSCT [165]. The severity of VOD/SOS ranges from mild to severe depending on the degree of hyperbilirubinemia, amount of fluid retention/weight gain, and pace of disease progression [166]. New grading criteria that are based on the severity of individual symptoms associated with VOD/SOS have recently been proposed [165].

The pathophysiology of VOD/SOS is complex and includes the contribution of dysregulated immune and coagulation pathways and underscores the importance of endothelial dysfunction in the hepatic sinusoids [165]. The inflammatory milieu contributes to a prothrombotic and hypofibrinolytic state. Microvascular clot formation developing from fibrin deposition and platelet aggregation, in conjunction with embolization of damaged ECs, results in sinusoidal narrowing, progressive blockage, and ultimately obstruction. This cascade of events culminates in the development of symptoms that characterize VOD/SOS and is believed to occur well before clinical (painful hepatomegaly, ascites, weight gain) and laboratory (hyperbilirubinemia and liver enzyme elevation) findings are obtained.

The treatment of VOD/SOS is multifaceted. The identification of patients at a high risk for disease development and careful monitoring early post-HSCT allow for early diagnosis and timely intervention. The primary goal in the management of VOD/SOS is to minimize extracellular fluid overload without worsening intravascular volume and renal perfusion. Hence, strict attention to fluid intake, salt load, urine output, and daily weights are the mainstays of supportive care. VOD/SOS that evolves to include pulmonary and renal dysfunction is associated with unacceptably high mortality rates [165, 167]. Those with MODS require a high level of intensive care. Some patients may experience renal compromise that leads to volume overload and ascites with or without pleural effusion, while others can develop pulmonary infiltrates and become hypoxemic. Pediatric patients with ascites associated with painful abdominal distention or pulmonary compromise may require the placement of a temporary peritoneal drain to facilitate serial, controlled, small-volume paracentesis (to maintain renal perfusion and adequate lung volumes). Continuous renal replacement therapy

(CRRT) is often necessary for patients who experience renal compromise or require more invasive methods to maintain euvolemia during the evolution of VOD/SOS [168]. Defibrotide is an agent approved by the US Food and Drug Administration and European Medicines Agency for the treatment of adults and children with VOD/SOS following HSCT with renal or pulmonary dysfunction and "severe" SOS/VOD, respectively. When used in this population, about 40–50% of patients are expected to be alive beyond day +100 [165].

## Critical Care Considerations for Pediatric HSCT Recipients

Critical care interventions are often necessary for pediatric HSCT recipients. The mortality rate of patients with pulmonary dysfunction remains high [169, 170], particularly those with GVHD or requiring mechanical ventilation, inotropic support, or CRRT [4, 171, 172]. The benefits of non-invasive, positive-pressure ventilation (NIPPV) have yet to be fully established [170, 173]. Similarly, the role of other lung protective strategies, including high-frequency oscillatory ventilation (HFOV), remains to be determined [174]. Increasing weight gain [175] and early warning scores [176] may identify HSCT patients at risk of respiratory failure and allow increased surveillance and early intervention. The importance of optimizing nutritional support in the HSCT patient has been recently recognized [177]. Enteral nutrition, which may modulate inflammation and minimize lung injury while preserving intestinal integrity, improves overall survival [178]. The ideal nutritional strategy likely includes optimized lipid formulations [179] along with supplemental vitamins and minerals [180–184]. Finally, the potential impact of prone positioning, inhaled nitric oxide, corticosteroids, combinatorial anti-cytokine approaches, and strategies to protect the pulmonary vascular endothelium remains to be investigated [6, 185].

The contribution of cardiac dysfunction to pediatric ARDS must also be considered. Right heart strain and alterations in pulmonary vascular resistance often accompany mechanical ventilation. Routine echocardiography can reveal abnormalities in 30% of patients as early as HSCT Day +7 with 13% having elevated right ventricular pressures. A trend toward decreased survival with any echocardiographic abnormality at Day +7 has been reported [186]. Among HSCT recipients requiring admission to the pediatric intensive care unit (ICU), one-third were found to have elevated right ventricular pressures [187]. Additionally, cardiac diastolic dysfunction is now being recognized more frequently in pediatric HSCT recipients as is the appreciation of its associated impact on outcomes [188].

Fluid overload and acute renal failure are associated with worse outcomes among ventilated pediatric HSCT recipients [189, 190]. ARDSNet fluid management studies demonstrated that conservative fluid management improved lung function and shortened mechanical ventilation and ICU days [189]. The potential impact of early CRRT has been recognized in pediatric HSCT recipients, [191, 192], specifically in the context of VOD/SOS [168], but remains understudied in PARDS [193]. Extracorporeal membrane oxygenation (ECMO) is being further explored in pediatric HSCT recipients [194, 195]. Recent promising survival rates using ECMO in a small subset of HSCT patients [196, 197] warrant further evaluation and have prompted studies to evaluate ECMO candidacy criteria and ultimately establish consensus criteria/recommendations for the use of ECMO for pediatric HSCT and cell therapy recipients [198, 199].

The suboptimal outcomes among pediatric HSCT recipients with ARDS underscore the need for early identification and mitigation of risk factors for critical illness and consideration of non-conventional therapies. The first study to match patients from two large databases, the Virtual Pediatric Systems (VPS, LLC) and the Center for International Blood and Marrow Transplant Research (CIBMTR), aimed to identify pediatric HSCT patients who ultimately required admission to intensive care units [172]. Five independent variables were incorporated into a multivariate model to establish quartiles of risk of ICU mortality. The findings underscored the value of establishing collaborative efforts between pediatric intensive care, HSCT, and multiple other subspecialties to identify and follow very high-risk patients.

## Conclusion

Pulmonary dysfunction along with TA-TMA and VOD/SOS remain common and life-threatening problems for pediatric and AYA HSCT recipients. While the HSCT field has evolved considerably over the last two decades, several challenges and unmet needs remain with respect to optimizing outcomes for these patients, especially those who ultimately require critical care. For example, there is a need to build, characterize, and study prospective, observational pediatric and AYA cohorts of patients. This effort should utilize, expand, and link existing databases to (1) develop a practical scoring system to assess the risk of lung dysfunction, (2) enhance deep phenotyping of pulmonary toxicities pre- and post-transplant, and (3) establish clinical laboratory biorepositories from which our understanding of transplant-related complications can be enhanced. There remains a continued need to advance the mechanistic understanding of pulmonary diseases in HSCT recipients and bring laboratory observations back to the clinic to improve outcomes; recent translational research efforts highlight the value of bench to bedside research through collaborative, multicenter, consortium studies [81]. The potential role of serum biomarkers, BAL findings, and novel imaging technologies to facilitate early diagnosis, characterize disease processes, and monitor the progression of pulmonary disease require further study. The complexity of advanced supportive care needs in patients who have progressed to MODS highlights the importance of a coordinated, multidisciplinary approach to care among pediatric HSCT and ICU teams along with medical and surgical subspecialists. Moreover, a team approach to research and clinical care, involving basic, translational, and clinician scientists, is essential to overcome existing clinical management challenges and improve outcomes for children and AYA patients requiring HSCT.

**Acknowledgments** YK and KRC completed literature review and wrote the manuscript. This work was supported by the Sea Dream Charitable Foundation, the Ashworth/Welch Charitable Fund, and Giant Food.

## References

1. Khandelwal P, Millard HR, Thiel E, Abdel-Azim H, Abraham AA, Auletta JJ, et al. Hematopoietic stem cell transplantation activity in pediatric cancer between 2008 and 2014 in the United States: a center for international blood and marrow transplant research report. Biol Blood Marrow Transplant. 2017;23(8):1342–9. https://doi.org/10.1016/j.bbmt.2017.04.018; Epub 2017/04/30.
2. Passweg JR, Baldomero H, Peters C, Gaspar HB, Cesaro S, Dreger P, et al. Hematopoietic SCT in Europe: data and trends in 2012 with special consideration of pediatric transplantation. Bone Marrow Transplant. 2014;49(6):744–50. https://doi.org/10.1038/bmt.2014.55; Epub 2014/03/19.
3. Upperman JS, Lacroix J, Curley MA, Checchia PA, Lee DW, Cooke KR, et al. Specific etiologies associated with the multiple organ dysfunction syndrome in children: part 1. Pediatr Crit Care Med. 2017;18(3_suppl Suppl 1):S50–S7. https://doi.org/10.1097/PCC.0000000000001048; Epub 2017/03/02.
4. Torres SF, Iolster T, Reyes Haczek PJ, Berro M, Longo PG, Siaba Serrate AJ, et al. Children admitted to a pediatric intensive care unit after hematopoietic stem cell transplantation: analysis of survival and predictors of mortality. Arch Argent Pediatr. 2021;119(4):230–7. https://doi.org/10.5546/aap.2021.eng.230; Epub 2021/07/27.
5. Zinter MS, Holubkov R, Steurer MA, Dvorak CC, Duncan CN, Sapru A, et al. Pediatric hematopoietic cell transplant patients who survive critical illness frequently have significant but recoverable decline in functional status. Biol Blood Marrow Transplant. 2018;24(2):330–6. https://doi.org/10.1016/j.bbmt.2017.10.036; Epub 2017/11/13.
6. Tamburro RF, Cooke KR, Davies SM, Goldfarb S, Hagood JS, Srinivasan A, et al. Pulmonary complications of pediatric hematopoietic cell transplantation. A national institutes of health workshop summary. Ann Am Thorac Soc. 2021;18(3):381–94. https://doi.org/10.1513/AnnalsATS.202001-006OT; Epub 2020/10/16.
7. Eikenberry M, Bartakova H, Defor T, Haddad IY, Ramsay NK, Blazar BR, et al. Natural history of pulmonary complications in children after bone marrow transplantation. Biol Blood Marrow Transplant. 2005;11(1):56–64. https://doi.org/10.1016/j.bbmt.2004.09.008; Epub 2004/12/31.

8. Panoskaltsis-Mortari A, Griese M, Madtes DK, Belperio JA, Haddad IY, Folz RJ, et al. An official American Thoracic Society research statement: noninfectious lung injury after hematopoietic stem cell transplantation: idiopathic pneumonia syndrome. Am J Respir Crit Care Med. 2011;183(9):1262–79. https://doi.org/10.1164/rccm.2007-413ST; Epub 2011/05/03.
9. Afessa B, Litzow MR, Tefferi A. Bronchiolitis obliterans and other late onset non-infectious pulmonary complications in hematopoietic stem cell transplantation. Bone Marrow Transplant. 2001;28(5):425–34. https://doi.org/10.1038/sj.bmt.1703142; Epub 2001/10/11.
10. Yousem SA. The histological spectrum of pulmonary graft-versus-host disease in bone marrow transplant recipients. Hum Pathol. 1995;26(6):668–75. https://doi.org/10.1016/0046-8177(95)90174-4; Epub 1995/06/01.
11. Fitch T, Myers KC, Dewan M, Towe C, Dandoy C. Pulmonary complications after pediatric stem cell transplant. Front Oncol. 2021;11:755878. https://doi.org/10.3389/fonc.2021.755878; Epub 2021/11/02.
12. Broglie L, Fretham C, Al-Seraihy A, George B, Kurtzberg J, Loren A, et al. Pulmonary complications in pediatric and adolescent patients following allogeneic hematopoietic cell transplantation. Biol Blood Marrow Transplant. 2019;25(10):2024–30. https://doi.org/10.1016/j.bbmt.2019.06.004; Epub 2019/06/16.
13. Kaya Z, Weiner DJ, Yilmaz D, Rowan J, Goyal RK. Lung function, pulmonary complications, and mortality after allogeneic blood and marrow transplantation in children. Biol Blood Marrow Transplant. 2009;15(7):817–26. https://doi.org/10.1016/j.bbmt.2009.03.019; Epub 2009/06/23.
14. van Gestel JP, Bollen CW, Bierings MB, Boelens JJ, Wulffraat NM, van Vught AJ. Survival in a recent cohort of mechanically ventilated pediatric allogeneic hematopoietic stem cell transplantation recipients. Biol Blood Marrow Transplant. 2008;14(12):1385–93. https://doi.org/10.1016/j.bbmt.2008.09.020; Epub 2008/12/02.
15. van Gestel JP, Bierings MB, Dauger S, Dalle JH, Pavlicek P, Sedlacek P, et al. Outcome of invasive mechanical ventilation after pediatric allogeneic hematopoietic SCT: results from a prospective, multicenter registry. Bone Marrow Transplant. 2014;49(10):1287–92. https://doi.org/10.1038/bmt.2014.147; Epub 2014/07/30.
16. Inaba H, Yang J, Pan J, Stokes DC, Krasin MJ, Srinivasan A, et al. Pulmonary dysfunction in survivors of childhood hematologic malignancies after allogeneic hematopoietic stem cell transplantation. Cancer. 2010;116(8):2020–30. https://doi.org/10.1002/cncr.24897; Epub 2010/02/27.
17. Kirkby J, Aurora P, Spencer H, Rees S, Sonnappa S, Stocks J. Stitching and switching: the impact of discontinuous lung function reference equations. Eur Respir J. 2012;39(5):1256–7. https://doi.org/10.1183/09031936.00173011; Epub 2012/05/02.
18. Kirkby J, Bonner R, Lum S, Bates P, Morgan V, Strunk RC, et al. Interpretation of pediatric lung function: impact of ethnicity. Pediatr Pulmonol. 2013;48(1):20–6. https://doi.org/10.1002/ppul.22538; Epub 2012/03/21.
19. Robinson PD, Spencer H, Aurora P. Impact of lung function interpretation approach on pediatric bronchiolitis obliterans syndrome diagnosis after lung transplantation. J Heart Lung Transplant. 2015;34(8):1082–8. https://doi.org/10.1016/j.healun.2015.03.010; Epub 2015/05/17.
20. Walkup LL, Higano NS, Woods JC. Structural and functional pulmonary magnetic resonance imaging in pediatrics-from the neonate to the young adult. Acad Radiol. 2019;26(3):424–30. https://doi.org/10.1016/j.acra.2018.08.006; Epub 2018/09/20.
21. Clark JG, Hansen JA, Hertz MI, Parkman R, Jensen L, Peavy HH. NHLBI workshop summary. Idiopathic pneumonia syndrome after bone marrow transplantation. Am Rev Respir Dis. 1993;147(6 Pt 1):1601–6. https://doi.org/10.1164/ajrccm/147.6_Pt_1.1601; Epub 1993/06/01.
22. Cooke KR, Yanik G. Lung injury following hematopoietic cell transplantation. In: Forman SJ, Nergin R, Antin JH, Appelbaum F, editors. Thomas's hematopoietic cell transplantation. 5th ed. Hoboken, NJ: Wiley-Blackwell; 2016. p. 1117–30.
23. Yanik G, Cooke KR. The lung as a target organ of graft-versus-host disease. Semin Hematol. 2006;43(1):42–52. https://doi.org/10.1053/j.seminhematol.2005.09.004; Epub 2006/01/18.
24. Seo S, Renaud C, Kuypers JM, Chiu CY, Huang ML, Samayoa E, et al. Idiopathic pneumonia syndrome after hematopoietic cell transplantation: evidence of occult infectious etiologies. Blood. 2015;125(24):3789–97. https://doi.org/10.1182/blood-2014-12-617035; Epub 2015/04/29.
25. Clark JG, Madtes DK, Martin TR, Hackman RC, Farrand AL, Crawford SW. Idiopathic pneumonia after bone marrow transplantation: cytokine activation and lipopolysaccharide amplification in the bronchoalveolar compartment. Crit Care Med. 1999;27(9):1800–6. https://doi.org/10.1097/00003246-199909000-00016; Epub 1999/10/03.
26. Kantrow SP, Hackman RC, Boeckh M, Myerson D, Crawford SW. Idiopathic pneumonia syndrome: changing spectrum of lung injury after marrow transplantation. Transplantation. 1997;63(8):1079–86. https://doi.org/10.1097/00007890-199704270-00006; Epub 1997/04/27.
27. Sakaguchi H, Takahashi Y, Watanabe N, Doisaki S, Muramatsu H, Hama A, et al. Incidence, clinical features, and risk factors of idiopathic pneumonia syndrome following hematopoietic stem cell transplantation in children. Pediatr Blood Cancer. 2012;58(5):780–4. https://doi.org/10.1002/pbc.23298; Epub 2011/09/17.

28. Sano H, Kobayashi R, Iguchi A, Suzuki D, Kishimoto K, Yasuda K, et al. Risk factor analysis of idiopathic pneumonia syndrome after allogeneic hematopoietic SCT in children. Bone Marrow Transplant. 2014;49(1):38–41. https://doi.org/10.1038/bmt.2013.123; Epub 2013/08/21.
29. Fukuda T, Hackman RC, Guthrie KA, Sandmaier BM, Boeckh M, Maris MB, et al. Risks and outcomes of idiopathic pneumonia syndrome after nonmyeloablative and conventional conditioning regimens for allogeneic hematopoietic stem cell transplantation. Blood. 2003;102(8):2777–85. https://doi.org/10.1182/blood-2003-05-1597; Epub 2003/07/12.
30. Wenger DS, Triplette M, Crothers K, Cheng GS, Hill JA, Milano F, et al. Incidence, risk factors, and outcomes of idiopathic pneumonia syndrome after allogeneic hematopoietic cell transplantation. Biol Blood Marrow Transplant. 2020;26(2):413–20. https://doi.org/10.1016/j.bbmt.2019.09.034; Epub 2019/10/13.
31. Lewis ID, DeFor T, Weisdorf DJ. Increasing incidence of diffuse alveolar hemorrhage following allogeneic bone marrow transplantation: cryptic etiology and uncertain therapy. Bone Marrow Transplant. 2000;26(5):539–43. https://doi.org/10.1038/sj.bmt.1702546; Epub 2000/10/06.
32. Kharbanda S, Panoskaltsis-Mortari A, Haddad IY, Blazar BR, Orchard PJ, Cornfield DN, et al. Inflammatory cytokines and the development of pulmonary complications after allogeneic hematopoietic cell transplantation in patients with inherited metabolic storage disorders. Biol Blood Marrow Transplant. 2006;12(4):430–7. https://doi.org/10.1016/j.bbmt.2005.12.026; Epub 2006/03/21.
33. Majhail NS, Parks K, Defor TE, Weisdorf DJ. Diffuse alveolar hemorrhage and infection-associated alveolar hemorrhage following hematopoietic stem cell transplantation: related and high-risk clinical syndromes. Biol Blood Marrow Transplant. 2006;12(10):1038–46. https://doi.org/10.1016/j.bbmt.2006.06.002; Epub 2006/10/28.
34. Jodele S, Laskin BL, Dandoy CE, Myers KC, El-Bietar J, Davies SM, et al. A new paradigm: diagnosis and management of HSCT-associated thrombotic microangiopathy as multi-system endothelial injury. Blood Rev. 2015;29(3):191–204. https://doi.org/10.1016/j.blre.2014.11.001; Epub 2014/12/09.
35. Jodele S, Davies SM, Lane A, Khoury J, Dandoy C, Goebel J, et al. Diagnostic and risk criteria for HSCT-associated thrombotic microangiopathy: a study in children and young adults. Blood. 2014;124(4):645–53. https://doi.org/10.1182/blood-2014-03-564997; Epub 2014/05/31.
36. Jodele S, Hirsch R, Laskin B, Davies S, Witte D, Chima R. Pulmonary arterial hypertension in pediatric patients with hematopoietic stem cell transplant-associated thrombotic microangiopathy. Biol Blood Marrow Transplant. 2013;19(2):202–7. https://doi.org/10.1016/j.bbmt.2012.08.022; Epub 2012/09/11.
37. Semple JW, Rebetz J, Kapur R. Transfusion-associated circulatory overload and transfusion-related acute lung injury. Blood. 2019;133(17):1840–53. https://doi.org/10.1182/blood-2018-10-860809.
38. Sanchez R, Toy P. Transfusion related acute lung injury: a pediatric perspective. Pediatr Blood Cancer. 2005;45(3):248–55. https://doi.org/10.1002/pbc.20395; Epub 2005/04/27.
39. Dotis J, Stabouli S, Violaki A, Vogiatzi L, Mitroudi M, Oikonomou M, et al. Transfusion-related acute lung injury management in a pediatric intensive care unit. Hippokratia. 2011;15(2):184–6; Epub 2011/11/24.
40. Cooke KR, Luznik L, Sarantopoulos S, Hakim FT, Jagasia M, Fowler DH, et al. The biology of chronic graft-versus-host disease: a task force report from the National institutes of health consensus development project on criteria for clinical trials in chronic graft-versus-host disease. Biol Blood Marrow Transplant. 2017;23(2):211–34. https://doi.org/10.1016/j.bbmt.2016.09.023; Epub 2016/10/08.
41. Barker AF, Bergeron A, Rom WN, Hertz MI. Obliterative bronchiolitis. N Engl J Med. 2014;370(19):1820–8. https://doi.org/10.1056/NEJMra1204664; Epub 2014/05/09.
42. Yoshihara S, Yanik G, Cooke KR, Mineishi S. Bronchiolitis obliterans syndrome (BOS), bronchiolitis obliterans organizing pneumonia (BOOP), and other late-onset noninfectious pulmonary complications following allogeneic hematopoietic stem cell transplantation. Biol Blood Marrow Transplant. 2007;13(7):749–59. https://doi.org/10.1016/j.bbmt.2007.05.001; Epub 2007/06/21.
43. Jagasia MH, Greinix HT, Arora M, Williams KM, Wolff D, Cowen EW, et al. National institutes of health consensus development project on criteria for clinical trials in chronic graft-versus-host disease: I. The 2014 diagnosis and staging working group report. Biol Blood Marrow Transplant. 2015;21(3):389–401.e1. https://doi.org/10.1016/j.bbmt.2014.12.001; Epub 2014/12/23.
44. Cheng GS, Campbell AP, Xie H, Stednick Z, Callais C, Leisenring WM, et al. Correlation and agreement of handheld spirometry with laboratory spirometry in allogeneic hematopoietic cell transplant recipients. Biol Blood Marrow Transplant. 2016;22(5):925–31. https://doi.org/10.1016/j.bbmt.2015.12.023; Epub 2016/01/10.
45. Bergeron A, Chevret S, Peffault de Latour R, Chagnon K, de Margerie-Mellon C, Riviere F, et al. Noninfectious lung complications after allogeneic haematopoietic stem cell transplantation. Eur Respir J. 2018;51(5):1702617. https://doi.org/10.1183/13993003.02617-2017; Epub 2018/04/14.
46. Cooke KR. A "window of opportunity" for patients with late-onset pulmonary dysfunction after allogeneic hematopoietic cell transplantation. Biol Blood Marrow Transplant. 2014;20(3):291–2.

https://doi.org/10.1016/j.bbmt.2014.01.008; Epub 2014/01/30.
47. Palmer J, Williams K, Inamoto Y, Chai X, Martin PJ, Tomas LS, et al. Pulmonary symptoms measured by the national institutes of health lung score predict overall survival, nonrelapse mortality, and patient-reported outcomes in chronic graft-versus-host disease. Biol Blood Marrow Transplant. 2014;20(3):337–44. https://doi.org/10.1016/j.bbmt.2013.11.025; Epub 2013/12/10.
48. Williams KM, Chien JW, Gladwin MT, Pavletic SZ. Bronchiolitis obliterans after allogeneic hematopoietic stem cell transplantation. JAMA. 2009;302(3):306–14. https://doi.org/10.1001/jama.2009.1018; Epub 2009/07/16.
49. Gassas A, Craig-Barnes H, Dell S, Doyle J, Schechter T, Sung L, et al. Chest health surveillance utility in the early detection of bronchiolitis obliterans syndrome in children after Allo-SCT. Bone Marrow Transplant. 2013;48(6):814–8. https://doi.org/10.1038/bmt.2012.228; Epub 2012/11/21.
50. Yoon JS, Chun YH, Lee JW, Chung NG, Cho B. Value of screening spirometry for early diagnosis of bronchiolitis obliterans syndrome in children after allogeneic hematopoietic stem cell transplantation. J Pediatr Hematol Oncol. 2015;37(8):e462–7. https://doi.org/10.1097/MPH.0000000000000421; Epub 2015/09/04.
51. Robson KS, West AJ. Improving survival outcomes in lung transplant recipients through early detection of bronchiolitis obliterans: daily home spirometry versus standard pulmonary function testing. Can J Respir Ther. 2014;50(1):17–22; Epub 2014/04/01.
52. Loiseau C, Lemonnier F, Randrianarivelo O, Itzykson R, Nguyen S, Becquemin MH, et al. Home spirometry in bronchiolitis obliterans after allogeneic haematopoietic cell transplant. Eur Respir J. 2018;52(1):1702328. https://doi.org/10.1183/13993003.02328-2017; Epub 2018/05/26.
53. Ginsberg JP, Aplenc R, McDonough J, Bethel J, Doyle J, Weiner DJ. Pre-transplant lung function is predictive of survival following pediatric bone marrow transplantation. Pediatr Blood Cancer. 2010;54(3):454–60. https://doi.org/10.1002/pbc.22337; Epub 2009/10/31.
54. Quigg TC, Kim YJ, Goebel WS, Haut PR. Lung function before and after pediatric allogeneic hematopoietic stem cell transplantation: a predictive role for DLCOa/VA. J Pediatr Hematol Oncol. 2012;34(4):304–9. https://doi.org/10.1097/MPH.0b013e3182346ed8; Epub 2012/01/17.
55. Lee HJ, Kim K, Kim SK, Lee JW, Yoon JS, Chung NG, et al. Hb-adjusted DLCO with GLI reference predicts long-term survival after HSCT in children. Bone Marrow Transplant. 2021;56(8):1929–36. https://doi.org/10.1038/s41409-020-01202-9; Epub 2021/03/31.
56. Parimon T, Madtes DK, Au DH, Clark JG, Chien JW. Pretransplant lung function, respiratory failure, and mortality after stem cell transplantation. Am J Respir Crit Care Med. 2005;172(3):384–90. https://doi.org/10.1164/rccm.200502-212OC; Epub 2005/05/17.
57. Srinivasan A, Sunkara A, Mitchell W, Sunthankar S, Kang G, Stokes DC, et al. Recovery of pulmonary function after allogeneic hematopoietic cell transplantation in children is associated with improved survival. Biol Blood Marrow Transplant. 2017;23(12):2102–9. https://doi.org/10.1016/j.bbmt.2017.08.025; Epub 2017/09/04.
58. Versluys AB, van der Ent K, Boelens JJ, Wolfs T, de Jong P, Bierings MB. High diagnostic yield of dedicated pulmonary screening before hematopoietic cell transplantation in children. Biol Blood Marrow Transplant. 2015;21(9):1622–6. https://doi.org/10.1016/j.bbmt.2015.06.002; Epub 2015/06/15.
59. Lahzami S, Schoeffel RE, Pechey V, Reid C, Greenwood M, Salome CM, et al. Small airways function declines after allogeneic haematopoietic stem cell transplantation. Eur Respir J. 2011;38(5):1180–8. https://doi.org/10.1183/09031936.00018311; Epub 2011/05/14.
60. Nyilas S, Baumeler L, Tamm M, Halter JP, Savic S, Korten I, et al. Inert gas washout in bronchiolitis obliterans following hematopoietic cell transplantation. Chest. 2018;154(1):157–68. https://doi.org/10.1016/j.chest.2017.12.009; Epub 2017/12/25.
61. Nyilas S, Carlens J, Price T, Singer F, Muller C, Hansen G, et al. Multiple breath washout in pediatric patients after lung transplantation. Am J Transplant. 2018;18(1):145–53. https://doi.org/10.1111/ajt.14432; Epub 2017/07/19.
62. Uhlving HH, Mathiesen S, Buchvald F, Green K, Heilmann C, Gustafsson P, et al. Small airways dysfunction in long-term survivors of pediatric stem cell transplantation. Pediatr Pulmonol. 2015;50(7):704–12. https://doi.org/10.1002/ppul.23058; Epub 2014/05/23.
63. Kerby GS, Rosenfeld M, Ren CL, Mayer OH, Brumback L, Castile R, et al. Lung function distinguishes preschool children with CF from healthy controls in a multi-center setting. Pediatr Pulmonol. 2012;47(6):597–605. https://doi.org/10.1002/ppul.21589; Epub 2011/11/15.
64. Kampschmidt JC, Brooks EG, Cherry DC, Guajardo JR, Wood PR. Feasibility of spirometry testing in preschool children. Pediatr Pulmonol. 2016;51(3):258–66. https://doi.org/10.1002/ppul.23303; Epub 2015/09/04.
65. Aurora P, Stocks J, Oliver C, Saunders C, Castle R, Chaziparasidis G, et al. Quality control for spirometry in preschool children with and without lung disease. Am J Respir Crit Care Med. 2004;169(10):1152–9. https://doi.org/10.1164/rccm.200310-1453OC; Epub 2004/03/19.
66. Bickel S, Popler J, Lesnick B, Eid N. Impulse oscillometry: interpretation and practical applications. Chest. 2014;146(3):841–7. https://doi.org/10.1378/chest.13-1875; Epub 2014/09/03.

67. Subbarao P, Milla C, Aurora P, Davies JC, Davis SD, Hall GL, et al. Multiple-breath washout as a lung function test in cystic fibrosis. A cystic fibrosis foundation workshop report. Ann Am Thorac Soc. 2015;12(6):932–9. https://doi.org/10.1513/AnnalsATS.201501-021FR; Epub 2015/06/16.
68. Galban CJ, Han MK, Boes JL, Chughtai KA, Meyer CR, Johnson TD, et al. Computed tomography-based biomarker provides unique signature for diagnosis of COPD phenotypes and disease progression. Nat Med. 2012;18(11):1711–5. https://doi.org/10.1038/nm.2971; Epub 2012/10/09.
69. Aliverti A, Pennati F, Salito C, Woods JC. Regional lung function and heterogeneity of specific gas volume in healthy and emphysematous subjects. Eur Respir J. 2013;41(5):1179–88. https://doi.org/10.1183/09031936.00050112; Epub 2012/08/11.
70. Walkup LL, Myers K, El-Bietar J, Nelson A, Willmering MM, Grimley M, et al. Xenon-129 MRI detects ventilation deficits in paediatric stem cell transplant patients unable to perform spirometry. Eur Respir J. 2019;53(5):1801779. https://doi.org/10.1183/13993003.01779-2018; Epub 2019/03/09.
71. Towe C, Chester Ogborn A, Ferkol T, Sweet S, Huddleston C, White F, et al. Bronchiolitis obliterans syndrome is not specific for bronchiolitis obliterans in pediatric lung transplant. J Heart Lung Transplant. 2015;34(4):516–21. https://doi.org/10.1016/j.healun.2014.10.004; Epub 2014/12/17.
72. Chellapandian D, Lehrnbecher T, Phillips B, Fisher BT, Zaoutis TE, Steinbach WJ, et al. Bronchoalveolar lavage and lung biopsy in patients with cancer and hematopoietic stem-cell transplantation recipients: a systematic review and meta-analysis. J Clin Oncol. 2015;33(5):501–9. https://doi.org/10.1200/JCO.2014.58.0480; Epub 2015/01/07.
73. Huaringa AJ, Leyva FJ, Signes-Costa J, Morice RC, Raad I, Darwish AA, et al. Bronchoalveolar lavage in the diagnosis of pulmonary complications of bone marrow transplant patients. Bone Marrow Transplant. 2000;25(9):975–9. https://doi.org/10.1038/sj.bmt.1702335; Epub 2000/05/09.
74. Jain P, Sandur S, Meli Y, Arroliga AC, Stoller JK, Mehta AC. Role of flexible bronchoscopy in immunocompromised patients with lung infiltrates. Chest. 2004;125(2):712–22. https://doi.org/10.1378/chest.125.2.712; Epub 2004/02/11.
75. Yanik G, Maslak J, Connelly J, Peres E, Mineishi S, Levine JE, et al. Impact of broncho-alveolar lavage on the diagnosis and management of pulmonary complicaitons post transplant. Biol Blood Marrow Transplant. 2008;14(2):suppl 33.
76. Shannon VR, Andersson BS, Lei X, Champlin RE, Kontoyiannis DP. Utility of early versus late fiberoptic bronchoscopy in the evaluation of new pulmonary infiltrates following hematopoietic stem cell transplantation. Bone Marrow Transplant. 2010;45(4):647–55. https://doi.org/10.1038/bmt.2009.203; Epub 2009/08/18.
77. Kasow KA, King E, Rochester R, Tong X, Srivastava DK, Horwitz EM, et al. Diagnostic yield of bronchoalveolar lavage is low in allogeneic hematopoietic stem cell recipients receiving immunosuppressive therapy or with acute graft-versus-host disease: the St. Jude experience, 1990-2002. Biol Blood Marrow Transplant. 2007;13(7):831–7. https://doi.org/10.1016/j.bbmt.2007.03.008; Epub 2007/06/21.
78. Dieffenbach BV, Madenci AL, Murphy AJ, Weldon CB, Weil BR, Lehmann LE. Therapeutic impact and complications associated with surgical lung biopsy after allogeneic hematopoietic stem cell transplantation in children. Biol Blood Marrow Transplant. 2019;25(11):2181–5. https://doi.org/10.1016/j.bbmt.2019.06.026; Epub 2019/07/01.
79. Seo S, Yu J, Jenkins IC, Leisenring WM, Steven-Ayers T, Kuypers JM, et al. Diagnostic and prognostic plasma biomarkers for idiopathic pneumonia syndrome after hematopoietic cell transplantation. Biol Blood Marrow Transplant. 2018;24(4):678–86. https://doi.org/10.1016/j.bbmt.2017.11.039; Epub 2017/12/11.
80. Yanik GA, Ho VT, Levine JE, White ES, Braun T, Antin JH, et al. The impact of soluble tumor necrosis factor receptor etanercept on the treatment of idiopathic pneumonia syndrome after allogeneic hematopoietic stem cell transplantation. Blood. 2008;112(8):3073–81. https://doi.org/10.1182/blood-2008-03-143412; Epub 2008/07/31.
81. Yanik GA, Grupp SA, Pulsipher MA, Levine JE, Schultz KR, Wall DA, et al. TNF-receptor inhibitor therapy for the treatment of children with idiopathic pneumonia syndrome. A joint pediatric blood and marrow transplant consortium and children's oncology group study (ASCT0521). Biol Blood Marrow Transplant. 2015;21(1):67–73. https://doi.org/10.1016/j.bbmt.2014.09.019; Epub 2014/10/02.
82. Schlatzer DM, Dazard JE, Ewing RM, Ilchenko S, Tomcheko SE, Eid S, et al. Human biomarker discovery and predictive models for disease progression for idiopathic pneumonia syndrome following allogeneic stem cell transplantation. Mol Cell Proteomics. 2012;11(6):M111.015479. https://doi.org/10.1074/mcp.M111.015479; Epub 2012/02/18.
83. Panoskaltsis-Mortari A, Taylor PA, Yaeger TM, Wangensteen OD, Bitterman PB, Ingbar DH, et al. The critical early proinflammatory events associated with idiopathic pneumonia syndrome in irradiated murine allogeneic recipients are due to donor T cell infusion and potentiated by cyclophosphamide. J Clin Invest. 1997;100(5):1015–27. https://doi.org/10.1172/JCI119612; Epub 1997/09/01.
84. Cooke KR, Krenger W, Hill G, Martin TR, Kobzik L, Brewer J, et al. Host reactive donor T cells are associated with lung injury after experimental allogeneic bone marrow transplantation. Blood. 1998;92(7):2571–80; Epub 1998/09/25.
85. Hildebrandt GC, Olkiewicz KM, Choi S, Corrion LA, Clouthier SG, Liu C, et al. Donor T-cell production of RANTES significantly contributes to the

development of idiopathic pneumonia syndrome after allogeneic stem cell transplantation. Blood. 2005;105(6):2249–57. https://doi.org/10.1182/blood-2004-08-3320; Epub 2004/11/18.
86. Hildebrandt GC, Duffner UA, Olkiewicz KM, Corrion LA, Willmarth NE, Williams DL, et al. A critical role for CCR2/MCP-1 interactions in the development of idiopathic pneumonia syndrome after allogeneic bone marrow transplantation. Blood. 2004;103(6):2417–26. https://doi.org/10.1182/blood-2003-08-2708; Epub 2003/11/15.
87. Hildebrandt GC, Corrion LA, Olkiewicz KM, Lu B, Lowler K, Duffner UA, et al. Blockade of CXCR3 receptor:ligand interactions reduces leukocyte recruitment to the lung and the severity of experimental idiopathic pneumonia syndrome. J Immunol. 2004;173(3):2050–9. https://doi.org/10.4049/jimmunol.173.3.2050; Epub 2004/07/22.
88. Choi SW, Hildebrandt GC, Olkiewicz KM, Hanauer DA, Chaudhary MN, Silva IA, et al. CCR1/CCL5 (RANTES) receptor-ligand interactions modulate allogeneic T-cell responses and graft-versus-host disease following stem-cell transplantation. Blood. 2007;110(9):3447–55. https://doi.org/10.1182/blood-2007-05-087403; Epub 2007/07/21.
89. Cooke KR, Hill GR, Gerbitz A, Kobzik L, Martin TR, Crawford JM, et al. Tumor necrosis factor-alpha neutralization reduces lung injury after experimental allogeneic bone marrow transplantation. Transplantation. 2000;70(2):272–9. https://doi.org/10.1097/00007890-200007270-00006; Epub 2000/08/10.
90. Gerbitz A, Nickoloff BJ, Olkiewicz K, Willmarth NE, Hildebrandt G, Liu C, et al. A role for tumor necrosis factor-alpha-mediated endothelial apoptosis in the development of experimental idiopathic pneumonia syndrome. Transplantation. 2004;78(4):494–502. https://doi.org/10.1097/01.tp.0000128839.13674.02; Epub 2004/09/28.
91. Hildebrandt GC, Olkiewicz KM, Corrion LA, Chang Y, Clouthier SG, Liu C, et al. Donor-derived TNF-alpha regulates pulmonary chemokine expression and the development of idiopathic pneumonia syndrome after allogeneic bone marrow transplantation. Blood. 2004;104(2):586–93. https://doi.org/10.1182/blood-2003-12-4259; Epub 2004/04/08.
92. Hildebrandt GC, Olkiewicz KM, Corrion L, Clouthier SG, Pierce EM, Liu C, et al. A role for TNF receptor type II in leukocyte infiltration into the lung during experimental idiopathic pneumonia syndrome. Biol Blood Marrow Transplant. 2008;14(4):385–96. https://doi.org/10.1016/j.bbmt.2008.01.004; Epub 2008/03/18.
93. Burman AC, Banovic T, Kuns RD, Clouston AD, Stanley AC, Morris ES, et al. IFNgamma differentially controls the development of idiopathic pneumonia syndrome and GVHD of the gastrointestinal tract. Blood. 2007;110(3):1064–72. https://doi.org/10.1182/blood-2006-12-063982; Epub 2007/04/24.
94. Mauermann N, Burian J, von Garnier C, Dirnhofer S, Germano D, Schuett C, et al. Interferon-gamma regulates idiopathic pneumonia syndrome, a Th17+CD4+ T-cell-mediated graft-versus-host disease. Am J Respir Crit Care Med. 2008;178(4):379–88. https://doi.org/10.1164/rccm.200711-1648OC; Epub 2008/05/31.
95. Varelias A, Gartlan KH, Kreijveld E, Olver SD, Lor M, Kuns RD, et al. Lung parenchyma-derived IL-6 promotes IL-17A-dependent acute lung injury after allogeneic stem cell transplantation. Blood. 2015;125(15):2435–44. https://doi.org/10.1182/blood-2014-07-590232; Epub 2015/02/13.
96. Yanik G, Hellerstedt B, Custer J, Hutchinson R, Kwon D, Ferrara JL, et al. Etanercept (Enbrel) administration for idiopathic pneumonia syndrome after allogeneic hematopoietic stem cell transplantation. Biol Blood Marrow Transplant. 2002;8(7):395–400; Epub 2002/08/13.
97. Cooke KR, Jannin A, Ho V. The contribution of endothelial activation and injury to end-organ toxicity following allogeneic hematopoietic stem cell transplantation. Biol Blood Marrow Transplant. 2008;14(1 Suppl 1):23–32. https://doi.org/10.1016/j.bbmt.2007.10.008; Epub 2008/01/01.
98. Hildebrandt GC, Chao N. Endothelial cell function and endothelial-related disorders following haematopoietic cell transplantation. Br J Haematol. 2020;190(4):508–19. https://doi.org/10.1111/bjh.16621; Epub 2020/04/23.
99. Carreras E, Barcelona ET. Vascular endothelial syndromes after HCT: 2020 update. Bone Marrow Transplant. 2020;55(10):1885–7. https://doi.org/10.1038/s41409-020-0852-2; Epub 2020/03/24.
100. Gerbitz A, Ewing P, Olkiewicz K, Willmarth NE, Williams D, Hildebrandt G, et al. A role for CD54 (intercellular adhesion molecule-1) in leukocyte recruitment to the lung during the development of experimental idiopathic pneumonia syndrome. Transplantation. 2005;79(5):536–42. https://doi.org/10.1097/01.tp.0000151763.16800.b0; Epub 2005/03/09.
101. Nieder ML, GB MD, Kida A, Hingorani S, Armenian SH, Cooke KR, et al. National cancer institute-national heart, lung and blood institute/pediatric blood and marrow transplant consortium first international consensus conference on late effects after pediatric hematopoietic cell transplantation: long-term organ damage and dysfunction. Biol Blood Marrow Transplant. 2011;17(11):1573–84. https://doi.org/10.1016/j.bbmt.2011.09.013; Epub 2011/10/04.
102. Bhargava M, Viken KJ, Dey S, Steinbach MS, Wu B, Jagtap PD, et al. Proteome profiling in lung injury after hematopoietic stem cell transplantation. Biol Blood Marrow Transplant. 2016;22(8):1383–90. https://doi.org/10.1016/j.bbmt.2016.04.021; Epub 2016/05/08.
103. Rowan CM, Smith L, Sharron MP, Loftis L, Kudchadkar S, Duncan CN, et al. A biomarker

panel for risk of early respiratory failure following hematopoietic cell transplantation. Blood Adv. 2022;6(6):1866–78. https://doi.org/10.1182/bloodadvances.2021005770; Epub 2022/02/10.
104. Sengsayadeth SM, Srivastava S, Jagasia M, Savani BN. Time to explore preventive and novel therapies for bronchiolitis obliterans syndrome after allogeneic hematopoietic stem cell transplantation. Biol Blood Marrow Transplant. 2012;18(10):1479–87. https://doi.org/10.1016/j.bbmt.2012.03.008; Epub 2012/03/28.
105. Martin PJ, Chien JW. What we know and mostly do not know about bronchiolitis obliterans syndrome. Bone Marrow Transplant. 2012;47(1):1–4. https://doi.org/10.1038/bmt.2011.38; Epub 2012/01/12.
106. Panoskaltsis-Mortari A, Tram KV, Price AP, Wendt CH, Blazar BR. A new murine model for bronchiolitis obliterans post-bone marrow transplant. Am J Respir Crit Care Med. 2007;176(7):713–23. https://doi.org/10.1164/rccm.200702-335OC; Epub 2007/06/19.
107. Strieter RM. What differentiates normal lung repair and fibrosis? Inflammation, resolution of repair, and fibrosis. Proc Am Thorac Soc. 2008;5(3):305–10. https://doi.org/10.1513/pats.200710-160DR; Epub 2008/04/12.
108. Wynn TA, Ramalingam TR. Mechanisms of fibrosis: therapeutic translation for fibrotic disease. Nat Med. 2012;18(7):1028–40. https://doi.org/10.1038/nm.2807; Epub 2012/07/10.
109. Srinivasan M, Flynn R, Price A, Ranger A, Browning JL, Taylor PA, et al. Donor B-cell alloantibody deposition and germinal center formation are required for the development of murine chronic GVHD and bronchiolitis obliterans. Blood. 2012;119(6):1570–80. https://doi.org/10.1182/blood-2011-07-364414; Epub 2011/11/11.
110. Flynn R, Du J, Veenstra RG, Reichenbach DK, Panoskaltsis-Mortari A, Taylor PA, et al. Increased T follicular helper cells and germinal center B cells are required for cGVHD and bronchiolitis obliterans. Blood. 2014;123(25):3988–98. https://doi.org/10.1182/blood-2014-03-562231; Epub 2014/05/14.
111. Dubovsky JA, Flynn R, Du J, Harrington BK, Zhong Y, Kaffenberger B, et al. Ibrutinib treatment ameliorates murine chronic graft-versus-host disease. J Clin Invest. 2014;124(11):4867–76. https://doi.org/10.1172/JCI75328; Epub 2014/10/02.
112. Flynn R, Allen JL, Luznik L, MacDonald KP, Paz K, Alexander KA, et al. Targeting Syk-activated B cells in murine and human chronic graft-versus-host disease. Blood. 2015;125(26):4085–94. https://doi.org/10.1182/blood-2014-08-595470; Epub 2015/04/09.
113. Verghese DA, Chun N, Paz K, Fribourg M, Woodruff TM, Flynn R, et al. C5aR1 regulates T follicular helper differentiation and chronic graft-versus-host disease bronchiolitis obliterans. JCI Insight. 2018;3(24):e124646. https://doi.org/10.1172/jci.insight.124646; Epub 2018/12/21.
114. Alexander KA, Flynn R, Lineburg KE, Kuns RD, Teal BE, Olver SD, et al. CSF-1-dependant donor-derived macrophages mediate chronic graft-versus-host disease. J Clin Invest. 2014;124(10):4266–80. https://doi.org/10.1172/JCI75935; Epub 2014/08/27.
115. Sime PJ, Marr RA, Gauldie D, Xing Z, Hewlett BR, Graham FL, et al. Transfer of tumor necrosis factor-alpha to rat lung induces severe pulmonary inflammation and patchy interstitial fibrogenesis with induction of transforming growth factor-beta1 and myofibroblasts. Am J Pathol. 1998;153(3):825–32. https://doi.org/10.1016/s0002-9440(10)65624-6; Epub 1998/09/15.
116. Miyazaki Y, Araki K, Vesin C, Garcia I, Kapanci Y, Whitsett JA, et al. Expression of a tumor necrosis factor-alpha transgene in murine lung causes lymphocytic and fibrosing alveolitis. A mouse model of progressive pulmonary fibrosis. J Clin Invest. 1995;96(1):250–9. https://doi.org/10.1172/JCI118029; Epub 1995/07/01.
117. Casadevall A, Pirofski LA. The damage-response framework of microbial pathogenesis. Nat Rev Microbiol. 2003;1(1):17–24. https://doi.org/10.1038/nrmicro732; Epub 2004/03/26.
118. Harris B, Morjaria SM, Littmann ER, Geyer AI, Stover DE, Barker JN, et al. Gut microbiota predict pulmonary infiltrates after allogeneic hematopoietic cell transplantation. Am J Respir Crit Care Med. 2016;194(4):450–63. https://doi.org/10.1164/rccm.201507-1491OC; Epub 2016/02/18.
119. Chien JW, Zhao LP, Hansen JA, Fan WH, Parimon T, Clark JG. Genetic variation in bactericidal/permeability-increasing protein influences the risk of developing rapid airflow decline after hematopoietic cell transplantation. Blood. 2006;107(5):2200–7. https://doi.org/10.1182/blood-2005-06-2338; Epub 2005/11/24.
120. Hildebrandt GC, Granell M, Urbano-Ispizua A, Wolff D, Hertenstein B, Greinix HT, et al. Recipient NOD2/CARD15 variants: a novel independent risk factor for the development of bronchiolitis obliterans after allogeneic stem cell transplantation. Biol Blood Marrow Transplant. 2008;14(1):67–74. https://doi.org/10.1016/j.bbmt.2007.09.009; Epub 2007/12/27.
121. O'Dwyer DN, Dickson RP, Moore BB. The lung microbiome, immunity, and the pathogenesis of chronic lung disease. J Immunol. 2016;196(12):4839–47. https://doi.org/10.4049/jimmunol.1600279; Epub 2016/06/05.
122. O'Dwyer DN, Ashley SL, Gurczynski SJ, Xia M, Wilke C, Falkowski NR, et al. Lung microbiota contribute to pulmonary inflammation and disease progression in pulmonary fibrosis. Am J Respir Crit Care Med. 2019;199(9):1127–38. https://doi.org/10.1164/rccm.201809-1650OC; Epub 2019/02/23.
123. Zhou X, O'Dwyer DN, Xia M, Miller HK, Chan PR, Trulik K, et al. First-onset herpesviral infection and lung injury in allogeneic hematopoietic cell transplantation. Am J Respir Crit Care Med. 2019;200(1):63–74. https://doi.org/10.1164/rccm.201809-1635OC; Epub 2019/02/12.

124. Versluys B, Bierings M, Murk JL, Wolfs T, Lindemans C, Vd Ent K, et al. Infection with a respiratory virus before hematopoietic cell transplantation is associated with alloimmune-mediated lung syndromes. J Allergy Clin Immunol. 2018;141(2):697–703.e8. https://doi.org/10.1016/j.jaci.2017.03.055; Epub 2017/07/19.
125. Mejias A, Dimo B, Suarez NM, Garcia C, Suarez-Arrabal MC, Jartti T, et al. Whole blood gene expression profiles to assess pathogenesis and disease severity in infants with respiratory syncytial virus infection. PLoS Med. 2013;10(11):e1001549. https://doi.org/10.1371/journal.pmed.1001549; Epub 2013/11/23.
126. Thomas NJ, Spear D, Wasserman E, Pon S, Markovitz B, Singh AR, et al. CALIPSO: a randomized controlled trial of calfactant for acute lung injury in pediatric stem cell and oncology patients. Biol Blood Marrow Transplant. 2018;24(12):2479–86. https://doi.org/10.1016/j.bbmt.2018.07.023; Epub 2018/07/31.
127. Keates-Baleeiro J, Moore P, Koyama T, Manes B, Calder C, Frangoul H. Incidence and outcome of idiopathic pneumonia syndrome in pediatric stem cell transplant recipients. Bone Marrow Transplant. 2006;38(4):285–9. https://doi.org/10.1038/sj.bmt.1705436; Epub 2006/07/05.
128. Tamburro RF, Kneyber MC, Pediatric Acute Lung Injury Consensus Conference G. Pulmonary specific ancillary treatment for pediatric acute respiratory distress syndrome: proceedings from the pediatric acute lung injury consensus conference. Pediatr Crit Care Med. 2015;16(5 Suppl 1):S61–72. https://doi.org/10.1097/PCC.0000000000000434; Epub 2015/06/03.
129. Tizon R, Frey N, Heitjan DF, Tan KS, Goldstein SC, Hexner EO, et al. High-dose corticosteroids with or without etanercept for the treatment of idiopathic pneumonia syndrome after Allo-SCT. Bone Marrow Transplant. 2012;47(10):1332–7. https://doi.org/10.1038/bmt.2011.260; Epub 2012/02/07.
130. Thompson J, Yin Z, D'Souza A, Fenske T, Hamadani M, Hari P, et al. Etanercept and corticosteroid therapy for the treatment of late-onset idiopathic pneumonia syndrome. Biol Blood Marrow Transplant. 2017;23(11):1955–60. https://doi.org/10.1016/j.bbmt.2017.07.019; Epub 2017/08/02.
131. Yanik GA, Horowitz MM, Weisdorf DJ, Logan BR, Ho VT, Soiffer RJ, et al. Randomized, double-blind, placebo-controlled trial of soluble tumor necrosis factor receptor: enbrel (etanercept) for the treatment of idiopathic pneumonia syndrome after allogeneic stem cell transplantation: blood and marrow transplant clinical trials network protocol. Biol Blood Marrow Transplant. 2014;20(6):858–64. https://doi.org/10.1016/j.bbmt.2014.02.026; Epub 2014/03/13.
132. Ueda N, Chihara D, Kohno A, Tatekawa S, Ozeki K, Watamoto K, et al. Predictive value of circulating angiopoietin-2 for endothelial damage-related complications in allogeneic hematopoietic stem cell transplantation. Biol Blood Marrow Transplant. 2014;20(9):1335–40. https://doi.org/10.1016/j.bbmt.2014.04.030; Epub 2014/05/07.
133. Rathi NK, Tanner AR, Dinh A, Dong W, Feng L, Ensor J, et al. Low-, medium- and high-dose steroids with or without aminocaproic acid in adult hematopoietic SCT patients with diffuse alveolar hemorrhage. Bone Marrow Transplant. 2015;50(3):420–6. https://doi.org/10.1038/bmt.2014.287; Epub 2014/12/23.
134. Heslet L, Nielsen JD, Nepper-Christensen S. Local pulmonary administration of factor VIIa (rFVIIa) in diffuse alveolar hemorrhage (DAH) - a review of a new treatment paradigm. Biol Theory. 2012;6:37–46. https://doi.org/10.2147/BTT.S25507; Epub 2012/03/16.
135. Park JA, Kim BJ. Intrapulmonary recombinant factor VIIa for diffuse alveolar hemorrhage in children. Pediatrics. 2015;135(1):e216–20. https://doi.org/10.1542/peds.2014-1782; Epub 2014/12/31.
136. Bergeron A, Cheng GS. Bronchiolitis obliterans syndrome and other late pulmonary complications after allogeneic hematopoietic stem cell transplantation. Clin Chest Med. 2017;38(4):607–21. https://doi.org/10.1016/j.ccm.2017.07.003; Epub 2017/11/13.
137. Yanik GA, Mineishi S, Levine JE, Kitko CL, White ES, Vander Lugt MT, et al. Soluble tumor necrosis factor receptor: enbrel (etanercept) for subacute pulmonary dysfunction following allogeneic stem cell transplantation. Biol Blood Marrow Transplant. 2012;18(7):1044–54. https://doi.org/10.1016/j.bbmt.2011.11.031; Epub 2011/12/14.
138. Williams KM, Cheng GS, Pusic I, Jagasia M, Burns L, Ho VT, et al. Fluticasone, azithromycin, and montelukast treatment for new-onset bronchiolitis obliterans syndrome after hematopoietic cell transplantation. Biol Blood Marrow Transplant. 2016;22(4):710–6. https://doi.org/10.1016/j.bbmt.2015.10.009; Epub 2015/10/18.
139. Cheng GS, Storer B, Chien JW, Jagasia M, Hubbard JJ, Burns L, et al. Lung function trajectory in bronchiolitis obliterans syndrome after allogeneic hematopoietic cell transplant. Ann Am Thorac Soc. 2016;13(11):1932–9. https://doi.org/10.1513/AnnalsATS.201604-262OC; Epub 2016/08/12.
140. Lam DC, Lam B, Wong MK, Lu C, Au WY, Tse EW, et al. Effects of azithromycin in bronchiolitis obliterans syndrome after hematopoietic SCT--a randomized double-blinded placebo-controlled study. Bone Marrow Transplant. 2011;46(12):1551–6. https://doi.org/10.1038/bmt.2011.1; Epub 2011/02/15.
141. Lemonnier F, Rivaud E, Neveu H, Catherinot E, Suarez F, Dhedin N, et al. Azithromycin in bronchiolitis obliterans syndrome after hematopoietic SCT. Bone Marrow Transplant. 2012;47(10):1374. https://doi.org/10.1038/bmt.2012.23; Epub 2012/03/01.
142. Bergeron A, Chevret S, Granata A, Chevallier P, Vincent L, Huynh A, et al. Effect of azithromycin on airflow decline-free survival after allogeneic hema-

topoietic stem cell transplant: the ALLOZITHRO randomized clinical trial. JAMA. 2017;318(6):557–66. https://doi.org/10.1001/jama.2017.9938; Epub 2017/08/09.
143. Vallet N, Le Grand S, Bondeelle L, Hoareau B, Corneau A, Bouteiller D, et al. Azithromycin promotes relapse by disrupting immune and metabolic networks after allogeneic stem cell transplantation. Blood. 2022;140(23):2500–13. https://doi.org/10.1182/blood.2022016926; Epub 2022/08/20.
144. Shamoun M, Braun T, Magenau JM, Choi SW, Reddy P, Pawarode A, et al. The effect of azithromycin on relapse in patients with moderate-severe chronic graft versus host disease. Biol Blood Marrow Transplant. 2019;25(3):s26–s7.
145. Cheng GS, Bondeelle L, Gooley T, He Q, Jamani K, Krakow EF, et al. Azithromycin use and increased cancer risk among patients with bronchiolitis obliterans after hematopoietic cell transplantation. Biol Blood Marrow Transplant. 2020;26(2):392–400. https://doi.org/10.1016/j.bbmt.2019.10.025; Epub 2019/11/05.
146. Patel B, Sheshardri A, Saliba RM, Rondon G, Ahmed T, Arain MH, et al. Azithromycin exposure following hematopoietic stem cell transplantation is associated with an increased risk of cancer relapse in acute leukemia. Biol Blood Marrow Transplant. 2019;25:S231.
147. Bergeron A, Chevret S, Chagnon K, Godet C, Bergot E, Peffault de Latour R, et al. Budesonide/formoterol for bronchiolitis obliterans after hematopoietic stem cell transplantation. Am J Respir Crit Care Med. 2015;191(11):1242–9. https://doi.org/10.1164/rccm.201410-1818OC; Epub 2015/04/04.
148. Miklos D, Cutler CS, Arora M, Waller EK, Jagasia M, Pusic I, et al. Ibrutinib for chronic graft-versus-host disease after failure of prior therapy. Blood. 2017;130(21):2243–50. https://doi.org/10.1182/blood-2017-07-793786; Epub 2017/09/20.
149. Streiler C, Shaikh F, Davis C, Abhyankar S, Brownback KR. Ruxolitinib is an effective steroid sparing agent in bronchiolitis obliterans due to chronic graft-versus-host-disease. Bone Marrow Transplant. 2019;55(6):1194–6. https://doi.org/10.1038/s41409-019-0662-6; Epub 2019/09/06.
150. Jain NA, Pophali PA, Klotz JK, Ito S, Koklanaris E, Chawla K, et al. Repair of impaired pulmonary function is possible in very-long-term allogeneic stem cell transplantation survivors. Biol Blood Marrow Transplant. 2014;20(2):209–13. https://doi.org/10.1016/j.bbmt.2013.10.025; Epub 2013/11/06.
151. Ruutu T, Barosi G, Benjamin RJ, Clark RE, George JN, Gratwohl A, et al. Diagnostic criteria for hematopoietic stem cell transplant-associated microangiopathy: results of a consensus process by an international working group. Haematologica. 2007;92(1):95–100. https://doi.org/10.3324/haematol.10699; Epub 2007/01/19.
152. Ho VT, Cutler C, Carter S, Martin P, Adams R, Horowitz M, et al. Blood and marrow transplant clinical trials network toxicity committee consensus summary: thrombotic microangiopathy after hematopoietic stem cell transplantation. Biol Blood Marrow Transplant. 2005;11(8):571–5. https://doi.org/10.1016/j.bbmt.2005.06.001; Epub 2005/07/26.
153. Dandoy CE, Rotz S, Alonso PB, Klunk A, Desmond C, Huber J, et al. A pragmatic multi-institutional approach to understanding transplant-associated thrombotic microangiopathy after stem cell transplant. Blood Adv. 2021;5(1):1–11. https://doi.org/10.1182/bloodadvances.2020003455; Epub 2021/02/12.
154. Jodele S, Laskin BL, Goebel J, Khoury JC, Pinkard SL, Carey PM, et al. Does early initiation of therapeutic plasma exchange improve outcome in pediatric stem cell transplant-associated thrombotic microangiopathy? Transfusion. 2013;53(3):661–7. https://doi.org/10.1111/j.1537-2995.2012.03776.x; Epub 2012/07/19.
155. Jodele S, Zhang K, Zou F, Laskin B, Dandoy CE, Myers KC, et al. The genetic fingerprint of susceptibility for transplant-associated thrombotic microangiopathy. Blood. 2016;127(8):989–96. https://doi.org/10.1182/blood-2015-08-663435; Epub 2015/11/26.
156. Jodele S. Complement in pathophysiology and treatment of transplant-associated thrombotic microangiopathies. Semin Hematol. 2018;55(3):159–66. https://doi.org/10.1053/j.seminhematol.2018.04.003; Epub 2018/07/24.
157. Jodele S, Fukuda T, Vinks A, Mizuno K, Laskin BL, Goebel J, et al. Eculizumab therapy in children with severe hematopoietic stem cell transplantation-associated thrombotic microangiopathy. Biol Blood Marrow Transplant. 2014;20(4):518–25. https://doi.org/10.1016/j.bbmt.2013.12.565; Epub 2013/12/29.
158. Jodele S, Dandoy CE, Lane A, Laskin BL, Teusink-Cross A, Myers KC, et al. Complement blockade for TA-TMA: lessons learned from a large pediatric cohort treated with eculizumab. Blood. 2020;135(13):1049–57. https://doi.org/10.1182/blood.2019004218; Epub 2020/01/15.
159. Jodele S, Fukuda T, Mizuno K, Vinks AA, Laskin BL, Goebel J, et al. Variable eculizumab clearance requires pharmacodynamic monitoring to optimize therapy for thrombotic microangiopathy after hematopoietic stem cell transplantation. Biol Blood Marrow Transplant. 2016;22(2):307–15. https://doi.org/10.1016/j.bbmt.2015.10.002; Epub 2015/10/13.
160. Corti P, Uderzo C, Tagliabue A, Della Volpe A, Annaloro C, Tagliaferri E, et al. Defibrotide as a promising treatment for thrombotic thrombocytopenic purpura in patients undergoing bone marrow transplantation. Bone Marrow Transplant. 2002;29(6):542–3. https://doi.org/10.1038/sj.bmt.1703414; Epub 2002/04/18.
161. McDonald GB, Sharma P, Matthews DE, Shulman HM, Thomas ED. Venocclusive disease of the liver after bone marrow transplantation: diagnosis, incidence, and predisposing factors. Hepatology.

1984;4(1):116–22. https://doi.org/10.1002/hep.1840040121; Epub 1984/01/01.
162. McDonald GB, Hinds MS, Fisher LD, Schoch HG, Wolford JL, Banaji M, et al. Veno-occlusive disease of the liver and multiorgan failure after bone marrow transplantation: a cohort study of 355 patients. Ann Intern Med. 1993;118(4):255–67. https://doi.org/10.7326/0003-4819-118-4-199302150-00003; Epub 1993/02/15.
163. Jones RJ, Lee KS, Beschorner WE, Vogel VG, Grochow LB, Braine HG, et al. Venoocclusive disease of the liver following bone marrow transplantation. Transplantation. 1987;44(6):778–83. https://doi.org/10.1097/00007890-198712000-00011; Epub 1987/12/01.
164. Bearman SI. The syndrome of hepatic veno-occlusive disease after marrow transplantation. Blood. 1995;85(11):3005–20; Epub 1995/06/01.
165. Cairo MS, Cooke KR, Lazarus HM, Chao N. Modified diagnostic criteria, grading classification and newly elucidated pathophysiology of hepatic SOS/VOD after haematopoietic cell transplantation. Br J Haematol. 2020;190(6):822–36. https://doi.org/10.1111/bjh.16557; Epub 2020/03/07.
166. Bearman SI, Anderson GL, Mori M, Hinds MS, Shulman HM, McDonald GB. Venoocclusive disease of the liver: development of a model for predicting fatal outcome after marrow transplantation. J Clin Oncol. 1993;11(9):1729–36. https://doi.org/10.1200/JCO.1993.11.9.1729; Epub 1993/09/01.
167. Coppell JA, Richardson PG, Soiffer R, Martin PL, Kernan NA, Chen A, et al. Hepatic veno-occlusive disease following stem cell transplantation: incidence, clinical course, and outcome. Biol Blood Marrow Transplant. 2010;16(2):157–68. https://doi.org/10.1016/j.bbmt.2009.08.024; Epub 2009/09/22.
168. Raina R, Abusin GA, Vijayaraghavan P, Auletta JJ, Cabral L, Hashem H, et al. The role of continuous renal replacement therapy in the management of acute kidney injury associated with sinusoidal obstruction syndrome following hematopoietic cell transplantation. Pediatr Transplant. 2018;22:2. https://doi.org/10.1111/petr.13139; Epub 2018/02/02.
169. Duncan CN, Lehmann LE, Cheifetz IM, Greathouse K, Haight AE, Hall MW, et al. Clinical outcomes of children receiving intensive cardiopulmonary support during hematopoietic stem cell transplant. Pediatr Crit Care Med. 2013;14(3):261–7. https://doi.org/10.1097/PCC.0b013e3182720601; Epub 2013/02/09.
170. Rowan CM, Smith LS, Loomis A, McArthur J, Gertz SJ, Fitzgerald JC, et al. Pediatric acute respiratory distress syndrome in pediatric allogeneic hematopoietic stem cell transplants: a multicenter study. Pediatr Crit Care Med. 2017;18(4):304–9. https://doi.org/10.1097/PCC.0000000000001061; Epub 2017/02/09.
171. Wosten-van Asperen RM, van Gestel JPJ, van Grotel M, Tschiedel E, Dohna-Schwake C, Valla FV, et al. PICU mortality of children with cancer admitted to pediatric intensive care unit a systematic review and meta-analysis. Crit Rev Oncol Hematol. 2019;142:153–63. https://doi.org/10.1016/j.critrevonc.2019.07.014; Epub 2019/08/14.
172. Zinter MS, Logan BR, Fretham C, Sapru A, Abraham A, Aljurf MD, et al. Comprehensive prognostication in critically ill pediatric hematopoietic cell transplant patients: results from merging the center for international blood and marrow transplant research (cibmtr) and virtual pediatric systems (vps) registries. Biol Blood Marrow Transplant. 2020;26(2):333–42. https://doi.org/10.1016/j.bbmt.2019.09.027; Epub 2019/09/30.
173. Rowan CM, Gertz SJ, McArthur J, Fitzgerald JC, Nitu ME, Loomis A, et al. Invasive mechanical ventilation and mortality in pediatric hematopoietic stem cell transplantation: a multicenter study. Pediatr Crit Care Med. 2016;17(4):294–302. https://doi.org/10.1097/PCC.0000000000000673; Epub 2016/02/26.
174. Rowan CM, Loomis A, McArthur J, Smith LS, Gertz SJ, Fitzgerald JC, et al. High-frequency oscillatory ventilation use and severe pediatric ARDS in the pediatric hematopoietic cell transplant recipient. Respir Care. 2018;63(4):404–11. https://doi.org/10.4187/respcare.05765; Epub 2017/12/28.
175. Rowan CM, Nitu ME, Moser EAS, Swigonski NL, Renbarger JL. Weight gain and supplemental O2: risk factors during the hematopoietic cell transplant admission in pediatric patients. Pediatr Blood Cancer. 2017;64(11):e26562. https://doi.org/10.1002/pbc.26561; Epub 2017/04/26.
176. Cater DT, Tori AJ, Moser EAS, Rowan CM. Modification and assessment of the bedside pediatric early warning score in the pediatric allogeneic hematopoietic cell transplant population. Pediatr Crit Care Med. 2018;19(5):483–8. https://doi.org/10.1097/PCC.0000000000001521; Epub 2018/03/10.
177. Pediatric Acute Lung Injury Consensus Conference G. Pediatric acute respiratory distress syndrome: consensus recommendations from the pediatric acute lung injury consensus conference. Pediatr Crit Care Med. 2015;16(5):428–39. https://doi.org/10.1097/PCC.0000000000000350; Epub 2015/02/04.
178. Valentine SL, Nadkarni VM, Curley MA, Pediatric Acute Lung Injury Consensus Conference G. Nonpulmonary treatments for pediatric acute respiratory distress syndrome: proceedings from the Pediatric acute lung injury consensus conference. Pediatr Crit Care Med. 2015;16(5 Suppl 1):S73–85. https://doi.org/10.1097/PCC.0000000000000435; Epub 2015/06/03.
179. Wilson B, Typpo K. Nutrition: a primary therapy in pediatric acute respiratory distress syndrome. Front Pediatr. 2016;4:108. https://doi.org/10.3389/fped.2016.00108; Epub 2016/10/30.
180. Marik PE, Khangoora V, Rivera R, Hooper MH, Catravas J. Hydrocortisone, vitamin C, and

thiamine for the treatment of severe sepsis and septic shock: a retrospective before-after study. Chest. 2017;151(6):1229–38. https://doi.org/10.1016/j.chest.2016.11.036; Epub 2016/12/13.
181. Carcillo JA, Dean JM, Holubkov R, Berger J, Meert KL, Anand KJS, et al. Interaction between 2 nutraceutical treatments and host immune status in the pediatric critical illness stress-induced immune suppression comparative effectiveness trial. JPEN J Parenter Enteral Nutr. 2017;41(8):1325–35. https://doi.org/10.1177/0148607116670377; Epub 2016/09/24.
182. Boudreault F, Pinilla-Vera M, Englert JA, Kho AT, Isabelle C, Arciniegas AJ, et al. Zinc deficiency primes the lung for ventilator-induced injury. JCI Insight. 2017;2(11):e86507. https://doi.org/10.1172/jci.insight.86507; Epub 2017/06/02.
183. Jafari B, Ouyang B, Li LF, Hales CA, Quinn DA. Intracellular glutathione in stretch-induced cytokine release from alveolar type-2 like cells. Respirology. 2004;9(1):43–53. https://doi.org/10.1111/j.1440-1843.2003.00527.x; Epub 2004/02/26.
184. Wallace G, Jodele S, Howell J, Myers KC, Teusink A, Zhao X, et al. Vitamin D deficiency and survival in children after hematopoietic stem cell transplant. Biol Blood Marrow Transplant. 2015;21(9):1627–31. https://doi.org/10.1016/j.bbmt.2015.06.009; Epub 2015/06/21.
185. Sipmann FS, Santos A, Tusman G. Heart-lung interactions in acute respiratory distress syndrome: pathophysiology, detection and management strategies. Ann Transl Med. 2018;6(2):27. https://doi.org/10.21037/atm.2017.12.07; Epub 2018/02/13.
186. Dandoy CE, Davies SM, Hirsch R, Chima RS, Paff Z, Cash M, et al. Abnormal echocardiography 7 days after stem cell transplantation may be an early indicator of thrombotic microangiopathy. Biol Blood Marrow Transplant. 2015;21(1):113–8. https://doi.org/10.1016/j.bbmt.2014.09.028; Epub 2014/10/11.
187. Dandoy CE, Jodele S, Paff Z, Hirsch R, Ryan TD, Jefferies JL, et al. Team-based approach to identify cardiac toxicity in critically ill hematopoietic stem cell transplant recipients. Pediatr Blood Cancer. 2017;64:10. https://doi.org/10.1002/pbc.26513; Epub 2017/03/09.
188. National Heart, Lung, Blood Institute Acute Respiratory Distress Syndrome Clinical Trials N, Wiedemann HP, Wheeler AP, Bernard GR, Thompson BT, et al. Comparison of two fluid-management strategies in acute lung injury. N Engl J Med. 2006;354(24):2564–75. https://doi.org/10.1056/NEJMoa062200; Epub 2006/05/23.
189. Michael M, Kuehnle I, Goldstein SL. Fluid overload and acute renal failure in pediatric stem cell transplant patients. Pediatr Nephrol. 2004;19(1):91–5. https://doi.org/10.1007/s00467-003-1313-z; Epub 2003/11/25.
190. Flores FX, Brophy PD, Symons JM, Fortenberry JD, Chua AN, Alexander SR, et al. Continuous renal replacement therapy (CRRT) after stem cell transplantation. A report from the prospective pediatric CRRT registry group. Pediatr Nephrol. 2008;23(4):625–30.https://doi.org/10.1007/s00467--007-0672-2; Epub 2008/01/30.
191. DiCarlo JV, Alexander SR, Agarwal R, Schiffman JD. Continuous veno-venous hemofiltration may improve survival from acute respiratory distress syndrome after bone marrow transplantation or chemotherapy. J Pediatr Hematol Oncol. 2003;25(10):801–5. https://doi.org/10.1097/00043426-200310000-00012; Epub 2003/10/07.
192. Elbahlawan L, West NK, Avent Y, Cheng C, Liu W, Barfield RC, et al. Impact of continuous renal replacement therapy on oxygenation in children with acute lung injury after allogeneic hematopoietic stem cell transplantation. Pediatr Blood Cancer. 2010;55(3):540–5. https://doi.org/10.1002/pbc.22561; Epub 2010/07/27.
193. Rajasekaran S, Jones DP, Avent Y, Shaffer ML, Elbahlawan L, Henderson N, et al. Outcomes of hematopoietic stem cell transplant patients who received continuous renal replacement therapy in a pediatric oncology intensive care unit. Pediatr Crit Care Med. 2010;11(6):699–706. https://doi.org/10.1097/PCC.0b013e3181e32423; Epub 2010/05/25.
194. Di Nardo M, Merli P, Cecchetti C, Pasotti E, Bertaina A, Locatelli F. Progressive increase in D-dimer levels during extracorporeal membrane oxygenation can predict membrane oxygenator failure in children given hematopoietic stem cell transplantation? J Crit Care. 2016;31(1):262–3. https://doi.org/10.1016/j.jcrc.2015.09.010; Epub 2015/10/20.
195. Maue DK, Hobson MJ, Friedman ML, Moser EA, Rowan CM. Outcomes of pediatric oncology and hematopoietic cell transplant patients receiving extracorporeal membrane oxygenation. Perfusion. 2019;34(7):598–604. https://doi.org/10.1177/0267659119842471; Epub 2019/04/26.
196. Klein OR, Bembea MM, McCloskey J, Wilkinson M, Chen AR, Gamper C, et al. Outcomes in pediatric bone marrow transplant patients undergoing extracorporeal membrane oxygenation. Biology of blood and marrow transplantation: journal of the American Society for Blood and Marrow. Transplantation. 2017;23(3, Supplement):S238.
197. Steppan DA, Coleman RD, Viamonte HK, Hanson SJ, Carroll MK, Klein OR, et al. Outcomes of pediatric patients with oncologic disease or following hematopoietic stem cell transplant supported on extracorporeal membrane oxygenation: The PEDECOR experience. Pediatr Blood Cancer. 2020;67:e28403. https://doi.org/10.1002/pbc.28403; Epub 2020/06/11.

198. Ghafoor S, Fan K, Di Nardo M, Talleur AC, Saini A, Potera RM, et al. Extracorporeal membrane oxygenation candidacy in pediatric patients treated with hematopoietic stem cell transplant and chimeric antigen receptor t-cell therapy: an international survey. Front Oncol. 2021;11:798236. https://doi.org/10.3389/fonc.2021.798236; Epub 2022/01/11.

199. Di Nardo M, Ahmad AH, Merli P, Zinter MS, Lehman LE, Rowan CM, et al. Extracorporeal membrane oxygenation in children receiving haematopoietic cell transplantation and immune effector cell therapy: an international and multidisciplinary consensus statement. Lancet Child Adolesc Health. 2022;6(2):116–28. https://doi.org/10.1016/S2352--4642(21)00336-9; Epub 2021/12/14.

# CAR T-Cell Therapy and Critical Care Considerations

32

Cristina Gutierrez, Oren Pasvolsky, and Partow Kebriaei

## Introduction

Immunotherapy has revolutionized oncological care and improved the prognosis of many refractory malignancies. As these therapies evolved and became widely used, a new range of complications that has made intensive care unit (ICU) staff rethink the way we diagnose, treat and think about the prognosis of critically ill cancer patients. Since the first trials of chimeric antigen receptor (CAR) cell therapy showing significant response rates, five CAR T-cell products have been approved for the treatment of refractory B-cell malignancies, such as acute lymphoblastic leukaemia (ALL), B-cell lymphoma and multiple myeloma [1–6]. About 50% to 80% of patients achieve remission after CAR T-cell therapy, with as many as 50–60% being free of disease at 12 months [1–6]. While these outcomes are impressive, it is important for the non-oncologist, and specifically for ICU staff, to understand the complications associated with these treatments and the prognosis they carry. Complications such as cytokine release syndrome (CRS), immune effector cell-associated neurotoxicity syndrome (ICANS) and hemophagocytic lymphohistiocytosis (HLH) are unique, relatively common and require staff to have an acute awareness to initiate rapid treatment (Fig. 32.1).

The objective of this chapter is to review the most common short- and long-term complications of CAR therapy that can lead to ICU admission or have implications when a patient is admitted to the ICU following the post-infusion phase. A better understanding of these complications can lead to better support and care of these patients who are known to have an excellent prognosis.

C. Gutierrez (✉)
Division of Anesthesiology, Critical Care and Pain Medicine, Department of Critical Care, The University of Texas M.D. Anderson Cancer Center, Houston, TX, USA
e-mail: CGutierrez4@mdanderson.org

O. Pasvolsky
Department of Stem Cell Transplant and Cellular Therapy, The University of Texas M.D. Anderson Cancer Center, Houston, TX, USA
Institute of Hematology, Davidoff Cancer Center, Rabin Medical Center, Petah-Tikva, Israel
e-mail: OPasvolsky@mdanderson.org

P. Kebriaei
Department of Stem Cell Transplant and Cellular Therapy, The University of Texas M.D. Anderson Cancer Center, Houston, TX, USA
e-mail: pkebriae@mdanderson.org


A. O. Soubani (ed.), *Pulmonary and Critical Care Considerations of Hematopoietic Stem Cell Transplantation*, https://doi.org/10.1007/978-3-031-28797-8_32

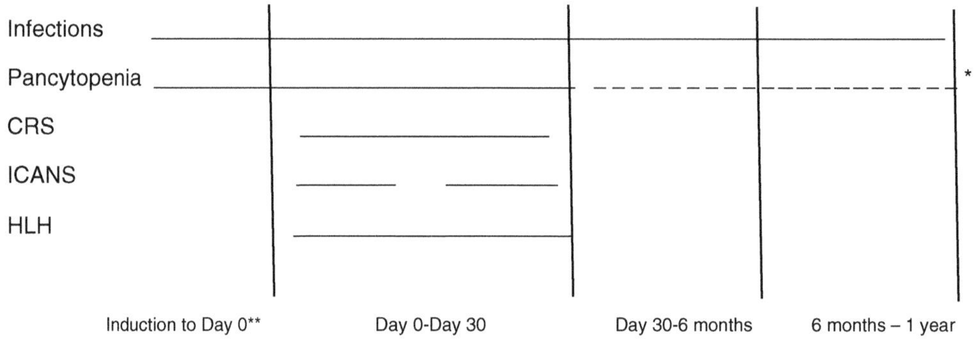


**Fig. 32.1** Complications of CAR-T therapy according to the timing of treatment. *with as many as 90% of patients having haematological toxicity after day 30. ** Day 0: day of CAR infusion. *CRS* cytokine release syndrome, *ICANS* immune effector cell-associated neurotoxicity syndrome, *HLH* hemophagocytic lymphohistiocytosis

# Overview of CAR Therapy

## Types of CAR, Indications and FDA Approval

Chimeric antigen receptor (CAR) T-cells are genetically modified T-cells that contain fusion proteins composed of an antigen-binding extracellular portion and an intracellular signalling portion derived from T-cell signalling proteins [7]. The CAR constructs contain additional varying costimulatory domains, such as CD28 and 4-1BB, and they can be produced from either patient-derived (autologous) or donor-derived (allogeneic) cytotoxic T-cells.

Autologous CD19 CAR T-cell therapy has yielded ground-breaking results in the field of haemato-oncology, providing durable remissions for many patients who had previously faced dismal prognosis. In 2017, axicabtagene ciloleucel became the first CAR T-cell approved by the FDA for clinical use, based on the results of the ZUMA-1 trial, which enrolled 111 patients with relapsed/refractory large B-cell lymphoma [1]. Subsequently, two other CAR-T therapies were approved by the FDA for several types of non-Hodgkin's lymphoma. Then, tisagenlecleucel and lisocabtagene maraleucel were also approved, following the JULIET and the TRANSCEND NHL001 trials, respectively [2, 4].

Tisagenlecleucel was the first CAR T-cell approved for B-cell acute lymphoblastic leukaemia (B-ALL) by the FDA, following the results of the phase II ELIANA trial, which included children and young adults [6]. The second CAR T-cell to be granted approval by the FDA for ALL was brexucabtagene autoleucel, based on results of the ZUMA-3 trial in adult patients [8]. Idecabtagene vicleucel is the first cellular therapy that received FDA approval for patients with multiple myeloma, following the positive results observed in the KarMMa trial [3].

## Cell Preparation, Apheresis, Lymphodepletion and Cell Infusion

The process of manufacturing autologous CAR T-cells begins with the collection of the patient's leukocytes through leukapheresis to obtain mononuclear cells (MNCs) [9]. Next, the collected cells are filtered to isolate specific T-cell subpopulations of interest and remove contaminants. The T-cells are then activated, and the CAR is inserted into the genome of the T-cells, usually via viral transduction [10]. The CAR product is then expanded using cell culture propagation. Finally, the CAR T-cells are washed, concentrated and cryopreserved in infusible cryomedia. The CAR T-cell is then delivered to the medical institute, thawed and infused to the patient following a lymphodepleting preparative regimen. Lymphodepletion with a combination of fludarabine and cyclophosphamide is considered to be optimal to enhance in vivo CAR T-cell expansion and persistence [11–13].

## Institutional Considerations

When implementing a CAR program within an institution, there are important aspects to consider. First, education of staff is one of the pillars of a successful CAR T-cell program [14]. The complications associated with this therapy and their clinical presentations can mimic common pathologies observed in cancer patients but require a unique approach and treatment. Quick recognition of these toxicities, early escalation of care and immediate treatment is extremely important to avoid worsening morbidity and mortality. Many subspecialties (e.g. neurology, cardiology and infectious diseases) and hospital areas (emergency rooms, ICUs, floors and step-down units) will support these patients; therefore, education and knowledge of when these patients receive treatment will ensure adequate care once complications arise. While staffing will depend on each institution, an initial core group to treat this patient population can be beneficial. As staff becomes more comfortable with treating these patients, the staffing and number of patients can expand. A slow approach can help the institution grow the program in a safe manner. Lastly, guidelines on how to monitor and treat these patients are extremely important to streamline their care [14–18]. High-risk patients, such as those with cardiac comorbidities, high disease burden and central nervous system (CNS) involvement, can be considered for telemetry beds [14, 17]. Lastly, published scores using common routine laboratory tests could help predict those patients who will develop severe toxicities and assist with triaging [19]. Close communication with the Intensive Care Unit (ICU) staff will be important as many as 40% of patients can require ICU admission due to severe toxicities after CAR infusion [20, 21].

## Acute Complications Post-Infusion

### Cytokine Release Syndrome

One of the most common complications post-CAR infusion is cytokine release syndrome, which presents as fever associated with either hypotension or hypoxemia [16] (Table 32.1). CRS is an inflammatory response led by the activation of CAR T-cells after recognition of the tumoral antigen. As CARs become activated and replicate, this leads to the activation of other inflammatory cells, such as macrophages, B-cells and T-cells, and a release of cytokines (IL-10, IL-6, IFNγ, TNFα, IL-1β) [16, 22, 23]. This exaggerated inflammatory response causes endothelial dysfunction and capillary leak syndrome and, if left untreated, can lead to multi-organ failure. While the clinical presentation and onset is similar within products (3–7 days post-infusion), its incidence and severity can vary [1, 3, 5, 17]. With axicabtagene, one of the first FDA-approved products, CRS occurs in as many as 90% of patients, and Grade 3 and 4 toxicity (hypotension that requires vasopressor support or hypoxemia requiring high-flow or invasive mechanical ventilation) is observed in 17% of patients [1]. Guidelines recommend all cases of Grade $\geq 3$ toxicity to be admitted to the ICU; however high-risk patients could be admitted earlier for close monitoring [14, 15, 17]. Despite the relatively high incidence of shock, recent data suggest that the requirement of vasopressors is usually short (median of 1 day), with 80% of patients requiring only one vasopressor [20]. Respiratory failure associated with CRS is rare, with less than 15% of patients requiring mechanical ventilation, high-flow nasal cannula or BiPAP [20]. Other organ toxicities that have been described with CRS include renal failure, electrolyte imbalances, non-ischemic cardiomyopathies, arrhythmias, liver dysfunction and coagulopathy [14, 24,

**Table 32.1** CRS grading as per ASTCT guidelines

| | Grade 1 | Grade 2 | Grade 3 | Grade 4 |
|---|---|---|---|---|
| CRS parameter | | | | |
| Fever[a] | Temperature ≥ 38 °C | Temperature ≥ 38 °C | Temperature ≥ 38 °C | Temperature ≥ 38 °C |
| With | | | | |
| hypotension | None | Not requiring vasopressors | Requiring a vasopressor ± vasopressin | Requiring multiple vasopressors (excluding vasopressin) |
| And/or[b] | | | | |
| hypoxia | None | Requiring low-flow nasal cannula (≤6 L/min) or blow-by | Requiring high-flow nasal cannula (>6 L/min), facemask, non-rebreather mask or venturi mask | Requiring positive pressure (e.g. CPAP, BiPAP, intubation and mechanical ventilation) |

*BiPAP* bilevel positive airway pressure, *CPAP* continuous positive airway pressure, *CRS* cytokine release syndrome, *ASTCT* American Society for Transplantation and Cellular Therapy
Lee et al. Biol Blood Marrow Transplant 2019 (25):625–638
[a]Fever may be absent in patients who have received tocilizumab and/or corticosteroids
[b]CRS grade is determined by the more severe event: hypotension or hypoxia

25]. The incidence of these complications is usually low, and they do not require invasive or life-saving interventions and resolve relatively quickly [20].

Treatment for CRS includes organ support, workup for infectious causes of fever and hypotension and immunomodulatory therapy. The first line of treatment for any grade of CRS is tocilizumab, a blocking interleukin-6 (IL-6) receptor monoclonal antibody. Earlier studies showed an early elevation of IL-6 in patients with CRS and that blockade of IL-6 leads to the resolution of CRS [26]. Corticosteroids, including dexamethasone or methylprednisolone, are reserved for patients with Grade 2–4 toxicities [17]. Initiation, dose, duration, and tapering recommendations can vary according to each CAR product [17, 27]. However, an approach that involves tapering and observation of the patient's clinical status is preferable. For rare refractory CRS, anakinra, an IL-1 receptor antagonist, has been utilized; however, data supporting its use are lacking [28]. ICU support is important for those patients who develop respiratory failure, shock and multi-organ failure, and most of these patients improve within 1 week of ICU admission [20]. However, if no improvement is seen in patients with severe CRS after corticosteroids and tocilizumab, sepsis needs to be considered as a cause for the ongoing organ failure [17]. Current interventions in the ICU are based on observations on other critically ill patients, and data specific to this patient population are still limited [20, 29].

## Immune Effector Cell-Associated Neurotoxicity Syndrome

The pathophysiology of ICANS is not as well understood as that of CRS; however a shared inflammatory process is thought to play a role. The initial inflammatory process led by CAR proliferation leads to endothelial dysfunction, increased permeability of the blood-brain barrier, and migration of inflammatory cells (including CARs) and cytokines into the central nervous system while activating local inflammatory cells such as microglia and astrocytes [17, 30–32]. The presentation of ICANS is unique and usually occurs on day 7 post-infusion, many times concomitantly with CRS [16] (Table 32.2). A second delayed presentation of ICANS, which usually presents alone, has also been described and occurs after 10 days of infusion. The prevalence of ICANS varies depending on the product, with some presenting in as many as 64% of patients (30% Grade ≥ 3) [1].

**Table 32.2** ICANS grading as per ASTCT guidelines

| Neurotoxicity domain[a] | Grade 1 | Grade 2 | Grade 3 | Grade 4 |
|---|---|---|---|---|
| ICE score | 7–9 | 3–6 | 0–2 | 0 (unarousable and unable to perform ICE) |
| Depressed level of consciousness | Awakens spontaneously | Awakens to voice | Awakens only to tactile stimulus | Unarousable or requiring vigorous or repetitive tactile stimuli to be aroused. Stupor or coma |
| Seizure | N/A | N/A | Any clinical seizure focal or generalized that resolves rapidly or nonconvulsive seizures on EEG that resolve with intervention | Life-threatening prolonged seizure (<5 min) or repetitive clinical or electrical seizures without returning to baseline in between |
| Motor findings | N/A | N/A | N/A | Deep focal motor weakness such as hemiparesis or paraparesis |
| Elevated ICP/ cerebral oedema | N/A | N/A | Focal/local oedema on neuroimaging | Diffuse cerebral oedema on neuroimaging; decerebrate or decorticate posturing; or cranial nerve VI palsy; or papilledema; or Cushing's triad |

*ICANS* immune effector cell-associated neurotoxicity syndrome, *ASTCT* American Society for Transplantation and Cellular Therapy, *EEG* electroencephalogram, *ICE* immune effector cell-associated encephalopathy, *ICP* intracranial pressure, *N/A* not applicable

Lee et al. Biol Blood Marrow Transplant 2019 (25):625–638

[a]ICANS grade is determined by the most severe event in the neurotoxicity domain

Patients with mild ICANS present with aphasia, headache, delirium, tremor and agraphia [16]. As the syndrome evolves, patients can develop global aphasia, seizures (non-convulsive are more common), status epilepticus, altered sensorium, and, in rare cases, motor deficits [16]. Cerebral edema has also been described in these patients. Focal edema is common in the basal ganglia, thalamus and brainstem, but cases of severe global cerebral edema leading to death have been reported [30, 32, 33]. Workup and supportive care in the ICU are important for patients with Grade 3 and 4 ICANS. Imaging, either CT or brain MRI, can be useful, especially to evaluate the severity of cerebral edema and to rule out other pathologies such as ischemic and haemorrhagic strokes. The role of lumbar puncture is limited but can be considered in those patients who are not improving or in those in whom concomitant infections are suspected. As with CRS, the treatment of ICANS focuses on organ support and immunomodulation with corticosteroids [17]. A slow taper observing the patient's clinical response to such treatments is recommended. The use of anti-IL-6 therapy is not recommended, and while anakinra can be considered for refractory cases, studies evaluating its efficacy are still needed [17, 34].

## Hemophagocytic Lymphohistiocytosis

While initially HLH was considered a rare complication in lymphoma patients treated with CD19 CARs, other products for the treatment of multiple myeloma and acute lymphoblastic leukaemia, have described higher incidences (15–30%) of this complication [3, 35, 36]. In the setting of CAR therapy, HLH presents as a spectrum of a prolonged and exaggerated inflammatory response after CRS occurs. Its clinical presentation and diagnostic profile are similar to malignancy-related HLH. Multi-organ failure, specifically liver failure and sometimes altered mentation, in the setting of elevated ferritin and triglyceride levels, liver function tests, coagulopathy, and rarely hemophagocytosis in bone marrow biopsy has been described [35, 36]. While infections should be considered during work-up, they are not a common cause of HLH in this patient population [35]. The pathophysiology of CAR-related HLH is thought to be related to a dysregulation between the ratio of NK, CAR and CD8 T-cells after CAR T-cell activation [36]. Response to therapy is variable, and treatment includes cytokine blockade with tocilizumab and anakinra, corticosteroids, and, in refractory cases, ruxolitinib and etoposide [37, 14, 17]. Risk factors still need to be identified, and clear diagnostic and treatment guidelines need to be created in this patient population, as their mortality continues to be high.

## Infectious Complications

Infectious complications after CAR therapy are common and can have a significant impact on patients' outcomes. While mortality due to CRS and ICANS is low (<1.5%), in the acute phase after CAR infusion, inpatient mortality is mainly due to infectious complications and progression of disease [20]. Due to the great similarity between CRS and sepsis, it is recommended to work up and treat patients for neutropenic sepsis once fever appears. Unfortunately, common markers used to guide antibiotic therapy such as CRP and pro-calcitonin may not be useful in this patient population [38]. Data regarding the validity of cytokine profiles to predict sepsis over CRS are scarce [39]. Most infections occur within 28 days after CAR T-cell infusion, of which more than 80% occur within 10 days [40, 41]. Some of the most common infections observed in the acute period after CAR infusion are bacteraemia and viral infections, while fungal infections are rare [40, 41]. Fortunately, life-threatening infections have been reported in only 2% of patients [40]. Risk factors associated with increased infectious complications include Grade $\geq$ 3 toxicities, prior haematopoietic stem cell transplant, corticosteroids, and an ANC < 500 cells/μL [38, 40, 41].

## Other Reasons for ICU Admission, Considerations and Resource Utilization

While mortality due to CRS and ICANS in the ICU is low, other reasons for ICU admission could carry a different prognosis [29]. CAR patients with critical illness can have underlying sepsis, multi-organ failure in the setting of disease progression, cardiac arrest, and tumour lysis, which can carry a significant morbidity and mortality [20, 29]. Close communication with the oncologist is necessary when evaluating the patient's cause of multi-organ failure to better guide treatment, workup and possibly discussion of goals of care.

Taking into consideration current staffing shortage and bed restriction in hospitals worldwide due to the COVID-19 pandemic, attention to bed utilization will be important when creating a new CAR T-cell program. Depending on the type of CAR product, their incidence of severe complications and the learning curve that occurs when first treating patients can help ICU staff prepare for an increase in ICU admissions. These patients, however, improve relatively quickly, have short ICU stays and require low organ support [20]. Creating a high-acuity step-down or specialized unit for CAR patients could also be considered to ease bed burden in the ICU.

# Long-Term Complications and Considerations Post CAR T-Cell Therapy

## Prolonged Cytopenias, Haematopoietic Failure and B-Cell Aplasia

Haematological toxicity is a common side effect of CAR T-cell therapy and can occasionally manifest as prolonged cytopenias. In one report, 93% of patients had haematological toxicity beyond day 21 [42]. The rates of late severe neutropenia (neutrophil count lower than 500/μL) and thrombocytopenia (platelet count lower than $50 \times 10^3$/

μL) were 34% and 21%, respectively [42]. The CAR-HEMATOTOX model identifies patients at risk for prolonged cytopenias after CAR T-cell according to baseline haematological reserve (neutrophil, haemoglobin and platelet counts) and inflammatory markers (C-reactive protein and ferritin) [43]. Additionally, almost 90% of patients have B-cell aplasia at 1 month after infusion, and in 40%, it persists for at least 1 year [44]. As observed by Logue et al., immunoglobulin G levels decrease to a nadir at 6 months post-CAR infusion, and median CD4 levels remain low at 1 year, further highlighting the delayed immune reconstitution in treated patients. The contributing factors to immunosuppression in these patients may include tumour-related effects, lymphodepletion chemotherapy, use of corticosteroids and cytokine effects. Such considerations of chronic immunosuppression are important for those patients admitted to the ICU with severe infections to further guide empiric therapy.

## Infectious Considerations and Prophylaxis

As described above, patients treated with CAR T for haematological malignancies face a prolonged period of immunosuppression, with attenuation of both the humoral and cellular arms of the immune system. In one study depicting infections in the real-world setting, 63% of patients experienced an infection in the first year after CAR T infusion. Bacteria were the most common pathogen identified, especially during the first month, followed by viral infections [38]. Approximately 30% of patients had severe bacterial infections, similar to results reported in the registration studies [1, 2]. Therefore, pre-emptive measures to avoid infections are widely employed.

Pretreatment screening for HIV and hepatitis B and C is recommended, with additional studies considered per medical facility preference and patient characteristics [45]. Recommendations regarding the use of antimicrobial prophylaxis are based largely on institutional preference and derived from experience in patients undergoing haematopoietic stem cell transplant (HSCT). Some centres initiate fluoroquinolone antibacterial prophylaxis when patients are severely neutropenic, although recent Spanish guidelines do not recommend routine use of antibacterial prophylaxis [45, 46]. The use of antiviral (acyclovir or valacyclovir), anti-Pneumocystis jiroveci pneumonia (PJP), and antifungal (such as fluconazole) prophylaxis agents is preferred [45, 46]. One should note that the Spanish guidelines recommend the use of antiviral agents only if the CAR T-cell recipient is herpes simplex virus (HSV) seropositive. The need for repeating basic immunizations following CAR T therapy is currently under investigation.

## Role of Haematopoietic Stem Cell Transplant After CAR Therapy

Although CAR T-cell therapy has provided remarkable response rates in B-ALL and B-cell lymphomas, remissions are often short-lived, and the role of allogeneic HSCT (allo-HSCT) for the consolidation of responses achieved by CAR therapy is an area of ongoing debate. Most data on the subject are derived from small numbers of patients who participated in the major CAR T registration studies and from retrospective reports. Nonetheless, for patients with B-ALL, most data suggest benefit of post-CAR T allo-HSCT, especially in paediatric patients who achieve MRD-negative complete remission [6, 47]. In adults the data have been more conflicting: Some reports suggest improved event-free survival with transplant consolidation, yet other analyses have not shown this outcome benefit [8, 48, 49]. For patients with B-cell lymphoma, there is even less long-term data, and recommendations published by the American Society for Transplantation and Cellular Therapy (ASTCT) state that for patients who achieve complete remission after CAR T, active surveillance is recommended, though allo-HSCT can be considered on an individual basis [50].

## Conclusion

The causes for ICU admission in patients after CAR T-cell therapy can vary according to the time lapsed from cell infusion. Acute complications include CRS and ICANS both with excellent outcomes, while infectious complications and HLH can have worse prognosis especially if they present with multi-organ failure. Prolonged cytopenias and B-cell aplasia make this patient population prone to infections, and therefore, a wide differential of infectious complications needs to be considered even 1 year after CAR infusion. As cell therapies continue to evolve and be widely utilized, the need for ICU support for this patient population will continue to be of extreme importance.

## References


1. Neelapu SS, Locke FL, Bartlett NL, et al. Axicabtagene ciloleucel CAR T-cell therapy in refractory large B-cell lymphoma. N Engl J Med. 2017;377(26):2531–44.
2. Schuster SJ, Bishop MR, Tam CS, et al. Tisagenlecleucel in adult relapsed or refractory diffuse large B-cell lymphoma. N Engl J Med. 2019;380(1):45–56.
3. Munshi NC, Anderson LD Jr, Shah N, et al. Idecabtagene vicleucel in relapsed and refractory multiple myeloma. N Engl J Med. 2021;384(8):705–16.
4. Abramson JS, Palomba ML, Gordon LI, et al. Lisocabtagene maraleucel for patients with relapsed or refractory large B-cell lymphomas (TRANSCEND NHL 001): a multicentre seamless design study. Lancet. 2020;396(10254):839–52.
5. Wang M, Munoz J, Goy A, et al. KTE-X19 CAR T-cell therapy in relapsed or refractory mantle-cell lymphoma. N Engl J Med. 2020;382(14):1331–42.
6. Maude SL, Laetsch TW, Buechner J, et al. Tisagenlecleucel in children and young adults with B-cell lymphoblastic leukemia. N Engl J Med. 2018;378(5):439–48.
7. June CH, O'Connor RS, Kawalekar OU, Ghassemi S, Milone MC. CAR T cell immunotherapy for human cancer. Science. 2018;359(6382):1361–5.
8. Shah BD, Ghobadi A, Oluwole OO, et al. KTE-X19 for relapsed or refractory adult B-cell acute lymphoblastic leukaemia: phase 2 results of the single-arm, open-label, multicentre ZUMA-3 study. Lancet. 2021;398(10299):491–502.
9. Smith JW. Apheresis techniques and cellular immunomodulation. Ther Apher. 1997;1(3):203–6.
10. Okuma A. Generation of CAR-T cells by lentiviral transduction. Methods Mol Biol. 2021;2312:3–14.
11. Gardner RA, Finney O, Annesley C, et al. Intent-to-treat leukemia remission by CD19 CAR T cells of defined formulation and dose in children and young adults. Blood. 2017;129(25):3322–31.
12. Kochenderfer JN, Somerville RPT, Lu T, et al. Lymphoma remissions caused by anti-CD19 chimeric antigen receptor T cells are associated with high serum Interleukin-15 levels. J Clin Oncol. 2017;35(16):1803–13.
13. Turtle CJ, Hanafi LA, Berger C, et al. CD19 CAR-T cells of defined CD4+:CD8+ composition in adult B cell ALL patients. J Clin Invest. 2016;126(6):2123–38.
14. Neelapu SS, Tummala S, Kebriaei P, et al. Chimeric antigen receptor T-cell therapy—assessment and management of toxicities. Nat Rev Clin Oncol. 2018;15(1):47–62.
15. Gutierrez C, McEvoy C, Mead E, et al. Management of the critically ill adult chimeric antigen receptor-T cell therapy patient: a critical care perspective. Crit Care Med. 2018;46(9):1402–10.
16. Lee DW, Santomasso BD, Locke FL, et al. ASTCT consensus grading for cytokine release syndrome and neurologic toxicity associated with immune effector cells. Biol Blood Marrow Transplant. 2019;25(4):625–38.
17. Maus MV, Alexander S, Bishop MR, et al. Society for immunotherapy of cancer (SITC) clinical practice guideline on immune effector cell-related adverse events. J Immunother Cancer. 2020;8(2):e001511.
18. Mahadeo KM, Khazal SJ, Abdel-Azim H, et al. Management guidelines for paediatric patients receiving chimeric antigen receptor T cell therapy. Nat Rev Clin Oncol. 2019;16(1):45–63.
19. Greenbaum U, Strati P, Saliba RM, et al. CRP and ferritin in addition to the EASIX score predict CAR-T-related toxicity. Blood Adv. 2021;5(14):2799–806.
20. Gutierrez C, Brown ART, May HP, et al. Critically ill patients treated for chimeric antigen receptor-related toxicity: a multicenter study. Crit Care Med. 2022;50(1):81–92.
21. Nastoupil LJ, Jain MD, Feng L, et al. Standard-of-care axicabtagene ciloleucel for relapsed or refractory large B-cell lymphoma: results from the US lymphoma CAR T consortium. J Clin Oncol. 2020;38(27):3119–28.
22. Hay KA, Hanafi LA, Li D, et al. Kinetics and biomarkers of severe cytokine release syndrome after CD19 chimeric antigen receptor-modified T-cell therapy. Blood. 2017;130(21):2295–306.
23. Teachey DT, Lacey SF, Shaw PA, et al. Identification of predictive biomarkers for cytokine release syndrome after chimeric antigen receptor T-cell therapy for acute lymphoblastic leukemia. Cancer Discov. 2016;6(6):664–79.

24. Steiner RE, Banchs J, Koutroumpakis E, et al. Cardiovascular events in patients treated with chimeric antigen receptor t-cell therapy for aggressive B-cell lymphoma. Haematologica. 2021;107:1555.
25. Wang J, Doran J. The many faces of cytokine release syndrome-related coagulopathy. Clin Hematol Int. 2021;3(1):3–12.
26. Grupp SA, Kalos M, Barrett D, et al. Chimeric antigen receptor-modified T cells for acute lymphoid leukemia. N Engl J Med. 2013;368(16):1509–18.
27. Oluwole OO, Bouabdallah K, Munoz J, et al. Prophylactic corticosteroid use in patients receiving axicabtagene ciloleucel for large B-cell lymphoma. Br J Haematol. 2021;194(4):690–700.
28. Giavridis T, van der Stegen SJC, Eyquem J, Hamieh M, Piersigilli A, Sadelain M. CAR T cell-induced cytokine release syndrome is mediated by macrophages and abated by IL-1 blockade. Nat Med. 2018;24(6):731–8.
29. Azoulay E, Castro P, Maamar A, et al. Outcomes in patients treated with chimeric antigen receptor T-cell therapy who were admitted to intensive care (CARTTAS): an international, multicentre, observational cohort study. Lancet Haematol. 2021;8(5):e355–64.
30. Strati P, Nastoupil LJ, Westin J, et al. Clinical and radiologic correlates of neurotoxicity after axicabtagene ciloleucel in large B-cell lymphoma. Blood Adv. 2020;4(16):3943–51.
31. Norelli M, Camisa B, Barbiera G, et al. Monocyte-derived IL-1 and IL-6 are differentially required for cytokine-release syndrome and neurotoxicity due to CAR T cells. Nat Med. 2018;24(6):739–48.
32. Gust J, Hay KA, Hanafi LA, et al. Endothelial activation and blood-brain barrier disruption in neurotoxicity after adoptive immunotherapy with CD19 CAR-T cells. Cancer Discov. 2017;7(12):1404–19.
33. Santomasso BD, Park JH, Salloum D, et al. Clinical and biological correlates of neurotoxicity associated with CAR T-cell therapy in patients with B-cell acute lymphoblastic leukemia. Cancer Discov. 2018;8(8):958–71.
34. Strati P, Ahmed S, Kebriaei P, et al. Clinical efficacy of anakinra to mitigate CAR T-cell therapy-associated toxicity in large B-cell lymphoma. Blood Adv. 2020;4(13):3123–7.
35. Hines MR, Keenan C, Maron Alfaro G, et al. Hemophagocytic lymphohistiocytosis-like toxicity (carHLH) after CD19-specific CAR T-cell therapy. Br J Haematol. 2021;194(4):701–7.
36. Lichtenstein DA, Schischlik F, Shao L, et al. Characterization of HLH-like manifestations as a CRS variant in patients receiving CD22 CAR T cells. Blood. 2021;138(24):2469–84.
37. Ahmed A, Merrill SA, Alsawah F, et al. Ruxolitinib in adult patients with secondary haemophagocytic lymphohistiocytosis: an open-label, single-centre, pilot trial. Lancet Haematol. 2019;6(12):e630–7.
38. Wudhikarn K, Palomba ML, Pennisi M, et al. Infection during the first year in patients treated with CD19 CAR T cells for diffuse large B cell lymphoma. Blood Cancer J. 2020;10(8):79.
39. Diorio C, Shaw PA, Pequignot E, et al. Diagnostic biomarkers to differentiate sepsis from cytokine release syndrome in critically ill children. Blood Adv. 2020;4(20):5174–83.
40. Hill JA, Li D, Hay KA, et al. Infectious complications of CD19-targeted chimeric antigen receptor-modified T-cell immunotherapy. Blood. 2018;131(1):121–30.
41. Vora SB, Waghmare A, Englund JA, Qu P, Gardner RA, Hill JA. Infectious complications following CD19 chimeric antigen receptor T-cell therapy for children, adolescents, and young adults. Open Forum Infect Dis. 2020;7(5):ofaa121.
42. Fried S, Avigdor A, Bielorai B, et al. Early and late hematologic toxicity following CD19 CAR-T cells. Bone Marrow Transplant. 2019;54(10):1643–50.
43. Rejeski K, Perez A, Sesques P, et al. CAR-HEMATOTOX: a model for CAR T-cell-related hematologic toxicity in relapsed/refractory large B-cell lymphoma. Blood. 2021;138(24):2499–513.
44. Logue JM, Zucchetti E, Bachmeier CA, et al. Immune reconstitution and associated infections following axicabtagene ciloleucel in relapsed or refractory large B-cell lymphoma. Haematologica. 2021;106(4):978–86.
45. Hill JA, Seo SK. How I prevent infections in patients receiving CD19-targeted chimeric antigen receptor T cells for B-cell malignancies. Blood. 2020;136(8):925–35.
46. Los-Arcos I, Iacoboni G, Aguilar-Guisado M, et al. Recommendations for screening, monitoring, prevention, and prophylaxis of infections in adult and pediatric patients receiving CAR T-cell therapy: a position paper. Infection. 2021;49(2):215–31.
47. Shah NN, Lee DW, Yates B, et al. Long-term follow-up of CD19-CAR T-cell therapy in children and young adults with B-ALL. J Clin Oncol. 2021;39(15):1650–9.
48. Park JH, Riviere I, Gonen M, et al. Long-term follow-up of CD19 CAR therapy in acute lymphoblastic leukemia. N Engl J Med. 2018;378(5):449–59.
49. Hay KA, Gauthier J, Hirayama AV, et al. Factors associated with durable EFS in adult B-cell ALL patients achieving MRD-negative CR after CD19 CAR T-cell therapy. Blood. 2019;133(15):1652–63.
50. Jain T, Bar M, Kansagra AJ, et al. Use of chimeric antigen receptor T cell therapy in clinical practice for relapsed/refractory aggressive B cell non-Hodgkin lymphoma: an expert panel opinion from the American Society for Transplantation and Cellular Therapy. Biol Blood Marrow Transplant. 2019;25(12):2305–21.

# 33 Critical Care Nursing of Haematopoietic Stem Cell Transplantation Patients

Stefano Botti and Matteo Seligardi

## Introduction

### Haematopoietic Stem Cell Transplantation

Haematopoietic stem cell transplantation (HSCT) is a standard therapy for malignant and non-malignant haematological diseases [1]. Patients undergoing allogeneic HSCT receive stem cells from related or unrelated donors, while those undergoing autologous HSCT receive their own stem cells [2]. Before stem cell infusion, recipients receive a conditioning regimen that includes combinations of chemotherapy, radiotherapy and/or immunotherapy with the aim of eradicating the underlying disease, creating space for cell engraftment and providing immunosuppression [3]. Following this conditioning regimen, patients risk developing insidious complications affecting body organs and tissues due to antineoplastic agent toxicity; these complications include gastrointestinal mucositis, sinusoidal obstruction syndrome, or other endothelial cell damage-related complications and renal insufficiency. After stem cell infusion, patients experience pancytopenia for 2 to 4 weeks, which puts them at a high risk of bacterial, viral and fungal infections as well as bleeding complications. After the cell engraftment, haematopoietic activity resumes. However, long-term immunosuppressive therapy to prevent and control graft-versus-host disease (GvHD) in allogeneic grafts is needed. GvHD is a transplant-related complication caused by the donor's lymphocyte-mediated immunological aggression of the recipient's tissues due to self-recognition failure [4]. It may lead to organ damage involving the skin, liver and bowel during the first 100 days post-transplant (acute-GvHD) and various other tissues, including mucous membranes, lungs, eyes, joints and genitalia after day +100 (chronic-GvHD). Several viral infections, such as cytomegalovirus (CMV), Epstein-Barr virus (EBV) and herpetic viruses [5], can affect the patients during the late post-transplant period due to immune recovery delay and the effects of the immunosuppressive therapy. In addition, a bidirectional relationship between the development of GvHD and CMV reactivation is posed [6]. In recent years, various factors, such as the improvements in antifungal prophylaxis and treatment, the introduction of the polymerase chain reaction (PCR) for CMV and Epstein-Barr virus (EBV) infection monitoring, the use of reduced-intensity or reduced-toxicity conditioning regimens and the introduction of alternative blood stem cell donors have made it possible to

S. Botti (✉)
Hematology Unit, Azienda USL-IRCCS di Reggio Emilia, Reggio Emilia, Italy
e-mail: stefano.botti@ausl.re.it

M. Seligardi
Intensive Care Unit, Azienda USL-IRCCS di Reggio Emilia, Reggio Emilia, Italy
e-mail: matteo.seligardi@ausl.re.it


A. O. Soubani (ed.), *Pulmonary and Critical Care Considerations of Hematopoietic Stem Cell Transplantation*, https://doi.org/10.1007/978-3-031-28797-8_33

extend the transplantation option to older recipients, to increase the number of transplants performed and to achieve better outcomes [7]. However, although HSCT yields improved long-term survival in patients with high-risk malignancies, it is still associated with high morbidity and mortality rates, and both patients and healthcare professionals (HCPs) consider it one of the most invasive and aggressive treatments provided in the haematology setting [5].

## ICU Admission of HSCT Patients

All the above conditioning- and /or transplant-related complications lead to severe or life-threatening conditions that require intensive care in 10–50% of cases [8]. While patients receiving autologous HSCT are no longer considered at a higher risk than the general ICU population, the ICU admission of allogeneic graft patients is still associated with higher mortality and morbidity rates [9, 10]. Pulmonary complications are the leading issue requiring intensive care (40–60% of ICU admissions) [11], followed by infectious complications such as sepsis or septic shock (30%) [12], neurological failure and renal insufficiency (15% each) [13, 14], while cardiac, hepatic and bleeding disorders and other conditions together cause less than 5% of ICU admissions [8]. Patients undergoing ICU life-sustaining therapies have high mortality rates: 21–72% of patients receive mechanical ventilation (MV), which is associated with 87% of deaths, increasing to 93% after 10 days. Renal replacement through haemodialysis (22–41%) and the use of vasopressors during sepsis (47–68%) are associated with 94% and 91% of deaths, respectively [8, 15, 16]. Multiple organ dysfunction (MOD) (especially when associated with MV), unresponsive GvHD, liver failure and renal insufficiency are other significant prognostic factors in both adult and paediatric patients [8, 17].

In addition to these aspects, it is essential to consider that the conditions of HSCT patients needing ICU and their organ dysfunctions are frequently determined by a combination of factors [5]. Furthermore, the mortality rate of patients admitted to ICU in the early post-transplant period appears to be similar to those admitted after HSCT unit discharge [16].

In the past, HCPs considered ICU admission of HSCT patients futile due to the high mortality rate [18, 19]. However, a progressive amelioration of outcomes in this setting has been observed over the last two decades, leading the scientific community to reflect on these themes [5]. This was primarily due to various factors, including the advances in transplant techniques detailed above, improvements in patient selection [20, 21], implementation of new ICU approaches such as early ICU management strategies and increased use of non-invasive ventilation [8]. Delays in ICU admission are due to various factors, including inadequate assessment and diagnostic issues, and are correlated both to a sudden evolution of the patient's clinical condition and to these patients' worse outcomes [22, 23]. The utility of ICU treatments for these patients could be perceived as uncertain because the mortality rate is high, especially in patients with impaired conditions and comorbidities. However, the improvements in transplantation and ICU techniques over the last few decades have demonstrated that these treatments are not futile [24]. The literature provides some decision-making protocols to transfer HSCT patients to the ICU [25–27], and some guideline recommendations on ICU admission of cancer patients are now available [28]. However, the proposed protocols were based on different strategies, and the available recommendations regard general cancer patients. This means that there is still no shared consensus among the scientific community concerning the strategies leading to HSCT patients' ICU admission [8].

## Collaboration Between Transplant and ICU HCPs

The latest edition of the FACT-JACIE International Standards [29] that assess the quality of haematopoietic cellular therapy processes requires that each transplant program have a readily accessible ICU or equivalent coverage for its patients, when needed. In addition, in order to facilitate clear communication between the transplant HCPs and intensivists, standard operating procedures (SOPs) on communication, patient monitoring, triage and decision-making for ICU transfer must be available. The ICUs collaborating with transplant programs are subject to inspection visit procedures, including SOP review, ICU HCP interviews and performance and quality parameter evaluations (e.g. how quickly the recipients are transferred to the ICU). A fundamental challenge for HSCT HCPs is the early involvement of other specialists in order to assess and manage the patients in a multidisciplinary manner [30]; various specialists, such as nephrologists, infectious disease specialists, pulmonologists, neurologists, psychologists, dietitians and nurse specialists, may together manage HSCT patients [31, 32], generally before intensive care HCPs are involved. This means that all the professionals involved should collaborate to assure the patient's safety by means of early recognition of organ dysfunction to avoid the patient's condition from worsening, resulting in unresponsive ICU conditions [10]. Timely and effective communication between the HCPs involved in the clinical pathway is fundamental, as is the planning of multiprofessional meetings to discuss and prioritize the treatment and care strategies [25, 33]. The collaboration between transplant and ICU nurses is essential [31, 32]; HSCT patient characteristics, such as immunosuppression, GvHD and specific conditioning-related toxicities, and the frequent need to begin intensive care techniques (e.g. non-invasive ventilation) before the patient's ICU transfer demand that these two areas of specialized nursing care share their respective knowledge and acquire new skills typical of each area.

The specificity of transplant-generated needs requires advanced skills to manage HSCT patients; these become fundamental during care transitions due to the patient's increased vulnerability [33]. Coordinated care and the development of adequate communication systems make it possible to clarify the objectives and improve both the continuity of care and the quality of the collaborative relationship [34]. The main topics for which shared ICU and HSCT nursing protocols should be adopted are as follows:

- Chemotherapy and immunotherapy administration
- Immunosuppressive medication administration
- Oral mucositis management
- Skin GvHD management
- Infection control and protective isolation management
- Non-invasive ventilation techniques
- Psychosocial support
- Patient and family education
- Palliative and end-of-life care

## Multidirectional Learning Process

Information-education and training processes have become fundamental: they make an adequate transition between the transplant ward and the ICU possible, they may limit patient and family anxiety, and they ensure patient safety. Information-educational processes involving the patients and their families should be put in place, and their outcomes should be assessed constantly. Training events for HSCT and ICU nurses should be planned regularly to maintain the acquired crossover skills. Scheduled meetings, journal clubs, lectures, educational programs and the shared implementation of research projects can support this.

ICU nurses do not receive training on the various care activities HSCT nurses typically provide to patients, for example, the use of strict protective isolation measures, the management and treatment of GvHD-related conditions and the administration of anticancer drugs. By the same token, HSCT nurses do not have enough skills regarding intensive care techniques, such as the management of non-invasive ventilation or the use of vasopressors. However, in real life, intensive care support of HSCT patients can begin before they are transferred to the ICU [35].

Other nursing activities may require collaborative decision-making to establish the goals and priorities of care. For example, oral hygiene practices for the prevention of ventilator-associated pneumonia (VAP) may not be adequate for the management of oral mucositis in HSCT patients undergoing orotracheal intubation.

Patients and their families must be adequately informed on the underlying malignant disease and its consequences, including treatment-related complications and care strategies. Information-education interventions should be carried out continuously during the HSCT patient's pathway [36].

## Nursing Management of HSCT Patients

Despite the continuous progress in the management of HSCT patients and the improvement in the standards of care, HSCT is a complex procedure with a high risk of mortality and morbidity. These patients' frailty and their immune impairments can result in various insidious clinical scenarios, which in turn determine the quantity and complexity of nursing care [37, 38]. Specific approaches to care, such as the application of dietary restrictions, isolation techniques and environmental hygiene practices [33], are thus fundamental to achieving good outcomes [39].

HSCT patients generally undergo strict monitoring protocols due to the consequences of both conditioning regimen and allograft. Nursing care during the various phases of the patient's pathway (pre-transplant risk assessment, conditioning regimen, transplant, early and late post-transplant periods) mainly focuses on infection prevention and control, conditioning and supportive therapy administration and management of toxic effects, adverse events and complications. In addition, nurses play a fundamental role in the information-educational process and in supporting patients with psychosocial issues [39].

A thorough pre-admission risk assessment and frequent monitoring during hospital stay are the basis for a proactive approach to patients' needs [40]. Early recognition of signs and symptoms through clinical observation, use of assessment tools and modulation of monitoring strategies according to a patient's risk and its evolution should be mandatory to intercept emerging complications and to ensure early access to ICU treatment [41]. HSCT patients should be transferred to the ICU promptly. However, depending on hospital policies, some ICU-supportive techniques, such as non-invasive ventilation (NIV), continuous vital signs monitoring, artery catheterization, tracheostomy and external drainage management, may be started while waiting for ICU transfer. This means that HSCT nurses must acquire and maintain the needed skills. HSCT nurses should be trained in the systematic use of tools evaluating patient's clinical evolution, such as early warning scores (Modified Early Warning Score—MEWS; Paediatric Early Warning Score—PEWS) [26]; the implementation of specific algorithms for ICU condition identification, such as the clinical criteria for sepsis and septic shock, based on the Sequential Organ Failure Assessment tool (SOFA) and its quick version [27]; and scoring systems with prognostic value, such as the European Blood and Marrow Transplantation (EBMT) severity grading of suspected sinusoidal obstruction syndrome (SOS) [42].

## Nursing Management of HSCT Patients in the ICU

The ICU requires skills to administer life-sustaining therapies to patients with deteriorating clinical conditions as well as to provide advanced support and monitoring using special equipment, such as telemetry, mechanical ventilator, arterial line transducer and pulmonary artery catheter, and aphaeretic procedures, including haemodialysis [33]. ICU admission is indicated for patients who have developed complications that can lead to organ failure [43].

Aside from the above-described issue of mortality, organ damage, its associated symptoms and the consequences of ICU-related cognitive (delirium, posttraumatic stress, depression) and physical (pain, immobility consequences) impairments may put the patient at a high risk of long-term disability [44]. Disability associated with ICU care and hospitalization is an unfortunately common occurrence, with significant consequences for patients and their caregivers [45].

Therefore, the presence of experienced intensive care professionals is essential, and the availability of facilities suitable for receiving transplant patients, with joint care provided by haematology and intensive care HCPs, and the development of SOPs for the management of the most frequent conditions (e.g. pulmonary insufficiency or hepato-renal impairment) are recommended [28]. A multi-professional team should guide HCPs with the aim of providing the right mix of evidence-based actions and personalized care, for example, by thinking about how to best reduce a patient's anxiety or discomfort during NIV management [46].

The ABCDEF bundle represents an evidence-based model to guide physicians and nurses to optimizing ICU patient recovery and outcomes. The ABCDEF bundle stands for *A*ssess, prevent and manage pain; *B*oth spontaneous awakening trials (SAT) and spontaneous breathing trials (SBT); *C*hoice of analgesia and sedation; *D*elirium assessment, prevention and management; *E*arly mobility and exercise; and *F*amily engagement and empowerment [47].

It may help HCPs adopt multidisciplinary approaches to care during a patient's ICU stay, thereby contributing to resource optimization and well-rounded patient care starting from the very beginning of the ICU pathway. The application of the bundle has been associated with reduced mortality and more ICU days without coma or delirium in a large "pre-post" cohort study [48]. The implementation and dissemination of the bundle and the best practices to conduct interprofessional team rounds are ongoing worldwide [49, 50].

This tool offers a new challenging paradigm to ICU nurses, providing them a modern vision of care management no longer based on a single (and frequently poorly linked) intervention or evaluation but on integrating nurses' experience, technical skills and competences in the use of assessment tools.

## The ABCDEF Bundle at the Bedside of the HSCT Patient: Implications for Nursing

### Assess, Prevent and Manage Pain

Pain is considered the major clinical symptom that requires a systematic approach to diagnosis and treatment in ICU patients [51]. It must be assessed regularly and as needed (e.g. prior to invasive procedures) using validated scoring systems; the tool used must be suitable to the patient's clinical condition. The Numerical Rating Scale (NRS) is considered the gold standard for pain self-reporting [52]. In patients with consciousness impairment, behavioural pain scales such as the Behavioral Pain Scale (BPS) and the Critical Care Pain Observation Tool (CPOT) may be used. Both scales provide guidance for pain treatment and the evaluation of its effectiveness [53, 54]. Opioids are the first-line therapy to control non-neuropathic pain in these patients [55]. Antiplatelet activity of analgesics such as non-steroidal anti-inflammatory drugs (NSAID) should be considered with caution prior to their use in HSCT patients; other drug-related adverse effects, such as opioid tolerance and the need for dose escalation over time, should be managed by nurses. Non-pharmacological interventions, such as mobilization and the use of heat or cold applications, could be useful to improve the patient's comfort [56].

### Both Spontaneous Awakening Trials (SAT) and Spontaneous Breathing Trials (SBT)

Practices such as daily SAT, minimization of sedative use and their titrating are associated with shorter duration of mechanical ventilation, shorter ICU stay and lower mortality [57]. Daily SBT associated with SAT seems to increase the time of spontaneous breathing, thereby reducing ventilator dependency as well as ICU and hospital stay [58]. ICU nurses are actively involved in these processes.

In addition, nurses are responsible for various activities that support patient's breathing and circulation. The evaluation of consciousness through the Glasgow Coma Scale (GCS) and the assessment of sedation status through the Richmond Agitation Sedation Scale (RASS) are recommended [55]. Nursing activities to check patients' natural and artificial airways, prevent $CO_2$ issues, manage tracheal aspiration and assure oral hygiene to prevent VAP contribute to airway patency. Respiratory dynamic monitoring, collection of respiratory parameters such as tissue oxygenation and blood gas tests, management of non-invasive and invasive ventilation methods, postural intervention and management of oxygen humidification are nursing actions that support patients' breathing. Nursing activities to support circulation include (1) assessment of circulation parameters, such as pulse and tissue/organ perfusion; (2) continuous monitoring of vital signs, including arterial pressure, mean arterial pressure, central venous pressure and electrocardiogram; (3) hemodynamic monitoring, including oxygen transport and cardiac output; (4) management of transduction circuits and vascular accesses; (5) management of vasoactive drug infusion, electrolyte and fluid balance, artificial nutrition and blood transfusions; (6) bleeding; (7) blood test sampling; and (8) other complex activities requiring advanced skills, such as continuous renal replacement treatment (CRRT), extracorporeal membrane oxygenation (ECMO) and intra-aortic balloon pump (IABP) monitoring.

## Choice of Analgesia and Sedation

As described above for pain management, the level of sedation, type of sedatives used, their dosage, blood concentration and subsequent discontinuation correlate with improved outcomes [59].

Nurses need to closely monitor patients' sedation level (RASS scale), train-of-four if on neuromuscular blocking agents, consciousness (GCS), cough reflex, pain, pupillary response and muscle strength and deficit. Compliance with endotracheal tube and nasogastric, vesical and faecal drainage catheters should be assured.

## Delirium Assessment, Prevention and Management

Severely ill patients admitted to the ICU are at a high risk of developing delirium, which correlates with poor outcomes such as longer hospital stay and increased morbidity and mortality [60, 61]. Delirium is frequently underrecognized by hospitals, and evidence on delirium prevention and treatment are poor and conflicting [62]. The few strategies suggested in the guidelines consist in preventing sleep disruption and the use of early and progressive mobilization [55]. However, routine delirium screening by the nursing staff is feasible using validated scales such as the Confusion Assessment Method for the Intensive Care Unit (CAM-ICU) and the Intensive Care Delirium Screening Checklist (ICDSC).

## Early Mobility and Exercise

Muscle weakness and weight loss due to immobility begin from the very first days in the ICU, resulting in short- and long-term disabilities and affecting primary outcomes [63, 64]. Nurses can assess muscle weakness using tools such as the Medical Research Council Scale for Muscle Strength [65]. Implementing a rehabilitation program for all ICU patients from their first days in the ICU appears to be safe and effective in minimizing disabilities due to prolonged immobility [66]. To optimize its positive effects on functional status and to define the best rehabilitation strategy during the ICU stay and after discharge, nurses, physiotherapists, and family caregivers must collaborate effectively [67]. During the patient's ICU stay, the nurses' role is fundamental to preventing postural lesions and pressure ulcers. Furthermore, nurses should receive wound care skills and training to be able to provide appropriate treatment of surgical wounds, drainage and vascular access insertion sites. The implementation of collaborative protocols to manage patients with extensive skin GvHD is mandatory, as is the involvement of specialists such as dermatologists and wound care nurses.

## Family Engagement and Empowerment

Decision-making regarding the most effective treatment plan may be very complex for clinicians responsible for HSCT patients in the ICU. Involving the patient (when feasible), family members or other authorized relatives is fundamental to reduce any misunderstanding concerning the patient's preferences and expectations and any family anxiety and conflicts as well as to provide clinicians with correct input [68]. Nurses are involved in the patient and family education process; they ensure safe ICU access to family members, recognize information gaps, manage relationship issues and assess the need for psychological support or cultural mediation.

**Acknowledgments** Many thanks to Jacqueline M. Costa for the English language editing.

## References


1. Balassa K, Danby R, Rocha V. Haematopoietic stem cell transplants: principles and indications. Br J Hosp Med (Lond). 2019;80(1):33–9. https://doi.org/10.12968/hmed.2019.80.1.33.
2. Copelan EA. Hematopoietic stem-cell transplantation. N Engl J Med. 2006;354(17):1813–26. https://doi.org/10.1056/NEJMra052638.
3. Zulu S, Kenyon M. Principles of conditioning therapy and cell infusion. In: Kenyon M, Babic A, editors. The European blood and marrow transplantation textbook for nurses: under the auspices of EBMT. Cham: Springer; 2017. p. 2018. Chapter 6.
4. Ferrara JL, Levine JE, Reddy P, Holler E. Graft-versus-host disease. Lancet. 2009;373(9674):1550–61. https://doi.org/10.1016/S0140-6736(09)60237-3.
5. Stecher SS, Stemmler HJ, Tischer J, von Bergwelt-Baildon M, Liebregts T, Fraccaroli A. Der knochenmarktransplantierte Patient auf der Intensivstation [Bone marrow transplantation patients in the intensive care unit]. Med Klin Intensivmed Notfmed. 2021;116(2):111–20. https://doi.org/10.1007/s00063-021-00782-8; German.
6. Cantoni N, Hirsch HH, Khanna N, Gerull S, Buser A, Bucher C, Halter J, Heim D, Tichelli A, Gratwohl A, Stern M. Evidence for a bidirectional relationship between cytomegalovirus replication and acute graft-versus-host disease. Biol Blood Marrow Transplant. 2010;16(9):1309–14. https://doi.org/10.1016/j.bbmt.2010.03.020.
7. Fraccaroli A, Prevalsek D, Fritsch S, Haebe S, Bücklein V, Schulz C, Hubmann M, Stemmler HJ, Ledderose G, Hausmann A, Schmid C, Tischer J. Sequential HLA-haploidentical transplantation utilizing post-transplantation cyclophosphamide for GvHD prophylaxis in high-risk and relapsed/refractory AML/MDS. Am J Hematol. 2018;93(12):1524–31. https://doi.org/10.1002/ajh.25281.
8. Saillard C, Blaise D, Mokart D. Critically ill allogeneic hematopoietic stem cell transplantation patients in the intensive care unit: reappraisal of actual prognosis. Bone Marrow Transplant. 2016;51(8):1050–61. https://doi.org/10.1038/bmt.2016.72.
9. Schellongowski P, Staudinger T, Kundi M, Laczika K, Locker GJ, Bojic A, Robak O, Fuhrmann V, Jäger U, Valent P, Sperr WR. Prognostic factors for intensive care unit admission, intensive care outcome, and post-intensive care survival in patients with de novo acute myeloid leukemia: a single center experience. Haematologica. 2011;96(2):231–7. https://doi.org/10.3324/haematol.2010.031583.
10. Azoulay E, Pène F, Darmon M, Lengliné E, Benoit D, Soares M, Vincent F, Bruneel F, Perez P, Lemiale V, Mokart D, Groupe de Recherche Respiratoire en Réanimation Onco-Hématologique (Grrr-OH). Managing critically ill hematology patients: time to think differently. Blood Rev. 2015;29(6):359–67. https://doi.org/10.1016/j.blre.2015.04.002.
11. Soubani AO, Kseibi E, Bander JJ, Klein JL, Khanchandani G, Ahmed HP, Guzman JA. Outcome and prognostic factors of hematopoietic stem cell transplantation recipients admitted to a medical ICU. Chest. 2004;126(5):1604–11. https://doi.org/10.1378/chest.126.5.1604.
12. Mayer S, Pastores SM, Riedel E, Maloy M, Jakubowski AA. Short- and long-term outcomes of adult allogeneic hematopoietic stem cell transplant patients admitted to the intensive care unit in the peritransplant period. Leuk Lymphoma. 2017;58(2):382–90. https://doi.org/10.1080/10428194.2016.1195499.
13. Escobar K, Rojas P, Ernst D, Bertin P, Nervi B, Jara V, Garcia MJ, Ocqueteau M, Sarmiento M, Ramirez P. Admission of hematopoietic cell transplantation patients to the intensive care unit at the Pontificia Universidad Católica de Chile hospital. Biol Blood Marrow Transplant. 2015;21(1):176–9. https://doi.org/10.1016/j.bbmt.2014.08.009.
14. Pène F, Aubron C, Azoulay E, Blot F, Thiéry G, Raynard B, Schlemmer B, Nitenberg G, Buzyn A, Arnaud P, Socié G, Mira JP. Outcome of critically ill allogeneic hematopoietic stem-cell transplantation recipients: a reappraisal of indications for organ failure supports. J Clin Oncol. 2006;24(4):643–9. https://doi.org/10.1200/JCO.2005.03.9073.

15. Boyacı N, Aygencel G, Turkoglu M, Yegin ZA, Acar K, Sucak GT. The intensive care management process in patients with hematopoietic stem cell transplantation and factors affecting their prognosis. Hematology. 2014;19(6):338–45. https://doi.org/10.1179/1607845413Y.0000000130.
16. Scales DC, Thiruchelvam D, Kiss A, Sibbald WJ, Redelmeier DA. Intensive care outcomes in bone marrow transplant recipients: a population-based cohort analysis. Crit Care. 2008;12(3):R77. https://doi.org/10.1186/cc6923.
17. An K, Wang Y, Li B, Luo C, Wang J, Luo C, Chen J. Prognostic factors and outcome of patients undergoing hematopoietic stem cell transplantation who are admitted to pediatric intensive care unit. BMC Pediatr. 2016;16(1):138. https://doi.org/10.1186/s12887-016-0669-8.
18. Azoulay E, Afessa B. The intensive care support of patients with malignancy: do everything that can be done. Intensive Care Med. 2006;32(1):3–5. https://doi.org/10.1007/s00134-005-2835-6.
19. Soares M, Salluh JI, Azoulay E. Noninvasive ventilation in patients with malignancies and hypoxemic acute respiratory failure: a still pending question. J Crit Care. 2010;25(1):37–8. https://doi.org/10.1016/j.jcrc.2009.04.001.
20. Sorror ML, Maris MB, Storb R, Baron F, Sandmaier BM, Maloney DG, Storer B. Hematopoietic cell transplantation (HCT)-specific comorbidity index: a new tool for risk assessment before allogeneic HCT. Blood. 2005;106(8):2912–9. https://doi.org/10.1182/blood-2005-05-2004.
21. Passweg JR, Baldomero H, Peters C, Gaspar HB, Cesaro S, Dreger P, Duarte RF, Falkenburg JH, Farge-Bancel D, Gennery A, Halter J, Kröger N, Lanza F, Marsh J, Mohty M, Sureda A, Velardi A, Madrigal A, European Society for Blood and Marrow Transplantation EBMT. Hematopoietic SCT in Europe: data and trends in 2012 with special consideration of pediatric transplantation. Bone Marrow Transplant. 2014;49(6):744–50. https://doi.org/10.1038/bmt.2014.55.
22. Azoulay E, Mokart D, Pène F, Lambert J, Kouatchet A, Mayaux J, Vincent F, Nyunga M, Bruneel F, Laisne LM, Rabbat A, Lebert C, Perez P, Chaize M, Renault A, Meert AP, Benoit D, Hamidfar R, Jourdain M, Darmon M, Schlemmer B, Chevret S, Lemiale V. Outcomes of critically ill patients with hematologic malignancies: prospective multicenter data from France and Belgium--a groupe de recherche respiratoire en réanimation onco-hématologique study. J Clin Oncol. 2013;31(22):2810–8. https://doi.org/10.1200/JCO.2012.47.2365.
23. Song JU, Suh GY, Park HY, Lim SY, Han SG, Kang YR, Kwon OJ, Woo S, Jeon K. Early intervention on the outcomes in critically ill cancer patients admitted to intensive care units. Intensive Care Med. 2012;38(9):1505–13. https://doi.org/10.1007/s00134-012-2594-0.
24. Lengline E, Darmon M, Azoulay E, Le Gall JR. Réanimation des patients d'onco-hématologie: nouvelles thérapeutiques, nouvelles complications, nouveaux contrats d'admission [Critical care of Onco-hematology patients: new therapeutic targets, new complications and new admission policies]. Bull Acad Natl Med. 2015;199(2–3):293–312; French.
25. Jenkins P, Johnston LJ, Pickham D, Chang B, Rizk N, Tierney DK. Intensive care utilization for hematopoietic cell transplant recipients. Biol Blood Marrow Transplant. 2015;21(11):2023–7. https://doi.org/10.1016/j.bbmt.2015.07.026.
26. Constantinescu C, Bodolea C, Pasca S, Teodorescu P, Dima D, Rus I, Tat T, Achimas-Cadariu P, Tanase A, Tomuleasa C, Einsele H. Clinical approach to the patient in critical state following immunotherapy and/or stem cell transplantation: guideline for the on-call physician. J Clin Med. 2019;8(6):884. https://doi.org/10.3390/jcm8060884.
27. Singer M, Deutschman CS, Seymour CW, Shankar-Hari M, Annane D, Bauer M, Bellomo R, Bernard GR, Chiche JD, Coopersmith CM, Hotchkiss RS, Levy MM, Marshall JC, Martin GS, Opal SM, Rubenfeld GD, van der Poll T, Vincent JL, Angus DC. The third international consensus definitions for sepsis and septic shock (Sepsis-3). JAMA. 2016;315(8):801–10. https://doi.org/10.1001/jama.2016.0287.
28. Kiehl MG, Beutel G, Böll B, Buchheidt D, Forkert R, Fuhrmann V, Knöbl P, Kochanek M, Kroschinsky F, La Rosée P, Liebregts T, Lück C, Olgemoeller U, Schalk E, Shimabukuro-Vornhagen A, Sperr WR, Staudinger T, von Bergwelt BM, Wohlfarth P, Zeremski V, Schellongowski P, Consensus of the German Society of Hematology and Medical Oncology (DGHO), Austrian Society of Hematology and Oncology (OeGHO), German Society for Medical Intensive Care Medicine and Emergency Medicine (DGIIN), and Austrian Society of Medical and General Intensive Care and Emergency Medicine (ÖGIAIN). Consensus statement for cancer patients requiring intensive care support. Ann Hematol. 2018;97(7):1271–82. https://doi.org/10.1007/s00277-018-3312-y.
29. FACT-JACIE International Standards for Hematopoietic Cellular Therapy Product Collection, Processing, and Administration. 8th ed. Version 8.1. 2021. https://www.ebmt.org/8th-edition-fact-jacie-standards. Accessed 27 Feb 2022.
30. Naeem N, Reed MD, Creger RJ, Youngner SJ, Lazarus HM. Transfer of the hematopoietic stem cell transplant patient to the intensive care unit: does it really matter? Bone Marrow Transplant. 2006;37(2):119–33. https://doi.org/10.1038/sj.bmt.1705222.
31. Rios M, Suzuki V, Magnum M, Caravia A, Roy J, Zanville N. Implementation of daily multidisciplinary rounds on an adult inpatient blood & marrow transplant unit: initial observations and future plans. Biol Blood Marrow Transplant. 2020;26(3, Supplement):S379–80. https://doi.org/10.1016/j.bbmt.2019.12.169.

32. Nakagaki M, Gavin NC, Hayes T, Fichera R, Stewart C, Naumann L, Brennan J, Perry N, Foley E, Crofton E, Brown C, Leutenegger J, Kennedy GA. Implementation and evaluation of a nurse-allied health clinic for patients after haematopoietic stem cell transplantation. Support Care Cancer. 2022;30(1):647–57. https://doi.org/10.1007/s00520-021-06461-w.
33. Young LK, Mansfield B, Mandoza J. Nursing care of adult hematopoietic stem cell transplant patients and families in the intensive care unit: an evidence-based review. Crit Care Nurs Clin North Am. 2017;29(3):341–52. https://doi.org/10.1016/j.cnc.2017.04.009.
34. Thomson B, Gorospe G, Cooke L, Giesie P, Johnson S. Transitions of care: a hematopoietic stem cell transplantation nursing education project across the trajectory. Clin J Oncol Nurs. 2015;19(4):E74–9. https://doi.org/10.1188/15.CJON.E74-E79.
35. Wermke M, Schiemanck S, Höffken G, Ehninger G, Bornhäuser M, Illmer T. Respiratory failure in patients undergoing allogeneic hematopoietic SCT--a randomized trial on early non-invasive ventilation based on standard care hematology wards. Bone Marrow Transplant. 2012;47(4):574–80. https://doi.org/10.1038/bmt.2011.160.
36. Cheron N, Riou M, Babouche I, Chevallier N, Aimee Dann MP, Delorme J, Denis V, Girard I, Godin S, Tardieu L, Yakoub-Agha I. Programme d'éducation thérapeutique du patient (ETP) faisant l'objet d'une allogreffe de cellules souches hématopoïétiques : recommandations de la Société francophone de greffe de moelle et de thérapie cellulaire (SFGM-TC) [Therapeutic education programs for the patient (ETP) undergoing an allogeneic hematopoietic cell transplantation: guidelines from the francophone Society of Bone Marrow Transplantation and Cellular Therapy (SFGM-TC)]. Bull Cancer. 2021;108(12S):S26–9. https://doi.org/10.1016/j.bulcan.2021.09.006; French.
37. Daniels P, Pate A, Flesch L, Teusink-Cross A, Matani H, Geiger A, Hayward M, Myers W, Schaefer S, Nelson A, Jodele S, Davies SM, Dandoy CE. Improving time to antibiotic administration for bone marrow transplant patients with first fever. Pediatrics. 2018;141(1):e20171549. https://doi.org/10.1542/peds.2017-1549.
38. Rodriguez JAP, Lacerda MR, Gomes IM, Paes MR, Ribeiro RP, Bonfim CMS. Clinical profile of children undergoing hematopoietic stem cell transplantation. Cogitare Enferm. 2019;24:e55967. https://doi.org/10.5380/ce.v24i0.55967.
39. Rodrigues JAP, Lacerda MR, Galvão CM, Gomes IM, Meier MJ, Caceres NTG. Nursing care for patients in post-transplantation of hematopoietic stem cells: an integrative review. Rev Bras Enferm. 2021;74(3):e20200097. https://doi.org/10.1590/0034-7167-2020-0097; English, Portuguese.
40. Blackburn G, Rasmussen B, Wynter K, Holton S. Proactive rounding: perspectives and experiences of nurses and midwives working in a large metropolitan hospital. Aust Crit Care. 2021;S1036-7314(21):00142–9. https://doi.org/10.1016/j.aucc.2021.09.006.
41. Botti S, Agreiter I, Orlando L, Gargiulo G, Bonifazi F, Banfi MM, Cappucciati L, Caffarri C, De Cecco V, Deiana GM, Gavezzotti M, Magarò A, Netti MG, Pignatelli AC, Rostagno E, Samarani E, Cardoso JS, Soave S, Valente CM, Vedovetto A, Zecca M, Luminari S, Merli F, Guberti M. Nursing role in the assessment and care of hepatic sinusoidal obstruction syndrome patients: a consensus paper by the "Gruppo Italiano Trapianto di Midollo Osseo". Support Care Cancer. 2020;28(11):5125–37. https://doi.org/10.1007/s00520-020-05353-9.
42. Mohty M, Malard F, Abecassis M, Aerts E, Alaskar AS, Aljurf M, Arat M, Bader P, Baron F, Bazarbachi A, Blaise D, Ciceri F, Corbacioglu S, Dalle JH, Dignan F, Fukuda T, Huynh A, Masszi T, Michallet M, Nagler A, NiChonghaile M, Okamoto S, Pagliuca A, Peters C, Petersen FB, Richardson PG, Ruutu T, Savani BN, Wallhult E, Yakoub-Agha I, Duarte RF, Carreras E. Revised diagnosis and severity criteria for sinusoidal obstruction syndrome/veno-occlusive disease in adult patients: a new classification from the European Society for Blood and Marrow Transplantation. Bone Marrow Transplant. 2016;51(7):906–12. https://doi.org/10.1038/bmt.2016.130.
43. Agarwal S, O'Donoghue S, Gowardman J, Kennedy G, Bandeshe H, Boots R. Intensive care unit experience of haemopoietic stem cell transplant patients. Intern Med J. 2012;42(7):748–54. https://doi.org/10.1111/j.1445-5994.2011.02533.x.
44. Pandharipande PP, Girard TD, Jackson JC, Morandi A, Thompson JL, Pun BT, Brummel NE, Hughes CG, Vasilevskis EE, Shintani AK, Moons KG, Geevarghese SK, Canonico A, Hopkins RO, Bernard GR, Dittus RS, Ely EW, BRAIN-ICU Study Investigators. Long-term cognitive impairment after critical illness. N Engl J Med. 2013;369(14):1306–16. https://doi.org/10.1056/NEJMoa1301372.
45. Covinsky KE, Pierluissi E, Johnston CB. Hospitalization-associated disability: "she was probably able to ambulate, but I'm not sure". JAMA. 2011;306(16):1782–93. https://doi.org/10.1001/jama.2011.1556.
46. Russo M, Bonanno C, Profazio C, La Foresta S, Faraone C, Lizio A, Vita GL, Sframeli M, Aricò I, Ruggeri P, Toscano A, Vita G, Lunetta C, Messina S. Which are the factors influencing NIV adaptation and tolerance in ALS patients? Neurol Sci. 2021;42(3):1023–9. https://doi.org/10.1007/s10072-020-04624-x.
47. Marra A, Ely EW, Pandharipande PP, Patel MB. The ABCDEF bundle in critical care. Crit Care Clin. 2017;33(2):225–43. https://doi.org/10.1016/j.ccc.2016.12.005.
48. Barnes-Daly MA, Phillips G, Ely EW. Improving hospital survival and reducing brain dysfunction at seven California community hospitals: implementing PAD guidelines via the ABCDEF bundle in 6,064

patients. Crit Care Med. 2017;45(2):171–8. https://doi.org/10.1097/CCM.0000000000002149.
49. Stollings JL, Devlin JW, Lin JC, Pun BT, Byrum D, Barr J. Best practices for conducting interprofessional team rounds to facilitate performance of the ICU liberation (ABCDEF) bundle. Crit Care Med. 2020;48(4):562–70. https://doi.org/10.1097/CCM.0000000000004197.
50. Balas MC, Pun BT, Pasero C, Engel HJ, Perme C, Esbrook CL, Kelly T, Hargett KD, Posa PJ, Barr J, Devlin JW, Morse A, Barnes-Daly MA, Puntillo KA, Aldrich JM, Schweickert WD, Harmon L, Byrum DG, Carson SS, Ely EW, Stollings JL. Common challenges to effective ABCDEF bundle implementation: the ICU liberation campaign experience. Crit Care Nurse. 2019;39(1):46–60. https://doi.org/10.4037/ccn2019927.
51. Chanques G, Viel E, Constantin JM, Jung B, de Lattre S, Carr J, Cissé M, Lefrant JY, Jaber S. The measurement of pain in intensive care unit: comparison of 5 self-report intensity scales. Pain. 2010;151(3):711–21. https://doi.org/10.1016/j.pain.2010.08.039.
52. Barr J, Fraser GL, Puntillo K, Ely EW, Gélinas C, Dasta JF, Davidson JE, Devlin JW, Kress JP, Joffe AM, Coursin DB, Herr DL, Tung A, Robinson BR, Fontaine DK, Ramsay MA, Riker RR, Sessler CN, Pun B, Skrobik Y, Jaeschke R, American College of Critical Care Medicine. Clinical practice guidelines for the management of pain, agitation, and delirium in adult patients in the intensive care unit. Crit Care Med. 2013;41(1):263–306. https://doi.org/10.1097/CCM.0b013e3182783b72.
53. Chanques G, Jaber S, Barbotte E, Violet S, Sebbane M, Perrigault PF, Mann C, Lefrant JY, Eledjam JJ. Impact of systematic evaluation of pain and agitation in an intensive care unit. Crit Care Med. 2006;34(6):1691–9. https://doi.org/10.1097/01.CCM.0000218416.62457.56.
54. Payen JF, Bosson JL, Chanques G, Mantz J, Labarere J, DOLOREA Investigators. Pain assessment is associated with decreased duration of mechanical ventilation in the intensive care unit: a post hoc analysis of the DOLOREA study. Anesthesiology. 2009;111(6):1308–16. https://doi.org/10.1097/ALN.0b013e3181c0d4f0.
55. Devlin JW, Skrobik Y, Gélinas C, Needham DM, Slooter AJC, Pandharipande PP, Watson PL, Weinhouse GL, Nunnally ME, Rochwerg B, Balas MC, van den Boogaard M, Bosma KJ, Brummel NE, Chanques G, Denehy L, Drouot X, Fraser GL, Harris JE, Joffe AM, Kho ME, Kress JP, Lanphere JA, McKinley S, Neufeld KJ, Pisani MA, Payen JF, Pun BT, Puntillo KA, Riker RR, Robinson BRH, Shehabi Y, Szumita PM, Winkelman C, Centofanti JE, Price C, Nikayin S, Misak CJ, Flood PD, Kiedrowski K, Alhazzani W. Clinical practice guidelines for the prevention and management of pain, agitation/sedation, delirium, immobility, and sleep disruption in adult patients in the ICU. Crit Care Med. 2018;46(9):e825–73. https://doi.org/10.1097/CCM.0000000000003299.
56. Erstad BL, Puntillo K, Gilbert HC, Grap MJ, Li D, Medina J, Mularski RA, Pasero C, Varkey B, Sessler CN. Pain management principles in the critically ill. Chest. 2009;135(4):1075–86. https://doi.org/10.1378/chest.08-2264.
57. Kress JP, Pohlman AS, O'Connor MF, Hall JB. Daily interruption of sedative infusions in critically ill patients undergoing mechanical ventilation. N Engl J Med. 2000;342(20):1471–7. https://doi.org/10.1056/NEJM200005183422002.
58. Girard TD, Kress JP, Fuchs BD, Thomason JW, Schweickert WD, Pun BT, Taichman DB, Dunn JG, Pohlman AS, Kinniry PA, Jackson JC, Canonico AE, Light RW, Shintani AK, Thompson JL, Gordon SM, Hall JB, Dittus RS, Bernard GR, Ely EW. Efficacy and safety of a paired sedation and ventilator weaning protocol for mechanically ventilated patients in intensive care (awakening and breathing controlled trial): a randomised controlled trial. Lancet. 2008;371(9607):126–34. https://doi.org/10.1016/S0140-6736(08)60105-1.
59. Ely EW, Truman B, Shintani A, Thomason JW, Wheeler AP, Gordon S, Francis J, Speroff T, Gautam S, Margolin R, Sessler CN, Dittus RS, Bernard GR. Monitoring sedation status over time in ICU patients: reliability and validity of the Richmond agitation-sedation scale (RASS). JAMA. 2003;289(22):2983–91. https://doi.org/10.1001/jama.289.22.2983.
60. Marcantonio ER. Delirium in hospitalized older adults. N Engl J Med. 2017;377(15):1456–66. https://doi.org/10.1056/NEJMcp1605501.
61. Schubert M, Schürch R, Boettger S, Garcia Nuñez D, Schwarz U, Bettex D, Jenewein J, Bogdanovic J, Staehli ML, Spirig R, Rudiger A. A hospital-wide evaluation of delirium prevalence and outcomes in acute care patients—a cohort study. BMC Health Serv Res. 2018;18(1):550. https://doi.org/10.1186/s12913-018-3345-x.
62. Winsnes K, Sochacki P, Eriksson C, Shereck E, Recht M, Johnson K, Loret De Mola R, Stork L. Delirium in the pediatric hematology, oncology, and bone marrow transplant population. Pediatr Blood Cancer. 2019;66(6):e27640. https://doi.org/10.1002/pbc.27640.
63. Sacanella E, Pérez-Castejón JM, Nicolás JM, Masanés F, Navarro M, Castro P, López-Soto A. Functional status and quality of life 12 months after discharge from a medical ICU in healthy elderly patients: a prospective observational study. Crit Care. 2011;15(2):R105. https://doi.org/10.1186/cc10121.
64. Herridge MS, Tansey CM, Matté A, Tomlinson G, Diaz-Granados N, Cooper A, Guest CB, Mazer CD, Mehta S, Stewart TE, Kudlow P, Cook D, Slutsky AS, Cheung AM, Canadian Critical Care Trials Group.

Functional disability 5 years after acute respiratory distress syndrome. N Engl J Med. 2011;364(14):1293–304. https://doi.org/10.1056/NEJMoa1011802.
65. Kleyweg RP, van der Meché FG, Schmitz PI. Interobserver agreement in the assessment of muscle strength and functional abilities in Guillain-Barré syndrome. Muscle Nerve. 1991;14(11):1103–9. https://doi.org/10.1002/mus.880141111.
66. Freeman R, Maley K. Mobilization of intensive care cardiac surgery patients on mechanical circulatory support. Crit Care Nurs Q. 2013;36(1):73–88. https://doi.org/10.1097/CNQ.0b013e31827532c3.
67. Dammeyer J, Dickinson S, Packard D, Baldwin N, Ricklemann C. Building a protocol to guide mobility in the ICU. Crit Care Nurs Q. 2013;36(1):37–49. https://doi.org/10.1097/CNQ.0b013e3182750acd.
68. Davidson JE, Powers K, Hedayat KM, Tieszen M, Kon AA, Shepard E, Spuhler V, Todres ID, Levy M, Barr J, Ghandi R, Hirsch G, Armstrong D, American College of Critical Care Medicine Task Force 2004-2005, Society of Critical Care Medicine. Clinical practice guidelines for support of the family in the patient-centered intensive care unit: American College of Critical Care Medicine Task Force 2004-2005. Crit Care Med. 2007;35(2):605–22. https://doi.org/10.1097/01.CCM.0000254067.14607.EB.

# 34 Nutritional Considerations of Critically Ill Hematopoietic Cell Transplantation Patients

Shigeo Fuji and Jessica Cheng

## Introduction

Patients after allogeneic hematopoietic cell transplantation (HCT) are at risk for severe complications requiring intensive care and prolonged nutritional support [1]. In such a situation, there is no doubt that patients require sophisticated nutritional support provided by a multidisciplinary nutritional support team to maintain their nutritional status [2]. Although there is no established specific nutritional support for allogeneic HCT recipients in the intensive care unit (ICU), we would like to summarize the relevant information on nutritional support for critically ill patients after allogeneic HCT.

S. Fuji (✉)
Department of Hematology, Osaka International Cancer Institute, Osaka, Japan

Nutrition Support WG, Asia-Pacific Blood and Marrow Transplantation Group, Chiang Mai, Thailand

J. Cheng (✉)
Nutrition Support WG, Asia-Pacific Blood and Marrow Transplantation Group, Chiang Mai, Thailand

Bone Marrow Transplant and Haematology, St Vincent's Public Hospital Sydney, Sydney, Australia
e-mail: Jessica.Cheng@svha.org.au

## Nutritional Issues in Allogeneic HCT Recipients in General

Allogeneic HCT recipients are at a high risk for malnutrition [3]. Notably, during the early period after allogeneic HCT, patients suffer from gastrointestinal complications such as mucositis and diarrhea. Therefore, patients require sophisticated nutritional support [4]. Enteral nutrition is a preferred route of nutritional support, but in patients with severe gastrointestinal complications, enteral nutrition (EN) could be difficult to achieve the target caloric intake [5]. In that case, parenteral nutrition (PN) is used as a route of nutritional support. The superiority of EN over PN has not yet been confirmed by a randomized controlled trial in this field [6, 7]. Patients after allogeneic HCT receive multiple drugs that are associated with hyperglycemia such as calcineurin inhibitors and corticosteroids. PN is also a risk factor for hyperglycemia. Thus, in patients who receive PN as nutritional support, it is mandatory to monitor the glucose level after allogeneic HCT. Additionally, further studies are needed to optimize nutritional support in the field of allogeneic HCT [8].



A. O. Soubani (ed.), *Pulmonary and Critical Care Considerations of Hematopoietic Stem Cell Transplantation*, https://doi.org/10.1007/978-3-031-28797-8_34

## Nutritional Support in Critically Ill HSCT Recipients

Critically ill patients after allogeneic HCT are almost always at a high risk for malnutrition [9]. Thus, it is reasonable to apply nutritional support for all patients in the ICU after allogeneic HCT (Table 34.1).

## Assessment of Nutritional Status

There is no established tool to assess the nutritional status in critically ill patients after allogeneic HCT. The clinical staff have to be careful in using laboratory tools to evaluate the nutritional status in critically ill patients, as the presence of inflammation could lead to the dynamic change in parameters such as albumin and pre-albumin levels: albumin and pre-albumin levels could be low values being a response to the inflammatory status [2]. In terms of the scores to assess the nutritional status, commonly used tools such as the subjective global assessment (SGA), mini-nutrition assessment (NMA), malnutrition screening tool (MST), or nutritional risk screening (NRS) 2002 could be used in critically ill patients, but there is no gold standard score to define patients at risk for malnutrition [9]. In general, all critically ill patients after allogeneic HCT are treated as being at a high risk for malnutrition.

**Table 34.1** Summary of nutritional support

| | |
|---|---|
| Estimation of caloric needs | Simplistic formulae (25–30 kcal/kg/day) can be used to estimate the caloric needs. Other formulas such as Harris Benedict formula or BASA-ROT table are also appropriate<br>In patients at a high risk for refeeding syndrome, caloric intake has to be gradually increased |
| Estimation of protein needs | Generally, 1.5–2.0 g/kg/day is recommended |
| Route of nutritional support | Oral intake>enteral nutrition>parenteral nutrition |
| Micronutrients | Vitamin and trace elements are generally recommended |
| Glucose control | Glucose level should be routinely monitored |

## Target Caloric Intake

Before administering nutrition in critically ill patients, it is crucial to assess the risk of refeeding syndrome (RFS), as patients in the ICU are at a high risk for RFS [10–12]. In the presence of severe underweight or weight loss and a prolonged fasting period before admission to ICU, the risk of RFS is particularly high [11]. In patients at a high risk for RFS, it is recommended to set initial target caloric intake at a low level such as 10 kcal/kg/day in high-risk cases or even lower such as 5 kcal/kg/day in extremely high-risk cases. Electrolytes including potassium, phosphate, and magnesium have to be closely monitored, and the target caloric intake could be slowly increased to meet the usual caloric intake in patients at a high risk for RFS. Clinicians also have to be aware of the risk of deficiency of nutrients such as thiamin or other vitamins. Thiamine deficiency is associated with the development of Wernicke's encephalopathy/Korsakoff psychosis. When patients are at a high risk for thiamine deficiency, thiamine supplementation should be considered.

When the risk of RFS is revealed to be low at admission or becomes low after the admission, the standard target caloric intake should be administered. It is recommended to gradually increase the administered dose of calorie in critically ill patients. The target caloric intake could be determined using simplistic formulae (25–30 kcal/kg/day), some predictive equations, or indirect calorimetry when available, although predictive equations were reported to be associated with significant inaccuracy [13]. Recent guidelines emphasized the importance of protein intake as several retrospective studies revealed that low protein intake was associated with higher ICU and in-hospital mortality [13]. The recommended protein intake is in general 1.5–2.0 g/kg/day [13].

## Route of Nutritional Support

Oral diet is the best route of nutritional support, when possible, even in critically ill patients. Although critically ill patients are not able to eat often, it is recommended to assess whether the patients tolerate oral diet or not. As the EFFORT trial demonstrated in medical inpatients, supplemental nutritional support using an oral supplement is highly beneficial [14]. In non-intubated patients not reaching the energy target with an oral diet, oral nutritional supplements should be considered first [9].

If oral intake is not possible, early EN in critically ill patients is generally recommended [15, 16]. Multiple meta-analyses of randomized controlled trials showed that early EN compared with late EN was associated with reduced infectious morbidity in ICU patients [17, 18]. Early EN is believed to prevent intestinal villi atrophy, enterocyte apoptosis, inflammatory infiltration, and dysbiosis [19]. An ancillary study of the NUTRIREA-2 trial which assessed the effect of the route of nutrition on the markers of enterocyte damage suggested that early EN was associated with a more rapid restoration of enterocyte than early PN [20]. However, the recommendation of early EN is under discussion as most studies were performed decades ago, and the design of trials had methodological limitations. Recent trials which assessed early EN vs. early PN did not show any difference in the rate of infectious diseases [21, 22]. Albeit such limitations, early EN is currently a standard of care in most countries when early EN is tolerable. At least, trophic EN should be started as early as possible. There are some cases when early EN should be carefully implemented. First, in critically ill patients after allogeneic HCT, intolerance could be a barrier to applying early EN. For instance, allogeneic HCT recipients sometimes have severe gut acute GVHD or gastroenteritis caused by bacteria such as clostridium difficile or viral infection such as cytomegalovirus. In such cases, it is reasonable to wait until the symptoms of diarrhea improve. Second, patients requiring vasopressor agents are at a high risk of gastrointestinal complications such as bowel ischemia. Thus, the clinicians have to carefully implement EN and slowly increase the dose of EN in patients requiring vasopressors. Other situations when EN should be delayed are reviewed elsewhere [9].

In case of contraindications to both oral nutrition and EN, PN should be implemented. PN is usually started within 3 to 7 days when oral diet or EN is not implemented [23]. As described above, EN is preferred over PN based on meta-analyses showing reduced infectious complications [9]. However, recent data from RCTs suggest that the addition of supplemental PN to EN does not necessarily result in increased rates of infectious complications [24, 25]. Thus, in patients who do not tolerate EN to meet the caloric intake, PN should not be withheld for a long duration [9].

## Special Considerations in Patients After Allogeneic HCT

Basically, the recommended nutrition support in critically ill patients is similar across the board [9]. However, some special considerations need to be taken into account for those patients who are acutely ill in ICU post-allogeneic HCT.

Post-allogeneic HCT patients are at a high risk for complications associated with PN. First, patients are at an increased risk for hyperglycemia after allogeneic HCT [2, 26–29]. There are various causes of hyperglycemia after allogeneic HCT as reviewed previously [28], such as the use of immunosuppressive drugs including systemic corticosteroid and calcineurin inhibitors.

In patients post-allogeneic HCT, they might have a complication relating to acute GVHD: skin rash, diarrhea, liver dysfunction. For instance, patients with acute GVHD of the gastrointestinal tract are intolerant to EN. In such cases, PN could be a realistic choice for nutritional support [30]. Patients with acute GVHD of the liver are at a high risk of liver failure. Thus, as recommended for patients with liver failure, EN is a preferred nutritional support [31].

Clinical evidence which suggests the relevance of microbiota in the field of allogeneic HCT is emerging [32–36]. Thus, intervention strategies targeting the intestinal microbiota, including the choice of antibiotics, use of prebiotics and probiotics, and fecal microbiota transplantation, are new potential options of nutritional support in patients post-allogeneic HCT.

## Conclusion

Critically ill patients post-allogeneic HCT are at a high risk for malnutrition. In such cases, sophisticated nutritional support by a multidisciplinary nutritional support care team is mandatory to mitigate the risk of malnutrition.

## References

1. Muscaritoli M, Arends J, Bachmann P, Baracos V, Barthelemy N, Bertz H, et al. ESPEN practical guideline: clinical nutrition in cancer. Clin Nutr. 2021;40(5):2898–913.
2. Fuji S, Einsele H, Savani BN, Kapp M. Systematic nutritional support in allogeneic hematopoietic stem cell transplant recipients. Biol Blood Marrow Transplant. 2015;21(10):1707–13.
3. Baumgartner A, Bargetzi A, Zueger N, Bargetzi M, Medinger M, Bounoure L, et al. Revisiting nutritional support for allogeneic hematologic stem cell transplantation-a systematic review. Bone Marrow Transplant. 2017;52(4):506–13.
4. Rzepecki P, Barzal J, Oborska S. Blood and marrow transplantation and nutritional support. Support Care Cancer. 2010;18(Suppl 2):S57–65.
5. Beckerson J, Szydlo RM, Hickson M, Mactier CE, Innes AJ, Gabriel IH, et al. Impact of route and adequacy of nutritional intake on outcomes of allogeneic haematopoietic cell transplantation for haematologic malignancies. Clin Nutr. 2019;38(2):738–44.
6. Lemal R, Cabrespine A, Pereira B, Combal C, Ravinet A, Hermet E, et al. Could enteral nutrition improve the outcome of patients with haematological malignancies undergoing allogeneic haematopoietic stem cell transplantation? A study protocol for a randomized controlled trial (the NEPHA study). Trials. 2015;16:136.
7. Baumgartner A, Bargetzi M, Bargetzi A, Zueger N, Medinger M, Passweg J, et al. Nutritional support practices in hematopoietic stem cell transplantation centers: a nationwide comparison. Nutrition. 2017;35:43–50.
8. Baumgartner A, Hoskin K, Schuetz P. Optimization of nutrition during allogeneic hematologic stem cell transplantation. Curr Opin Clin Nutr Metab Care. 2018;21(3):152–8.
9. Singer P, Blaser AR, Berger MM, Alhazzani W, Calder PC, Casaer MP, et al. ESPEN guideline on clinical nutrition in the intensive care unit. Clin Nutr. 2019;38(1):48–79.
10. De Silva A, Nightingale JMD. Refeeding syndrome: physiological background and practical management. Frontline Gastroenterol. 2020;11(5):404–9.
11. da Silva JSV, Seres DS, Sabino K, Adams SC, Berdahl GJ, Citty SW, et al. ASPEN consensus recommendations for refeeding syndrome. Nutr Clin Pract. 2020;35(2):178–95.
12. McKnight CL, Newberry C, Sarav M, Martindale R, Hurt R, Daley B. Refeeding syndrome in the critically ill: a literature review and Clinician's guide. Curr Gastroenterol Rep. 2019;21(11):58.
13. De Waele E, Jakubowski JR, Stocker R, Wischmeyer PE. Review of evolution and current status of protein requirements and provision in acute illness and critical care. Clin Nutr. 2021;40(5):2958–73.
14. Schuetz P, Fehr R, Baechli V, Geiser M, Deiss M, Gomes F, et al. Individualised nutritional support in medical inpatients at nutritional risk: a randomised clinical trial. Lancet. 2019;393(10188):2312–21.
15. Preiser JC, Arabi YM, Berger MM, Casaer M, McClave S, Montejo-González JC, et al. A guide to enteral nutrition in intensive care units: 10 expert tips for the daily practice. Crit Care. 2021;25(1):424.
16. Tian F, Heighes PT, Allingstrup MJ, Doig GS. Early enteral nutrition provided within 24 hours of ICU admission: a meta-analysis of randomized controlled trials. Crit Care Med. 2018;46(7):1049–56.
17. Reintam Blaser A, Starkopf J, Alhazzani W, Berger MM, Casaer MP, Deane AM, et al. Early enteral nutrition in critically ill patients: ESICM clinical practice guidelines. Intensive Care Med. 2017;43(3):380–98.
18. Taylor BE, McClave SA, Martindale RG, Warren MM, Johnson DR, Braunschweig C, et al. Guidelines for the provision and assessment of nutrition support therapy in the adult critically ill patient: Society of Critical Care Medicine (SCCM) and American Society for Parenteral and Enteral Nutrition (A.S.P.E.N.). Crit Care Med. 2016;44(2):390–438.
19. McClave SA, Lowen CC, Martindale RG. The 2016 ESPEN Arvid Wretlind lecture: the gut in stress. Clin Nutr. 2018;37(1):19–36.
20. Piton G, Le Gouge A, Brulé N, Cypriani B, Lacherade JC, Nseir S, et al. Impact of the route of nutrition on gut mucosa in ventilated adults with shock: an ancillary of the NUTRIREA-2 trial. Intensive Care Med. 2019;45(7):948–56.
21. Reignier J, Boisramé-Helms J, Brisard L, Lascarrou JB, Ait Hssain A, Anguel N, et al. Enteral versus parenteral early nutrition in ventilated adults with shock: a randomised, controlled, multicentre, open-label, parallel-group study (NUTRIREA-2). Lancet. 2018;391(10116):133–43.

22. Harvey SE, Parrott F, Harrison DA, Bear DE, Segaran E, Beale R, et al. Trial of the route of early nutritional support in critically ill adults. N Engl J Med. 2014;371(18):1673–84.
23. Fuentes Padilla P, Martinez G, Vernooij RW, Urrutia G, Roque IFM, Bonfill CX. Early enteral nutrition (within 48 hours) versus delayed enteral nutrition (after 48 hours) with or without supplemental parenteral nutrition in critically ill adults. Cochrane Database Syst Rev. 2019;2019(10):CD012340.
24. Ridley EJ, Davies AR, Parke R, Bailey M, McArthur C, Gillanders L, et al. Supplemental parenteral nutrition versus usual care in critically ill adults: a pilot randomized controlled study. Crit Care. 2018;22(1):12.
25. Wischmeyer PE, Hasselmann M, Kummerlen C, Kozar R, Kutsogiannis DJ, Karvellas CJ, et al. A randomized trial of supplemental parenteral nutrition in underweight and overweight critically ill patients: the TOP-UP pilot trial. Crit Care. 2017;21(1):142.
26. Welsch S, Sawadogo K, Brichard B, de Ville de Goyet M, Van Damme A, Boulanger C, et al. Characterization and risk factors of hyperglycaemia during treatment of childhood hematologic malignancies. Diabet Med. 2021;39:e14720.
27. Fuji S, Kim SW, Mori S, Fukuda T, Kamiya S, Yamasaki S, et al. Hyperglycemia during the neutropenic period is associated with a poor outcome in patients undergoing myeloablative allogeneic hematopoietic stem cell transplantation. Transplantation. 2007;84(7):814–20.
28. Fuji S, Rovo A, Ohashi K, Griffith M, Einsele H, Kapp M, et al. How do I manage hyperglycemia/post-transplant diabetes mellitus after allogeneic HSCT. Bone Marrow Transplant. 2016;51(8):1041–9.
29. Kawajiri A, Fuji S, Tanaka Y, Kono C, Hirakawa T, Tanaka T, et al. Clinical impact of hyperglycemia on days 0-7 after allogeneic stem cell transplantation. Bone Marrow Transplant. 2017;52(8):1156–63.
30. McMillen KK, Coghlin-Dickson T, Adintori PA. Optimization of nutrition support practices early after hematopoietic cell transplantation. Bone Marrow Transplant. 2021;56(2):314–26.
31. Bischoff SC, Bernal W, Dasarathy S, Merli M, Plank LD, Schütz T, et al. ESPEN practical guideline: clinical nutrition in liver disease. Clin Nutr. 2020;39(12):3533–62.
32. Peled JU, Gomes ALC, Devlin SM, Littmann ER, Taur Y, Sung AD, et al. Microbiota as predictor of mortality in allogeneic hematopoietic-cell transplantation. N Engl J Med. 2020;382(9):822–34.
33. Konishi T, Kusakabe S, Hino A, Inamoto K, Yoshifuji K, Kiridoshi Y, et al. Low diversity of gut microbiota in the early phase of post-bone marrow transplantation increases the risk of chronic graft-versus-host disease. Bone Marrow Transplant. 2021;56(7):1728–31.
34. Lin D, Hu B, Li P, Zhao Y, Xu Y, Wu D. Roles of the intestinal microbiota and microbial metabolites in acute GVHD. Exp Hematol Oncol. 2021;10(1):49.
35. Masetti R, Zama D, Leardini D, Muratore E, Turroni S, Brigidi P, et al. Microbiome-derived metabolites in allogeneic hematopoietic stem cell transplantation. Int J Mol Sci. 2021;22(3):1197.
36. Skaarud KJ, Hov JR, Hansen SH, Kummen M, Valeur J, Seljeflot I, et al. Mortality and microbial diversity after allogeneic hematopoietic stem cell transplantation: secondary analysis of a randomized nutritional intervention trial. Sci Rep. 2021;11(1):11593.

# Critically Ill Hematopoietic Stem Cell Transplantation Patient: Provider Burnout and Support

35

Nancy Cruz Sitner, Caroll C. Tipian, Ann A. Jakubowski, and Stephen M. Pastores

## Introduction

Burnout among healthcare professionals is widely recognized as an organizational problem in health care that needs to be addressed [1]. The US Surgeon General has identified this as an urgent issue because of the increased demand for healthcare providers to meet the needs of an aging population [2]. Burnout was initially described as a manifestation of physical, mental, and emotional exhaustion [3]. Although definitions of burnout have varied over the years, especially in oncology, Maslach and Jackson, experts in this area who have conducted studies since 1973, defined burnout as "a syndrome of emotional exhaustion and cynicism that frequently occurs among individuals who do people-work of some kind" [4]. Three domains have traditionally characterized the burnout syndrome: depersonalization (callous, seeing others as objects), inefficacy or moral distress (diminished sense of accomplishment), and emotional exhaustion (overwhelmed, drained, and unable to meet demands) (Fig. 35.1). The Maslach Burnout Inventory (MBI) [4, 5] is a 22-item questionnaire considered the "gold standard for measuring burnout." In a recent systematic review and meta-analysis by Ahola et al. [6], the MBI was the most utilized burnout measurement tool.

These three dimensions of burnout exist along a spectrum in which emotional exhaustion may trigger cynicism and detachment, leading to decreased professional performance [7]. Burnout is distinguishable from compassion fatigue. It is distinctly associated with a person's relationship to work [8], primarily recognized as an occupational-related condition by the World Health Organization [9]. Compassion fatigue can occur concurrently with burnout in the work set-

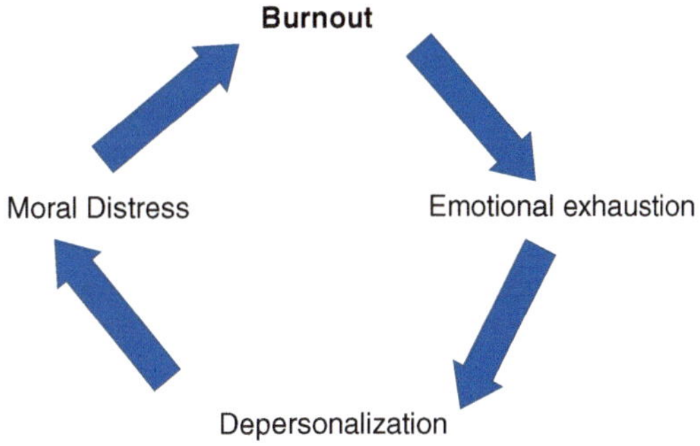


**Fig. 35.1** Three distinct dimensions of burnout

N. C. Sitner · C. C. Tipian
Adult Bone Marrow Transplant Service, Memorial Sloan Kettering Cancer Center, New York, NY, USA
e-mail: cruzsitn@mskcc.org; tipianc@mskcc.org

A. A. Jakubowski
Adult Bone Marrow Transplant Service, Department of Medicine, Memorial Sloan Kettering Cancer Center, New York, NY, USA
e-mail: jakubowa@mskcc.org

S. M. Pastores (✉)
Critical Care Center, Department of Anesthesiology and Critical Care Medicine, Memorial Sloan Kettering Cancer Center, New York, NY, USA
e-mail: pastores@mskcc.org



A. O. Soubani (ed.), *Pulmonary and Critical Care Considerations of Hematopoietic Stem Cell Transplantation*, https://doi.org/10.1007/978-3-031-28797-8_35

ting, with a more rapid onset and inability to feel empathy due to secondary trauma from stressful patient events. Burnout, in contrast, is a comprehensive concept with a slow onset and can result from numerous stressors [10]. Burnout contributes to turnover intention and patient dissatisfaction [11]. Therefore, it is imperative to understand job-related outcomes and the factors contributing to burnout.

There is a high prevalence of burnout in oncology. Specifically, in hematopoietic stem cell transplantation (HSCT), the overall prevalence of burnout in HSCT health professionals, including nurse practitioners (NPs) and physician assistants (PAs), also known as advanced practice providers (APPs), nurses, physicians, and pharmacists, was reported as 40% [12]. This chapter describes the causes of burnout, the signs and symptoms, and individual and possible organizational interventions to potentially mitigate burnout among providers of critically ill HSCT patients.

## Background

To address burnout of providers caring for critically ill HSCT patients and its impact on care, one needs to understand the care and complications associated with this treatment. HSCT is a uniquely challenging targeted intervention for a range of complex conditions associated with high mortality in high-risk patients. Patients who receive HSCT undergo a rigorous treatment course that can span months, transitioning between inpatient and outpatient settings during the many phases of transplant (pre-transplant workup, conditioning chemotherapy, inpatient admission/transplant/engraftment, outpatient recovery, and readmission complications). The consequences of these phases of HSCT can lead to significant stressors for the patients, caregivers, and healthcare providers.

Conditioning therapy to treat residual disease with consequent bone marrow and immune suppression renders patients susceptible to developing critical illness [13]. Over the past few decades, HSCT outcomes (mainly transplant-related mortality [TRM] and overall survival) have substantially improved due to reduced-intensity conditioning therapy and improved prophylactic, diagnostic, and therapeutic management of infectious complications [14]. However, more intensive myeloablative transplants with increased risks of complications have continued in specific disease settings. The increasing number of older adults with a more significant number of comorbidities continues to place patients at risk of critical illness.

HSCT is associated with complications that may require admission to an intensive care unit (ICU) [15–17]. The early complications of HSCT (Day 30–100) are predominantly infectious in nature with or without graft-versus-host disease (GVHD). Saillard et al. reported that approximately 15% of post-HSCT patients require critical care [16]. The most common reasons for ICU admission after HSCT are respiratory failure and septic shock [17]. Even though ICU outcomes have improved over the last few decades, ICU admission after an HSCT continues to be associated with poor prognosis with an average mortality rate of 50% [16, 17].

In addition, HSCT patients can have prolonged hospitalizations, adding to providers' chronicity burden. A recent study of patients undergoing allogeneic HSCT from 2002 to 2015 showed that infections, acute GVHD, acute kidney injury (AKI), and the use of total body irradiation (TBI) in conditioning therapy were predictors for longer hospital length of stay (LOS) [18]. The median LOS in the entire cohort was 25.8 days. The median age was 50 years, with 37% of the patients falling into the age group of 18–45 years; 54%, 45–65 years; and then 9%, >65 years. Cohorts by stem-cell source were peripheral blood (PB; 80%), bone marrow (BM; 15%), and cord blood (CB; 5%). The oldest age group (>65 years) had a shorter LOS than the 18–65-year age group. This variation could be due to the type of stem-cell source used, intensity of the preparative regimen (greater use of reduced-intensity and non myeloablative regimens in older adults), or subsequent risk for complications. Additionally, increased LOS is directly associated with increased mortality.

Approximately 10% of patients who underwent HSCT had a LOS of greater than 50 days [18].

Acute and chronic GVHD is an immunologically mediated disease caused by donor-origin T-cells recognizing recipient tissues as foreign and instigating an immune response against the recipient. Acute GVHD frequently occurs within the first 100 days after transplant and can affect the skin, mucosa, intestinal tract, and liver. It often occurs during the transplant hospitalization and can contribute to prolonged LOS. Grading is based on the severity of clinical symptoms. A conceptual model proposed by the National Institutes of Health Chronic GVHD workgroup divides the pathophysiology of chronic GVHD into three phases: early inflammation (phase 1), followed by chronic inflammation and dysregulated B-cell and T-cell immunity (phase 2), and then tissue repair with fibrosis (phase 3) [19]. The consequences of fibrosis in the skin, musculoskeletal system, and lungs can be quite debilitating. Chronic immunosuppression results in frequent infections. The course and potential lengthy treatment of acute and chronic GVHD, with the need for frequent follow-up visits and changes in therapy, can cause feelings of frustration and helplessness in patients, caregivers, and healthcare providers. While GVHD can often be effectively treated, it can be lethal on occasion.

Disease relapse remains the most significant cause of mortality following HSCT. Significant early and late TRM may occur depending on the status of the disease, comorbidities, and patient age. Relapse, infections, toxicity, and GVHD are the leading causes of death. Nearly 50% of mortality cases following HSCT occur within the first 6 months after transplant [20]. A critical factor in HSCT end-of-life care patterns is the ambiguity of predicting timeframes for patients and caregivers.

Patients undergoing HSCT and their families are exposed to significant physical and psychological stressors during this potentially life-threatening treatment. The burden of unmet psychological needs such as anxiety, depression, psychological distress (including worry, uncertainty, and fear of recurrence), post-traumatic stress disorder, treatment-related financial burden, and cognitive impairment remains high [21–23]. The feelings of disappointment, frustrations, and helplessness of the critically ill patients and their caregivers, who entered the transplant with the intention of cure, contribute significantly to the stress and burnout of the healthcare providers.

## HSCT and Provider Burnout

The clinical team composed of APPs, nurses, physicians, pharmacists, and social workers plays a crucial role in the HSCT setting. Their responsibilities include supporting patients and families throughout the procedure and the recovery phase, monitoring changes in the patients' condition and any developing complications, and managing and planning a range of therapeutic interventions. HSCT providers must have highly skilled critical thinking, clinical judgment, and superior knowledge as comprehensive assessment and rapid management of complications are critical to ensuring the success of HSCT. Caring for HSCT patients demands that healthcare providers also be competent in providing emotional comfort, especially in end-of-life situations [12], in addition to clinical care.

Burnout among HSCT providers is a multifactorial and multilayered paradigm. The critical complexity of patients can lead to stress, burnout, and, ultimately, poor staff retention. Critical illness or acuity of patients was reported as the most stressful factor for HSCT clinicians [24]. The intense focus on cure and survival that patients and caregivers have when entering the HSCT process extends the lengths to which HSCT providers might go to prolong life. This can displace attention on other important outcomes, such as symptom control and preparation for the end of life [25]. The failure of treatment and the loss of patients can be complicated for providers to manage. In addition, HSCT providers are often faced with challenges in recognizing ethically appropriate decisions related to end-of-life care. For example, the ethical basis of clinical decision-making such as introducing multiple lines of therapies for severe GVHD that is not responding, more chemotherapy treatments in the setting of relapsed disease, or when to stop blood transfusions for patients who endured critical illness but whose condition has declined can lead to feelings of moral distress among providers.

There are organizational factors that contribute to burnout among HSCT providers. There is a growing demand from institutions, payors, and patients to deliver high-quality, cost-effective care. Additional factors such as heavy workloads [26], role ambiguity [27], and lack of autonomy [28] contribute to the high levels of burnout that are being reported separately in recent studies of physicians [29], nurses [6], and NPs [30].

While the burnout rate has increased nationally across various clinical specialties and practice settings, there is a scarcity of studies about burnout among HSCT providers. Therefore, data showing high levels of burnout among oncology and critical care providers can be extrapolated to HSCT. In the most extensive study of burnout in oncologists conducted in the United States, 44.7% of oncologists were found to experience symptoms of burnout before the COVID-19 pandemic [31]. A few critical components identified for causes of burnout included teamwork and organizational leadership deficiencies. These factors are at the core of developing successful multidisciplinary team collaboration in oncology and place providers at a higher risk of developing burnout [32]. One study found that approximately 35% of oncology PAs and 31% of oncology NPs reported burnout [33].

In 2018, Neumann and colleagues published the first study that specifically evaluated the prevalence of and factors contributing to work-related distress, namely, burnout and moral distress, in HSCT healthcare professionals [12]. Emotional exhaustion appeared to be the prevalent cause of burnout across disciplines. Pharmacists had the highest level of burnout, with 53% self-identifying as having symptoms of burnout. When the subscales of the MBI were examined, APPs had an overall prevalence of 45%, followed by physicians with a rate of 41%. Moreover, about 38% of nurse respondents reported experiencing burnout, and 30% of social workers felt symptoms of burnout. This study was pivotal in determining the contributors to burnout among HSCT providers at a multidiscipline level, such as decreased work-life balance and career satisfaction for all disciplines.

It is challenging to gauge how much burnout affects patient care. Multiple studies have linked burnout to lower quality of care [34]. However, many of those studies mainly relied on subjective measures, such as patient surveys and self-reporting by nurses and physicians, making it difficult to draw a cause-and-effect relationship. Nevertheless, burnout has been associated with increased patient safety incidents, including medical errors, reduced patient satisfaction, and poorer safety and quality ratings [1].

## Signs and Symptoms

The signs and effects of burnout may build gradually over time, making it harder for an individual to recognize them when present [7]. The literature shows that even indirect exposure to trauma and suffering creates risks of significant emotional, cognitive, and behavioral changes in the clinician [35]. There are many degrees of burnout, and they may be different for everyone. Burnout may appear in physical, mental, or emotional ways. The physical signs and symptoms observed may be headaches, muscle tension, lowered immunity, feeling sick, appetite changes, sleep patterns, chest pain, shortness of breath, or palpitations. Emotional signs and symptoms may include feeling overwhelmed and cynical, frustrated, and unfulfilled with any experience, "Sunday night blues" before work, sense of apathy or "over complaining," feeling depleted after work, irritability, decreased satisfaction, and decreased sense of accomplishment. The complexity of these symptoms of burnout may exist along a continuum with the progression of distinctly unique symptoms or overlap of symptoms, hindering the ability to recognize burnout.

## Interventions

Evidence-based domains and promising practices may decrease clinician burnout across multi-center guided interventions. Burnout interventions may be focused at the individual or organizational level. Identifying the root causes of burnout and recognizing its signs is the first step to addressing and managing the symptoms and promoting resilience. The ramifications of feelings of burnout may lead to potential medical errors, increased turnover, poor workplace environment, lack of teamwork, and lack of commitment [26]. Institutions can use these metrics to begin measuring the potential magnitude of burnout in their organization. With the metrics in hand, it becomes imperative that healthcare organizations develop innovative methods to help HSCT and critical care clinicians cope with the day-to-day challenges of caring for these complex patients. Many groups and organizations have taken up the call to address burnout among healthcare professionals [1] through burnout surveys and the creation of employee wellness committees.

Organizational interventions have focused on improving the practice environment, increasing professional engagement, and team building [12]. Adopting well-being as an organizational value can normalize and support expressions of wellness-promoting behaviors [36]. The Mayo Clinic produced a detailed guide for implementing organizational strategies to prevent and reduce burnout by addressing individual, work unit, organizational, and national factors across seven domains [26]. These domains involve workload and job demands, efficiency and resources, meaning in work, culture and values, control and flexibility, social support and community at work, and work-life integration. Within the ICU setting, prospective analyses of interventions to decrease burnout among physicians and APPs are limited and focus primarily on novel approaches to staffing such as expanded roles for APPs and night coverage; strategies for handling ICU surge in volume and acuity; optimization of team culture, collaboration, and communication; addressing causes of moral distress; and enhancement of personal resilience and emotional intelligence [37].

Committing to a transformational leadership culture through the organizations' strategic planning can improve and sustain professional well-being [38]. Adopting team-based care through an interprofessional approach is now advocated and could help burnout. There is also some evidence suggesting that models where the palliative care specialist is integrated into the HSCT team could also increase the capacity of non-palliative specialist team members to offer interventions such as goals of care discussions [39]. Practice standards can help organizations in a stepwise approach to selecting and implementing interventions to improve clinician well-being [38]. Some of the recommended practice standards include (1) organization assessment of burnout; (2) identification of interventions through a quality improvement project that aligns with organizations' mission, vision, and strategic plan; (3) engagement of clinicians; (4) piloting of interventions; and (5) evaluation of metrics and objectives to evaluate the effectiveness of interventions.

Several strategies have been developed to combat burnout at an individual level, such as identifying the cause, creating balanced emotional intelligence, and being active in self-awareness, self-regulation, motivation, and empathy [40]. Following Maslow's Hierarchy of Needs, basic requirements such as rest and security must be met before a person can move on to addressing the psychological, relationship, and self-esteem needs, and ultimately self-fulfillment. Individuals with higher levels of well-being have enhanced outlook on life, live longer, perceive themselves to be in a better health, engage in healthy behaviors, have fewer mental and physical illnesses, feel more socially connected, and are more productive at work and home [41]. Furthermore, strengthening workforce relationships, optimizing workload, practicing autonomy, and improving physical health with sleep and physical activity have also been applied. Communication skills training has been an effective mechanism for communicating feelings of frustration, anger, sadness, and grief to avoid the buildup of these emotions [42].

It is noteworthy that burnout symptoms were not systematically alleviated by individually focused interventions, which are the type that have most often been evaluated [6]. Because most known risk factors for burnout occur at the organization level, it is not surprising that a pre-pandemic meta-analysis of interventions for physicians found that organizational interventions were more effective than individual interventions [43]. Neumann et al. emphasized that addressing burnout entails a multifaceted approach that integrates the provider, the institution, and the support of professional organizations [12]. For example, A Well-Being Task Force within the American Society of Oncology was created to guide committees, initiatives, members, and the cancer organization to address oncology burnout [42]. Its mission is to improve the quality, safety, and value of cancer care by enhancing oncology clinician well-being and practice sustainability within oncology clinicians and cancer organizations. Table 35.1 lists the burnout domains and selected individual and organizational interventions focused on improving provider well-being.

**Table 35.1** Burnout domains and the individual and organization-level interventions

| Burnout domains | Individual interventions | Organization-level interventions |
|---|---|---|
| Critical illness and complexity of patients | Ongoing education, training, workshops | Promoting mentorship |
| Challenging end-of-life and ethical situations | Creation of balanced emotional intelligence and coping mechanisms | Structural psychosocial promoting behaviors |
| Emotional burden of patient care | Wellness-promoting behaviors | Fostering an environment of self-awareness |
| Heavy workloads | Optimizing autonomy | Optimizing workload |
| Deficiencies in teamwork | Enhancing work relationships | Team building activities and building of team structures |
| Lack of organizational leadership and support | Increasing professional engagement and job satisfaction | Transformational leadership framework |

## Impact of COVID-19 on HSCT Providers

Before the coronavirus disease 2019 (COVID-19) pandemic, oncology clinicians were at risk of burnout due to the increasing demands on clinical time, productivity, and evolving medical landscape with limited control over daily responsibilities and endless electronic documentation. Research on the mental health implications among healthcare workers during the COVID-19 response is still emerging. However, the pandemic exacerbated underlying oncologist burnout, creating stress associated with disruptions in care, education, research, financial practice, personal health, and telemedicine [42].

Between May 28 and Oct. 1, 2020, using the AMA Coping with COVID-19 for Caregivers Survey, 42 healthcare organizations across the United States assessed their healthcare workers' stress during the pandemic [44]. This survey revealed a 55% prevalence of burnout across multiple disciplines (physicians, APPs, nurses, social workers, and rehabilitation therapists) in healthcare. The survey revealed that 61% felt intense fear of exposing themselves or their families to COVID-19, while 38% self-reported experiencing anxiety or depression. Data from multiple surveys showed that healthcare workers responsible for providing direct care to COVID-19 patients are more likely to have depression, anxiety, and mental distress. These mental health issues may be related to psychological distress from witnessing COVID-19-related deaths, extra-long work hours, and work-life imbalance.

Risk factors for burnout have been multifactorial throughout the COVID-19 pandemic, with isolation, loss of safety net services, family stressors and trauma, and deferred care and services compounding this issue across communities worldwide. Furthermore, it has been magnified by high demands, lack of control, resource scarcity, and ethical dilemmas. Among HSCT providers, burnout was further heightened by concerns about the high susceptibility to opportunistic and community-acquired infections and the increased mortality rate in this unique population [45]. The COVID-19 mortality in HSCT patients was 19%, significantly higher than the observed case fatality ratio of 1.6% in the general US population [46].

## Implications

This chapter highlights the multifaceted nature of burnout among HSCT providers. Although there is a significant amount of literature on the cause and effect of burnout across multiple disciplines of medicine, that which relates to prevention, intervention, and recovery from burnout is much more limited. Robust longitudinal surveys of cancer center care team members are necessary to enhance understanding of the relationship between team members, burnout, and quality of patient care [42]. These studies could provide insightful information in creating a comprehensive, holistic approach to improving oncology providers' well-being. Furthermore, efforts to reduce burnout need to be tailored to the individual provider's specialized practice settings. It will be essential to evaluate the link between HSCT providers' burnout and patient outcomes and design preventive interventions in this clinical setting.

Healthcare providers must engage in designing preventive interventions planned by their organizations and seek to implement one or more of the evidence-based strategies used by their peers [38]. Retention of all providers is necessary to enhance the delivery and quality of care, as access to care remains challenging. Research on the effects of burnout interventions would benefit from consensus guidelines for defining and assessing burnout [6]. Studies that examine intervention sustainability and those focused on developing personal and professional resilience are also needed [47].

## References


1. AHRQ. 2019. https://psnet.ahrq.gov/primer/burnout. Accessed 14 Mar 2022.
2. Frieden J. Surgeon general concerned about physician burnout—if physicians aren't happy, they can't heal others. 2016. https://www.medpagetoday.com/publichealthpolicy/generalprofessionalissues/57280. Accessed 14 Mar 2022.
3. Freudenberger HJ. Staff burnout. Aust J Soc Issues. 1974;30:159–65.
4. Maslach C, Jackson SE, Leiter MP, Schaufeli WB, Schwab RL. Maslach burnout inventory, vol. 21. Palo Alto, CA: Consulting Psychologists Press; 1986. p. 3463–4.
5. Schaufeli WB, Leiter MP, Maslach C. Burnout: 35 years of research and practice. Career Dev Int. 2009;14(3):204–20.
6. Ahola K, Toppinen-Tanner S, Seppänen J. Interventions to alleviate burnout symptoms and support return to work among employees with burnout: systematic review and meta-analysis. Burn Res. 2017;4:1–11.
7. Zhang JQ, Riba L, Magrini L, Fleishman A, Ukandu P, Alapati A, James TA. Assessing burnout and professional fulfillment in breast surgery: results from a national survey of the American Society of Breast Surgeons. Ann Surg Oncol. 2019;26(10):3089–98.
8. Klein CJ, Weinzimmer LG, Cooling M, Lizer S, Pierce L, Dalstrom M. Exploring burnout and job stressors among advanced practice providers. Nurs Outlook. 2020;68(2):145–54.
9. World Health Organization. International statistical classification of diseases and related health problems. 11th ed. Geneva: World Health Organization; 2020.
10. Negash S, Sahin S. Compassion fatigue in marriage and family therapy: implications for therapists and clients. J Marital Fam Ther. 2011;37(1):1–13.
11. Lee HF, Kuo CC, Chien TW, Wang YR. A meta-analysis of the effects of coping strategies on reducing nurse burnout. Appl Nurs Res. 2016;31:100–10.
12. Neumann JL, Mau LW, Virani S, et al. Burnout, moral distress, work-life balance, and career satisfaction among hematopoietic cell transplantation professionals. Biol Blood Marrow Transplant. 2018;24(4):849–60.
13. McArdle JR. Critical care outcomes in the hematologic transplant recipient. Clin Chest Med. 2009;30:155–67.
14. Gooley TA, Chien JW, Pergam SA, et al. Reduced mortality after allogeneic hematopoietic-cell transplantation. N Engl J Med. 2010;363(22):2091–101.
15. Kew AK, Couban S, Patrick W, Thompson K, White D. Outcome of hematopoietic stem cell transplant recipients admitted to the intensive care unit. Biol Blood Marrow Transplant. 2006;12(3):301–5.
16. Saillard C, Darmon M, Bisbal M, et al. Critically ill allogeneic HSCT patients in the intensive care unit: a systematic review and meta-analysis of prognostic factors of mortality. Bone Marrow Transplant. 2018;53:1233–41.
17. Bayraktar UD, Nates JL. Intensive care outcomes in adult hematopoietic stem cell transplantation patients. World J Clin Oncol. 2016;7(1):98–105.
18. Godara A, Siddiqui NS, Munigala S, Dhawan R, Kansagra AJ, Rapoport AP, Yared JA, Dahiya S. Length of stay and hospital costs for patients undergoing allogeneic stem-cell transplantation. JCO Oncol Pract. 2021;17(3):e355–68.

19. Cooke KR, Luznik L, Sarantopoulos S, et al. The biology of chronic graft-versus-host disease: a task force report from the National Institutes of Health consensus development project on criteria for clinical trials in chronic graft-versus-host disease. Biol Blood Marrow Transplant. 2017;23(2):211–34.
20. Busemann C, Jülich A, Buchhold B, Schmidt V, Schneidewind L, Pink D, Schmidt CA, Neumann T, Krüger WH. Clinical course and end-of-life care in patients who have died after allogeneic stem cell transplantation. J Cancer Res Clin Oncol. 2017;143(10):2067–76.
21. Epstein AS, Goldberg GR, Meier DE. Palliative care and hematologic oncology: the promise of collaboration. Blood Rev. 2012;26(6):233–9.
22. Barata A, Wood WA, Choi SW, Jim HS. Unmet needs for psychosocial care in hematologic malignancies and hematopoietic cell transplant. Curr Hematol Malig Rep. 2016;11(4):280–7.
23. Rueda-Lara M, Lopez-Patton MR. Psychiatric and psychosocial challenges in patients undergoing haematopoietic stem cell transplants. Int Rev Psychiatry. 2014;26(1):74–86.
24. Gallagher R, Gormley DK. Perceptions of stress, burnout, and support systems in pediatric bone marrow transplantation nursing. Clin J Oncol Nurs. 2009;13(6):681–5.
25. Levine DR, Baker JN, Wolfe J, Lehmann LE, Ullrich C. Strange bedfellows no more: how integrated stem-cell transplantation and palliative care programs can together improve end-of-life care. J Oncol Pract. 2017;13(9):569–77.
26. Shanafelt TD, Noseworthy JH. Executive leadership and physician well-being: nine organizational strategies to promote engagement and reduce burnout. Mayo Clin Proc. 2017;92(1):129–46.
27. Klein CJ, Dalstrom M, Lizer S, Cooling M, Pierce L, Weinzimmer L. Advanced practice provider perspectives on organizational strategies for work stress reduction. West J Nurs Res. 2020;42(9):708–17. https://doi.org/10.1177/0193945919896606.
28. Hagan J, Curtis DL Sr. Predictors of nurse practitioner retention. J Am Assoc Nurse Pract. 2018;30(5):280–4.
29. West CP, Dyrbye LN, Shanafelt TD. Physician burnout: contributors, consequences, and solutions. J Intern Med. 2018;283(6):516–29.
30. Dyrbye L, Johnson P, Johnson LM, Halasy MP, Gossard AA, Satele D, Shanafelt T. Efficacy of the well-being index to identify distress and stratify well-being in nurse practitioners and physician assistants. J Am Assoc Nurse Pract. 2019;31(7):403–12.
31. Shanafelt TD, Raymond M, Kosty M, et al. Satisfaction with work-life balance and the career and retirement plans of US oncologists. J Clin Oncol. 2014;32:1127–35.
32. Tetzlaff ED, Hylton HM, DeMora L, Ruth K, Wong YN. National study of burnout and career satisfaction among physician assistants in oncology: implications for team-based care. J Oncol Pract. 2018;14(1):e11–22.
33. Bourdeanu L, Zhou QP, DeSamper M, Pericak KA, Pericak A. Burnout, workplace factors, and intent to leave among hematology/oncology nurse practitioners. J Adv Pract Oncol. 2020;11(2):141–8.
34. Dewa CS, Loong D, Bonato S, et al. The relationship between physician burnout and quality of healthcare in terms of safety and acceptability: a systematic review. BMJ Open. 2017;7(6):e015141.
35. Bride BE. Prevalence of secondary traumatic stress among social workers. Soc Work. 2007;52(1):63–70.
36. Peck JL, Sonney J. Exhausted and burned out: COVID-19 emerging impacts threaten the health of the pediatric advanced practice registered nursing workforce. J Pediatr Health Care. 2021;35(4):414–24.
37. Pastores SM, Kvetan V, Coopersmith CM, et al. Workforce, workload, and burnout among intensivists and advanced practice providers: a narrative review. Crit Care Med. 2019;47:550–7.
38. Sinsky CA, Biddison LD, Mallick A, Dopp AL, Perlo J, Lynn L, Smith CD. Organization evidence-based and promising practices for improving clinician well-being. NAM Perspect. 2020;2020:10.31478/202011a; Discussion paper, National Academy of medicine, Washington, DC.
39. Szekendi MK, Vaughn J, McLaughlin B, Mulvenon C, Porter-Williamson K, Sydenstricker C, Williamson M. Integrating palliative care to promote earlier conversations and increase the skill and comfort of non-palliative care clinicians: lessons learned from an interventional field trial. Am J Hosp Palliat Care. 2018;35(1):132–7.
40. Panagioti M, Panagopoulou E, Bower P, Lewith G, Kontopantelis E, Chew-Graham C, Esmail A. Controlled interventions to reduce burnout in physicians: a systematic review and meta-analysis. JAMA Intern Med. 2017;177(2):195–205.
41. Song Z, Baicker K. Effect of a workplace wellness program on employee health and economic outcomes: a randomized clinical trial. JAMA. 2019;321(15):1491–501.
42. Hlubocky FJ, Shanafelt TD, Back AL, et al. Creating a blueprint of well-being in oncology: an approach for addressing burnout from ASCO's clinician well-being taskforce. Am Soc Clin Oncol Educ Book. 2021;41:e339–53.
43. West CP, Dyrbye LN, Erwin PJ, Shanafelt TD. Interventions to prevent and reduce physician burnout: a systematic review and meta-analysis. Lancet. 2016;388(10057):2272–81.
44. Prasad K, McLoughlin C, Stillman M, et al. Prevalence and correlates of stress and burnout among US healthcare workers during the COVID-19 pandemic: a national cross-sectional survey study. EClinicalMedicine. 2021;35:100879.
45. Samaha R, Kattan J. Hematopoietic stem cell transplantation dilemma during the COVID-19 era. Future Oncol. 2020;16(22):1569–73.
46. Medicine Johns Hopkins University. Mortality analyses. 2021. https://coronavirus.jhu.edu/data/mortality. Accessed 14 Mar 2022.
47. Lin L, He G, Yan J, Gu C, Xie J. The effects of a modified mindfulness-based stress reduction program for nurses: a randomized controlled trial. Workplace Health Saf. 2019;67(3):111–22.

# 36 Multidisciplinary Care and ICU Organization for Hematopoietic Stem Cell Transplantation Patients

Sarah Hemstetter, Rachael A. Fornwalt, and R. Scott Stephens

## Introduction

Hematopoietic stem cell transplant (HSCT) is a complex and resource-intensive therapeutic modality that is potentially curative for a spectrum of malignant and non-malignant hematologic diseases. Approximately 15% of HSCT patients still require critical care, with an associated intensive care unit (ICU) mortality of approximately 50% [1]. Respiratory failure and septic shock are the most common reasons for ICU admission after HSCT, but life-threatening HSCT complications can affect any organ system. Accordingly, access to critical care support is recognized as an essential component for HSCT programs [2]. Like HSCT itself, critical care is complex and resource-intensive. Both HSCT and critical care require substantial expertise and experience from a multidisciplinary team. This need for diverse expertise informs both staffing and organizational considerations for HSCT ICUs.

## Multidisciplinary Care

Critical care is increasingly recognized as a team effort, with input and actions from multiple disciplines. The intensivist is the nominal "leader" of the team, but each member of the team is equally essential [3]. Recognition of each discipline's specific expertise and optimization of communication between team members are essential to good ICU outcomes,

S. Hemstetter · R. A. Fornwalt · R. S. Stephens (✉)
Division of Pulmonary and Critical Care Medicine, Department of Medicine, Johns Hopkins University, Baltimore, MD, USA

Oncology Intensive Care Unit, Johns Hopkins Sidney Kimmel Comprehensive Cancer Center, Johns Hopkins Hospital, Baltimore, MD, USA
e-mail: rsteph13@jhmi.edu


A. O. Soubani (ed.), *Pulmonary and Critical Care Considerations of Hematopoietic Stem Cell Transplantation*, https://doi.org/10.1007/978-3-031-28797-8_36

especially in complex HSCT patients [4, 5]. There are few data guiding optimum staffing patterns for HSCT ICUs, and achieving adequate staffing is a challenge for many institutions. Distress and burnout among healthcare workers caring for HSCT patients are well documented and should be considered in staffing decisions [6, 7].

## ICU Providers

### Intensivists

Intensivist involvement has been shown to improve outcomes in critically ill patients, including patients with cancer [8–10]. While this relationship has not been specifically shown in HSCT patients, many of the critical illnesses faced by HSCT patients such as acute hypoxemic respiratory failure and septic shock are areas of expertise for most intensivists. Still, the profound immunosuppression after HSCT requires somewhat different considerations than the same problems in non-HSCT patients. Indeed, some have advocated for oncologic critical care (including HSCT) to be an identified subspecialty of critical care medicine [11]. While no specific training content has yet been supported in the literature, intensivists caring for HSCT patients should be familiar with the treatment of neutropenic sepsis, acute respiratory failure in the immunocompromised host, acute graft-versus-host disease (GVHD), and other HSCT-specific conditions [3, 12–14].

### Hematologists/Oncologists

Even though patients may require critical care under the direction of an intensivist, the input of the hematologist/oncologist remains essential. Hematologists/oncologists can provide disease-specific prognostic information and input on treatment- or disease-related toxicities. Additionally, and perhaps most importantly, the hematologist/oncologist has a long-standing relationship with the patient and family. This connection is vital both to assuring trust in the ICU team and facilitating difficult decisions regarding goals of care. Accordingly, the hematologist/oncologist should be involved in ICU admission decisions and participate in daily rounds or communication with the ICU team [12].

### Advanced Practice Providers

Advanced practice providers (APPs; nurse practitioners and physician assistants) provide critical care [15]. APPs have demonstrated efficacy in oncology and hematopoietic stem cell transplantation, but utilization of APPs to the fullest scope of their practice in acute care settings has been slow [16–18]. Integration of APPs in the ICU has repeatedly demonstrated outcomes similar to their physician peers [19, 20]. Care provided by APPs in the ICU decreased hospital and ICU length of stay (LOS), adverse events, time on mechanical ventilation, unexpected hospital and ICU readmissions, procedural complication rates, costs, and sepsis-related hospital mortality, improved patient/family satisfaction, and increased the use of clinical practice guidelines [21–23]. Similarly, APP-led rapid response teams reduced time to ICU transfer [22]. In the face of rotating physician schedules, APPs also provide continuity of care and rapport with core ICU staff, facilitating communication among the multidisciplinary team members [22]. APPs also serve as valuable educators, assisting with procedural training and bridging knowledge gaps on HSCT-specific critical care [24].

Basic acute care nurse practitioner (NP) and physician assistant (PA) educational curricula and clinical practicum focus on the preparation for general hospital-based acute care. This is typically inadequate for complex, specialized critical care [25, 26]. The transition to a competent critical care provider requires an extended orientation period [26], and many centers have developed post-graduate APP critical care fellowships [25]. However, the specialized care required by critically ill HSCT patients is typically not covered in these fellowships. This knowledge gap can be bridged with didactic lectures focused on HSCT specific care and the utilization of other members of the multidisciplinary care team. The key areas of competency for APPs in the HSCT ICU are listed in Table 36.1.

**Table 36.1** Key competencies for advanced practice providers in the HSCT ICU

| Care facilitation | Procedures | Care coordination | Education |
|---|---|---|---|
| – Obtaining histories<br>– Physical exams<br>– Participating in daily rounds<br>– Prescribing and titrating medications<br>– Documenting progress notes and procedures<br>– Managing mechanical ventilation<br>– Reassessing interventions | – Vascular access (central, arterial, and dialysis access)<br>– Pleural procedures (thoracentesis, small-core chest tube placement)<br>– Paracentesis<br>– Intubation<br>– Lumbar puncture<br>– Skin biopsy<br>– Bronchoscopy<br>– Feeding tube placement<br>– Point-of-care ultrasound | – Participating in multidisciplinary rounds<br>– Care coordination with transplant teams and consultants<br>– Communication with patients and families<br>– Critical care consult/ evaluation for ICU upgrade<br>– Rapid response<br>– Discharge planning | – Supervising procedures<br>– Precept students (APP and medical)<br>– Educate nursing staff<br>– Quality/ performance improvement projects<br>– Clinical research |

## Nursing

Nurses working on HSCT critical care units may possess a variety of educational and training backgrounds, clinical skills, and certifications. Regardless of background, knowledge and skill are key to successful HSCT care across the spectrum of acuity. HSCT ICU nurses must be familiar with the care of critically ill patients, including titration of vasopressors and fluids, care of the mechanically ventilated patient, and other fundamental critical care skills. The key areas of nursing care include not only administration of medications but prevention and recognition of life-threatening complications such as bleeding (due to thrombocytopenia) and sepsis [27]. HSCT care necessarily includes administration of chemotherapy, and while HSCT preparative regimens are almost never administered to a critically ill patient, it is useful for critical care nurses caring for HSCT patients to be familiar with the HSCT process, including BMT preparative regimens, GVHD prophylactic regimens, handling/sequelae of chemotherapy, blood administration protocols, and common complications of HSCT [2]. In the United States, HSCT ICU nurses may hold a variety of national credentials, including Adult Critical Care Nurse (CCRN) certification, Oncology Nursing (OCN) certification, and Blood and Marrow Transplant Nursing (BMTCN) certification. Certified nurses have typically been active in the field for at least 2 years in their specialty and have demonstrated their expertise and leadership in their specialty [28–30]. For all three certifications, the nurse must successfully pass a certification exam, followed by mandatory continuing education and regular recertification.

## Respiratory Therapists

Respiratory therapists are experts in the management and use of respiratory support devices, including mechanical ventilators, non-invasive ventilation, and heated humidified high-flow oxygen. They may also administer nebulized medications, including bronchodilators, mucolytics, and antibiotics. Though few data exist specifically in HSCT ICU patients, respiratory therapist-driven protocols have been shown to improve compliance with low tidal volume ventilation, decrease duration of high-flow nasal cannula support, and decrease length of stay in general ICU patients [31–33].

## Pharmacists

Clinical pharmacists are integral and invaluable members of multidisciplinary ICU teams [34]. Providing insight and pharmacotherapy guidance regarding antimicrobial selection and dosing, anticoagulation, sedation, analgesia, and drug interactions and integrated ICU clinical pharmacists have been shown to reduce overall medication errors and improve patient outcomes, including mortality [34, 35]. In addition to standard critical care pharmacotherapy expertise, the clinical pharmacist supporting HSCT ICUs must be able to provide guidance and assistance regarding common toxicities of chemotherapy conditioning regimens, antimicrobial prophylaxis strategies and drug-level monitoring, and drug-drug interactions, especially those regarding immunosuppressive agents used for GVHD prophylaxis (e.g., tacrolimus) [36]. The involvement of clinical pharmacists in HSCT patient care (including critically ill patients) has been shown to result in a higher proportion of therapeutic tacrolimus and cyclosporine levels, increased empiric dose adjustments to account for drug interactions, overall reduced incidence of adverse events, and increased patient satisfaction [36–38].

## Nutritionists/Dieticians

Inadequate nutritional intake is a serious problem in critically ill patients, increasing the risk of complications such as poor wound healing, impaired immune function, diminished gut barrier function, increased sepsis risk, muscle wasting, immobilization, and overall increased LOS and mortality [39, 40]. As part of the multidisciplinary ICU team, a registered dietician can assist with the evaluation of nutritional status, identification of patients with caloric deficit or malnutrition, and development of a nutritional care plan [39]. HSCT patients are often malnourished at admission and are at a high risk of not taking sufficient oral intake to meet nutritional/caloric needs [41, 42]. HSCT patients with malnutrition are at an increased risk of delayed engraftment, relapse, and overall mortality [42]. Unlike the general ICU population, there is no clear consensus on optimal timing of enteral or parenteral nutrition in HSCT ICU patients [42]. Current guidelines suggest a preference for enteral over parenteral nutrition unless precluded by severe mucositis, intractable vomiting, ileus, severe malabsorption, protracted diarrhea, or symptomatic GVHD of the gut [41, 43].

## Physical and Occupational Therapists

Physical therapy and rehabilitation have established benefits within both the critical care and bone marrow transplant populations, and rehabilitation therapists are necessary members of the multidisciplinary ICU team [44–46]. HSCT patients frequently require prolonged hospitalizations (or intensive outpatient treatment) and rapidly become deconditioned, lose muscle mass, and develop decreased exercise tolerance [46]. Treatment toxicities such as chemotherapy-induced fatigue, steroid myopathy, and GVHD may further potentiate this decrease in physical conditioning. Early consultation by physical and occupational therapists may improve overall physical function, reduce fatigue, and facilitate a faster return to pre-transplant functional status [46, 47]. Multidisciplinary exercise and activity programs improve patient activity and participation in physical therapy in pediatric and young adult patients undergoing HSCT [48, 49]. Occupational therapy was shown to improve strength, coordination, and independence among pediatric patients undergoing HSCT, particularly upper-extremity strength [50]. Though a platelet count of less than 20,000 cells/mm$^3$ has been thought of as a relative contraindication to physical therapy, evidence suggests that exercises supervised by experienced occupational and physical therapists are safe in HSCT patients [47].

## Consultants

The complex nature of HSCT critical care mandates that the entire spectrum of additional consultant specialists, besides intensivists and hematologist/oncologists, will be required to manage the breadth of medical problems that may arise. Several are particularly worth mentioning, as their involvement in HSCT ICU patients is (or should be) nearly ubiquitous. Infectious disease specialists with experience and training in transplant/oncology infectious disease are essential to the care of HSCT ICU patients, who frequently develop complicated and unusual infectious complications. Nephrologists (and the accompanying ability to provide renal replacement therapy) are specifically mentioned in the Foundation for Accreditation of Cellular Therapy Standards. Dermatologists are frequently asked to assist in the management of severe GVHD. Finally, palliative and supportive care consultation has been shown to improve quality of life and symptom burden in HSCT patients and should be integrated into the HSCT ICU environment [51–53].

## Intensive Care Unit Organization

The association of earlier ICU admission with improved survival demonstrates the need for adequate HSCT critical care facilities [54, 55]. However, there are few data to guide specific organizational recommendations for HSCT ICUs. While many high-volume transplant centers utilize "general" ICUs for HSCT critical care, some centers have developed specialty HSCT ICUs or embed critical care or high-level intermediate care capability in their HSCT ICUs. While specialty HSCT ICUs have a number of potential benefits, there are few data to support (or dissuade) their development. Development of best practices for HSCT critical care, including optimum ICU organization, is a key target for future study [56].

## Unit Model

ICUs can be organized in several different ways. Many of these may be adaptable to HSCT critical care if the requisite expertise can be brought to bear. Generally, there are several venues in which HSCT critical care could be provided (Fig. 36.1). First, critically ill HSCT patients could be transferred to a "general" ICU, usually a medical intensive care unit (MICU). Second, HSCT patients could be transferred to a specialty HSCT ICU which only (or predominantly) cares for critically ill HSCT patients. Third, HSCT patients could be transferred to a specialty "oncology ICU," which also cares for patients undergoing other oncologic/hematologic therapies (e.g., leukemia, solid tumors). Finally, HSCT patients may be cared for on an "adaptable acuity" unit, which cares for patients for the duration of their hospitalization regardless of acuity. In this model, critical care technology/expertise is brought to the patient on an as-needed basis [57].

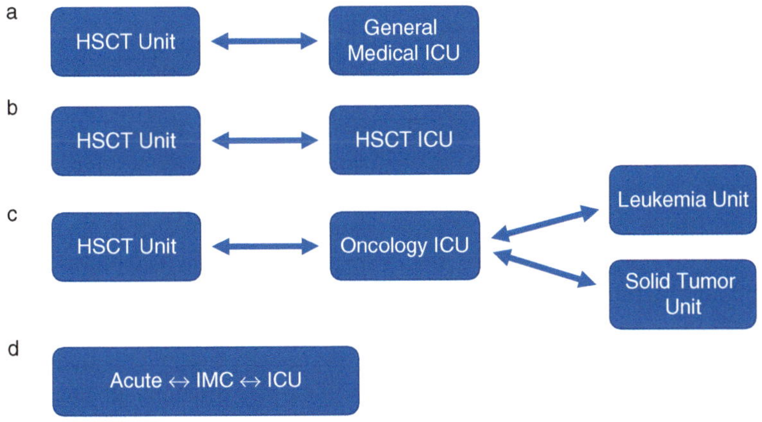


**Fig. 36.1** Organizational models of HSCT critical care. (**a**) Critically ill HSCT patients are transferred to a general medical intensive care unit. (**b**) Critically ill HSCT patients are transferred to a specialty HSCT ICU. (**c**) Critically ill HSCT patients are transferred to a specialty oncology ICU which also cares for critically ill hematologic malignancy and solid tumor patients. (**d**) Critically ill HSCT patients are cared for in an acuity-adaptable HSCT unit

There are no HSCT-specific data to support any of these models over another. Most of the data regarding acuity-adaptable units comes from studies of cardiac surgical patients. Acuity-adaptable units have been reported to provide some cost savings, predominantly by decreasing length of stay and improving some outcomes and patient satisfaction [58–60]. The advantage of an acuity-adaptable model primarily lies in the decrease in transitions of care between units and care teams [61]. It is worth noting that acuity-adaptable units are primarily described in cardiac surgical patients who tend to have a more protocolized, predictable, and consistent hospital course than HSCT patients [61, 62]. Acuity-adaptable units demand careful attention not only to unit design but to nursing staffing and skill mix to allow care of the entire spectrum of patients [63].

The potential benefits of an acuity-adaptable unit stand in contrast to the proven benefits of a "closed" ICU model, in which critical care is provided in a designated space by a dedicated team under the direction of an intensivist. Compared to an "open" ICU model, in which care is provided by the same primary team regardless of the patient's condition (i.e., the HSCT team cares for the patient for the duration of hospitalization), closed ICUs have been shown to improve outcomes including decreased infectious complications [64–66]. Thus, of the different potential models, the closed ICU model is supported by the most robust outcome data.

An additional consideration is whether HSCT patients should be cared for in a HSCT-only specialty ICU, a more broad-based "oncology" ICU (HSCT, hematologic malignancies, solid tumors), or a general ICU. There are few data to guide this decision. Boarding of critically ill patients in different subspecialty ICUs is associated with increased mortality, suggesting a benefit of ICU specialization [67]. However, other studies have suggested that specialty ICUs do not improve outcomes in common critical care conditions [68]. It is unknown whether HSCT patients benefit from specialty ICU admission.

## Physical Plant Considerations

Because of the severely immunocompromised state of critically ill HSCT patients, infection control and prevention is a major consideration in HSCT ICU space. The Foundation for the Accreditation of Cellular Therapies (FACT) standards recommend high-efficiency particulate air (HEPA) filtration with positive pressure for HSCT patient rooms [69]. This means that air entering patient rooms is HEPA-filtered and that the air pressure in a patient room is greater than the adjoining hallway, preventing potentially contaminated hallway air from entering the patient room. Easy access to sinks for hand hygiene should be provided, both inside and outside the room. Ample space for life support equipment, such as mechanical ventilators, high-flow oxygen, and continuous dialysis machines, should be available, as well as adequate oxygen, medical air, vacuum, and power sources. Space should also be sufficient to allow for rehabilitation work and equipment, including cycle ergometers, tilt tables, and ambulation. Finally, as family presence may have benefit in critically ill patients, accommodations should be made for family presence, including chairs, couches, and convertible beds [70].

## Unit Leadership

Unit leadership is a key aspect of developing and maintaining a successful and high-performing ICU. One approach to unit leadership is the development of a nurse manager-physician medical director dyad. This joint ownership model attempts to ensure that nursing and physician expertise informs unit protocols and that multidisciplinary concerns are recognized and acted upon [71]. Though the appeal of this approach is clear, there are few data demonstrating the efficacy of this structure. Regardless of the leadership model, the leaders of HSCT ICUs (or ICUs caring for HSCT patients) must have strong lines of communication with hospital and cancer center leadership. This includes the provision of adequate resources to care for critically ill HSCT patients.

In addition to the unit manager and medical director, there are other key leadership roles in a successful ICU on both the provider and nursing side. These may include lead APPs and lead clinical nurses or nurse educators who can serve as a resource to other staff. Especially in non-specialized ICUs, it may be helpful to have an APP and a senior nurse developed focused expertise in HSCT critical care to help ensure that high standards are maintained when HSCT patients are admitted to the ICU.

## Quality Assurance and Outcome Metrics

No discussion of ICU organization would be complete without mentioning quality improvement and outcome metrics. Important aspects of a quality assurance program include key (and agreed-upon) performance metrics, standardization of care when possible, and continuous review of outcomes. The Center for International Blood and Marrow research (CIBMTR) provides survival statistics for HSCT programs in the United States, as well as causes of death [72]. However, these lack some of the granularity needed for a continuous quality assurance program. Some disciplines, like cardiac surgery, have established publicly reported outcome metrics [73]. For the HSCT ICU, important metrics for continuous monitoring and quality assurance might include hospital-acquired infection rates, duration of mechanical ventilation, and rates of renal replacement therapy. Other metrics for consideration might be rates of respiratory failure and sepsis after HSCT as well as mortality from these complications. It is important to note that both neutropenic sepsis and respiratory failure are inherent and often unavoidable complications after HSCT. It is important to consider not only the occurrence of these complications but also the rates of mortality, or "failure to rescue," from these complications [74]. In many cases, high-performing ICUs will be able to "rescue" patients from complications which might otherwise have been fatal. The rate of failure to rescue is increasingly recognized as an important quality metric in many disciplines, but as yet have not been applied to HSCT ICU care.

## Conclusion

HSCT ICU care is a complex endeavor that requires input, care, and cooperation from numerous clinical disciplines. There are few data to guide optimum organization of HSCT ICUs and quality assurance. These are key targets for future outcomes and cost-effectiveness research.

## References

1. Saillard C, Darmon M, Bisbal M, Sannini A, Chow-Chine L, Faucher M, et al. Critically ill allogeneic HSCT patients in the intensive care unit: a systematic review and meta-analysis of prognostic factors of mortality. Bone Marrow Transplant. 2018;53(10):1233–41.
2. Pasquini MC, Srivastava A, Ahmed SO, Aljurf M, Atsuta Y, Doleysh C, et al. Worldwide network for blood and marrow transplantation (WBMT) recommendations for establishing a hematopoietic cell transplantation program (part I): minimum requirements and beyond. Hematol Oncol Stem Cell Ther. 2020;13(3):131–42.
3. Meert AP, Wittnebel S, Holbrechts S, Toffart AC, Lafitte JJ, Piagnerelli M, et al. Critically ill cancer patient's resuscitation: a Belgian/French societies' consensus conference. Intensive Care Med. 2021;47(10):1063–77.
4. Turkelson C, Aebersold M, Redman R, Tschannen D. Improving nursing communication skills in an intensive care unit using simulation and nursing crew resource management strategies: an implementation project. J Nurs Care Qual. 2017;32(4):331–9.
5. Haerkens MH, Kox M, Lemson J, Houterman S, van der Hoeven JG, Pickkers P. Crew resource management in the intensive care unit: a prospective 3-year cohort study. Acta Anaesthesiol Scand. 2015;59(10):1319–29.
6. Grulke N, Larbig W, Kachele H, Bailer H. Distress in patients undergoing allogeneic haematopoietic stem cell transplantation is correlated with distress in nurses. Eur J Oncol Nurs. 2009;13(5):361–7.

7. Neumann JL, Mau LW, Virani S, Denzen EM, Boyle DA, Boyle NJ, et al. Burnout, moral distress, work-life balance, and career satisfaction among hematopoietic cell transplantation professionals. Biol Blood Marrow Transplant. 2018;24(4):849–60.
8. Song JH, Kim S, Lee HW, Lee YJ, Kim MJ, Park JS, et al. Effect of intensivist involvement on clinical outcomes in patients with advanced lung cancer admitted to the intensive care unit. PloS One. 2019;14(2):e0210951.
9. Pronovost PJ, Angus DC, Dorman T, Robinson KA, Dremsizov TT, Young TL. Physician staffing patterns and clinical outcomes in critically ill patients: a systematic review. JAMA. 2002;288(17):2151–62.
10. Hawari FI, Al Najjar TI, Zaru L, Al Fayoumee W, Salah SH, Mukhaimar MZ. The effect of implementing high-intensity intensive care unit staffing model on outcome of critically ill oncology patients. Crit Care Med. 2009;37(6):1967–71.
11. von Bergwelt-Baildon M, Hallek MJ, Shimabukuro-Vornhagen AA, Kochanek M. CCC meets ICU: redefining the role of critical care of cancer patients. BMC Cancer. 2010;10:612.
12. Kiehl MG, Beutel G, Boll B, Buchheidt D, Forkert R, Fuhrmann V, et al. Consensus statement for cancer patients requiring intensive care support. Ann Hematol. 2018;97(7):1271–82.
13. Kochanek M, Schalk E, von Bergwelt-Baildon M, Beutel G, Buchheidt D, Hentrich M, et al. Management of sepsis in neutropenic cancer patients: 2018 guidelines from the infectious diseases working party (AGIHO) and intensive care working party (iCHOP) of the German Society of Hematology and Medical Oncology (DGHO). Ann Hematol. 2019;98(5):1051–69.
14. Azoulay E, Mokart D, Lambert J, Lemiale V, Rabbat A, Kouatchet A, et al. Diagnostic strategy for hematology and oncology patients with acute respiratory failure: randomized controlled trial. Am J Respir Crit Care Med. 2010;182(8):1038–46.
15. Kreeftenberg HG, Pouwels S, Bindels A, de Bie A, van der Voort PHJ. Impact of the advanced practice provider in adult critical care: a systematic review and meta-analysis. Crit Care Med. 2019;47(5):722–30.
16. Bruinooge SS, Pickard TA, Vogel W, Hanley A, Schenkel C, Garrett-Mayer E, et al. Understanding the role of advanced practice providers in oncology in the United States. J Oncol Pract. 2018;14(9):e518–e32.
17. Shah NN, Kucharczuk CR, Mitra N, Hirsh R, Svoboda J, Porter D, et al. Implementation of an advanced practice provider service on an allogeneic stem cell transplant unit: impact on patient outcomes. Biol Blood Marrow Transplant. 2015;21(9):1692–8.
18. Austin A, Jeffries K, Krause D, Sugalski J, Sharrah K, Gross A, et al. A study of advanced practice provider staffing models and professional development opportunities at national comprehensive cancer network member institutions. J Adv Pract Oncol. 2021;12(7):717–24.
19. Scherzer R, Dennis MP, Swan BA, Kavuru MS, Oxman DA. A comparison of usage and outcomes between nurse practitioner and resident-staffed medical ICUs. Crit Care Med. 2017;45(2):e132–e7.
20. Costa DK, Wallace DJ, Barnato AE, Kahn JM. Nurse practitioner/physician assistant staffing and critical care mortality. Chest. 2014;146(6):1566–73.
21. Landsperger JS, Semler MW, Wang L, Byrne DW, Wheeler AP. Outcomes of nurse practitioner-delivered critical care: a prospective cohort study. Chest. 2016;149(5):1146–54.
22. Kleinpell RM, Grabenkort WR, Kapu AN, Constantine R, Sicoutris C. Nurse practitioners and physician assistants in acute and critical care: a concise review of the literature and data 2008-2018. Crit Care Med. 2019;47(10):1442–9.
23. Kapu A. Origin and outcomes of acute care nurse practitioner practice. J Nurs Adm. 2021;51(1):4–5.
24. Paton A, Stein DE, D'Agostino R, Pastores SM, Halpern NA. Critical care medicine advanced practice provider model at a comprehensive cancer center: successes and challenges. Am J Crit Care. 2013;22(5):439–43.
25. Grabenkort WR, Meissen HH, Gregg SR, Coopersmith CM. Acute care nurse practitioners and physician assistants in critical care: transforming education and practice. Crit Care Med. 2017;45(7):1111–4.
26. D'Agostino R, Halpern NA. Acute care nurse practitioners in oncologic critical care: the memorial Sloan-Kettering cancer center experience. Crit Care Clin. 2010;26(1):207–17.
27. Babic A, Murray J. Role of nursing in HSCT. In: Carreras E, Dufour C, Mohty M, Kroger N, editors. The EBMT handbook: hematopoietic stem cell transplantation and cellular therapies. Cham: Springer; 2019. p. 237–43.
28. Lim F, Chen L, Salina A. CCRN® certification: why it matters. Nurs Crit Care. 2020;15(3):38–41.
29. McMillan SC, Heusinkveld K, Chai S, Miller Murphy C, Huang CY. Revising the blueprint for the oncology certified nurse (OCN) examination: a role delineation study. Oncol Nurs Forum. 2002;29(9):E110–7.
30. https://www.oncc.org/certifications/blood-marrow-transplant-certified-nurse-bmtcn.
31. Donadee C, Cohen-Melamed M, Delgado E, Gunn SR. Improving delivery of low tidal volume ventilation in 10 ICUs. BMJ Open Qual. 2022;11(1):e001343.
32. Peterson RJ, Hassumani DO, Hole AJ, Slaven JE, Tori AJ, Abu-Sultaneh S. Implementation of a high-flow nasal cannula management protocol in the pediatric ICU. Respir Care. 2021;66(4):591–9.
33. Miller AG, Haynes KE, Gates RM, Zimmerman KO, Heath TS, Bartlett KW, et al. A respiratory therapist-driven asthma pathway reduced hospital length of stay in the pediatric intensive care unit. Respir Care. 2019;64(11):1325–32.
34. Lee H, Ryu K, Sohn Y, Kim J, Suh GY, Kim E. Impact on patient outcomes of pharmacist par-

ticipation in multidisciplinary critical care teams: a systematic review and meta-analysis. Crit Care Med. 2019;47(9):1243–50.
35. Preslaski CR, Lat I, MacLaren R, Poston J. Pharmacist contributions as members of the multidisciplinary ICU team. Chest. 2013;144(5):1687–95.
36. Gawedzki P, Collins J. Impact of the implementation of a pharmacist-driven immunosuppression drug monitoring protocol for hematopoietic stem cell transplant recipients. J Oncol Pharm Pract. 2021;27(8):1907–13.
37. Correa PM, Zuckermann J, Fischer GB, Castro MS. Immunosuppressive serum levels in allogeneic hematopoietic stem cell transplantation: pharmaceutical care contribution. Pharm Pract (Granada). 2016;14(2):683.
38. Andrick B, Tusing L, Jones LK, Hu Y, Sneidman R, Gregor C, et al. The impact of a hematopoietic cellular therapy pharmacist on clinical and humanistic outcomes: a RE-AIM framework analysis. Transplant Cell Ther. 2022;28:334.e1.
39. Lee JS, Kang JE, Park SH, Jin HK, Jang SM, Kim SA, et al. Nutrition and clinical outcomes of nutrition support in multidisciplinary team for critically ill patients. Nutr Clin Pract. 2018;33(5):633–9.
40. De Waele E, Jakubowski JR, Stocker R, Wischmeyer PE. Review of evolution and current status of protein requirements and provision in acute illness and critical care. Clin Nutr. 2021;40(5):2958–73.
41. Muscaritoli M, Arends J, Bachmann P, Baracos V, Barthelemy N, Bertz H, et al. ESPEN practical guideline: clinical nutrition in cancer. Clin Nutr. 2021;40(5):2898–913.
42. Andersen S, Banks M, Brown T, Weber N, Kennedy G, Bauer J. Nutrition support during allogeneic stem cell transplantation: evidence versus practice. Support Care Cancer. 2020;28(11):5441–7.
43. McMillen KK, Coghlin-Dickson T, Adintori PA. Optimization of nutrition support practices early after hematopoietic cell transplantation. Bone Marrow Transplant. 2021;56(2):314–26.
44. Schweickert WD, Pohlman MC, Pohlman AS, Nigos C, Pawlik AJ, Esbrook CL, et al. Early physical and occupational therapy in mechanically ventilated, critically ill patients: a randomised controlled trial. Lancet. 2009;373(9678):1874–82.
45. Tipping CJ, Harrold M, Holland A, Romero L, Nisbet T, Hodgson CL. The effects of active mobilisation and rehabilitation in ICU on mortality and function: a systematic review. Intensive Care Med. 2017;43(2):171–83.
46. Mohananey D, Sarau A, Kumar R, Lewandowski D, Abreu-Sosa SM, Nathan S, et al. Role of physical activity and cardiac rehabilitation in patients undergoing hematopoietic stem cell transplantation. JACC CardioOncol. 2021;3(1):17–34.
47. Mohammed J, Smith SR, Burns L, Basak G, Aljurf M, Savani BN, et al. Role of physical therapy before and after hematopoietic stem cell transplantation: white paper report. Biol Blood Marrow Transplant. 2019;25(6):e191–e8.
48. Shaw AM, Robert R, Kresta K, Andersen CR, Lewis B, Maetzold B, et al. Totally excited about moving mobility and exercise (TEAM M (e)): a successful multidisciplinary exercise quality improvement initiative for pediatric and young adult oncology and stem cell transplant inpatients. Children (Basel). 2022;9(2):186.
49. Gonzales A, Gates E, Bhunia N, Mehyar L, Hashem H, Stanek JR, et al. Transplant energize me patient outcome (TEMPO): a quality improvement project that maintains functional mobility in pediatric patients admitted for allogeneic hematopoietic cell transplantation. Biol Blood Marrow Transplant. 2019;25(9):1779–85.
50. Colman J, Casto SC, Wisner E, Stanek JR, Auletta JJ. Improving occupational performance in pediatric hematopoietic cell transplant recipients. Am J Occup Ther. 2020;74(5):7405205020p1–p11.
51. Uber A, Ebelhar JS, Lanzel AF, Roche A, Vidal-Anaya V, Brock KE. Palliative care in pediatric oncology and hematopoietic stem cell transplantation. Curr Oncol Rep. 2022;24(2):161–74.
52. Gemmell R, Halley A, Stevens AM, Allam A, Perkins M, Ethell M, et al. Palliative care for patients around the time of haematopoietic stem cell transplant: a qualitative study of patients' perceptions and experiences of unmet need and attitudes towards palliative care involvement. Support Care Cancer. 2022;30(3):2253–61.
53. Nelson AM, Johnson PC, Kavanaugh AR, Jackson VA, Jagielo AD, Fenech AL, et al. Palliative care for patients undergoing stem cell transplant: intervention components and supportive care measures. Bone Marrow Transplant. 2021;56(8):1971–7.
54. Azoulay E, Mokart D, Pene F, Lambert J, Kouatchet A, Mayaux J, et al. Outcomes of critically ill patients with hematologic malignancies: prospective multicenter data from France and Belgium--a groupe de recherche respiratoire en reanimation onco-hematologique study. J Clin Oncol. 2013;31(22):2810–8.
55. Azoulay E, Pene F, Darmon M, Lengline E, Benoit D, Soares M, et al. Managing critically ill hematology patients: time to think differently. Blood Rev. 2015;29(6):359–67.
56. Azoulay E, Schellongowski P, Darmon M, Bauer PR, Benoit D, Depuydt P, et al. The intensive care medicine research agenda on critically ill oncology and hematology patients. Intensive Care Med. 2017;43(9):1366–82.
57. Drexler D, Newman N. Acuity adaptable nursing units in oncology. Oncol Nurs Forum. 2011;38(3): 263–6.
58. Emaminia A, Corcoran PC, Siegenthaler MP, Means M, Rasmussen S, Krause L, et al. The universal bed model for patient care improves outcome and lowers cost in cardiac surgery. J Thorac Cardiovasc Surg. 2012;143(2):475–81.
59. Kitchens JL, Fulton JS, Maze L. Patient and family description of receiving care in acuity adaptable care model. J Nurs Manag. 2018;26(7):874–80.

60. Chindhy SA, Edwards NM, Rajamanickam V, Lushaj EB, Lozonschi L, De Oliveira NC, et al. Acuity adaptable patient care unit system shortens length of stay and improves outcomes in adult cardiac surgery: University of Wisconsin experience. Eur J Cardiothorac Surg. 2014;46(1):49–54.
61. Zimring C, Seo HB. Making acuity-adaptable units work: lessons from the field. HERD. 2012;5(3):115–28.
62. Stephens RS, Whitman GJ. Postoperative critical care of the adult cardiac surgical patient. Part I: routine postoperative care. Crit Care Med. 2015;43(7):1477–97.
63. Brown KK, Gallant D. Impacting patient outcomes through design: acuity adaptable care/universal room design. Crit Care Nurs Q. 2006;29(4):326–41.
64. El-Kersh K, Guardiola J, Cavallazzi R, Wiemken TL, Roman J, Saad M. Open and closed models of intensive care unit have different influences on infectious complications in a tertiary care center: a retrospective data analysis. Am J Infect Control. 2016;44(12):1744–6.
65. Garland A, Gershengorn HB. Staffing in ICUs: physicians and alternative staffing models. Chest. 2013;143(1):214–21.
66. Treggiari MM, Martin DP, Yanez ND, Caldwell E, Hudson LD, Rubenfeld GD. Effect of intensive care unit organizational model and structure on outcomes in patients with acute lung injury. Am J Respir Crit Care Med. 2007;176(7):685–90.
67. Stretch R, Della Penna N, Celi LA, Landon BE. Effect of boarding on mortality in ICUs. Crit Care Med. 2018;46(4):525–31.
68. Lott JP, Iwashyna TJ, Christie JD, Asch DA, Kramer AA, Kahn JM. Critical illness outcomes in specialty versus general intensive care units. Am J Respir Crit Care Med. 2009;179(8):676–83.
69. Therapy FftAoC. International standards for hematopoietic cellular therapy product collection, processing, and administration: accreditation manual. 8th ed. Version 8.2. 2021.
70. Davidson JE, Aslakson RA, Long AC, Puntillo KA, Kross EK, Hart J, et al. Guidelines for family-centered care in the neonatal, pediatric, and adult ICU. Crit Care Med. 2017;45(1):103–28.
71. McGonigal M, Snyder A. Institute to frontline ICU quality. Crit Care Nurs Q. 2021;44(3):293–300.
72. Phelan R, Arora M, Chen M. Current use and outcome of hematopoietic stem cell transplantation: CIBMTR US summary slides, 2020. p. 2020.
73. Stephens RS, Whitman GJ. Postoperative critical care of the adult cardiac surgical patient: part II: procedure-specific considerations, management of complications, and quality improvement. Crit Care Med. 2015;43(9):1995–2014.
74. Ahmed EO, Butler R, Novick RJ. Failure-to-rescue rate as a measure of quality of care in a cardiac surgery recovery unit: a five-year study. Ann Thorac Surg. 2014;97(1):147–52.

# Long Term Survivors of Hematopoietic Stem Cell Transplantation: The Role of the Pulmonologist

# 37

Guang-Shing Cheng

## Introduction

The primary role of the pulmonologist in the long-term care of HSCT recipients is to provide expert consultation for the diagnosis and management of late-onset lung complications. As HSCT continues to grow as an accepted modality for the treatment of hematologic malignancies and other conditions worldwide, the need for pulmonary expertise has become more apparent for caregivers of HSCT survivors. Lung complications of HSCT have emerged as a legitimate field of clinical expertise within the discipline of pulmonary medicine. This chapter offers a perspective of the multi-faceted role of pulmonologists in the care of patients after HSCT.

## The Historical Context

Dr. E. Donnall Thomas, who pioneered the transplantation of HLA-matched sibling donor bone marrow into leukemia patients in the late 1970s, recognized that the long-term success of this procedure depended as much on preventing and mitigating acute organ toxicities as did the appropriate donor matching and conditioning regimen for graft survival. To that end, Dr. Thomas and his team in Seattle assembled specialty clinician scientists, such as gastrointestinal and infectious diseases specialists, to run care services specifically for HSCT recipients. The addition of pulmonary/critical care as a subspecialty service was a response to devastating acute lung injury syndromes such as CMV pneumonitis and diffuse alveolar hemorrhage, which were a major cause of early non-relapse mortality. The meticulous specialty care has contributed greatly to progress in survivorship, as well as to our understanding of organ toxicities and biology of processes beyond the HSCT context.

In the past two decades, less toxic conditioning regimens and infectious prophylaxis have significantly reduced the incidence of infectious and noninfectious acute lung injury syndromes, resulting in improved short-term outcomes [1, 2]. In parallel, the role of the pulmonary/critical care specialist has shifted from predominantly early post-transplant acute care to long-term needs of HSCT survivors. Pulmonary care in the contemporary era is ambulatory and longitudinal and can extend to the end of life.

The acute and chronic lung conditions that afflict HSCT recipients also occur in other clinical settings. Thus, pulmonologists draw upon knowledge from broader contexts within chest medicine for the evaluation and management of

G.-S. Cheng (✉)
Clinical Research Division, Fred Hutchinson Cancer Center and Division of Pulmonary, Critical Care and Sleep Medicine, Department of Medicine, University of Washington School of Medicine, Seattle, WA, USA
e-mail: gcheng2@fredhutch.org


A. O. Soubani (ed.), *Pulmonary and Critical Care Considerations of Hematopoietic Stem Cell Transplantation*, https://doi.org/10.1007/978-3-031-28797-8_37

post-HSCT lung disease. Idiopathic pneumonia syndrome is a form of acute lung injury in an early posttransplant context and is considered a regimen-related toxicity [3]. Obliterative bronchiolitis is seen in the general population as a rare sequelae of viral infection, rheumatoid arthritis, and inhalational toxins and, more commonly, in the setting of lung transplantation [4]. Different forms of well-defined interstitial lung disease (ILD) have been found post-HSCT [5].

The challenge for pulmonologists lies in understanding the post-HSCT context that affects the clinical presentation and trajectory of the lung disease [6]. The approach towards an HSCT recipient with lung disease is sufficiently unique that this can be considered a subspecialty within pulmonary medicine. Bronchiolitis obliterans syndrome (BOS) is a well-recognized complication that has been formally designated as an organ-specific manifestation of chronic graft-versus-host disease (cGVHD) [7]. There is growing speculation that restrictive lung disease entities including ILD are manifestations of alloimmunity, but much work needs to be done to clarify the epidemiologic association with cGVHD and to clarify specific chronic lung disease phenotypes after HSCT [8]. It may be convenient to consider "lung GVHD" as analogous to chronic lung allograft dysfunction (CLAD) after lung transplantation, which encompasses both BOS and restrictive allograft syndrome; however the triggers and trajectories of lung disease in these two clinical contexts may manifestly differ [9]. Understanding interstitial lung disease in the context of cGVHD is likely to provide insight into the pathogenesis of lung fibrosis and potentially new biologic pathways for targeted treatment.

## The Burden of Late-Onset Lung Disease

Compared with non-HSCT cancer patients, HSCT recipients experience greater long-term morbidities—respiratory morbidity was second only to infectious diseases in a Washington state registry survey of 2-year cancer survivors [10]. Bergeron and colleagues showed that the incidence of late-onset noninfectious pulmonary complications was nearly 20% in a prospective cohort of 200 allogeneic HSCT recipients and was a major contributor to non-relapse mortality [11]. As early HSCT outcomes improve, the incidence of cGVHD has increased [12]; hence the overall burden of lung disease has also likely increased. Recent advances in the prophylaxis of cGVHD have the potential to reduce the proportion of individuals affected by cGVHD, but the numbers of patients who receive allogeneic HSCT around the world continues to increase annually; therefore the overall burden of lung disease and respiratory impairment is expected to remain steady. Lung-specific prophylactic and preemptive therapies remain a significant gap in the care of HSCT survivors.

## Models of Long-Term Care

Managing lung disease after HSCT requires a multidisciplinary approach. A transplant patient's primary medical provider is usually a hematologist. As an organ specialist, the pulmonologist is positioned to provide consultative care. However, given the complexity of posttransplant care, the pulmonologist may ultimately serve as the patient's point of contact if the medical needs are primarily due to lung impairment. Importantly, the pulmonary expertise that is developed at transplant centers of excellence is a necessary resource for community providers who provide ongoing longitudinal care posttransplant.

In large-volume stand-alone cancer centers, pulmonary subspecialists may be integrated with the faculty that cares exclusively for cancer patients. At tertiary academic medical centers that offer all disciplines of medicine, pulmonologists belong to a larger division of pulmonary/critical care faculty within an internal medicine department and thus carry a wider scope of practice. Specific expertise may be developed within one individual or a group of interested pulmonologists. Clinics focused on pulmonary complications after HSCT, such as lung GVHD, can be established when the pulmonologist is not

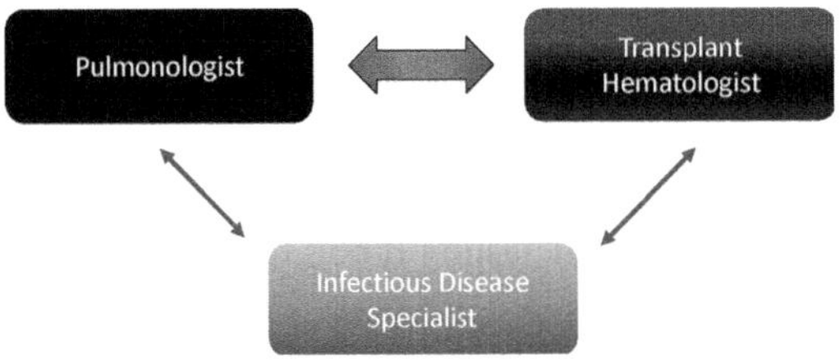


**Fig. 37.1** Model of multidisciplinary care for posttransplant pulmonary complications. The pulmonary/transplant hematology dyad is central to this model. The ideal situation is a trio of expertise that includes infectious diseases

embedded within a cancer center. In either model, expertise with posttransplant complications develops when there are collaborative and collegial relationships resulting in a pulmonologist/transplant hematologist dyad. In addition, the relationship between pulmonary and infectious diseases is crucial given the relative frequency and morbidity of opportunistic lung infections in survivors who remain at a high risk for opportunistic infections due to immunosuppressive treatments for cGVHD [13]. The ideal situation is the availability of this trio of expertise between the pulmonologist, infectious disease expert, and hematologist (Fig. 37.1).

## Early Diagnosis of BOS After HSCT

One of the most common posttransplant pulmonary consult requests is the evaluation of suspected BOS and other noninfectious pulmonary complications. This consult is often prompted by new-onset respiratory symptoms and/or PFT changes. Timely recognition of BOS depends on the primary physician's clinical suspicion and subsequent prompt referral. A patient referred for suspected BOS should be seen within 1–2 weeks, as the progression of lung function can occur over a brief time frame of weeks in some instances [6, 14]. For the most efficient evaluation, patients should arrive to the initial visit with a full set of PFTs (including spirometry with bronchodilator response, lung volumes, and diffusing capacity) and a non-contrast high-resolution chest CT with inspiratory and expiratory phases. An inventory of the transplant history, including history of early posttransplant complications; cGVHD manifestations; recent respiratory infections; tobacco and marijuana use, including vaping; and prior lung disease, should be taken. Specific symptoms of conditions that can potentially trigger BOS should be elicited (Table 37.1).

**Table 37.1** Diagnostic elements required for an efficient pulmonary consultation

| Diagnostic element required | Comments |
|---|---|
| Pulmonary function tests | Prior to visit: recent study with 2 weeks that includes spirometry (ideally with bronchodilator response), lung volumes, and DLCO |
| | Prior PFTs including pretransplant baseline and any immediate prior PFTs |
| Chest CT | Prior to visit: high resolution with inspiratory and expiratory cuts to assess for air trapping and parenchymal abnormalities |
| | Application of parametric response mapping may be helpful for the detection of small airway disease if this modality is clinically available |
| Clinical history | Smoking and vaping history |
| | History of preexisting lung disease and autoimmune disease |
| | Early posttransplant complications including lung infections, acute lung injury syndromes |
| | Chronic GVHD: timing of onset, manifestations, course of systemic treatment |
| | Recent respiratory viral illness or sick contacts |
| Symptoms | Cough |
| | Exertional dyspnea |
| | Wheezing |
| | Upper respiratory viral illness symptoms |
| | Gastrointestinal reflux symptoms |
| | Post-nasal drip, sinus congestion, and other symptoms of sinus disease |

*DLCO* diffusing capacity for carbon monoxide, *GVHD* graft-versus-host disease, *PFTs* pulmonary function tests

Detection of BOS at early stages and mild lung impairment offers the greatest opportunity to modify disease trajectory [6, 15]. However, patients are often referred to a pulmonologist when severe irreversible lung impairment already exists [16], which can occur rapidly over a matter of weeks in some cases. The working definition for BOS proposed by the 2014 NIH guidelines do not encourage early detection, because the spirometric criteria employ a specific FEV1 percent predicted cut-off of 75% rather than assessment of the trajectory of FEV1 impairment compared with prior lung function [17]. If PFTs are prompted only at the time of symptoms, FEV1 impairment is already likely to be advanced and largely irreversible. Hence, the implementation routine PFT screening is crucial for early detection and intervention.

The diagnosis of BOS is often confounded by consideration of other processes that cause airflow decline. A history of a recent upper respiratory viral infection or pneumonia may delay a formal diagnosis of BOS. Atypical spirometric patterns and concomitant restrictive processes also complicate the recognition of BOS. An atypical pattern on spirometry suggests restriction but may indicate incomplete exhalation due to small airway obstruction, manifesting as increased air trapping and elevated residual volume but with a preserved total lung capacity [18]. Therefore it is essential to obtain lung volumes with PFTs to ascertain whether there is a "preserved ratio impaired spirometry" [19] phenotype, or a restrictive process. The workup of PFT abnormalities or new respiratory symptoms will also reveal non-BOS processes, which may occur concomitantly with BOS. Organizing pneumonia may present acutely or subacutely and can manifest with restrictive, obstructive, or a mixed PFT pattern [20]. In addition to ILDs, restriction on PFTs may reflect extrathoracic truncal sclerosis, which is a complication of cGVHD, or respiratory muscle weakness, which may be a consequence of cGVHD myositis or chronic steroid use.

The pulmonologist needs to advocate and facilitate PFT screening, which can directly impact the outcomes for survivors. Despite multiple guidelines on post-HSCT care, PFT screening is not consistently implemented in the United States, largely owing to the perceived burden of testing for the patient [14]. The presence of a dedicated pulmonologist with expertise in HSCT care can help overcome the barriers of implementing PFT screening. The 2020 NIH Chronic GVHD Consensus guidelines on early diagnosis recommend PFT testing for all transplant recipients at pretransplant and every 3 month spirometry through 1 year posttransplant and yearly thereafter. The landmark timepoints for full PFTs (including lung volumes and DLCO) are pretransplant, Day 100, and yearly; limited spirometry is acceptable for other timepoints. High-risk individuals, such as those with active cGVHD, should have more frequent spirometry every 3 months. Those with documented respiratory viral infection should also be considered for more frequent interval monitoring [21]. While FEV1 and FEF25–75 impairment at Day 80–100 has been shown to be a risk factor for the later development of BOS [11, 22, 23], this has not been implemented as a criterion for screening. An important role of the pulmonologist is to educate hematology and primary care providers on the need for interval PFTs while facilitating the implementation of PFT screening. If routine PFTs at pretransplant, Day 80–100, and 1 year are not already standard practice, it behooves the pulmonologist to initiate a conversation with the transplant physician group.

Alternatives or adjuncts to laboratory-based PFTs include handheld home spirometry and the 6-min walk test (6MWT). The advent of smartphones and wireless telecommunications, i.e., Wi-Fi, has enabled home health telemonitoring of spirometry in which the data is transmitted wirelessly from the patient's smartphone to a clinician-accessed web portal. Recent work demonstrates that wireless home spirometry is feasible in HSCT survivors [24]. In a population enriched for lung GVHD, home spirometry can identify antecedent FEV1 changes [25]. There are now a number of commercially available wireless home spirometers with cloud-based monitoring portals that are easily accessed by a clinicians and PFT technicians. It is reasonable to anticipate that home spirometry monitoring for high-risk HSCT recipients will become standard care in some centers. Pulmonologists will be instrumental in implementing this monitoring modality. The 6MWT may provide prognostic value in addition to, or in lieu of, spirometry, as it is a test of functionality that does not always correlate with the degree of FEV1 impairment [26, 27]. More research needs to be done to assess the utility of 6MWT in pre- and posttransplant individuals.

The role of chest imaging for the early diagnosis of BOS and other noninfectious pulmonary complications is an area of active investigation. A European prospective cohort of 200 allogeneic HSCT recipients showed that nodular ground-glass opacities on chest computed tomography (CT) at the Day 100 landmark time point was predictive of later development of a noninfectious pulmonary complication [11]. As with other diagnostic modalities in the pulmonologist's toolbox, novel imaging techniques developed in other lung disease contexts are readily applicable to the HSCT context. Parametric response mapping, a quantitative voxel-based method that can distinguish small airway pathology from emphysema, has a prognostic value as an imaging biomarker in lung transplant [28, 29] and has diagnostic discrimination in lung GVHD [30, 31]. Hyperpolarized-xenon MRI can demonstrate ventilation defects of BOS without the ionizing radiation, which is advantageous in children [32]. These techniques are being studied for early detection, when subclinical lung function changes are not yet apparent. Machine learning techniques have also been applied in the context of BOS [33] and will continue to be developed to help identify patients at risk for BOS.

Bronchoscopy at the initial evaluation of BOS can be performed to assess for exacerbating factors and concomitant infections, i.e., viral infection, that might be triggers of lung function decline. An important aspect of longitudinal care is close attention to infectious exacerbations of BOS and chronic ILDs. There should be a low threshold for timely bronchoscopy in a patient with new radiographic findings suspicious for fungal disease or lung opacities, the latter of which could represent infection or organizing pneumonia. At a minimum, patients with classic chest imaging findings and compatible PFTs should have a noninvasive workup for respiratory viruses and bronchodilator testing. In individuals where the pathologic diagnosis of BOS or ILD is required for the purposes of enrolling into a clinical trial, referral to a thoracic surgery for lung biopsy may be appropriate.

Longitudinal follow-up for a patient with BOS or other lung complication should include close interval spirometry, assessment of the need for systemic corticosteroids, and evaluation of FEV1 decline (Fig. 37.2).

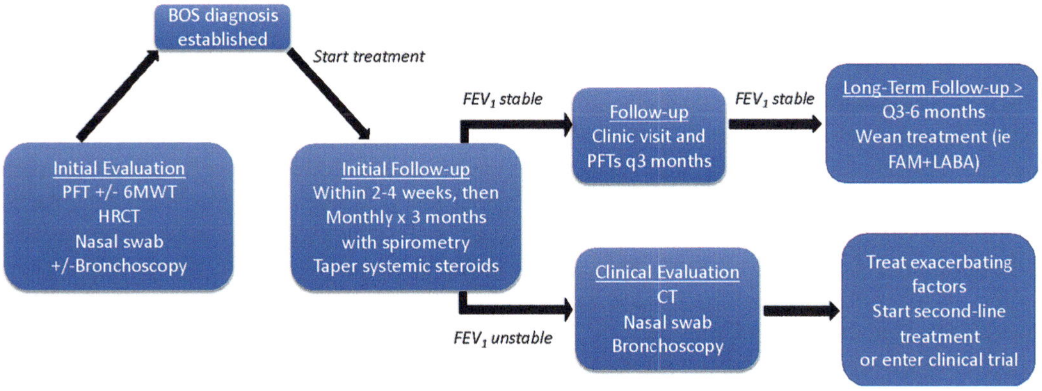


**Fig. 37.2** Suggested initial evaluation and longitudinal follow-up of a patient with BOS after HSCT. Initial treatment may include inhaled corticosteroids with or without long-acting beta-agonist as well as prednisone and other oral agents (e.g., azithromycin and montelukast as part of the FAM regimen). Second-line treatments include extracorporeal photopheresis and newer agents directed at cGVHD, such as ruxolitinib, and pulmonary anti-fibrotics, such as pirfenidone. Participation in a clinical trial, if one is available, is strongly encouraged

## Treatment of BOS After HSCT

The treatment of post-HSCT BOS draws upon the pulmonologist's armamentarium for chronic airway diseases. Inhaled corticosteroids, with or without a long-acting bronchodilator, is often the first-line therapy, based on an RCT in which patients with newly diagnosed BOS after HSCT were given budesonide/formoterol without the addition of systemic corticosteroids. Patients randomized to the treatment arm showed modest FEV1 improvement of 200 cc/12% after 1 month [34], suggesting that for patients whose disease was recognized at moderate impairment, there was still a reversible inflammatory component that could be ameliorated with topical steroids. The fluticasone, azithromycin, montelukast (FAM) cocktail was first used as a steroid-sparing approach at the Fred Hutchinson Cancer Center by pulmonologist Dr. Jason Chien [35]. A subsequent Phase II single-arm trial showed that FAM was well tolerated and that FEV1 remained stable [36]. Whether this is due to the natural history of the disease or whether the FAM modified FEV1 decline remains unknown [14].

Given the low side effect profile, FAM has been adopted in many centers and is currently recommended by some non-pulmonary professional societies [37]. However a consensus from pulmonologists on first-line therapy, including the use of systemic corticosteroids, remains a matter of debate [15]. The use of azithromycin has recently been called into question due to the early termination of a randomized clinical trial of azithromycin prophylaxis in allogeneic HSCT recipients in which the treatment arm had an unexpected increase in deaths due to hematologic relapse compared with placebo [38]. A subsequent analysis of patients who were exposed to azithromycin for BOS treatment showed an increased risk of subsequent neoplasms, rather than hematologic relapse, but without a negative effect on survival. In fact, those patients with BOS who had taken azithromycin had a decreased cause-specific hazard of death free from malignancy [39]. Taken together, these studies suggest that the immunomodulatory effect of azithromycin has unintended consequences for immune cancer surveillance that manifests differently depending on the stage of posttransplant survivorship. It must be noted, however, that there are no studies that convincingly demonstrate a benefit of azithromycin on lung function in patients with BOS after HSCT [15, 40]. Therefore, the use of azithromycin should take into consideration the risks and benefits for an individual's clinical situation.

In recognition of the irreversible fibrotic lesion of obliterative bronchiolitis, which renders lung impairment in BOS irreversible, pulmonologists now have anti-fibrotic agents in the armamentarium to consider for the treatment of progressive BOS. Pirfenidone and nintedanib are FDA-approved for the treatment of idiopathic pulmonary fibrosis (IPF) and related interstitial lung diseases. It remains unclear if there is a benefit of these antifibrotic agents, especially when given as second- or third-line therapy for already established disease with fixed severe FEV1 impairment (i.e., <35% predicted), given their modest efficacy in moderate IPF. In a phase I study in BOS after HSCT, pirfenidone was tolerable, and a subset of patients had demonstrable FEV1 improvement [41]. A European randomized clinical trial of pirfenidone in BOS after lung transplant did not demonstrate efficacy [42]. Nonetheless, these agents highlight the notion that novel agents that are being developed for and tested in IPF should be considered for use in BOS after HSCT.

## Quality of Life and End of Life

For patients with chronic lung disease for which there are a paucity of disease-modifying therapies, the pulmonologist provides important longitudinal supportive care to optimize quality of life. For those with irreversible lung dysfunction, care is focused on symptom management. This comes in the form of bronchodilators or nebulizer therapy, oxygen supplementation, and cough suppression. Pulmonary rehabilitation has been shown to provide benefit for dyspnea, patient-reported outcomes, and exercise tolerance [43, 44]. Patients who progress to chronic respiratory failure may require noninvasive ventilatory support such as BiLevel positive airway pressure (BIPAP) for nocturnal home use.

Lung transplantation may be considered for individuals in which BOS or ILD is the primary organ complication of HSCT. Case series have shown that outcomes for HSCT recipients who receive a lung allograft are generally comparable to other indications [45, 46]. However, because most HSCT recipients have a history of hematologic malignancy, certain criteria need to be considered prior to referral to a lung transplantation center. Candidates should be at least >5 years from the HSCT for their underlying malignancy and should not have active cGVHD or significant extrapulmonary organ dysfunction due to cGVHD or other posttransplant complications [47].

Unfortunately, lung transplantation is not a feasible option for most individuals, and a significant proportion of patients will experience progressive chronic respiratory failure as their primary posttransplant morbidity and cause of death. In a multicenter retrospective cohort of 316 patients with BOS, respiratory causes including primary respiratory failure and infections accounted for nearly 50% of deaths [39]. Naturally, it often falls upon the pulmonologist to address end-of-life issues, which in many instances occurs out of necessity when the patient is admitted to the intensive care unit for mechanical ventilatory support. The pulmonologist who provides longitudinal care should address code status and palliative care in the ambulatory setting, when severe functional and physiologic decline is evident. For patients with BOS, the trajectory of FVC is more prognostic of death within 2 years than the trajectory of FEV1 or the severity of FEV1 impairment [14]. With supportive care such as supplemental oxygen, some individuals can survive for >20 years with very severe but stable FEV1 impairment, i.e., <35%, reflecting end-organ sequelae of cGVHD rather than active disease. On the other hand, FVC decline may also reflect extraparenchymal processes, such as pulmonary cachexia, truncal sclerosis due to cGVHD, or generalized neuromuscular weakness from chronic corticosteroid exposure. It is appropriate at this juncture not only to address further ventilatory decline medically but also to recommend palliative care over aggressive life support if an acute decompensation occurs.

## Pediatric Considerations

Significant long-term effects of HSCT on lung health remain a major concern for this population for whom many years of life are anticipated after a curative transplant. Although cGVHD is less common in pediatric allogeneic HSCT recipients compared with adults, lung manifestations may affect a greater proportion of those who do have cGVHD [48]. Lung function decline is very common: 62% of patients in longitudinal pediatric cohort ages 6–16 years experienced a > 10% decline in a lung function parameter between 3 and 9 months posttransplant and was associated with acute and chronic GVHD [49]. The impact of BOS remains devastating when a child develops progressive lung impairment leading to death. Living-donor lobar lung transplantation has been performed on pediatric patients for BOS after HSCT [45]. On the other hand, unlike adults, a proportion of young children with moderate lung impairment at BOS diagnosis are able to recover FVC, owing to continued lung growth during childhood [50]. This is also observed in longitudinal cohorts of lung impairment in pediatric HSCT in general and portends better long-term outcomes [51].

The diagnosis of late-onset lung disease is challenging in young children, and the NIH criteria for BOS perform poorly in this population [48]. Routine screening for BOS is also challenging in children, as reliable spirometry is not generally thought to be feasible for children ages 7 and younger [21]. Routine procedures for adults such as high-resolution CT and diagnostic bronchoscopy in children may require sedation and general anesthesia to allow for tolerability. Alternative methods of diagnosis such as hyperpolarized-xenon MRI and multiple breath washout (for lung clearance index) are being explored.

## Education, Training, and Research

The educational role of the pulmonologist goes hand-in-hand with clinical care of HSCT survivors. Open discussion with patients about the diagnosis, prognosis, and treatment of chronic lung disease is an assumed requirement for a therapeutic longitudinal relationship with a patient. It is worth emphasizing again that a successful collaborative dyad of the pulmonologist and the HSCT physician involves a two-way conversation about best practices based on recent scientific evidence, particularly with regard to the early detection of BOS with PFTs. The pulmonologist's expertise in lung physiology and other lung diseases should be shared; pulmonologists may also be called upon to explain atypical PFT or radiographic findings. The education of transplant and allied subspecialty providers should be integral to a pulmonologist's practice and can take the form of formal teaching conferences (such as morbidity and mortality conferences), in addition to ad hoc teaching over a specific patient case. Pulmonologists at academic centers who see a critical mass of patients with HSCT complications should also be available to advise and educate community physicians who encounter these conditions rarely. The education of pulmonologists-in-training through clinical exposure and didactics is equally important in light of the growing numbers of HSCT survivors.

Lastly, and importantly, pulmonologists can advance scientific knowledge of chronic lung diseases after HSCT by advocating for and participating in research. The need for pulmonologists to conduct research is highlighted in a 2018 National Institutes of Health-sponsored workshop on pulmonary complications of pediatric HSCT recipients [52]. The 2020 NIH consensus guidelines for chronic GVHD included organ specialists, including pulmonologists, in the discussion of knowledge gaps and highest priorities in the highly morbid manifestations guidelines [8]. Given the general rarity of late lung complications, multi-institutional collaborations of pulmonary researchers, in collaboration with transplant researchers, will be necessary for the understanding of the natural history of lung GVHD and testing novel treatments. This is particularly relevant for the conduct of randomized clinical trials, as the lessons learned from clinical trials in IPF can be applied to BOS and ILD manifestations of cGVHD.

## Summary

Pulmonologists are critical providers of long-term care for HSCT recipients. The collaborative dyad of pulmonology and transplant hematology should be established for optimal clinical care. Not only do pulmonologists provide expertise in the diagnosis and management of late-onset pulmonary complications, they are also in a position to educate transplant providers and to advocate for early detection of BOS through PFT screening. The accumulated experience in the clinical care and scientific knowledge of late-onset lung complications of HSCT has established these conditions as a field of expertise within pulmonary medicine; thus pulmonologists are poised to advance best clinical practices through advocacy and research.

## References

1. Gooley TA, Chien JW, Pergam SA, Hingorani S, Sorror ML, Boeckh M, et al. Reduced mortality after allogeneic hematopoietic-cell transplantation. N Engl J Med. 2010;363(22):2091–101.
2. McDonald GB, Sandmaier BM, Mielcarek M, Sorror M, Pergam SA, Cheng GS, et al. Survival, nonrelapse mortality, and relapse-related mortality after allogeneic hematopoietic cell transplantation: comparing 2003-2007 versus 2013-2017 cohorts. Ann Intern Med. 2020;172(4):229–39.
3. Panoskaltsis-Mortari A, Griese M, Madtes DK, Belperio JA, Haddad IY, Folz RJ, et al. An official American Thoracic Society research statement: noninfectious lung injury after hematopoietic stem cell transplantation: idiopathic pneumonia syndrome. Am J Respir Crit Care Med. 2011;183(9):1262–79.
4. Barker AF, Bergeron A, Rom WN, Hertz MI. Obliterative bronchiolitis. N Engl J Med. 2014;370(19):1820–8.
5. Schlemmer F, Chevret S, Lorillon G, De Bazelaire C, Peffault de Latour R, Meignin V, et al. Late-onset noninfectious interstitial lung disease after allogeneic

hematopoietic stem cell transplantation. Respir Med. 2014;108(10):1525–33.
6. Bergeron A, Cheng GS. Bronchiolitis obliterans syndrome and other late pulmonary complications after allogeneic hematopoietic stem cell transplantation. Clin Chest Med. 2017;38(4):607–21.
7. Jagasia MH, Greinix HT, Arora M, Williams KM, Wolff D, Cowen EW, et al. National institutes of health consensus development project on criteria for clinical trials in chronic graft-versus-host disease: I. the 2014 diagnosis and staging working group report. Biol Blood Marrow Transplant. 2015;21(3):389–401.e1
8. Wolff D, Radojcic V, Lafyatis R, Cinar R, Rosenstein RK, Cowen EW, et al. National institutes of health consensus development project on criteria for clinical trials in chronic graft-versus-host disease: IV. The 2020 highly morbid forms report. Transplant Cell Ther. 2021;27(10):817–35.
9. Glanville AR. Bronchiolitis obliterans syndrome after lung or haematopoietic stem cell transplantation: current management and future directions. ERJ Open Res. 2022;8:00185–2022.
10. Chow EJ, Cushing-Haugen KL, Cheng GS, Boeckh M, Khera N, Lee SJ, et al. Morbidity and mortality differences between hematopoietic cell transplantation survivors and other cancer survivors. J Clin Oncol. 2017;35(3):306–13.
11. Bergeron A, Chevret S, Peffault de Latour R, Chagnon K, de Margerie-Mellon C, Riviere F, et al. Noninfectious lung complications after allogeneic haematopoietic stem cell transplantation. Eur Respir J. 2018;51(5):1702617.
12. Arai S, Arora M, Wang T, Spellman SR, He W, Couriel DR, et al. Increasing incidence of chronic graft-versus-host disease in allogeneic transplantation: a report from the center for international blood and marrow transplant research. Biol Blood Marrow Transplant. 2015;21(2):266–74.
13. Foord AM, Cushing-Haugen KL, Boeckh MJ, Carpenter PA, Flowers MED, Lee SJ, et al. Late infectious complications in hematopoietic cell transplantation survivors: a population-based study. Blood Adv. 2020;4(7):1232–41.
14. Cheng GS, Storer B, Chien JW, Jagasia M, Hubbard JJ, Burns L, et al. Lung function trajectory in bronchiolitis obliterans syndrome after allogeneic hematopoietic cell transplant. Ann Am Thorac Soc. 2016;13(11):1932–9.
15. Bondeelle L, Bergeron A. Managing pulmonary complications in allogeneic hematopoietic stem cell transplantation. Expert Rev Respir Med. 2019;13(1):105–19.
16. Palmer J, Williams K, Inamoto Y, Chai X, Martin PJ, Tomas LS, et al. Pulmonary symptoms measured by the national institutes of health lung score predict overall survival, nonrelapse mortality, and patient-reported outcomes in chronic graft-versus-host disease. Biol Blood Marrow Transplant. 2014;20(3):337–44.
17. Paczesny S, Hakim FT, Pidala J, Cooke KR, Lathrop J, Griffith LM, et al. National institutes of health consensus development project on criteria for clinical trials in chronic graft-versus-host disease: III. The 2014 biomarker working group report. Biol Blood Marrow Transplant. 2015;21(5):780–92.
18. Bergeron A, Godet C, Chevret S, Lorillon G, Peffault de Latour R, de Revel T, et al. Bronchiolitis obliterans syndrome after allogeneic hematopoietic SCT: phenotypes and prognosis. Bone Marrow Transplant. 2013;48(6):819–24.
19. Wan ES, Balte P, Schwartz JE, Bhatt SP, Cassano PA, Couper D, et al. Association between preserved ratio impaired spirometry and clinical outcomes in US adults. JAMA. 2021;326(22):2287–98.
20. Freudenberger TD, Madtes DK, Curtis JR, Cummings P, Storer BE, Hackman RC. Association between acute and chronic graft-versus-host disease and bronchiolitis obliterans organizing pneumonia in recipients of hematopoietic stem cell transplants. Blood. 2003;102(10):3822–8.
21. Kitko CL, Pidala J, Schoemans HM, Lawitschka A, Flowers ME, Cowen EW, et al. National Institutes of Health consensus development project on criteria for clinical trials in chronic graft-versus-host disease: IIa. The 2020 clinical implementation and early diagnosis working group report. Transplant Cell Ther. 2021;27(7):545–57.
22. Jamani K, He Q, Liu Y, Davis C, Hubbard J, Schoch G, et al. Early post-transplantation spirometry is associated with the development of bronchiolitis obliterans syndrome after allogeneic hematopoietic cell transplantation. Biol Blood Marrow Transplant. 2019;26(5):943–8.
23. Duque-Afonso J, Ihorst G, Waterhouse M, Zeiser R, Wasch R, Bertz H, et al. Impact of lung function on bronchiolitis obliterans syndrome and outcome after allogeneic hematopoietic cell transplantation with reduced-intensity conditioning. Biol Blood Marrow Transplant. 2018;24(11):2277–84.
24. Sheshadri A, Alousi A, Bashoura L, Stolar K, Baghaie S, Arain MH, et al. Feasibility and reliability of home-based spirometry telemonitoring in allogeneic hematopoietic cell transplant recipients. Ann Am Thorac Soc. 2020;17:1329.
25. Turner J, He Q, Baker K, Chung L, Lazarevic-Fogelquist A, Bethune D, et al. Home spirometry telemonitoring for early detection of bronchiolitis obliterans syndrome in patients with chronic graft-versus-host disease. Transplant Cell Ther. 2021;27(7):616.e1–6.
26. Nathan SD, Shlobin OA, Reese E, Ahmad S, Fregoso M, Athale C, et al. Prognostic value of the 6 min walk test in bronchiolitis obliterans syndrome. Respir Med. 2009;103(12):1816–21.
27. Fakhro M, Ingemansson R, Algotsson L, Lindstedt S. Impact of forced expiratory volume in 1 second (FEV1) and 6-minute walking distance at 3, 6, and 12 months and annually on survival and occurrence

of bronchiolitis obliterans syndrome (BOS) after lung transplantation. Ann Transplant. 2017;22:532–40.
28. Belloli EA, Degtiar I, Wang X, Yanik GA, Stuckey LJ, Verleden SE, et al. Parametric response mapping as an imaging biomarker in lung transplant recipients. Am J Respir Crit Care Med. 2017;195(7):942–52.
29. Belloli EA, Gu T, Wang Y, Vummidi D, Lyu DM, Combs MP, et al. Radiographic graft surveillance in lung transplantation: prognostic role of parametric response mapping. Am J Respir Crit Care Med. 2021;204(8):967–76.
30. Cheng GS, Selwa KE, Hatt C, Ram S, Fortuna AB, Guerriero M, et al. Multicenter evaluation of parametric response mapping as an indicator of bronchiolitis obliterans syndrome after hematopoietic stem cell transplantation. Am J Transplant. 2020;20:2198.
31. Galban CJ, Boes JL, Bule M, Kitko CL, Couriel DR, Johnson TD, et al. Parametric response mapping as an indicator of bronchiolitis obliterans syndrome after hematopoietic stem cell transplantation. Biol Blood Marrow Transplant. 2014;20(10):1592–8.
32. Walkup LL, Roach DJ, Hall CS, Gupta N, Thomen RP, Cleveland ZI, et al. Cyst ventilation heterogeneity and alveolar airspace dilation as early disease markers in lymphangioleiomyomatosis. Ann Am Thorac Soc. 2019;16(8):1008–16.
33. Sharifi H, Lai YK, Guo H, Hoppenfeld M, Guenther ZD, Johnston L, et al. Machine learning algorithms to differentiate among pulmonary complications after hematopoietic cell transplant. Chest. 2020;158:1090.
34. Bergeron A, Chevret S, Chagnon K, Godet C, Bergot E, Peffault de Latour R, et al. Budesonide/formoterol for bronchiolitis obliterans after hematopoietic stem cell transplantation. Am J Respir Crit Care Med. 2015;191(11):1242–9.
35. Norman BC, Jacobsohn DA, Williams KM, Au BK, Au MA, Lee SJ, et al. Fluticasone, azithromycin and montelukast therapy in reducing corticosteroid exposure in bronchiolitis obliterans syndrome after allogeneic hematopoietic SCT: a case series of eight patients. Bone Marrow Transplant. 2011;46(10):1369–73.
36. Williams KM, Cheng GS, Pusic I, Jagasia M, Burns L, Ho VT, et al. Fluticasone, azithromycin, and montelukast treatment for new-onset bronchiolitis obliterans syndrome after hematopoietic cell transplantation. Biol Blood Marrow Transplant. 2016;22(4):710–6.
37. Penack O, Marchetti M, Ruutu T, Aljurf M, Bacigalupo A, Bonifazi F, et al. Prophylaxis and management of graft versus host disease after stem-cell transplantation for haematological malignancies: updated consensus recommendations of the European Society for Blood and Marrow Transplantation. Lancet Haematol. 2020;7(2):e157–e67.
38. Bergeron A, Chevret S, Granata A, Chevallier P, Vincent L, Huynh A, et al. Effect of azithromycin on airflow decline-free survival after allogeneic hematopoietic stem cell transplant: the ALLOZITHRO randomized clinical trial. JAMA. 2017;318(6):557–66.
39. Cheng GS, Bondeelle L, Gooley T, He Q, Jamani K, Krakow EF, et al. Azithromycin use and increased cancer risk among patients with bronchiolitis obliterans after hematopoietic cell transplantation. Biol Blood Marrow Transplant. 2020;26(2):392–400.
40. Yadav H, Peters SG, Keogh KA, Hogan WJ, Erwin PJ, West CP, et al. Azithromycin for the treatment of obliterative bronchiolitis after hematopoietic stem cell transplantation: a systematic review and meta-analysis. Biol Blood Marrow Transplant. 2016;22(12):2264–9.
41. Matthaiou EI, Sharifi H, O'Donnell C, Chiu W, Owyang C, Chatterjee P, et al. The safety and tolerability of pirfenidone for bronchiolitis obliterans syndrome after hematopoietic cell transplant (STOP-BOS) trial. Bone Marrow Transplant. 2022;57:1319.
42. Perch M, Besa V, Corris PA, Iversen M, Kneidinger N, Leuckfeld I, et al. A European multi-center, randomized, double-blind trial of Pirfenidone in bronchiolitis-obliterans-syndrome grade 1-3 in lung transplant recipients (European trial of Pirfenidone in BOS (EPOS)). J Heart Lung Transplant. 2020;39(4S):S12.
43. Tran J, Norder EE, Diaz PT, Phillips GS, Elder P, Devine SM, et al. Pulmonary rehabilitation for bronchiolitis obliterans syndrome after hematopoietic stem cell transplantation. Biol Blood Marrow Transplant. 2012;18(8):1250–4.
44. Choi HE, Lim SN, Lee JH, Park SH. Comprehensive pulmonary rehabilitation in patients with bronchiolitis obliterans syndrome: a case series. Respir Med Case Rep. 2020;31:101161.
45. Cheng GS, Edelman JD, Madtes DK, Martin PJ, Flowers ME. Outcomes of lung transplantation after allogeneic hematopoietic stem cell transplantation. Biol Blood Marrow Transplant. 2014;20(8):1169–75.
46. Greer M, Berastegui C, Jaksch P, Benden C, Aubert J, Roux A, et al. Lung transplantation after allogeneic stem cell transplantation: a pan-European experience. Eur Respir J. 2018;51(2):1701330.
47. Leard LE, Holm AM, Valapour M, Glanville AR, Attawar S, Aversa M, et al. Consensus document for the selection of lung transplant candidates: an update from the International Society for Heart and Lung Transplantation. J Heart Lung Transplant. 2021;40(11):1349–79.
48. Cuvelier GDE, Nemecek ER, Wahlstrom JT, Kitko CL, Lewis VA, Schechter T, et al. Benefits and challenges with diagnosing chronic and late acute GVHD in children using the NIH consensus criteria. Blood. 2019;134(3):304–16.
49. Uhlving HH, Bang CL, Christensen IJ, Buchvald F, Nielsen KG, Heilmann CJ, et al. Lung function after allogeneic hematopoietic stem cell transplantation in children: a longitudinal study in a population-based cohort. Biol Blood Marrow Transplant. 2013;19(9):1348–54.
50. Walther S, Rettinger E, Maurer HM, Pommerening H, Jarisch A, Sorensen J, et al. Long-term pulmonary function testing in pediatric bronchiolitis obliterans syndrome after hematopoietic stem cell transplantation. Pediatr Pulmonol. 2020;55(7):1725–35.

51. Srinivasan A, Sunkara A, Mitchell W, Sunthankar S, Kang G, Stokes DC, et al. Recovery of pulmonary function after allogeneic hematopoietic cell transplantation in children is associated with improved survival. Biol Blood Marrow Transplant. 2017;23(12):2102–9.
52. Tamburro RF, Cooke KR, Davies SM, Goldfarb S, Hagood JS, Srinivasan A, et al. Pulmonary complications of pediatric hematopoietic cell transplantation. A National Institutes of Health workshop summary. Ann Am Thorac Soc. 2021;18(3):381–94.

# Index





A. O. Soubani (ed.), *Pulmonary and Critical Care Considerations of Hematopoietic Stem Cell Transplantation*, https://doi.org/10.1007/978-3-031-28797-8

GPSR Compliance

*The European Union's (EU) General Product Safety Regulation (GPSR) is a set of rules that requires consumer products to be safe and our obligations to ensure this.*

*If you have any concerns about our products, you can contact us on ProductSafety@springernature.com*

In case Publisher is established outside the EU, the EU authorized representative is:

Springer Nature Customer Service Center GmbH
Europaplatz 3
69115 Heidelberg, Germany

**Batch number: 10732807**

Printed by Printforce, the Netherlands